Materia Medica
Clinical Manifestations
Affinities
Biological Profiles
and
Characteristics
of

# REPTILES

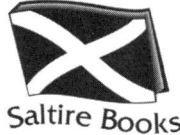
Saltire Books

Saltire Books Limited, Glasgow, Scotland

Materia Medica
Clinical Manifestations
Affinities
Biological Profiles
and
Characteristics
of

# REPTILES

## FRANS VERMEULEN

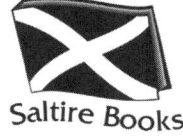
Saltire Books Limited, Glasgow, Scotland

Published by Saltire Books Ltd

18–20 Main Street, Busby, Glasgow G76 8DU, Scotland
books@saltirebooks.com   www.saltirebooks.com

Text © Frans Vermeulen
Cover, Design, Graphics and Layout © Saltire Books Ltd 2020

 is a registered trademark

First published in 2020

Typeset by Type Study, Scarborough, UK in 9.5/12pt Stone Serif
Printed and bound in the UK by TJ International Ltd, Padstow, Cornwall

ISBN 978-1-908127-35-8

*For Saltire Books*
Project Development: Lee Kayne
Editorial: Steven Kayne
Design: Phil Barker

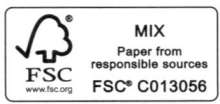

MIX
Paper from
responsible sources
FSC® C013056

# CONTENTS

alligators. Weak link in the armoured chain of events. Wishing fertility & power. You are what eats you.

*Surviving the Death Roll*

## Crocodilians in homeopathy    31

*Alligator mississippiensis – American alligator*
    Systematics. Biological profile. Filling a yawning vacancy. Guarding the nest. Calling out in distress. Shifting about or staying put. Materia medica [++]. Summary of proving.

*Alligator sinensis – Chinese alligator*
    Systematics. Biological profile. Materia Medica [–].

*Crocodylus acutus – American crocodile*
    Systematics. Biological profile. Worse from cold. Guarding & responding. Materia Medica [–].

*Crocodylus novaeguineae – New Guinea crocodile*
    Systematics. Biological profile. Helping each other. Creation myths. Marks of the crocodile. Crocodile sorcerers. Materia Medica [–].

## Dinosaurs    43

### Dinosaurs in Homeopathy    43

*Maiasaura lapidea – fossilized dinosaur bone*
    Systematics. Biological profile. Herds of good mothers. Materia Medica [++].

*Siroccopteryx moroccoensis – pterosaur dinosaur*
    Systematics. Biological profile. Materia Medica [–].

*Tyrannosaurus rex – T-rex*
    Systematics. Biological profile. Materia Medica [+]. Case observations. General concept of T-rex.

## Lizards    51

*Biological Profile*

*Listing Lizards*
    Agamids. Anguids. Beaded lizards. Chameleons. Flap-foots. Geckos. Girdled lizards. Iguanids. Monitor lizards. Skinks. Teiids & whiptails. Wall or true lizards. Remarkable lizards.

*Lizards from Head to Tail*
    Diversity of lizards. Scales & skin. Shedding & sloughing. Shape & size. Tongue 'n teeth. Tail. Limbs & locomotion. Anoxia. Lizards loved or loathed.

CONTENTS

*for Linda,*
*wholly and evermore*

# ACKNOWLEDGEMENTS

No list of acknowledgements in a book concerning homeopathy is complete without Samuel Hahnemann at its head. As the Founding Father, his contribution is undisputed. Worthy of praise are also the Founding Followers to which Hering, Lippe, Hale, Boenninghausen, Boericke, T.F. Allen, the Wesselhoefts, Clarke, Boger, Kent and Mezger belong. Additionally, I extend my appreciation to all the people cited in the reference list. The work of each of these researchers, clinicians and authors has beneficially contributed to my understanding and made this book possible.

My full heart-felt appreciation goes to our hard-working publishers, Steven and Lee Kayne of Saltire Books. Their ideas, support and thorough professionalism throughout the painstaking stages of the publication process have been responsible for being able to offer you this book. The layout, graphics, paper, fonts and other stylistic considerations do play an important part in producing a book not only aesthetically pleasing but also easy to read and making the information available to the reader. The Kaynes and their staff have exceeded all expectations in achieving a very high quality in every regard.

# ABOUT THE AUTHOR

Born in Den Helder, Holland, Frans taught at an elementary school from 1970 to 1978. From 1976 to 1983 he pursued his homeopathic education, while beginning his own practice in 1979. At this time, he had begun to translate homeopathic books by masters such as Kent, Allen, Tyler, Vithoulkas, and others. In 1985 he wrote Kindertypes in de Homoeopathie (Children types in Homeopathy), based on his experiences as both a teacher and a homeopath.

Recognised throughout the homeopathic world as an author, lecturer and authority on materia medica, Frans Vermeulen will have been 44 years involved in homeopathy in 2020. The first 20 years concerned homeopathic education and a busy practice. The second half focused on materia medica research and writing.

Each of the many books he has authored makes a contribution of major significance to our understanding of substances and materia medica. His lectures are inspiring and appreciated for their liveliness, depth of knowledge and breadth of factual information.

Major works published with Saltire in 2011–19 include *Plants* [a 4-volume work co-authored by his wife, Linda Johnston, MD], *Concordant Reference 2nd ed.* [1284 remedies, including Allen's Handbook and Allen's Encyclopedia], *Synoptic Reference 1* [505 remedies], *Synoptic Reference 2* [606 remedies], *Prisma Reference* [222 remedies with full and brief cases], and now *Reptiles* [snakes, lizards, worm lizards, turtles, crocodilians].

Earlier works are *Kingdom Monera and Viruses* [2005] about nosodes, followed by *Kingdom Fungi* in 2007.

Electronic works include *Source & Substance* [identification and detailed description of 4250+ substances used in homeopathy], *Vista Vintage* [6000 original case reports, clinical observations, provings, poisonings and self-experimentations, collected from journals, transactions and other publications from the period 1820 to 1920], and *Vista Views* [original articles by the old masters on philosophy, methodology, posology, etc., from the period 1820–1920].

# PREFACE

Reptiles hold a particular and inexplicable fascination or repugnance for us. From the Garden of Eden to a professor of herpetology in an obscure university, we are both inescapably drawn to or repulsed by them. Either way, it can be said that we are mesmerized by them. This is especially true of the largest grouping, the snakes.

It is an interesting twist of lexicography that the phenomenon of an invisible natural force given off by the animate and inanimate, known as animal magnetism, would be called mesmerism after its namesake, the German doctor Franz Friedrich Anton Mesmer [1734–1815]. Essentially he is given credit for a characteristic that is a natural part of the essence of snakes. As attested by the ubiquitous presence of all manner of reptiles, particularly snakes, in mythology, folklore, cultural traditions, movies and literature, reptiles are interwoven into our consciousness. Has it all been due to their animal magnetism? In what other ways do reptiles play a part in our lives, either consciously or subconsciously? For homeopaths, that question includes asking in what ways reptiles assist in healing.

Homeopaths are far from immune to the allure of reptiles and their mesmerizing capacity. It is hardly a coincidence that more homeopathic books have been written on snakes than any other remedy grouping. I am adding my contribution to the mix. However, with this book, I offer a more comprehensive listing and description of members of this fascinating and eminently useful class of animals. Although snakes are the most well-known, this book covers the entire class, including turtles, lizards, worm lizards, dinosaurs and crocodilians. Pardoning the mixed metaphor, with the remedies here described you can spread your wings and start to think past Lachesis and Crotalus.

To gather information about the reptiles in this book hundreds of articles and medical reports have been reviewed and extracted, resulting in the symptoms included [see the Reference list]. These have predominantly been the clinical manifestations from envenomations. This wealth of information provides sufficient basis for the prescription of yet another 60 reptiles.

Homeopaths tend to understand snakes by putting them all into a single group. Aside from it being a huge mistake, this has hindered the proper use of the extent of possibilities that this wide range of snakes really has to offer. We would no more think of grouping all trees, or all mammals together, yet we do so with snakes. We recognize that a whale is very different from a fox or a pine tree from an apple tree. Why then don't we acknowledge that Naja tripudians, Crotalus horridus and Boa constrictor are equally different from each other?

The answer to that question is because we have not had proper classification or enough information to discern important differences. In *Reptiles*, I have corrected those deficiencies. To date, this book is the only homeopathic resource that classifies the snakes into their proper zoological families while providing detailed information, thereby opening up our ability to use these remedies with greater precision and success.

Using and prescribing the reptiles for which as yet no symptoms are recorded or known, can be based upon the additional information provided, such as behavior, temperament, biological profile, folklore, associations, environment, as is done for other substances in our Materia Medica.

Causative links of certain reptiles to specific medical conditions, pathologies or target organs will also be useful indicators to their use. For instance: lactic acidosis; Lyme disease; hyponatremia; hypernatremia; hypokalemia; renal dysfunction; multiple sclerosis; Guillain-Barré syndrome; intense pain; ischemic stroke; hemorrhagic stroke; clotting disorders; haemorrhages; heart conditions; muscle weakness; paralysis; breast cancer.

The Class Reptilia – air-breathing, ectothermic [cold-blooded], scaled animals – comprises 4 orders of living reptiles. The extinct superorder of the dinosaurs is generally also included with the reptiles, although they are now thought to have been endothermic [warm-blooded].

The 4 orders include Crocodilia [23 species, including crocodiles, caimans, alligators, and gharials]; Rhynchocephalia [1 species of tuatara]; Squamata [9000+ species of lizards, snakes, and worm lizards]; and Testudines [300 species of turtles, terrapins and tortoises].

In *traditional* homeopathy [up to the year 1900] the reptile group was represented by 12 snakes, 2 lizards, 1 worm lizard and 1 unknown turtle species:

*Lachesis muta* – introduced by Hering in 1828, when he lived in Suriname. Hering conducted a self-experimentation with the 1st and 2nd trituration of the venom. In about 1834 or 1835, after he had moved to America in 1833, Hering organized a full proving with the 30th dilution involving 17 male provers and 3–4 female patients. Lachesis is the oldest and by far the largest snake remedy in homeopathy, with an estimated 12,000+ symptoms in repertoriums and materia medica.

*Crotalus horridus* – proving by Hering in c. 1836 with the 1st and 2nd triturations of the venom involving 4 male provers. Crotalus horridus is currently the second largest snake in the materia medica, with about 3000 symptoms.

*Vipera berus* [under the old name Vipera torva], *Vipera aspis* and *Vipera redi* [now known as Vipera aspis francisciredi]. No provings. All symptoms from effects of bites [envenomations], reported / collated by various authors, among them Hering in his *Wirkungen des Schlangengiftes* [Effects of snake venoms], 1837. Symptoms listed in Allen's Encyclopedia under the genus name Vipera. Vipera berus has about 1100 symptoms in current repertoriums.

*Crotalus cascavella* – introduced by Mure in Brazil in 1843; 1 male and 1 female prover. Current symptoms: c. 1500.

*Elaps corallinus* – introduced by Mure in Brazil in c. 1845; symptoms from a proving with the 3c trituration [number of provers unknown] and some clinical observations. Current symptoms: c. 1800.

*Amphisbaena vermicularis* – introduced by Mure in Brazil in c. 1847. Unknown how symptoms were obtained. Current symptoms: 200.

*Naja tripudians* – provings by Stokes [England] on himself and his future wife, 19-yr-old Rosa with 1st, 2nd, 4th and 6th dilutions of venom, 1852–53; and by Russell [England], with 1x, 2x, 3x dilutions and triturations, involving 2 female and 8 male provers, 1853. Current symptoms: c. 2000.

*Bothrops lanceolatus* – introduced by Ozanam [France], collection of cases and general observations on effects of bite, quoted from Rufz, 1859. Current symptoms: c. 450.

*Lachesis acrochorda*, under the name *Acrochordon chocoe* – effects of bite, recorded by Higgins in Colombia in c. 1873. Current symptoms: 0.

*Bothrocophias colombianus* [bile of the Colombian toad-headed pit viper], under the misnomer *Vipera lachesis fel* – proving by Berridge [England] on himself, with repeated doses of CM, and another man, who 'took 6 globules without knowing the name of medicine'; c. 1874.

*Cenchris contortrix* – proving by Kent [USA] with 6c, 30c and 10M; c. 1888; 3 female and 2 male provers. Current symptoms: c. 1200.
Hering's planned proving in the early 1830s with a lizard believed to be venomous by the local population in Suriname never came to fruition. Hering gave it the name *Askalabotes laevis* or *laevigatus*, mixing some of the then current scientific names – Ascalabotes surinamensis, Gecko laevis, Thecadactylus laevis – for a lizard now known as Thecadactylus rapicauda, the smooth or turnip-tailed gecko.

*Heloderma suspectum* – self-experimentation by Boocock [USA] with 6x and 30x in 1892–93. Boocock misnamed the lizard and thus the remedy Heloderma horridus, which has led to a lot of confusion. Current symptoms: c. 800.

It didn't end well for the only turtle listed in the traditional homeopathic literature. It was introduced by Jacob Jeanes, an associate of Hering in Philadelphia, under the name *Cholos terrapini* and consisted of the potentized bile of an unnamed species of turtle.
Since the 1930s provings have been conducted with 30 more reptiles [1 crocodilian; 1 dinosaur; 1 lizard; 2 turtles; 25 snakes], all fully included in *Reptiles*:

Bothrops atrox [USA; 1930s].
Hydrophis cyanocinctus [UK; 1958]
Vipera aspis [France; 1970]
Bothrops jararacussu [Brazil; 1990s]
Maiasaura lapidea [USA; 1990s].
Python reticulatus [India; 1990s]

Dendroaspis polylepis [India; 1994]
Boa constrictor [Austria; 1996]
Agkistrodon piscivorus [India; 1996]
Vipera berus [Austria; 1998]
Bitis arietans [South Africa, 1998; India, 2003]
Python regius [Germany; 1999]
Cerastes cerastes [Austria; 2000]
Alligator mississippiensis [USA; 2001].
Bungarus fasciatus [India; 2002]
Bitis gabonica [South Africa; 2004]
Chelydra serpentina [USA; 2004]
Echis carinatus [India; 2004]
Naja mossambica [South Africa; 2004]
Oxyuranus scutellatus [India; 2005]
Chamaeleo dilepis [South Africa; 2006]
Geochelone sulcata [USA; 2006]
Hemachatus haemachatus [South Africa; 2007]
Naja haje [India; 2009]
Naja pallida [India; 2009]
Ophiophagus hannah [India; 2009]
Dendroaspis angusticeps [South Africa; 2010]
Natrix natrix [Germany, 2003; UK, 2011]
Bitis atropos [South Africa; 2013]
Pseudonaja textilis [Australia; 2013]

My wish is that with this book you will gain even more proficiency and skill in more precisely using the remedies made from the animals in this fascinating, or shall I say mesmerizing, group.

Sapere aude.

**Frans Vermeulen**
*Texas, February, 2020*

# INDEX REPTILES COMMON NAMES

# INDEX REPTILES REMEDIES

INDEX REPTILES REMEDIES

# CLASS REPTILIA – REPTILES

## CROCODILES, ALLIGATORS & CAYMANS
*Alligator mississippiensis* – American alligator
*Alligator sinensis* – Chinese alligator
*Crocodylus acutus* – American crocodile
*Crocodylus novaeguineae* – New Guinea crocodile

## DINOSAURS [extinct]
*Maiasaura lapidea* – fossilized dinosaur bone
*Siroccopteryx moroccoensis* – pterosaur dinosaur
*Tyrannosaurus rex* – T-rex

## LIZARDS
*Anguis fragilis* – Slow-worm
*Askalabotes laevis* – Smooth gecko
*Basiliscus basiliscus* – Common basilisk
*Basiliscus vittatus* – Brown basilisk
*Chamaeleo chamaeleon* – Common chameleon
*Chamaeleo dilepis* – Flap-necked chameleon
*Chamaeleo zeylanicus* – Indian chameleon
*Chlamydosaurus kingii* – Frill-necked lizard
*Elgaria coerulea* – Northern alligator lizard
*Elgaria kingii* – Madrean alligator lizard
*Furcifer oustaleti* – Giant Madagascar chameleon
*Heloderma horridum* – Mexican beaded lizard
*Heloderma suspectum* – Gila monster
*Hemidactylus flaviviridis* – House lizard [gecko]
*Iguana iguana* – Green iguana
*Lacerta agilis* – Sand lizard
*Lacerta muralis* – Common wall lizard
*Lacerta vivipara* – Viviparous lizard
*Pogona vitticeps* – Central bearded dragon
*Sceloporus occidentalis* – Western fence lizard
*Varanus komodoensis* – Komodo dragon

## SNAKES

- Family Boidae – Constrictors
  *Antaresia perthensis* – Pygmy python

*Boa constrictor* – Boa constrictor
*Corallus hortulanus* – Amazon tree boa
*Eunectes murinus* – Green anaconda
*Eunectes notaeus* – Yellow anaconda
*Morelia spilota variegata* – Carpet python
*Morelia viridis* – Green tree python
*Python molurus* – Indian python
*Python regius* – Ball python
*Python reticulatus* – Reticulated python

- Family Colubridae – Colubrids
*Cyclagras* [= Hydrodynastes] *gigas* – False water cobra
*Dispholidus typus* – Boomslang
*Drymarchon corais* – Yellowtail cribo
*Drymarchon couperi* – Eastern indigo snake
*Elaphe guttata* – Corn snake
*Elaphe longissima* – Aesculapian snake
*Lampropeltis calligaster calligaster* – Prairie kingsnake
*Lampropeltis calligaster rhombomaculata* – Mole kingsnake
*Lampropeltis getula californiae* – California kingsnake
*Lampropeltis triangulum* – Milk snake
*Natrix natrix* – Grass snake
*Pantherophis obsoletus* – Texas ratsnake
*Thamnophis sirtalis sirtalis* – Eastern garter snake
*Vipera acuaticus carinata* – Chironius carinatus [Amazonian whipsnake]

- Family Elapidae – Elapids
*Bungarus caeruleus* – Common krait
*Bungarus candidus* – Blue krait
*Bungarus fasciatus* – Banded krait
*Bungarus multicinctus* – Many-banded krait
*Dendroaspis angusticeps* – Eastern green mamba
*Dendroaspis polylepis* – Black mamba
*Dendroaspis viridis* – Western green mamba
*Elaps* [= Micrurus] *corallinus* – Brazilian coral snake
*Hemachatus haemachatus* – Rinkhals
*Maticora bivirgata* – Blue Malayan coral snake
*Micrurus lemniscatus* – South American coral snake
*Naja anchietae* – Anchieta's cobra
*Naja annulifera* – Snouted cobra
*Naja haje* – Egyptian cobra
*Naja kaouthia* – Monocled cobra
*Naja melanoleuca* – Forest cobra
*Naja mossambica* – Mozambique spitting cobra
*Naja nigricollis* – Black-necked spitting cobra
*Naja nivea* – Cape cobra

*Naja [mossambica] pallida* – Red spitting cobra
*Naja tripudians* – Indian cobra
*Notechis scutatus occidentalis* – Western tiger snake
*Notechis scutatus scutatus* – Eastern tiger snake
*Ophiophagus hannah* – King cobra
*Oxyuranus microlepidotus* – Inland taipan
*Oxyuranus scutellatus* – Coastal taipan
*Pseudonaja textilis* – Eastern brown snake

- Family Hydrophiidae – Sea snakes
*Hydrophis cyanocinctus* – Annulated sea snake
*Laticauda colubrina* – Banded sea krait
*Pelamis platurus* – Yellow-bellied sea snake

- Family Viperidae – subfamily Crotalinae – Pit vipers
*Acrochordon chocoe* [= Lachesis acrochorda] – Chocoan bushmaster
*Ancistrodon piscivorus* [= Agkistrodon piscivorus] – Cottonmouth
*Bothriechis schlegelii* – Eyelash pit viper
*Bothrocophias colombianus* – Toad-headed pit viper
*Bothrops alternatus* – Crossed pit viper
*Bothrops asper* – Asper
*Bothrops atrox* – Common lancehead
*Bothrops caribbaeus* – St. Lucia pit viper
*Bothrops colombiensis* = Bothrops atrox
*Bothrops insularis* – Golden lancehead
*Bothrops jararaca* – Jararaca
*Bothrops jararacussu* – Jararacussu
*Bothrops lanceolatus* – Fer-de-lance
*Bothrops neuwiedi urutu* – Neuwied's lancehead
*Cenchris* [= Agkistrodon] *contortrix* – Copperhead
*Crotalus adamanteus* – Eastern diamondback rattlesnake
*Crotalus atrox* – Western diamondback rattlesnake
*Crotalus cascavella* – South American rattlesnake
*Crotalus cerastes cerastes* – Mojave Desert rattlesnake
*Crotalus enyo* – Baja California rattlesnake
*Crotalus horridus* – Timber rattlesnake
*Crotalus lepidus* – Rock rattlesnake
*Crotalus mitchellii* – Speckled rattlesnake
*Crotalus molossus [oaxacus]* – Black-tailed rattlesnake
*Crotalus polystictus* – Mexican lance-headed rattlesnake
*Crotalus viridis viridis* – Prairie rattlesnake
*Deinagkistrodon acutus* – Sharp-nosed pit viper
*Lachesis acrochorda* – Chocoan bushmaster
*Lachesis muta* – Bushmaster
*Sistrurus catenatus catenatus* – Eastern massasauga
*Sistrurus miliarius barbouri* – Dusky pygmy rattlesnake

*Trimeresurus* [= Protobothrops] *flavoviridis* – Habu
*Trimeresurus* [= Protobothrops] *mucrosquamatus* – Brown spotted pit viper
*Trimeresurus puniceus* – Flat-nosed pit viper
*Trimeresurus purpureomaculatus* – Mangrove pit viper
*Trimeresurus stejnegeri* – Green tree viper
*Trimeresurus* [= Tropidolaemus] *wagleri* – Temple pit viper
*Vipera lachesis fel* – bile of toad-headed pit viper

- Family Viperidae – subfamily Viperinae – True vipers
  *Atheris squamigera* – African bush viper
  *Bitis arietans* – Puff adder
  *Bitis atropos* – Berg adder
  *Bitis caudalis* – Horned adder
  *Bitis gabonica* – Gaboon viper
  *Bitis nasicornis* – Rhinoceros viper
  *Cerastes cerastes* – Horned viper
  *Daboia russelii* – Russell's viper
  *Daboia siamensis* – Eastern Russell's viper
  *Echis carinatus* – Saw-scaled viper
  *Proatheris superciliaris* – Swamp viper
  *Vipera ammodytes meridionalis* – Eastern nose-horned viper
  *Vipera aspis* – Asp viper
  *Vipera berus* – Common European viper
  *Vipera daboia* [= Daboia russelii] – Russell's viper
  *Vipera* [= Macrovipera] *lebetina* – Blunt-nosed viper
  *Vipera* [= Daboia] *palaestinae* – Palestine viper
  *Vipera redi* [= Vipera aspis francisciredi] – Central Italian asp viper
  *Vipera russelii siamensis* [= Daboia siamensis] – Eastern Russell's viper
  *Vipera torva* [= Vipera berus] – Common European viper
  *Vipera* [= Montivipera] *xanthina* – Ottoman viper

## TURTLES & TORTOISES

*Chelonia mydas* – Green turtle
*Chelydra serpentina* – Snapping turtle
*Cholos terrapini* [Cholas terrapina in Boericke] – bile of freshwater turtles
*Eretmochelys imbricata* – Hawksbill turtle
*Geochelone sulcata* – African spurred tortoise
*Lepidochelys olivacea* – Olive Ridley turtle
*Terrapene carolina* – Eastern box turtle
*Testudo hermanni* – Hermann's tortoise
*Trachemys scripta elegans* – Red-eared slider

## WORM LIZARDS

*Amphisbaena alba* – White worm lizard
*Amphisbaena vermicularis* – Wagler's worm lizard

# REPTILIAN TRAITS

## Shared characteristics

*History*
Two specialisations in particular characterise snakes: extreme elongation of the body and accompanying displacement and rearrangement of internal organs; and specialisations for eating large prey. Some reptiles are at home in aquatic environments; e.g. crocodilians, aquatic snakes, and sea turtles.

## Reproduction
Development in reptiles is direct, without larval forms as in amphibians. Female reptiles produce shelled, amniotic eggs, which contains nourishment and protective membranes for supporting embryonic development. They lay their eggs in sheltered locations on land. The young hatch as lung-breathing juveniles. Reptiles have some form of copulatory organs, permitting internal fertilisation, and obviously a requirement for a shelled egg.

In some turtle families, as in all crocodilians and some lizards, the nest temperature determines the sex of the hatchlings. In turtles, low temperatures during incubation produce males and high temperatures produce females.

## Temperature Regulation
Reptiles must adjust their body temperature to their environment. They use outside energy sources to regulate body temperature for metabolism and regulatory functions.

Being ectothermic, misleadingly called cold-blooded, reptiles lack the ability to regulate their metabolic heat [heat derived from the oxidation, or 'burning' of food and from other processes] for the production of sustained body warmth and a constant body temperature.

Because cold-bloodedness is a misleading term, biologists employ 2 others instead, describing reptiles as poikilothermic and ectothermic. Poikilothermy refers to the condition in which body temperature varies with the temperature of the environment; it is contrasted with homeothermy, a characteristic of birds and mammals, in which body temperature remains essentially the same through a wide range of environmental temperatures.

Ectothermy refers to the condition in which an animal depends on an external source, such as the sun, rather than its own metabolism, for body warmth. Birds and mammals, which use their internal metabolic heat for body warmth, are referred to as endothermic.

Reptilian thermoregulatory activities include [1] panting [evaporative cooling], [2] basking, [3] movement, [4] shivering, [5] reduction of blood flow to avoid heat loss, and [6] chromatophores.

When the temperature is not conducive to a reptile, they can go into a state of hibernation and wait until the weather is right for them to be active. Hibernating reptiles reduce individual heat loss by reducing total surface area. Unlike true hibernators, the body temperature of reptiles in torpor is not regulated; if the winter is too cold or the retreat too shallow, the animal can freeze and die. Cold death is an important source of mortality for temperate reptiles.

### Surviving on Very Little

'It is worth making the point here that, although ectothermy is often looked upon as a limitation, or as evidence of a primitive, poorly developed life-style, nothing could be further from the truth. Indeed, reptiles owe their success in many parts of the world, where they are the dominant group of vertebrates, to ectothermy.

'Warm-blooded, or endothermic, animals such as mammals and birds rely heavily on heat produced via their metabolic processes. In other words, a large proportion of their food [perhaps as much as 90%] is diverted away from growth, maintenance, and reproduction, and channeled into heat production. For this reason, they need to feed frequently and so are restricted to places where they can be sure of a regular food supply. Reptiles, including snakes, on the other hand, require food only to maintain themselves and to grow and reproduce if possible. This enables them to survive on a small fraction of the food that would be required by a bird or mammal of the same body weight. . . .

'Although snakes' low metabolic rates help them to survive on very little food, there is a trade-off in terms of energy. Endotherms, with their high metabolic rates are able to sustain work over a long period because their breathing and heart rates can continually supply oxygen to the muscles. Only after a relatively long period of exertion do the muscles build up an oxygen debt. Snakes, on the other hand, with their low metabolic rates, build up an oxygen debt very quickly. Although they can continue to operate by breaking down stored chemicals in the muscle cells [anaerobic metabolism] this will also be of limited duration because there is only a limited amount of material that can be processed. For this reason, they may be capable of *short bursts of activity*, when chasing prey or escaping from predators for instance, but they soon "*burn out*" and must rest until they have replenished their systems. In practice, snakes overcome this problem by rarely venturing far from their retreats and, in particular, only the most active species are seen out in the open, away from suitable cover.' [Mattison, 2002]

### Digestive Tract

Most reptiles are carnivores and have rather simple and not overly long guts, meat being fairly simple to break down and digest. Digestion is slower than in mammals, reflecting both the fact that they cannot divide and masticate their food like mammals do, and their lower metabolism. Being ectothermic their energy requirement is about a 5th to a 10th of that of a mammal of the same size. Large reptiles like crocodiles and the large constrictors can basically live from a single large meal for months, digesting it slowly.

## Brain & Sense Organs

The reptile's brain is small, but the cerebrum is larger relative to the rest of the brain. The increased size of cerebrum and the enlarged optic lobes result in improved sense of smell, increased reliance on vision and better coordination of muscle function. *Vision is the dominant sense.* Due to a great number of cones in retina, most reptiles have a well-developed colour vision. With the exception of blind snakes, reptiles rely more heavily on vision than on any other sense to detect objects in their surroundings. Snakes lack middle ear cavity and tympanic membrane, detecting vibrations through the jaw instead.

## Circulatory System

Reptiles have 2 aortic arches [blood vessels] carrying blood from the heart to the body; mammals have only one aorta, the left; birds also have but one, the right. Except for crocodilians, which have a four-chambered heart, all reptiles have a three-chambered heart consisting of 2 atrial chambers, separated by a complete septum, and a single ventricle.

The cardiac anatomy of crocodilians is very different from other reptiles but similar to that of birds and mammals. Crocodilians have 2 completely separated ventricles; in other reptiles the ventricle is incompletely separated. The morphology of the reptilian heart results in the mixing of oxygenated returning from the lungs and deoxygenated blood returning from the systemic circuit [cardiac shunts] owing to their undivided ventricle. Under different conditions, deoxygenated blood can be shunted back to the body or oxygenated blood can be shunted back to the lungs. This variation in blood flow has been hypothesized to allow more effective thermoregulation and longer diving times for aquatic species.

## Respiration

All reptiles breathe with lungs and depend almost exclusively on lungs for gas exchange, supplemented by respiration through the pharyngeal membranes in some aquatic turtles. Some file snakes, family Acrochordidae, and sea snakes, family Hydrophiidae, as well as the soft-shelled turtle, Trionyx, can use their skin for respiration when submerged. Reptiles suck air into the lungs by enlarging the pleural cavity, either by expanding the rib cage [snakes and lizards] or by movement of internal organs [turtles and crocodilians].

Reptiles except for crocodilians have no muscular diaphragm, a structure found in mammals. In snakes, presumably as an adaptation to their long, thin bodies, the left lung is reduced in size or entirely lacking.

In squamates, the lungs are ventilated almost exclusively by the axial musculature, the same musculature as is used during locomotion. Because of this constraint, most squamates are forced to hold their breath during intense runs. Some, however, have found a way around it. Varanids, and a few other lizard species, employ buccal pumping as a complement to their normal 'axial breathing'. This allows the animals to completely fill their lungs during intense locomotion, and thus remain aerobically active for a long time.

In many reptiles, particularly many turtles and crocodilians, lung ventilation is intermittent, wherein brief ventilatory periods are interspersed among apnoeas of variable duration. These apnoeic periods can be associated with quiet breathing or with diving in semi-aquatic species.

## Urinary Tract

Reptiles have kidneys with far fewer nephrons than higher vertebrates, as well as a poorly developed renal pelvis, and lacking a loop of Henle [long loop in the medulla of the kidney from which water and salts are resorbed into the blood]. To remove salts from the blood, many reptiles have salt glands located near the nose or eyes [in the tongue of saltwater crocodiles], which secrete a salty fluid that is strongly hyperosmotic to the body fluids.

Among reptiles the form taken by nitrogenous wastes, resulting from the oxidation of proteins, is closely related to the habits and habitat of the animal. Aquatic reptiles tend to excrete a large proportion of these wastes as ammonia in aqueous solution. Terrestrial reptiles must conserve body water and they convert their nitrogenous wastes to insoluble, harmless uric acid, which forms a more or less solid mass in the cloaca. Turtles, like mammals, mainly excrete urea.

The cloaca, whose name comes from the Latin word for sewer, is a body chamber leading to the outside and into which empty the excretory products of the kidneys, the waste products of the intestines, and the reproductive products of the testes and ovaries. The reptilian ureter empties into the cloaca, and if a bladder is present it receives and holds the urine overflow.

Renal disease is a major cause of mortality in captive lizards and snakes.

## Skeleton

Reptilian jaws are efficient for crushing or gripping prey. The specialised mobility of the reptilian skull enables lizards to seize and manipulate their prey. It also increases the effective closing force of the jaw musculature. The skull of snakes is even more kinetic than that of lizards. Such exceptional skull mobility enables snakes to eat animals much bigger than themselves.

## Skin

Tough, dry skin with scales, reptilian skin provides protection against desiccation and physical injury. Scales are largely formed of keratin. In snakes and lizards, new scales grow beneath the old, which are shed periodically. Since blood does not extend to the epidermis in snakes and lizards, cells lose contact with blood supply and die. Moult [shedding of outer covering] is usually initiated in the head region.

In snakes the old skin [epidermis and scales] is turned inside out when discarded; lizards split out of the old skin leaving it mostly intact and right side out or it may slough off in pieces. In turtles and crocodilians the large epidermal scales [scutes] are not moulted but are retained throughout life and are enlarged and thickened by additional layers of keratin from beneath; the uppermost layers of the scutes may be lost through wear or other factors.

Chromatophores present in dermis function much like amphibians: cryptic colouration, mimicry; colour and colour changes function in sex recognition and thermoregulation.


## Those Crawly Things

*Bans & Fans*

Herpetology is the study of reptiles *and* amphibians. Herpeton derives from Greek *herpein,* to crawl or creep. The name and classification come from Linnaeus [1707–1778], the Swedish physician-naturalist whose divinely inspired ambition it was to classify every living thing on Earth, like a second Adam. Unwitting of the enormous diversity, Linnaeus lumped reptiles and amphibians together as herpetons. Linnaeus combined his mission to name all things with an active relationship to God and Nature as God's creation. Linnaeus himself coined the phrase: 'God created, Linnaeus classified.'

Modesty was not one of Linnaeus' qualities. He wrote five autobiographies, in one of them writing about himself in the elevated third person as that 'God has permitted him to see more of his created work than any mortal before him.' This most likely inspired his lowly vision on crawly things: 'These foul and loathsome animals have a single ventricle and auricle, doubtful lungs, and a double penis. Most are abhorrent because of their cold body, pale colour, cartilaginous skeleton, filthy skin, fierce aspect, calculating eye, offensive smell, harsh voice, squalid habitation, and terrible venom; and so their Creator has not exerted his powers to make many of them.'

By contrast, eastern belief systems like Buddhism and Hinduism are unabashed fans, painting the snake as wise, benevolent, even revered as a deity. Many indigenous peoples have creation myths involving reptiles and amphibians [snakes figure most heavily], and ancient animism is rife with snake iconography.


## The Obnoxious Duty to Denote Blame

'A reptile is not, perhaps, an amiable thing. Its name "that which creeps" prejudices some of us against it. Nor is there anything thoroughly unjustifiable in this. The necessities of speech require a word that shall compendiously express the idea of the contemptible and crawling, and at the same time the potentially hurtful.

'And "reptile" fulfils this obnoxious duty. So when Beattie applies this term of reproach to a servile poet, or Byron to a mean critic, they are not to be found fault with. The sycophant in Shelley, the slave in Montgomery, even man – "the poor reptile man and heir of woe" himself – in loftily moralizing Greene, are metaphorically rendered, and not unfairly, by a term that zoologically implies either a turtle, a crocodile, a frog, a lizard, or a snake. Southey brings some priests under the same category and scattered up and down in verse will be found scores of individuals whom the poets, anxious to stigmatize as despicably base, denominate "reptiles."

'Now all this is perfectly fair. We have attached to a certain word a certain metaphorical meaning, which is a very odious one. Bismarck called the Secret Service Vote "the Reptile Fund," and the Man of Iron [Bismarck] includes in it all such miserable creatures as venal editors and spies. The self-seeking parasite, the insidious hypocrite, the cringing slave, deserve the worst we can say of them, and as we have decided that there is nothing worse to be said of such than "reptile" reptiles let them be.

'But, setting logic aside, I contend that it is infinitely unjust to speak ill of an immense number of creatures, nearly all of which are either beautiful, directly useful to man, or harmless, simply because, in our usual high-handed way of dealing with the helpless, we have borrowed their collective names as figures of speech. Yet this is what most poets habitually do. Their toads are loathsome and their frogs obscene. Their chameleons are turncoats, and their scorpions' traitors. Their snakes are utterly abominable.

'Now I fail to see any justification for this. It strikes me as thoroughly immoral. Even snakes, against which human prejudice cites Scriptural authority, are admirable. They are one of the most splendid parables in all nature. Nothing that breathes less deserves the title of reptile – meaning by that word a despicable cowardly thing – than the creature that stands in Holy Writ itself as the semblance of a power that could defy Heaven and challenge terms with Omnipotence.' [Robinson, 1893]

## Nature's Regrettable Moments of Creation

'. . . those revolting forms that Nature would seem to have created in some regrettable moment of boundless vindictiveness, for the express purpose of surrounding the beautiful and useful members of the animal creation with the ever-present risk of a ghastly death by constriction, venom, or drowning. Were there traceable in this incomprehensible dispensation any beneficial or indeed intelligible purpose, any advantage to the many in the sacrifice of the few, the horrible mission of the reptiles might be understood and, to some slight extent perhaps, respected. But there is none whatsoever.

'When one comes to reflect upon the immense and lamentable loss of human and animal life caused by the vast numbers of reptiles by which Africa is infested – a loss of life uncompensated by any single discoverable advantage, unrequited by the smallest benefit to those who survive – one fails hopelessly to comprehend their inclusion in the scheme of Nature, or to feel anything regarding them other than vain regret that their numbers and varieties should today be to all intents and purposes just as great and numerous as at any period regarding which we possess reliable data. Another singular and incomprehensible fact connected with this subject is the length of the period of life assigned to certain members of the reptile families in comparison with that which the mammals enjoy.' [Maughan, 1914]

## Fear, Fascination & Freaks

Snakes have fascinated and frightened humans for thousands of years. Some cultures still worship snakes, seeing them as creators and protectors. Other cultures fear snakes as devils and symbols of death.

'Ophidiophobia refers to the fear of snakes. Fear of snakes is sometimes called by a more general term, herpetophobia, fear of reptiles. It is one of the most common zoophobias [animal phobias]. Care must also be taken to differentiate people who do not like snakes or fear them for their venom or the inherent danger involved. A typical ophidiophobic would not only fear them when in live contact but also dreads to think about them or even see them on TV or in pictures. Recent studies conducted have theorised that humans may have an innate reaction to snakes, which was vital for the survival of humankind as it allowed such dangerous threats to be identified immediately.' [Wikipedia]

For many of the same reasons that people hate snakes, there are people that love snakes [ophiophilia]. An increasing number of people are keeping snakes as pets. Children show no fear of snakes or most things for that matter and are taught to fear snakes and other animals by their parents.

'Reptiles and amphibians embody all the subconscious elements at play in human attraction: fascination, repulsion, desire, fear. Strange habits and a primitive look, colourful geometries and ornamental postures, ornery disposition and death-dealing abilities add up to the perfect animal storm – an irresistible draw for would-be herpers, who, unlike bird-watchers, are not at all content to simply watch. . . . Uncharitable though the term [freak factor] may be, no other way exists to describe the eccentrics lurking outside herpetology's scientific core hoping for coattail identity, meaning, or membership. The Cult of Herps. Symbologists. Occultists. A bike gang's club anaconda. A stripper's phallic boa constrictor prop. Breeders playing god, looking to create their own decorative reptilian tapestries.

'Searchers, emulators, obsessors, and the truly confused – caught in the mental crossfire between good and evil, between a higher calling and a lower fate; where anything and everything in life's identity roulette becomes horribly and brutally syncretic. . . . Unique in its susceptibility to being hijacked, making us all guilty by association, modern herpetology finds itself in constant struggle to wash off the taint of the damned. . . . It didn't matter because whether you worked with turtles, lizards, frogs, or salamanders, you were doomed by association with the snake guys; a Faustian bargain with Cobras 'R Us that many herpetologists – nerds, freaks, and misfits that they were – wore as a badge of honour. Or a belt. Like punk rockers flaunting "individuality" with Mohawks and safety-pin uniforms, many drawn to herpetology feel a need to look the part. Thus, an inordinate number of bikers, strippers, and other fringe types count herpetology among their hobbies and aren't shy about it. Then again, neither are some science-minded practitioners: snakeskin boots, poison arrow frog T-shirts, and necklaces of crocodile teeth long flourished at meetings of the good ol' boy Herpetologists' League.' [Anthony, 2008]

## Immortality Lost

African traditions blame the loss of human immortality on the dim-witted chameleon. [See Chamaeleo chamaeleon]. The chameleon is not the only reptile being accused of causing man's mortality. Whereas this was due to the chameleon's slowness and apparent laziness, the snake did something much worse – it stole the immortality originally intended for man.

'After comparing many stories in which the snake by chance or design obtains man's immortality, Sir James Frazer came to the conclusion that the story of the Fall in the third chapter of Genesis is incomplete and perhaps originally ran as follows. The serpent was sent as a messenger to the Garden of Eden, where they grew 2 wondrous trees, to warn Adam and Eve that the fruit of one of these trees would bring death to the eater while the fruit of the other would ensure eternal life. The wily serpent decided that he would like to live forever so he perverted God's message, persuading Eve to eat the fatal fruit from the tree of death. The wily serpent meanwhile ate from the tree of life and so became immortal.' [Morris, 1968]

Alternatively, the snake sometimes is supposed to have become immortal because of its alert wakefulness. When God came to ask men and the animals if they wished to live forever, all were asleep, with the exception of the snake, which of course never shuts its eyes.

## Reptiles as Sex Symbols

Scottish chemist and scientist James Ballantyne Hannay [1855–1931] authored a pioneer work on sexual symbolism in religion in the 1920s. After reiterating the ancient but threadbare notion of reptiles as sexual symbols, he comes up with the intriguing twist that Jehovah in sentencing the snake makes sexual passion a sin and institutes venereal disease, particularly syphilis, as a punishment.

Hannay writes: 'Now the serpent is *the universal symbol* for the phallus or for sexual passion. . . . The Tortoise or Turtle is a complete phallic or creative symbol – "the world rests on a Tortoise" – its head when protruded being a model of the phallus, while its oval shell or carapace represents the female. . . . By its rounded form it represents the Dome or D'Om [place of the womb] of our churches, like Minerva's shield with its serpents. The serpent was introduced because religious prostitution caused syphilis to be rampant, and the Cobra not only erects itself, but its bite is fatal like syphilis, so the Cobra represented the "evil" side of "Adam's first transgression" better than the tortoise. In fact, the 2 incurable things were the serpent's bite and syphilis; . . . the latter was rampant where temple women were kept.'

Notwithstanding the belief of syphilis being a relatively recent disease, arriving in Europe with the return of Columbus from America in 1493, Hannay argues that the disease 'visiting the sins of the fathers upon the children to the third and fourth generation' could have been no other than syphilis. [Hannay, 1922]

## Reptilians

*The Reptilian Brain*

According to the famous triune brain theory developed by Paul MacLean, 3 distinct brains co-inhabit the human skull: the reptilian brain, the limbic brain, and the neo-cortex. MacLean called it the tri-une [three-one] brain because the 3 formations constitute an amalgamation of 3 brains in one.

Our reptilian brain includes the main structures found in a reptile's brain: the brainstem and the cerebellum. The brain stem is the smallest region of the human brain. Various clumps of cells in the brain stem determine the brain's general level of alertness. Reliable but tending to be somewhat rigid, compulsive and highly resistant to change, the reptilian brain is 'preverbal' and controls life functions such as autonomic brain, breathing, heart rate and the execution of the fight or flight response in stress. Lacking language, its impulses are instinctual and ritualistic. It is concerned with fundamental needs such as survival, physical maintenance, hoarding, dominance, preening and mating. It is also found in lower life forms such as lizards, crocodiles, and birds.

The 'reptilian in us' controls our instinctual drives that are least subject to conscious control – sex, sustenance, survival, and safety.

According to Skip Largent, 'First and foremost among the traits generated through the reptilian brain is the drive to establish and defend territory. This is fueled by an extremely potent "will-to-power," exemplified among lizards by the ritual behaviour of 2 rainbow lizards competing for dominance. These animals have beautiful colours and like many lizards, use head-bobbing and push-ups in assertive, aggressive courtship and greeting displays. In a contest, once the gauntlet is thrown down, the aggressive displays give way to violent combat, and the struggle is unrelenting. In victory, they are tyrannical dictators in the extreme. In defeat, they lose their majestic colours, lapse into a kind of depression, and die 2 weeks later.

'At least 5 human behaviours originate in the reptilian brain. These have been denoted as isopraxic, preservative, re-enactment, tropistic, and deceptive. Without defining them, I shall simply say that in human activities they find expression in: obsessive-compulsive behaviour; personal day-to-day rituals and superstitious acts; slavish conformance to old ways of doing things; ceremonial re-enactments; obeisance to precedent, as in legal, religious, cultural, and other matters; responding to partial representations [colouration, "strangeness," certain ways of moving, images of certain kinds, etc.], whether alive or inanimate; and all manner of deception.

'All movies and television likely are a projection of the reptilian brain. . . . Movies and television [video games, etc.] are all undeniably dreamlike, not only in their presentation of symbolic reality, but also in that humans experiencing movies, etc. have the same brain wave patterns as when they are dreaming. And guess where dreaming originates in your head? In the reptilian brain [although other parts of our brains are involved].

'The "language" of the reptilian brain is visual imagery. Most communications transferred by reptiles are done so by visual symbolic representations, each having specific meaning. Mammals and birds do dream, but reptiles do not dream. Why? Because the reptilian mind is still operating in them and we humans call that mental state "dreaming." There is no "dream state" in reptiles because this mentality is their waking state. It is repressed during our waking hours [but still functioning – it never sleeps] by chemicals released neo-cortically – then the reptilian is allowed to function during sleep and dream, when the left hemisphere is in turn repressed. But obviously, the reptilian brain is not satisfied being relegated to the "night-watch" of an inert body. It wants far more than that.

'. . .We have excellent duplication of the reptilian mindset with movies and television, etc. – which by some estimates, occupies up to 16–18 hours of our time per day, when you add in sleep-dream time. . . . The reptilian brain is a powerful source of human behaviour – primarily because it is hidden. It is deceptive. It is a secret from our conscious. But we do "know" it emotionally, intuitively. It is the slithering serpent in darkness! It is The Unconscious.' [www.paleoart.com]

*Reptilian Humanoids*
'Reptilian humanoids are a common theme in fiction, whether fantasy or science fiction. Because of the aversion that many people have for reptiles in general, reptile-like aliens are often the villain in such works. Human-like reptiles have appeared in various popular treatments, from early pulp short stories and novellas, to full novels, comic books, television features, films, and the gaming industry. For example, the television show Doctor Who featured several reptilian humanoid races, including the Mars-dwelling Ice Warriors, the alien Draconians, the marine Sea Devils and the land-based Silurians. The sleestaks from Land of the Lost are villainous lizard creatures.' [Wikipedia]

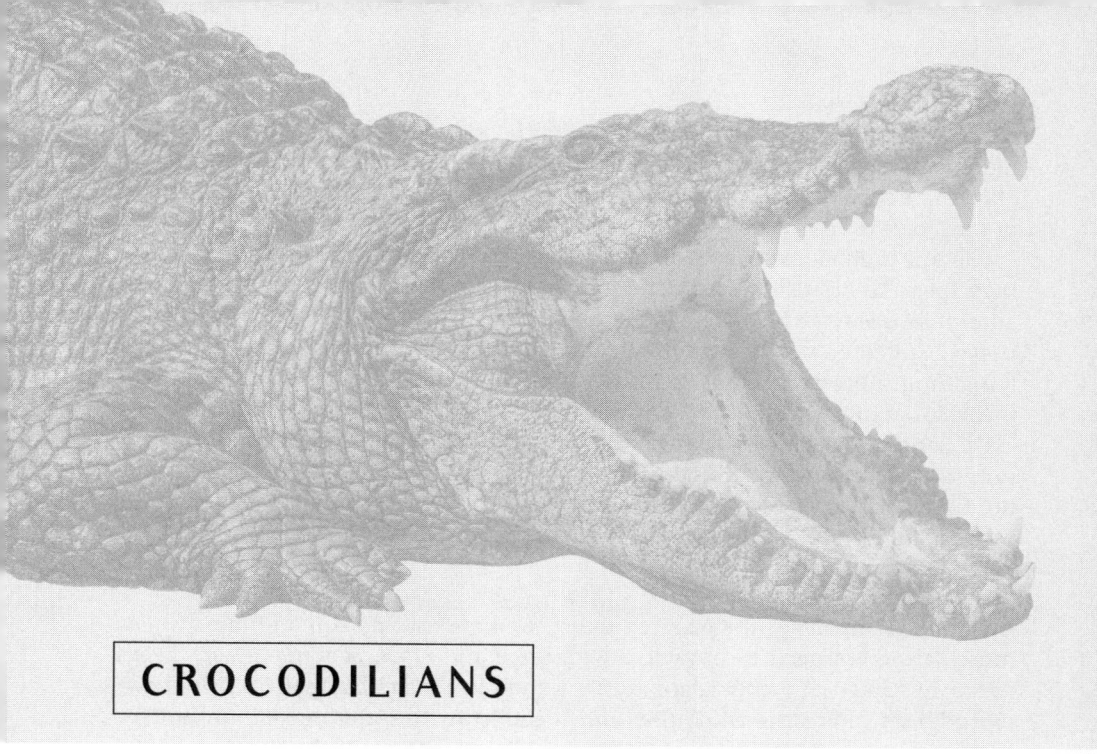

# CROCODILIANS

## BIOLOGICAL PROFILE

### Diversity of Crocodilians

According to the most widely used taxonomic classification [King & Burke, 1997], there are 23 extant crocodilian species, divided over 3 families: Alligatoridae, Crocodylidae and Gavialidae.

1 Alligatoridae [alligator and caiman family] comprises 4 genera: Alligator [2 species]; Caiman [2–3 species]; Melanosuchus [black caiman; 1 species]; and Paleosuchus [dwarf caiman; 2 species]. This family is found almost exclusively in the New World, with the sole exception of the Chinese alligator, which is found in eastern China.

2 Crocodylidae [crocodile family] holds 2 genera: Crocodylus [true crocodiles; 11–12 species] and Osteolaemus [dwarf crocodile; 1 species]. Only a few members of this family are native to the Americas, the rest is found throughout Africa, India and Asia.

3 Gavialidae [gavial family] consists of 2 genera: Gavialis [gavial, also known as gharial; 1 species] and Tomistoma [false gharial, also known as false gavial; 1 species]. The gavial is from India and the false gharial is from Malaysia and Indonesia.

## Distribution & Habitat

Crocodilians are generally found in tropical regions, being unable to survive and reproduce successfully in cold climates. The American alligator and the Chinese alligator are the most cold-tolerant and are both found in the highest latitudes of any species.

Water is their element, where they procreate, hunt and feed; dry land is where they spend to bask in the sun. The form of most crocodilians is adapted to their amphibious way of life. The elongated body with its long, muscular paddletail is well suited to rapid swimming. Air-breathers, crocodilians are capable of remaining submerged for as much as an hour.

Alligators prefer freshwater; crocodiles like brackish water and even saltwater.

Crocodiles also have special glands in their tongues that can get rid of excess salt, so they tend to live in saltwater habitats. Alligators have these glands, too, but they don't work as well as the crocodiles', so alligators prefer to live in fresh-water habitats.

## Physical Features

All crocodilians have an elongate, robust, well-reinforced skull and massive jaw musculature arranged to provide a wide gape and *rapid, powerful closure*. Teeth are set in sockets. Another adaptation is a complete secondary palate. This allows crocodilians to breathe when the mouth is filled with water or food [or both].

The estuarine crocodile [Crocodylus porosus], found in southern Asia, and the Nile crocodile [C. niloticus] grow to great size [adults weighing 1000 kg have been reported] and are swift and aggressive. Crocodiles are known to attack animals as large as cattle and deer.

'The crocodilian's body is joined to the powerful tail so inconspicuously that, were it not for the hind legs, one might have trouble telling where the body ends and the tail begins. Apart from being all-important in the crocodilian's undulatory swimming motions, the tail is also a powerful weapon of defence. A swift sideswipe of the heavy tail sweeps a man off his feet at the moment when a similar sideswipe of the open jaws has put the crocodilian in a position to take the best advantage of the blow by the tail.

Despite being thought of as living fossils, 'the crocodilian's body is not without its modern developments. The heart, for example, has 4 chambers, the teeth are in separate sockets, and the body is divided by a diaphragm or muscle that is used in breathing. These "living fossils" can thus look down their long noses at other reptiles and justly claim to be ahead of them in those important improvements that were only later developed by the mammals themselves.' [Pope, 1971]

## Digestive Tract & Metabolism

'Many crocodilians are found to have empty stomachs because they use the energy in the food they eat *more efficiently than almost any other animal*. They manage this partly by the way they obtain their food, partly by being cold-blooded, and partly from the thoroughness with which food is digested. . . .

'The crocodilian digestive system is remarkable for several reasons. Firstly, the stomach is the *most acidic recorded for any vertebrate*, allowing the crocodilian to digest all the bone it consumes. Secondly, about 60% of the energy contained in the food it eats is stored away as fat in the tail, in mesenteric organs in the abdomen, along the back, and almost anywhere it can be stored. Even some of the energy contained in *protein is converted to fat* in crocodilians. This allows crocodilians to survive for exceptionally long periods with no food at all.

'A newly hatched crocodile can survive for more than 4 months without eating, by using the fat from the remains of the yolk sac tucked away in its belly. A large crocodile, which may weigh more than 1 ton, can probably last for up to 2 years between meals. Alligators and some crocodiles regularly fast through the cooler months but the larger animals probably need to eat little even during the summer, provided they do not waste too much energy on breeding.

'Naturally, there are costs of such efficient metabolism. The first cost is the rate of growth. When food is constantly available crocodiles can grow nearly half a metre a year but in the wild this growth rate is often much lower. Because the young are storing so much of their food as fat, in case they have to go for a long time with none, fewer resources are directed into increasing length and muscle size.

'The other cost comes when crocodilians have to expend energy quickly, as when they capture food. Using energy requires oxygen in the blood but, because the crocodilian system is geared to using energy slowly, it can never get much oxygen in the blood at any one time. Without oxygen, exertion produces lactic acid, which gradually breaks down after activity ceases and more oxygen becomes available.

'The levels of lactic acid in the blood that can be tolerated by crocodilians have astonished researchers; their blood reaches an acidity level that would easily kill most other animals. However, it also means that crocodilians are easily exhausted and take a long time to recover from exercise of any kind.' [Garnett, 1989]

## Lactic Acidosis

'The languid existence of crocodiles can be punctuated by fierce activity during predation, defence and escape. Crocodiles often feed on large terrestrial animals that they pull into the water and drown. Thus, they must be capable of powerful physical activity and they must also be adequate divers. Both intense activity and diving behaviour promote a reliance on anaerobic metabolism. The magnitude of anaerobiosis in reptiles may exceed that of any other animal group and the build-up of lactate and protons in muscle and blood can lead to severe acid-base disturbance. Extreme exertion is done anaerobically [without oxygen] and must be followed by a period of rest so that the 'oxygen debt' can be repaid to their muscles.

The result of anaerobic activity is a build-up of lactic acid in the blood. A drop in pH follows a rise in lactic acid; the lactate produced in mild excitement displaces, equivalent for equivalent, bicarbonate ions in the extracellular fluids. Periods of apnoea may contribute to the fall in pH. Although crocodiles can withstand higher levels of blood acidity than other animals, sometimes it can be fatal. In particular, during the capture of large crocodiles, the animals' use of their glycolytic muscles often alters the blood's pH to a point where they are *unable to respond to stimuli or move.* Cases are recorded in which particularly large crocodiles that put up extreme resistance to capture later died of the resulting pH imbalance.

### Heart like Mammals

Crocodilians have a 4-chambered heart, in contrast to lizards, turtles and snakes, which have a 3-chambered heart. Despite the 4 partitions, the crocodilian heart is relatively small, its mass making approximately 0.15% up of their body mass. In mammals the heart mass is 0.4 to 0.7% of body mass. Moreover, crocodilians have a relatively low systemic blood pressure.

The crocodilian heart has a specialisation not found in any other animal. There is a connection, known as the foramen of Panizza, between the right [pulmonary] side and the left [systemic] side of the heart, allowing mixing of deoxygenated and oxygenated blood, similar to other reptiles and amphibians. This right-to-left shunt reduces aerobic efficiency and would seem a disadvantage. However, crocodilian hearts have a special added feature: a valve in the right ventricle called cog-tooth valve. Crocodilians can actively regulate this valve, enabling them to block the pulmonary circuit, bypassing the lungs, and increase shunting to send more hypoxic blood to the tissues, inducing a hypometabolic state. And a hypometabolic state, in addition to a heart rate of 1 or 2 beats per minute, is just perfect for crocodilians in underwater resting or lurking mode.

The *hypo state can be reversed into a hyper state in a flash.* The valve is opened, the shunting ceased; the *heart is up to speed in seconds* and the full supply of energy-giving oxygenated blood is being pumped out to the muscles and tissues. Thus when active, the heart of a crocodile functions like a mammalian heart in that blood from the systemic circulation is kept separate from the blood in the pulmonary circulation.

Crocodilians have 2 main physiological responses for adjusting peripheral blood flow. They can speed up [tachycardia] or slow down [bradycardia] their heart rate, and/or they can widen [vasodilate] or narrow [vasoconstrict] their blood vessels.

### Lungs like Birds

'In addition to the completely divided heart, . . . other curiously sophisticated properties of the crocodile [include]. They have complex, bird-like lung structure, and birds are the pulmonary champions among the vertebrates, with amazingly efficient respiratory surfaces. They have muscular specialisations for lung inflation during active locomotion, which seem superfluous in a sit-and-wait ambush predator. Their bones have the characteristic richly vascularised structure of fibro-lamellar bone, one of the hallmarks of endothermy and one of the pieces of evidence that dinosaurs were warm-blooded. Interestingly, one bit of counter evidence used against the hot-blooded dino hypothesis was the fact that crocodilians have the same structure . . . maybe there's another reason for the similarity that crocs are also descended from hot-blooded ancestors.' [Myers, 2005]

## Death Roll to Subdue & Dismember Prey

Crocodilians perform a spinning maneuver to subdue and dismember prey. The spinning maneuver, which is referred to as the 'death roll', involves rapid rotation about the longitudinal axis of the body. For aquatic predators with teeth and jaws that lack specialised cutting dentition, having no shearing or grinding action, this method of twisting and gulping is a highly efficient way of overcoming prey.

'Fearsome as they are, the teeth of crocodilians are ill-suited for tearing their prey apart or even for chewing. Combined with the awesome closing power of the jaws, they are, however, perfect for clamping onto and holding their victims. Small prey is swallowed whole, but larger animals are often dragged underwater and stashed there until decay begins to soften the skin and flesh. The crocodile butchers its prey by clamping onto a piece of flesh and violent twisting over and over until a mouthful is torn loose from the carcass. Lacking a tongue, it must engulf its food with a series of jerks and tosses of the head.' [Nagami, 2004]

[It is often mistakenly assumed that crocodilians don't have tongues. They do have a fleshy tongue that is attached along its length between the lower jaws.]

## Downward Movement

Most of the crocodilian's *power is contained in downward movement*. The death roll is an essentially downward movement and so is the clamping down on prey. Crocodiles have powerful muscles for closing their jaws and holding them shut. Large crocodilians can pulverise turtle shells or the skulls of their prey in a single crushing movement of their jaws. No other animal has such bite force as crocodilians. But the muscles for opening their jaws are weak. It is relatively easy to keep a crocodilian's massive jaws closed; a strong rubber band is all that is needed.

Equally downward is the tremendous pounding force with which fighting crocodiles come down upon each other, like tons of bricks.

## Senses

Crocodilians are efficient hunters, and their senses are more powerful than those of most other reptiles. They have excellent hearing, having slits on their heads that lead to a well-developed inner ear and the slits close up when they dive to keep water out. Crocodilians can hear their young calling from inside their eggshells.

They also have keen eyesight above water, similar to an owl's. Their eyes are placed on top of their heads so they can see well as they cruise the water looking for prey. They can probably see some colour and they have good night vision because their vertical pupils can open wider than our round ones to let in more light.

Crocodilians have taste buds to taste their food and special organs in their snouts give them a great sense of smell. Both crocodiles and alligators have dotted sensory pits along the upper and lower jaws. The exact function of these pits hasn't been conclusively determined as yet, but it is thought they detect slight changes in water pressure, possibly to help the animals locate underwater prey, and perhaps changes in salinity. The sensory pits go under a number of different names, incl. integumentary sense organs [ISOs] and dermal pressure receptors [DPRs]. In alligators and caimans they are restricted to the head – upper jaw, nose, around the eyes, lower jaw, even the upper palate – whereas crocodiles and gharials have them on the head as well as all over the body.

## Territorial Tiffs

'Crocodilians are the most efficient predators in their ecosystems, and they guard their territories jealously. Saltwater crocodiles are the most territorial of all crocodilians and their territory in the wild can range from a few hundred metres to several kilometres in length. Both male and female adults will *see off intruders*. An adult female will often drive other females away from the nesting ground she has selected. She will defend her nest sites vigorously, going without food if necessary. As her eggs will take between 70 and 95 days to hatch, a nesting female can lose a lot of condition.

'Dominant crocodilian males will not tolerate intruders in their territories. Battles commence with a series of displays and rituals. The dominant animal will raise its body out of the water, trying to intimidate its challenger. Submissive animals will raise their heads at a steep angle, offering their throats to the dominant male. They will sometimes also vocalize their submission. . . . Should the intimidatory display fail, however, the dominant male becomes more intent on punishing the presumptuous intruder. Lifting its head and body from the water, the attacker smashes down onto the head or body of its opponent, often at an angle with jaws open. This crashing blow from a head solid with reinforced bone and jaws full of strong sharp teeth can do great damage. Bones are smashed, skin is ripped and teeth fly. Another strategy is to try and bite their opponent on the body, tail or limbs, occasionally holding on and spinning the body to inflict damage.' [Kelly, 2006]

## Social Behaviour

On the *reptilian scale of sociability, snakes rank lowest and crocodilians highest.* To be regarded as social, behaviour must involve the tendency to associate with others and to form social groups, which includes social recognition, communication, parental care, territorial aggression, and social bonding.

Crocodilians are unusual among reptiles in being able to make definite vocalisations. Male alligators can give loud bellows in the mating season. Alligators are notably the most vocal and are renowned for the bellowing choruses of breeding males and females that reverberate through the marshes and swamps in late spring. Non-vocal methods of communication include head-slapping – a loud noise made by snapping the jaws together just at the surface of the water – and tail thrashing.

Kin selection is fundamental for cooperation in many animal societies, and so it is in crocodilians. 'Crocodilians differ from all other reptiles by showing a complex social behaviour. They communicate with sounds, postures, motions, odours, and touch. As explained by Lang, communication starts in the egg and continues throughout life. Embryos near hatching time possibly may vocalise to synchronise the hatching of the clutch. Hatchlings and young may vocalise to maintain group cohesion or, in a dangerous situation, to alert others and attract the attention of adults. Typically, adults react by attacking the possible predator.' [Fowler, 2001]

Head-slapping and associated behaviours such as head submergence and the production of copious bubbles from around the head is an instant attention getter and announces the presence and location of its performer. 'Head-slapping is a contagious activity, and an initial head-slap is usually answered almost immediately by head-slaps from other individuals nearby. . . . Animals emerge from underwater, those in the water respond by approaching or retreating, and those on land move into the water. Head-slapping, like bellowing, is associated with establishing and maintaining long-term social relationships and is most obvious during seasonal reproductive activities. In captivity, loud noises and disturbances, such as vehicle backfiring or a gunshot, sometimes elicit head-slaps.'

[Wilfred T. Neill [1971] was of the exact opposite opinion that 'the chief function of the bellow is to keep individuals apart, not bring them together. . . . Bellowing is not followed by combat, and bellowers remain in the position they were occupying when a chorus began. Bellowing functions to reveal the location of the caller to others of the same species.'] . . .

'Body posture [in and out of the water] and specific movements are the principal visual communicating signals. In all species, the exposure of the head, back, and tail above the water surface conveys important information about an individual's social status and intent. Dominant animals advertise their large size by swimming boldly at the surface. Conversely, submissive individuals usually expose only the head and readily retreat by submerging underwater. In many species, a threatening individual inflates the body and assumes an erect, static posture to exaggerate body size. . . . In breeding enclosures, adult crocodilians exhibit many behaviours that strongly suggest that odours may be an important mode of communication. . . .

'Hatchlings frequently remain in the vicinity of the nest site in crèches and nurseries where they form social groups or pods. Although this behaviour is usually associated with the presence of a parent or other adults nearby, hatchling groups persist in assembling even when adults are not present. Presumably, group living decreases an individual's risk of predation and it is therefore not surprising that such behaviour is pronounced in hatchlings, which are especially vulnerable to predation. . . .

'Juveniles and adults are less gregarious than hatchlings, but they also associate in loosely organised social groups.' [J.W. Lang, in Garnett 1989]

## Courting & Mating

'Crocodilian males fight not only for territory, but also for the right to impregnate the local females. All crocodilian species are *polygamous,* and the dominant male will mate with all the sexually mature females in his territory. The sexual maturity of crocodilians is quoted in body length not age, because growth rates depend on the resources available. . . .

'Mating behaviour varies between species from the very formalised, predictable rituals of the American crocodile to the fairly flexible rituals and unpredictable success in mating of the American alligator. Behaviour includes snout contact and lifting, head and body rubbing, body riding, circling and swimming displays. Given the size of the larger crocodilians, the actual act of mating takes place in the water.

'Crocodilians have a much more acute sense of hearing than other reptiles, and sound plays a large part in the mating rituals of a number of crocodilian species. . . . American alligators bellow loudly during the courting and mating seasons. This bellowing can be so strong that the alligators vibrate along the entire length of their bodies. Once an individual starts, a whole group can bellow and vibrate in chorus – a truly alarming sound and sight for the unwary, but obviously intoxicating to those taking part. Other crocodilian males rumble, cough or bark to attract their females.' [Kelly, 2006]

## Maternal Care

Alligators and crocodiles are oviparous. Crocodiles lay their eggs in mud or sand nests near brackish water, while alligators and caimans make their nests out of mounds of vegetation surrounding freshwater.

Females lay 20 to 50 hard-shelled white eggs and *protect their eggs fiercely* for the 8 to 14 weeks before hatching. The mother hears vocalisations from the hatching young and responds by opening the nest to allow the hatchlings to escape. As with many turtles and some lizards, the incubation temperature of the eggs determines the sex ratio of the offspring. However, unlike turtles low nest temperatures produce only females, while high nest temperatures produce only males.

'For such ancient, ferocious-looking animals, crocodilian moms take really good care of their hatchlings! Crocs are one of the few reptiles that watch out for and protect their young until they are old enough to be on their own. The cow [female croc] looks for just the right place to build a nest to lay her eggs.

'Some species make a mound nest out of soil and vegetable material; others dig a hole in the sandy beach for their nest. The mama croc then settles in nearby to guard the eggs from predators that might try to dig them up and eat them. When the babies are ready to hatch, they make grunting or barking noises from inside the egg and use a short little tooth on the end of their snouts called an "egg tooth" to start breaking out of the leathery shell. Some croc moms even help by gently biting the egg to open it up more easily.

'After the young have hatched, the mom carries them to the water in her mouth [except for gharials, which have mouths that are too narrow], then guards them for most of the first year of their lives. Sometimes the hatchlings get to ride on her back, too. She will threaten or attack any predator that lurks too close, and in some species she will call the hatchlings to swim into her mouth for protection – making it look like she's swallowed them!' [website San Diego Zoo]

## Anti-bacterial Properties – Putting the Bite on Germs

Crocodiles fight a lot and *inflict horrendous wounds upon each other*, wounds that would be fatal to mammals, either through blood loss or infection from the bacteria-infested, muddy water in which crocodilians live. Three-legged or tailless crocodilians are not an uncommon sight in tropical swamps, the missing limb or appendage having been torn off by a combatant.

Despite serious injuries and giant bleeding wounds, *no infection occurs*. Apart from inherent toughness, their survival of highly traumatic events has been attributed to a special wound-healing compound in their system. It was discovered that crocodilians have a peptide in their blood that appears to function as an antibiotic, which was named 'crocodillin'. Researcher Gill Diamond, who isolated the peptide from the blood of Crocodylus porosus, claims that crocodillin 'blows away' bacteria, and can even kill resistant bacteria. It seems furthermore that bacteria have a hard time developing resistance against it.

The discovery prompted scientists to sink their teeth into the anti-bacterial properties of other crocodilians.

'Treatment of alligator [Alligator mississippiensis] and human serum samples with Escherichia coli resulted in a time- and concentration-dependent inhibition of bacterial proliferation. When inoculated with E. coli, alligator serum exhibited 10-fold lower bacterial survival rates after 1 hour than human serum. In addition, the antibacterial spectrum of alligator serum was shown to be much broader than that of human serum, with growth inhibition occurring in 100% of bacterial strains tested [compared to only 35% for human serum]. Additional results showed that the antimicrobial activities of alligator serum could be completely inhibited by pre-incubation with proteases, indicating the proteinaceous nature of the antimicrobial activities.

'Furthermore, incubation of alligator serum at 56°C [132.8°F] for 30 min [classical human serum complement inactivation conditions] obliterated all antimicrobial properties of the alligator serum. The antibacterial activities occurred relatively quickly in vitro, with significant activity occurring within 5 min of inoculation with E. coli and maximal activity at 20 min. Also, the antimicrobial activity exhibited temperature dependence, with a substantial decrease in activity below 15 degrees C. These data suggest that the antimicrobial properties of alligator serum may be due to an active serum complement system.' [Merchant, 2003]

Subsequent studies by Merchant showed that the alligator's unusually strong immune system is very different from that of humans. Unlike people, alligators can fight microorganisms such as fungi, viruses, and bacteria without having prior exposure to them. According to Merchant, 'there's a real possibility that you could be treated with an alligator blood product one day.' If studies continue to show promise, the drugs could land on pharmacy shelves in another 7 to 10 years, he estimated in 2008.

## Differences between Crocodiles & Alligators

Crocodiles have a very long, narrow, V-shaped snout, while the alligator's snout is wider and U-shaped. Because of the wide snout of the alligator it packs more *crushing power* to eat prey like turtles that constitute part of its diet. The narrow crocodile snout, although still very powerful, is not really suited for prey like turtles but is very versatile for fish and mammals.

The upper and lower jaws of crocodiles are nearly the same width, so that the teeth are exposed all along the jaw line in an interlocking pattern. Alligators have a wider upper jaw, so that when its mouth is closed the teeth in the lower jaw fit into sockets of the upper jaw, hidden from view. Only the teeth of the upper jaw are exposed along the lower jaw line. The 4th tooth on the lower jaw sticks up over the upper lip in crocodiles, so you can see it when their mouths are closed. In alligators, this 4th tooth is covered up.

### Differences in Temper & Activity

'To the observer who is familiar with fair-sized alligators, but has never been properly introduced to a crocodile, the writer would say a few words of caution. There is about as much difference in temper and activity between an alligator and a crocodile, as between a tortoise and a snapping turtle. An enraged alligator will throw its head from side to side, bang the jaws together sonorously and violently swish the tail, but a man with steady nerves may approach within a few feet of the animal, throw a noose over the head, tie the jaws together, push a pole toward the body – then, by successive nooses pulled backward over the head and forward over the tail, splint the animal to the pole so it is entirely powerless.

'On one of a number of occasions, involving transferring alligators, operating upon them and the like, the writer, assisted by one man, in this way completely overpowered a vigorous, 12-foot example. Throughout the process the big saurian hissed, grunted, snapped from side to side and made swings with his tail that would have knocked a man off his feet – but the animal *remained in the same spot*.

'Such proceedings would have been abruptly terminated with a crocodile. The writer well remembers his first acquaintance with a big fellow from Florida. Driven out of the crate the crocodile looked the picture of good nature. Standing away from what he thought to be the reach of his tail, the writer prodded the apparently sluggish brute with a stick to start it for the tank. Several things happened in quick order. With a crescentic twist of the body utterly beyond the power of an alligator, the brute dashed its tail at the writer, landing him such a powerful blow that he was lifted completely from the ground.

'As he left *terra-firma*, an almost involuntary inclination caused him to hurl his body away from a pair of widely-gaping, tooth-studded jaws swinging perilously near. Landing with a thud on one shoulder, though otherwise unhurt, the writer threw himself over and over, rolling from the dangerous brute that was actually pursuing him on the run, body raised high from the ground. For an instant it seemed as if the crocodile would win. As the writer suddenly sprang to his feet and glanced backward, he beheld the brute throw itself flat on its belly, open the jaws widely, then remain motionless as a statue.

'Such is the average crocodile – *an active, vicious and, above all, treacherous brute*. When the keepers of the reptile house in the New York Zoological Park clean out the big pool for crocodilians, they actually walk over the backs of some of the big 'gators, so tame are these. They never become unduly familiar with the crocodiles, finding it necessary to pen the latter behind heavy barred gates – and in the process the men are often chased from the enclosure.' [Ditmars, 1910]

## CROCODILIAN CONNOTATIONS

### Amazingly Stealthy
'Crocodiles are *stealthy* – amazingly so, for such large beasts. When stalking terrestrial victims at the water's edge, they remain invisible underwater until the last second. Strong as they are, quick as they are, they take people by surprise, not just by quickness and strength.' [Quammen, 2003]

### Amphibious Ambiguity
'This amphibiousness of crocodiles is a most influential component of their symbolism. To be amphibious is to be ambiguous; neither one thing nor the other, unpredictable, obscure, and therefore dangerous. Such ambivalence has *Jekyll/Hyde qualities* – the calm, peaceful exterior concealing a vicious, raging other self; it equals treachery, a crocodile "characteristic" typically invoked to rationalise the dreadful humiliation of being attacked unawares.' [Graham, 1973]

### Brutal Force
'These are the facts of life among crocodiles. So long as one is constantly threatened by savage brutes one is to some extent *bound in barbarism*; they hold you down. For this reason there is in man a cultural instinct to separate himself from and destroy wild beasts such as crocodiles. It is only after a period of civilisation free of wild animals that man again turns his attention on them, seeking in them qualities to cherish.' [Graham, 1973]

### Burdened with Malice
'Given their proximity to people along lakes and rivers, and their genuine menace, crocodiles almost inevitably became burdened with imputations of *malice and depravity*.' [Graham, 1973]

### Crocodilian Character
Mabuiag is one of the many islands of the Torres Strait Island group, between Papua New Guinea and northern Australia. In Mabuiag the clansmen of the crocodile are said to have the temperament of the crocodile: they are proud, cruel, always ready to fight.

### Devil's Mafia
'For all of us, crocs symbolise evil. They are the sentinels of evil – the devil's mafia – who carry out assaults, murders, intimidations, acts of vengeance, and other unspeakable crimes. Above all they stand for violence [often sexual violence]. Huge ravening predators, armed with massive, teeth-studded jaws;

strong, unrestainable, indestructible and destructive. . . . What is about them that strikes the human unconscious as evil? . . . By far the most potent is the fact of *eating*. Medieval bestiaries depicted crocs as "hell-mouths," the portals of irrevocable, despicable bestiality. A crocodile is a consuming, ravenous, *raging* beast.' [Graham, 1973]

## Devouring
'The crocodile stands as a primitive symbol that conflates the terrible "maw of war," devouring the youth of Europe, and the "ma of war," the castration-anxiety producing mother, who symbolises both womb and tomb according to a familiar formulation, both the source of the soldier's "homesickness" and emblem of the war's terrible toll in human life.' [Linville, 2004]

## Distinguishing between Right & Wrong
'In some parts of Africa crocodiles were looked upon as judges. On the White Nile at Malaka, the Shilluk tribe allowed men accused of adultery to swim the river. If they were attacked, they were deemed guilty and the crocodile was the executioner.

'On the island of Madagascar similar beliefs called Tangem-voay were held. Here crocodiles were known as "voay" and credited with the ability to distinguish between right and wrong. It was said that they never attacked anyone with a clear conscience. Many times an accused, in the heat of a legal debate would rise up and shout "May the voay eat me if, if I have done what I am accused of" and make for the nearest river. In one case a girl was said to be having an affair with a slave and was condemned to trial by voay. On a full moon night she entered a river close to an island inhabited by voay then submerged herself 3 times. She was not attacked, and her accuser was ordered to pay heavy indemnity.' [blog Richard Freeman, Crocodile Cults]

## Evil Outsiders
'There is nothing romantic about crocs, nothing cuddly. The potent symbolism of evil and terror that they hold for most people makes them outsiders.' [Graham, 1973]

## Fear of Emasculation
Courting alligators will try to force each other underwater as a test of strength. The male alligator must show the female that he can restrain her before she becomes receptive to mating. A likely link exists with the unifying motif for crocodilians in American Indian folklore with the vagina dentata, the toothed vagina, and its South-American variety of referring to the female organ as the 'crocodile's mouth'. No choice of beast as menace personified could convey more graphically woman's threat to man and man's fear of emasculation.

## Growing Largest from the Smallest Beginning
'Of all the mortal creatures of which we have knowledge this grows to the greatest bulk from the smallest beginning; for the eggs that she produces are not

much larger than those of geese and the newly-hatched young one is in proportion to the egg, but as he grows he becomes as much as 17 cubits [7.77 m] long and sometimes yet larger.' [Herodotus, Greek historian, c. 484–c. 425]

## Hell's Entrance
'Christian symbolism never showed any sympathy for this evilly disposed creature and made it the personification of hell itself, doubtless because of the immense size of its gullet, which engulfs the small animals and fish on which it feeds. The artists in stained glass, the illuminators, and the first wood-engravers before the Renaissance often depicted the entrance to hell as the gaping maw of a dragon-like monster in which the demons roasted the condemned souls; and the dragon is nothing else but the crocodile endowed with wings.' [Charbonneau-Lassay, 1991]

## Hideous Blot
'Take for example that hideous blot upon the creation, the crocodile.' [Maughan, 1914]

## Inverted Aggression & Crippling Sentiment
'The blind preservation of wildlife is too irrational, too much a part of neurotic compulsions arising out of inverted aggression and crippling sentiment to be a realistic justification for "saving" crocodiles. The adoration of nature, conveniently packaged as it is today, is too often the worship of a lost childhood by disillusioned adults whose struggles toward a regained naïveté are often grotesquely successful.' [Graham, 1973]

## Quick to Learn & Adapt
'The adaptability of their behaviour is something that may play into their survival. It certainly has in modern times. We haven't lost a species of crocodile to extinction since humans have been dominant on the planet, even in the last few hundred years when our impact has been appalling. The reason appears to be in large part because crocodiles learn quickly and adapt to changes in their situation. They particularly learn to avoid dangerous situations very quickly. For research purposes, we find that we often have to change capture techniques, because it's very hard to catch them with the same trick twice.' [James Ross, croc researcher]

## Sluggish Pretense of Humility
'"The crocodile, the dragon of the waters, In iron panoply fell as the plague, And merciless as famine," is obviously a creature that no poet can be expected to admire. And it would perhaps be stretching sentiment too far to expect them to do so. It is not a lovable beast. I have seen them, huge ones, lying on a mudbank, "like a forest-tree, basking in the sun," as Mary Howitt says, or crawling through reeds, and there was something in the demeanour of the thing that always made me long to kill it. It lay flat, with a *sluggish affectation of humility* that exasperated me, and bestirred itself with an air of helplessness that was positively monstrous.' [Robinson, 1893]

## Tainted with Sin
Unlike the Turkana tribe of Kenya, who believe that a clean conscience precludes from crocodile attack, the Ba-Kuena or crocodile clan of South Africa believe that any clan member surviving crocodilian assault is more crocodile than human, tainted with sin, and thus to be ostracised from the clan.

## Tears of a Crocodile
'And also, for this purpose, because he knows that he is not able to overtake a man in his course or chase, he takes a great deal of water in his mouth, and casts it in the pathways, so that when they endeavour to run from the crocodile, they fall down in the slippery path, and are overtaken and destroyed by him. The common proverb also, Crocodili lachrimae, the Crocodile's tears, justifies the treacherous nature of this beast, for there are not many brute beasts that can weep, but such is the nature of the Crocodile that to get a man within his danger [reach], he will sob, sigh, and weep, as though he were in extremity, but suddenly he destroys him.' [Topsell, 1608]

## Top of the Chain
'A croc is like the CEO of an organisation – remove him and the organisation is in shambles. The croc is like that; top of the food chain in his environment. If you remove him, you've got troubles.' [Greg Parker, cited in Kelly, 2006]

## Typical Bully
'The crocodile's reputation for ferocity has little justification, for, in reality, it is a great coward and extremely timid, a typical bully that rarely takes the offensive unless all the odds are in its favour.' [Charles Pitman, Uganda's first Game Warden]

## Up to our Rears in Alligators
The aphorism 'We were up to our rears in alligators when we realised that our main mission was to drain the swamps,' is sporadically quoted to illustrate that we are often diverted from our main mission because of nuances, unexpected occurrences.

## Weak Link in the Armoured Chain of Events
'In addition to an ability to take care of itself by using the jaws and tail, the crocodilian is well protected on the back by a tough coat of hard, horny scales reinforced by little plates of bone. The horny scales are set in rows and have keels that form continuous ridges. The resulting armour is so tough that it might be described as impenetrable, remembering, of course, that all such terms are relative.

'In some crocodilians, even the belly scales are reinforced with bone and the massive skull is so bony that *no vulnerable spot* can be found by an enemy. In spite of this formidable armour, the crocodilian, like the turtle, has a weak link in the chain of its existence. While developing in the egg and just after hatching, it is *dependent upon its mother for protection*. The eggs are easily found and are relished by various mammals, and the hatchlings are comparatively defenceless.' [Pope, 1971]

Crocodilian hatchlings have at most 1% chance of reaching maturity.

## Wishing Fertility & Power
At the Berending and Kachikalli Crocodile Pools in Gambia wishes for fertility and power have been made and granted for more than 500 years. Women who have trouble in conceiving bathe in the pools, protected from the crocodiles by wooden screens. If she conceives, she will bring her child back to the pool and show it to the crocodiles whist thanking them for their help. Wrestlers hoping to win a championship also visit the pools, as do businessmen before important transactions.

Similar things take place in Bazoulé, the Village of Sacred Crocodiles in Burkina Faso. Here more than 100 crocodiles are living in a pond. They are venerated, touched and admired as part of the cultural and traditional environment of the village. Inhabitants, visitors, and others come to appeal to the crocodiles for fertility, happiness, success, fortune, or social protection in return for cloth, kola nuts or a cash donation to the elders of the families that guard the pools.

## You Are What Eats You
The fear of crocodilian and other man-eaters in Graham's view is entangled with the fear of becoming a man-eater oneself. 'One of civilisation's imperative taboos is against cannibalism; little else arouses such fear or loathing. And we do not easily distinguish, emotionally, between a human eating a human and an animal eating a human. Such fears generate volcanoes of rage and terror. Nor should we be so culturally arrogant as to suppose ourselves too far removed from cannibalism. Given the conditions of physical and mental anarchy that accompany war, for example, or other cataclysms, cannibalism soon reappears. It was almost inevitable that crocodiles should have such notions of purely *human* evil projected onto them. They are too well placed, too inviting, and altogether too guilty to evade such typecasting in what humans call "nature's plan." It is around the matter of cannibalism that the symbolism of crocodiles twists and writhes. To be eaten by a croc is to be consumed forever *by evil*. One forfeits all hope of immortality. One's soul is irrevocably Satan's, one's body is dung. Now, to be enveloped by evil, in the nursery logic of our unconscious, is to *be* evil, for all practical purposes.' [Graham, 1973]

## Surviving the Death Roll
In February 1985 Val Plumwood was paddling a canoe in the East Alligator River, Kakadu National Park, Australia, looking for aboriginal rock art. By the early afternoon she got 'a strong feeling of being watched and suddenly the canoe seemed flimsy.' Shortly after, she is under crocodilian attack. 'For the first time, it came to me fully that I was prey.' When she tries to jump into a tree growing from the water near the bank, the crocodile bursts from the water, its jaws agape, 'a flash of teeth', and:

'Then I was seized between the legs in a red-hot pincer grip and whirled into the suffocating wet darkness. . . .

[I thought] 'This is not really happening. This is a nightmare from which I will soon awake. This desperate delusion split apart as I hit the water. In that flash, I glimpsed the world for the first time "from the outside," as a world no longer my own, an unrecognizable bleak landscape composed of raw necessity, indifferent to my life or death. Few of those who have experienced the crocodile's death roll have lived to describe it.

'It is, essentially, an experience beyond words of total terror. The crocodile's breathing and heart metabolism are not suited to prolonged struggle, so the roll is an intense burst of power designed to overcome the victim's resistance quickly. The crocodile then holds the feebly struggling prey underwater until it drowns. The roll was a centrifuge of boiling blackness that lasted for an eternity, beyond endurance, but when I seemed all but finished, the rolling suddenly stopped. My feet touched bottom, my head broke the surface, and, coughing, I sucked at air, amazed to be alive. The crocodile still had me in its pincer grip between the legs. I had just begun to weep for the prospects of my mangled body when the crocodile pitched me suddenly into a second death roll.

'When the whirling terror stopped again, I surfaced again, still in the crocodile's grip next to a stout branch of a large sandpaper fig growing in the water. I grabbed the branch, vowing to let the crocodile tear me apart rather than throw me again into that spinning, suffocating hell. For the first time I realised that the crocodile was growling, as if angry. I braced myself for another roll, but then its jaws simply relaxed; I was free. I gripped the branch and pulled away, dodging around the back of the fig tree to avoid the forbidding mud bank, and tried once more to climb into the paperbark tree.

'As in the repetition of a nightmare, the horror of my first escape attempt was repeated. As I leapt into the same branch, the crocodile seized me again, this time around the upper left thigh, and pulled me under. Like the others, the third death roll stopped, and we came up next to the sandpaper fig branch again. I was growing weaker, but I could see the crocodile taking a long time to kill me this way. I prayed for a quick finish and decided to provoke it by attacking it with my hands. Feeling back behind me along the head, I encountered 2 lumps. Thinking I had the eye sockets, I jabbed my thumbs into them with all my might. They slid into warm, unresisting holes [which may have been the ears, or perhaps the nostrils], and the crocodile did not so much as flinch. In despair, I grabbed the branch again. And once again, after a time, I felt the crocodile jaws relax, and I pulled free.' [Plumwood, 2000]

| Homeopathic name | Common name | Abbreviation | Symptoms |
|---|---|---|---|
| Alligator mississippiensis | American alligator | Allig-mi. | ++ |
| Alligator sinensis sebum | Chinese alligator [sebum] | Allig-sin-seb. | – |
| Crocodylus acutus | American crocodile | Croc-ac. | – |
| Crocodylus novaeguineae | New Guinea crocodile | Croc-nov. | – |

# ALLIGATOR MISSISSIPPIENSIS

## Systematics
- Scientific name: Alligator mississippiensis [Daudin, 1802].
- Synonyms: Crocodilus mississipiensis [Daudin, 1802]. Crocodilus lucius [Cuvier, 1807]. Alligator lucius [Duméril & Bibron, 1836].
- Common names: American alligator. Florida alligator. Mississippi alligator. Louisiana alligator. Gator.
- Family: Alligatoridae.

## Biological Profile
- Robust crocodilian, olive brown to almost black in colour, with an average length of 3 m [females] to 4–4.5 m [males], and a record length of 5.84 m [19 ft 2 in]. Distinguished by the broad, rounded snout, without conspicuous teeth protruding while the mouth is closed [esp. the lower 4th tooth]. Eyes silverish in colour.
- Range: SE USA, from coastal North Carolina south to southern Florida and the Keys, and westward through the Deep South to central Texas and extreme southeastern Oklahoma.
- Habitat: Aquatic, omni-carnivorous reptile capable of living in many types of waterways, both natural and man-made, and feeding upon almost any fauna it can catch.
- Construction of burrows is well documented in this species. The burrows are used for shelter and hibernation when the seasonal temperatures fall. Deep holes with connecting dens are dug that can remain filled with water during droughts, thus maintaining an aquatic environment for indigenous fauna.
- Oviparous; up to 45 eggs per clutch.
- Females exhibit varying degrees of parental care by guarding the nest, releasing hatchlings from the nest and eggs, and transporting them to water in her mouth. Young may remain in a protective crèche with the mother and sometimes other adults for a considerable length of time, sometimes for several seasons.
- Tends to stay in family groups for years.

## Filling a Yawning Vacancy

'The name alligator is of Spanish origin, *el lagarto*, the lizard, and was given by the early Spanish explorers of our Southern States because this was the greatest lizard they had ever seen.

'This American crocodile, the alligator, is one of the best-known creatures in the world. Being easily caught, and easily reared, it is seen in the cheapest shows, museums, and menageries, and in many public aquariums and zoological gardens. . . . The adult alligator is easily taken prisoner by being seized from behind as it lies basking; its legs are securely bound, its mouth muzzled, and then – away to a showman's cage! . . .

'While an alligator basking on a log in hot sunshine, deep water close at hand to slip into for safety, is a picture of intense lazy enjoyment, an alligator blinking at an electric light in an aquarium, a chilly beast stretched upon wet stones, seems in his stillness a picture of apathetic misery. . . .

'The alligator's bill of fare is not confined to living creatures . . . as furnishing its favourite food. Alert for its breakfast, this pirate of the lagoons and bayous gathers up fish, flesh, and fowl for its table, but swallows, as a condiment, whatever comes handy. An old rubber shoe floating in the water, an empty soda-water bottle, a lost jack-knife, a battered tin can, a stone as big as an orange, part of a broken lamp, – any of these are welcomed as serving to fill the yawning vacancy in its stomach, and to aid in grinding up more digestible food.

'Baby alligators make rather amusing pets for a number of months, before they begin to exhibit hereditary traits, when they at once fail to be agreeable. They will eat eggs, raw or cooked meat, rats, mice, birds, frogs, toads. They learn to come when they are called, enjoy hearing a whistle, and, on rare occasions, show some slight degree of gratitude and affection, *amiable characteristics, which they speedily outgrow*. When these baby alligators are a few months old, they must be killed or put back into the water where their relatives live.

'Alligators are usually silent animals, but in the spring, when the eggs are being laid, they all become noisy and excited, and bellow like buffaloes. A number of adult alligators roaring together make a sound like distant heavy thunder.' [McNair Wright, 1895]

## Guarding the Nest

'The female normally remains with her nest while the eggs are developing. Usually the guardian female rests with her throat on the nest, although at intervals she may lie about 5 to 10 feet away. If alligators are frequently hunted, they will become shy, and the females may no longer guard the nest, at least against man. Also, captive females may become inured to the presence of a keeper and may lose the guarding impulse. However, under normal conditions the female will guard her nest even against man. The guarding behaviour looks like an attack, but it is not. As a person approaches the nest, the guardian female rises, turns rather slowly toward the intruder, and begins to inflate with air. If the person halts about 20 feet from the nest, the female may do nothing but hiss.

'If the person continues to approach, however, the reptile will lunge open-mouthed in his direction. The open mouth is aimed upward, toward the person's face. The lunge is accompanied by a loud hiss. In this lunge, the alligator does not actually attempt to bite. If the person steps back a pace or 2, the alligator advances and repeats its threatening gesture. If the person turns and flees, the alligator will follow for a short distance. In other words, the guarding behaviour is a series of stereotyped actions, which cause the alligator's potential enemy to retreat from the vicinity of the nest. . . . It is by no means certain that a guardian female would actually bite a person if he failed to retreat. It may be significant that, while adult alligators have been known to attack swimmers in the water, there is no report of anyone having been bitten by a female alligator defending her nest.

'It is certain that the female gives the intruder ample opportunity to escape. Ritualised confrontation, without actual bloodshed, is widespread among animals.' [Neill, 1971]

## Calling Out in Distress

'When an alligator reaches a length of about 4 feet, it ceases to grunt, or to "shriek" when seized, and begins to bellow for the first time. Concomitantly, some other behaviour patterns of the alligator change completely. Grunting and shrieking in distress are pre-pubertal activities of the alligator, activities lost with the attainment of sexual maturity. When an alligator becomes an adult, and loses the impulse to voice the distress call, it develops the impulse to react to the distress call of another and younger individual.

'Although the grunting of an alligator is an activity that has a very low threshold, the voicing of the distress call is an activity with a very high threshold. Nothing will stimulate the juvenile to give the distress call except actual seizure, and rough painful seizure at that. Many living things go through certain defensive actions only when seized roughly, perhaps actually hurt, as though by the teeth or claws of some predator. The alligator's distress call, louder and sharper than the grunt, is given over and over again in rapid succession. The young alligator continues to shriek as long as it is under attack. Adult alligators, if not rendered unnaturally shy by man's activities, are galvanised into activity by the distress call. The action of an adult alligator in response to the juvenile's distress call is not a ritual confrontation but a true attack; and the would-be predator is bitten if it does not flee.' [Neill, 1971]

## Shifting About or Staying Put

'After mating, a male alligator sometimes establishes itself in the same area it had occupied the previous year. A large alligator in an undisturbed tract may reappear, year after year, in about the same location. But most alligators are growing, changing rapidly in their requirements and abilities; most environments change, too. Thus, an alligator may shift its area, not only from year to year but even every few months. A female, when her nest-guarding urge has waned, may change or enlarge her area of activity. Thus, during the summer the adults are moving about quite a bit, each one advertising its whereabouts by an occasional bellow. . . .

'When an ousted adult finds no area that it can dominate within a given swamp, marsh, or stretch of river, it leaves that expanse of habitat; and by so doing, it has at least some chance of finding some area it can pre-empt. Once established in an area, the adult alligator will confront not only another adult of its kind, but any large animal that appears on the scene, except, of course, an animal that is identified as potential prey, to be seized rather than confronted ritualistically.

'The juvenile alligators are not affected by the adult's partitioning of the biotope into individual areas. The juveniles cruise about and forage in the territory of any adult. Their occasional grunts alert the adult to their nearby presence; and if one of the juveniles runs afoul of a predator, its distress cry brings the adult promptly not to confront the predator ritualistically but to attack it directly. Otherwise, the juveniles are ignored until they are in their 4th year. Then they become adults, begin to join in bellowing choruses, and are moved to stay out of an area that is already occupied by an adult. Some alligators, newly turned adult, can find a pre-emptable area, but many cannot. Accordingly, those in their 4th year are the ones that most often travel overland, with a chance of finding a swamp or marsh in which they can take up residence.' [Neill, 1971]

## MATERIA MEDICA ALLIGATOR MISSISSIPPIENSIS

### Sources
1 Proving Todd Rowe [USA], 15 provers [8 females, 7 males], 30c; 2001.

### Mind
∞ Confident and self-reliant [5 pr.]; vital and powerful; does not care what other people think.
∞ Irritable, impatient, intolerant, snappish, uptight, tense, going through the roof from little things; fear not being able to control anger; feeling could destroy everything around.
∞ Irritability from lack of common sense, lack of manners, and stupidity of others; from people not being considerate; from people complaining and presenting themselves as victims.
∞ Enjoying the night, feeling free; enjoying being by oneself at night.
∞ Sensitive to noise, esp. rustling paper and voices; voices echo and vibrate and can't be shut out.
∞ Attracted to water and fountains; calming effect.
∞ Darkness > [2 pr.].
∞ Desires death [2 pr.].
∞ Anxiety from motion.
∞ Anxiety from noise. Irritability from noise [3 pr.].
∞ Anxiety > walking.
∞ Fears: when alone; of death; poverty; robbers.
∞ Desires to go home.

## Dreams

∞ Cats, leopards, lions, pumas.
∞ Conspiracies, persecution, being killed.
∞ Crocodiles, alligators, lizards.
∞ Dead bodies; dead cows; dead people.
∞ Dinosaurs.
∞ Fish.
∞ Insects.
∞ Large animals.
∞ Swimming.
∞ Water, rivers, ocean.

## Generals

∞ Explosive, abrupt, sudden – headache, nausea, diarrhoea; waking from sleep; anger.
∞ Swelling – of eyes in morning; of feet and legs below knees;
∞ Left side more affected [3 pr.].
∞ Morning on waking < [5 pr.].
∞ Anorexia during day; increased or voracious appetite in evening.
∞ Craving for fish and seafood, particularly salmon [3 pr.]; chicken and protein; cheese.
∞ Aversion to bread, coffee, meat, milk.

## Sensations

∞ Needle in throat.
∞ Frog in throat.
∞ Splinters in stomach.
∞ Left thumb as if dislocated.
∞ Hips and legs stiff, metallic difficulty in moving.
∞ Bones as if metallic.

## Locals

∞ Dizziness in morning, > eating.
∞ Great deal of acid like acid reflux; burning in stomach extending to mouth; like a needle or splinter.
∞ Pain in anus extending up intestines.
∞ Pain in kidneys > lying on back.
∞ Pain right hip pain and right thigh < walking; pinched feeling; > sitting; < driving; < right side; 'got so bad that I thought I might need hip surgery; at times the pain was threatening but if I avoided any twisting motion I could avoid the pain.'

## Summary of proving

'The central issue of Alligator mississippiensis has to do with power. Self-confidence and self- assertion were some of the strongest themes in the proving. Many of the provers described a feeling of self-reliance and an ability to do things that they felt uncomfortable with before. This was associated with a feeling of increased alertness. There was a strong feeling of freedom, fearlessness, majesty and beauty associated with that power.

'There was also a feeling that there were no limits to what one could do. This was experienced by some provers as a mania, while other provers experienced significant depression, even to the point of feeling that life was not worth living. This remedy has been demonstrated to be effective in bipolar illness.

'The negative side of this power issue came out in the form of greed and anger. The greed was best exemplified through themes pertaining to stealing and theft. There were strong fears of robbers, dreams of robbers, dreams of espionage, dreams of crime families and urges to steal coupled with a lack of remorse.

'Mythologically, the crocodilians have been associated with greed and hypocrisy, as well as judges of guilt and innocence. The opposite side of this issue had to do with the need for increased security.

'The anger could be intense and sudden. Mostly it manifested as irritability, coupled with intolerance and impatience. Several described it as a "chip on their shoulder." The anger was easily triggered, especially by noise. Much of the issues here relate to feeling attacked and having to defend oneself, especially from others "stupidity." Several described it as being "touchy" and "snappish".

'Many of the provers described a strong connection to death. . . . Crocodilians are mythologically connected to the underworld and to death. Sobek was the crocodilian God directly related to Set, the God of darkness and death. They were described as ferryman for departed souls as well as judges of the dead. This also took the form during the proving of reconnecting to that which had been lost.

'The energy of the proving was often intense, sudden and violent. It was described by many as a feeling of panic or terror, which was intense and overwhelming. This was described as being similar to how it felt when suddenly abandoned as a small child.

'There were many animal themes present in the proving. In addition to the themes of attack and defence, many of the provers experienced increased sexuality and themes of competition. There were many experiences and dreams of animals throughout the proving. In particular large animals were a recurrent theme.

'Water themes were strongly present throughout the proving. This manifested through images of diving, swimming, floating and fish. Many of the provers had a strong craving for fish and in particular salmon. Provers spoke of feeling peaceful and at home in the water.

'The sensitivity to noise in many of the provers was fairly profound. This produced significant irritability and was strongest with voices. Crocodilians have a very fine sense of hearing.

'Opposed to the violence and rage was also a feeling of peace. This seemed particularly associated with water and darkness, floating and creeping slowly along. Several of the provers who were not particularly comfortable with darkness noted that they felt increasing comfort with this during the proving. The peace with darkness also manifested with making peace with death.

CROCODILIANS

'Strong general themes include better exertion, icy coldness, worse afternoon, stitching pains, left sidedness and craving for fish. The amelioration from exercise is interesting in that crocodilians have extremely high levels of exercise and take a long time to recover from any exertion.

'Strong physical characteristics included lack of appetite during the day but dramatically increased appetite at night, explosive frontal headaches accompanied by nausea, dryness of the throat and throat pain, nausea, diarrhoea, neck pain, increased sex drive, deep sleep, itching of the lower extremities, acid reflux, sprain of left groin muscle, pinching hip pain better sitting, sensation of dislocation in left thumb, difficulty falling asleep and restless sleeplessness.

'In regard to the acid reflux, crocodilians are noted to have the most acid stomachs of any vertebrates. The increased appetite at night is related to the nocturnal activities and feeding of most alligators. Several provers described a feeling of enormous weight and pressure on their shoulders [crocodilians are said to carry the world on their back in Aztec mythology].' [Todd Rowe]

# ALLIGATOR SINENSIS

## Systematics
- Scientific name: Alligator sinensis [Fauvel, 1879].
- Synonym: Caigator sinensis [Deraniyagala, 1947].
- Common names: Chinese alligator. T'o. Yow Lung. Yangtze alligator.
- Family: Alligatoridae.

## Biological Profile
- Critically endangered, yellowish-grey alligator with upturned snout, long, thick tail and pronounced black spotting of lower jaw. Four short claw-tipped limbs with 5 partially webbed toes on each limb.
- Average length males 1.5 m, maximum 2.2 m; females average 1.4 m, maximum 1.7 m.
- Osteoderms, dermal bone lying over the epidermis used as armour, covering both the back and underside of the body [the American alligator has no bony belly plates].
- Bony plate in upper eyelid, unlike their closest relative, American alligator [Alligator mississippiensis].
- Range: Formerly widespread in lower Yangtse River system, now appears restricted to southeastern Anhui Province of China. Possibly very low numbers in Zhejiang and Jiangsu Provinces.
- Habitat: Wetlands and swamps, ponds, lakes, freshwater rivers and streams.
- Nocturnal, carnivorous; preys mostly on fish, snails, clams, crustaceans, small mammals and waterfowl.
- Secretive; spends a large part of the year in complex networks of underground burrows containing above and below-ground pools of water.
- Burrow may house more than one alligator.

- Male polygamous, will fertilize several females in one mating season. Female monogamous.
- Oviparous; 10–40 eggs per clutch. Female guards the nest and helps the hatchlings break out of their egg shells. Male has no paternal involvement.
- Female stays together with her young through the first winter.
- Young vocalize to bring the group together and maintain its cohesion, while adults respond to juvenile distress calls. Bellowing occurs among males and females during the breeding season. Nest mates may spend weeks to years together in the protection of the mother.
- Both sexes may react very aggressively to one another, esp. in first encounter situations.
- Thought to be the most docile of the crocodilians.

### Materia Medica
- No symptoms.

# CROCODYLUS ACUTUS

### Systematics
- Scientific name: Crocodylus acutus [Cuvier, 1807].
- Synonyms: Lacerta hispaniolica [Shaw & Nodder, 1806]. Crocodilus pacificus [Duméril & Bocourt, 1870]. Crocodilus floridanus [Hornaday, 1875].
- Common name: American crocodile.
- Family: Crocodylidae.

### Biological Profile
- One of the largest crocodilian species, greyish-olive to dull yellowish-green in colour, belly white or yellow, averaging 3.65 m in length at maturity, with a maximum length of about 6 m. Males larger than females, weighing an average of up to 350 kg [maximum 1000 kg according to some sources]. Young crocodiles 20 to 25 cm when hatching. Can reach 60 to 70 years of age, with rare instances documented up to 100 years.
- Range: Neotropics, from S Florida to Venezuela; largest populations found in extreme south of Florida and the Dominican Republic.
- Habitat: Mostly freshwater or brackish water coastal habitats such as the saltwater sections of rivers, coastal lagoons, and mangrove swamps; occasionally freshwater areas located well inland.
- Characterised by the most reduced and irregular dorsal armour [osteoderms] of any crocodilian, and a very long, narrow snout [hence the specific epithet acutus].
- Digs burrows to escape the summer heat and will travel long distances on land if its waterhole dries up. Active at night, basking near water in daytime.
- Reaches breeding maturity at about 8 to 13 years of age, at which time it is about 2.5 m long.

- Females occupy mostly non-saline waters in non-breeding season, moving to saline waters when breeding and building a nest of loose dirt in a mound by the water's edge. Females lay 20 to 50 white, goose-egg-sized eggs and guard their nest. When eggs hatch, females help carry their young to the water, but, unlike the alligator, they *will not continue to care* for their young.
- Preys primarily on fish, small mammals, birds, and crabs. Principal food is fish, for the pursuit of which it is anatomically and behaviourally adapted. Juveniles feed on insects, snails, frogs, small fish, and crabs. Its slow digestive rate during cold weather allows it to go for months without food.
- Hunts by remaining completely motionless in the water; attacks when prey is close enough, grabbing and drowning it. May also regurgitate bits of food to attract fish.
- Swallows rocks, which stay inside the stomach and grind up its food. Some scientists believe rocks give the crocodile stability when swimming.
- Can move with extreme speed for its size and can easily outrun or outswim a person.
- Produces a commercially valuable hide and the principal reason for past declines in population size can be attributed to the extensive commercial over-exploitation that occurred from the 1930s into the 1960s.

## Worse from Cold

The American crocodile is unable to live for long in cold water. If kept in water with a temperature below about 65°F [18.3°C], the crocodile becomes torpid, sinks to the bottom, and eventually drowns. 'It may be mentioned in passing that 65°F is approximately the body temperature below which tropical reptiles in general are likely to be killed outright or weakened and rendered susceptible to respiratory infections.' [Neill, 1971]

## Guarding & Responding

'The female crocodile guards her nest; but being very shy, she will not guard it against man. If a person is in the vicinity, the nesting female will slip away to hide in the water nearby. Nevertheless, it is easy to prove that she remains with her nest, for her fresh tracks are usually to be seen at the edge of it. On one occasion, a wire fence was erected around a crocodile's nest in the wild, with the hope of containing the hatchlings when they appeared; but during the night the female not only tore away the fence but also twisted it into a veritable wire rope. The female crocodile may have to travel 20 yards or more from water to find a sandy nesting ground; and her movements, between the nest and the water, may produce a well-worn trail.

'The small American crocodile voices the juvenile grunt, which like the alligator's is occasionally given even before hatching. If mauled by some predator, the small crocodile voices the juvenile distress call, a repetitive note much like the alligator's distress call but higher in pitch. The adult crocodile is more rapidly galvanised into action by the distress call of its young than is the adult alligator under comparable conditions. Even a freshly caught crocodile, which would normally stay hidden for weeks in the mud and water of its pen, will charge at an imitation of the distress cry and can be made to leap or scramble over a fence that would contain the reptile at other times. If someone is skilled at imitating crocodilian distress calls, he can rouse an American crocodile without evoking any response from an alligator.' [Neill, 1971]

## Materia Medica
• No symptoms.

# CROCOCYLUS NOVAEGUINEAE

## Systematics
• Scientific name: Crocodylus novaeguineae [Schmidt, 1928].
• Synonym: Philas novaeguineae [Wells & Wellington, 1984].
• Common name: New Guinea crocodile.
• Family: Crocodylidae.

## Biological Profile
• Small to medium-sized crocodile with a tapered snout; 3.5 m maximum length in males, 2.7 m maximum in females but generally smaller. Colouration brownish to grey with black to dark brown bands on tail and bands or spots on body.
• Range: Papua New Guinea and Indonesia [province Irian Jaya].
• Habitat: Freshwater – swamps, marshes, lakes.
• Primarily nocturnal, preying on fish, waterbirds, amphibians, and smaller reptiles.
• Oviparous; 22–45 eggs per clutch. Parental care has been observed; both parental male and female have been observed to open the nest and carry the young to water.

## Helping Each Other
'While staff at a crocodile farm in Papua New Guinea were walking around the breeding pens of freshwater New Guinea crocodiles [C. novaeguineae] they heard a stray hatchling calling along a fence line. After some searching they found and picked up the hatchling. It called loudly, and immediately the previously quiet pond nearby erupted with the frantic activity of some 20 adults plunging into the water and swimming in the direction of the staff and hatchling. The dominant male responded by dashing to their corner of the enclosure. He head-slapped repeatedly in the water at the base of the bank and then charged out of the water straight into the chain-link fence where they were standing. Females swam nervously about, vocalised with deep guttural calls, and also head-slapped frequently.

'Several nights later, the "experiment" was repeated by approaching other pens with a calling young in hand. In an enclosure containing a female and her young from 2 previous years, the calls from the hand-held captive readily elicited lower frequency calls from juveniles throughout the pen. In a nearby rearing pen full of juveniles, the hatchling's calls were immediately answered by a loud syn-chronous chorus of grunts.' [Lang, in Garnett, 1989]

## Creation Myths

'The Kikori people from the south of Papua New Guinea tell of the creation of the land by the New Guinea freshwater crocodile.

'In the beginning the world was just water. In the water there lived a huge crocodile and he was God. When God gave birth to man and woman, there was no land on which they could live. The only place they could make their home was on his back. They bred in such great numbers that soon there was no room left on his back. The crocodile ordered them to leave his back. There was no land but there were great islands of crocodile dung. The people made their home on these islands. There they were able to grow all they required for the land was very fertile. They could fish the ocean and farm the land, and thus there was an abundance of food. These were the islands of Papua New Guinea where all of mankind started.' [Kelly, 2006]

'The image most frequently seen in both East and West Timorese textiles is the crocodile, a creature of central importance in Timorese ancestral legends. The whole form of the animal may be shown on the textile, or in some cases, the texture of its skin may be represented in a geometric design.

The crocodile is here used as a symbol for the new nation of East Timor. There is a traditional story in East Timor told about a boy and a crocodile: "According to this creation story, a young boy came across a sick crocodile, burning in the sun. The boy took pity on the crocodile and carried it to the sea. To repay the boy's kindness, the crocodile took the boy, as was his wish, on many long journeys across the sea, carrying the boy on his back. Despite being tempted to eat the boy, the crocodile kept his promise and let the boy ride safely. They journeyed until the crocodile became old. When he realised he was dying, the crocodile said to the boy 'I will change into a land where you and your descend-ants will live from my fruits, as payment for your kindness.' And according to Timorese tradition, that crocodile became the island of Timor, and the Timorese are the descendants of that boy."' [Wise, 2001]

## Marks of the Crocodile

'Tribes in the East Sepik province of Papa New Guinea to this day still practice an ancient initiation ceremony. A way of testing and introducing adolescents into manhood, the ceremony is a strenuous and painful process, that leaves the men's skins scarred all over; the effect resembling the crocodile scales.

'The meaning behind this ceremony has deeply spiritual and symbolic conno-tations. The tribe's people believe that the scars are crocodile teeth that have swallowed the adolescents and morphed them into "crocodile men." The event culminates as the tribe's celebration of the return of the ancestral crocodiles: legend has it, that when they migrated through the Sepik river, the crocodiles established a human population.

'As well as a celebration, the ceremony is very important in establishing disci-pline and testing the strength of the young males. Their backs, buttocks and chest all receive multiple lacerations with bamboo sticks, creating scars that when healed form keloids.

'Scarification is also common amongst other equatorial tribes. It is often practiced on females whose scars are considered to be sexually arousing in a similar way to the act of tribal tattooing. Scarification for equatorial tribes is a way to strengthen one's identity, position and religion within a clan.' [When Men Become Crocodiles: Extreme Tribal Scars; scribal.com]

## Crocodile Sorcerers

'The following is an instance of the power ascribed to and claimed by a sorcerer, which is generally accepted by the natives as true. Some sorcerers possess the power of transmitting their spirits to a crocodile, whereupon the crocodile becomes a devil with power to assume the shape of any person known to the sorcerer; the devil-crocodile then, at the instigation of the sorcerer, waits near a village, until it sees the man against whom it is to act, go alone down a track or to a garden; then it assumes the shape of a young married woman or girl well known to the intended victim, and follows him.

'Upon a sufficiently secluded spot being reached, the sorcerer-cum-crocodile-cum-girl approaches the man and endeavours to induce him to have sexual inter-course; should he do so, he will not discover his error until evening, when he will feel a desire to go to the river, there to vanish forever. It is not until the sorcerer claims the result as his work that the people know what has become of him and that he has fallen a prey to the crocodile. Sometimes the shape assumed by the witch-crocodile is that of a well-known and good-looking young man, and then a young married woman or girl is seduced. In such case the woman's first male child will be taken by the crocodile and the disembowelled body be later discovered floating in the water. Occasionally, I have been told, the most careful of persons and the most moral are entrapped by the actual shape of husband or wife being assumed by the crocodile; and so anyone may be tricked to his or her death.' [Monckton, 1921]

## Materia Medica
• No symptoms.

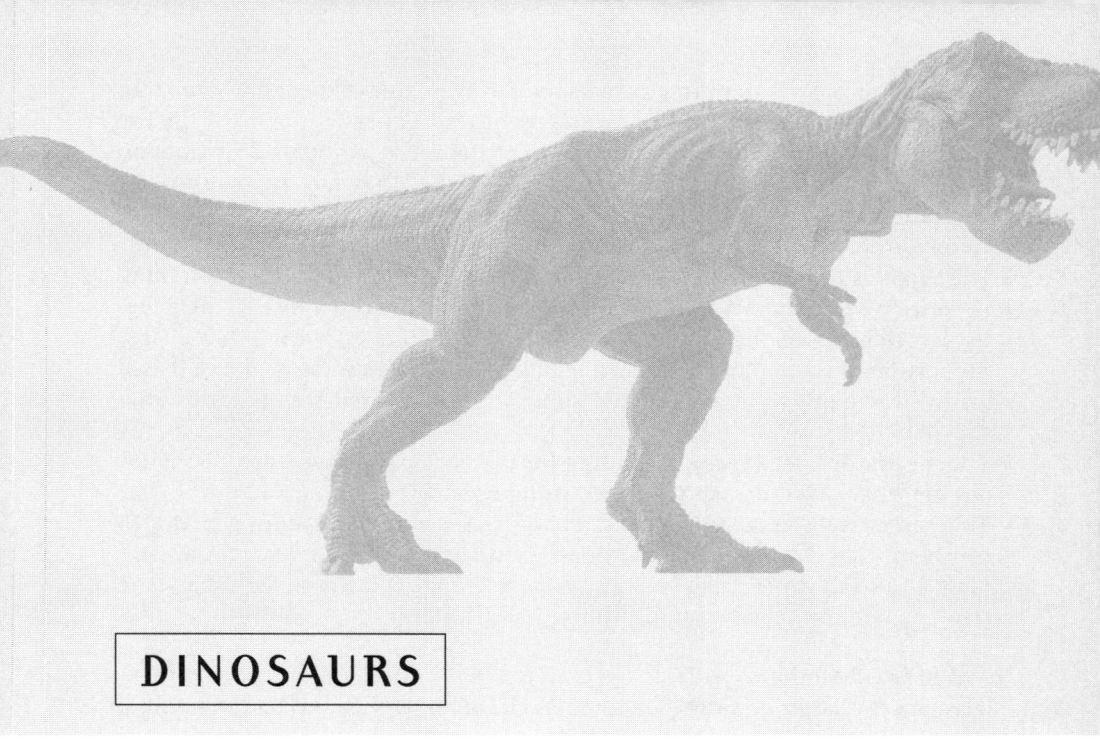

# DINOSAURS

## DINOSAURS IN HOMEOPATHY

| Homeopathic name | Common name | Abbreviation | Symptoms |
|---|---|---|---|
| Maiasaura lapidea | Good-mother lizard | Maias-l. | ++ |
| Siroccopteryx moroccoensis | Moroccon pterosaur | Siroc-mo. | – |
| Tyrannosaurus rex | T-rex | Tyran-rex. | + |

# MAIASAURA LAPIDEA

### Systematics
- Scientific name: Maiasaura peeblesorum [Horner & Makela, 1979].
- Common name: Good mother lizard.
- Family: Hadrosauridae.
- Group: Hadrosaurs ['bulky lizards'].

### Biological Profile
- Large dinosaur of about 9 m long and 5 tons in weight.
- Range and habitat: Plains of western North America.

- Belonged to the group of the hadrosaurs, 4-legged, duck-billed dinosaurs that in many respects can be considered the prehistoric equivalent of cattle. By the end of the Cretaceous, the hadrosaurs were the most populous dinosaurs on earth, an important part of the food chain in that they ate the overflowing vegetation and were eaten in turn by carnivores.
- Herbivorous.
- The remains of more than 200 Maiasaura have been found at 'Egg Mountain' in western Montana, USA, in the late 1970s; their close proximity to their eggs [which were about the same size as modern ostrich eggs] means that a large proportion of them must have been female. Also, there's some evidence [based on fossil remains of juveniles] that adult Maiasaura cared for their kids after they hatched.
- The specific epithet *lapidea*, meaning 'stony', is not part of the scientific name, but appears to refer to the fossilised, stony remains.
- The source substance for making the remedy was found during a dig in southern New Mexico and identified as originating from Maiasaura. This identification is questionable since, as far as could be ascertained, Maiasaura remains have only been found in Montana.

### Herds of Good Mothers

'Maiasaura was large, attaining an adult length of about 9 m and had the typical hadrosaurid flat beak and a thick nose. It had a small, spiky crest in front of its eyes. The crest may have been used in head-butting contests between males during the breeding season.

'This dinosaur was herbivorous. It walked both on 2 [bipedal] or 4 [quadrupedal] legs and appeared to have no defence against predators, except, perhaps, its heavy muscular tail and its herd behaviour. These herds were extremely large and could have comprised as many as 10,000 individuals.

'Maiasaura lived in herds and it raised its young in nesting colonies. The nests in the colonies were packed closely together, like those of modern seabirds, with the gap between the nests being around 7 m; less than the length of the adult animal. The nests were made of earth and contained 30 to 40 eggs laid in a circular or spiral pattern. The eggs were about the size of ostrich eggs.

'The eggs were incubated by the heat resulting from rotting vegetation placed into the nest by the parents, rather than a parent sitting on the nest. Upon hatching, fossils of baby Maiasaura show that their legs were not fully developed and thus they were incapable of walking. Fossils also show that their teeth were partly worn, which means that the adults brought food to the nest.

'The hatchlings grew from a size of 41 to 150 cm long in the span of their first year. At this point, or perhaps after another year, the animal left the nest. This high rate of growth may be evidence of warm bloodedness. The hatchlings had different facial proportions from the adults, with larger eyes and a shorter snout. These features are associated with cuteness and are common among animals that are dependent on their parents for survival during the early stages of life.' [Wikipedia]

## MATERIA MEDICA MAIASAURA LAPIDEA

### Sources
1 Proving Nancy Herrick [USA], 7 provers [3 females, 4 males], 30c; *c.* 1997.
2 Degroote, Dream Repertory.

### Mind
∞ Accident-prone.[1]
∞ Anticipation, sensation of impending evil, of any unusual ordeal.[1]
∞ Anxiety as if not having done one's duty.[1]
∞ Anxiety, gloomy forebodings.[1]
∞ Anxiety about heart.[1]
∞ Anxiety as if going to be ill.[1]
∞ Delusion going to have a fatal accident.[1]
∞ Delusion devoured by animals.[1]
∞ Delusion of danger to one's life.[1]
∞ Delusion becoming insane.[1]
∞ Delusion going to be robbed.[1]
∞ Fears – impending danger.[1]
∞ Forebodings of evil.[1]
∞ Desire to curse, swear.[1]
∞ Dishonest, lying.[2]
∞ Time as if passing too quickly.[2]
∞ Trifles seem important.[2]

### Dreams
∞ Abused, scolded, being.[2]
∞ Accidents; in car.[1]
∞ Attacked from above.[1]
∞ Bears biting off people's heads.[1]
∞ Chaotically, everything goes.[2]
∞ Children, something has happened to the.[2]
∞ Dangerous amusement park rides.[1]
∞ Darkness and danger.[1]
∞ Dead bodies, searching for.[2]
∞ Desolate landscape.[1]
∞ Destructive behaviour.[2]
∞ Disputes about money.[1]
∞ Eating.[1]
∞ Exam, missing an.[2]
∞ Excrements.[2]
∞ Fights.[1]
∞ Flying.[1]
∞ Helping people.[1]
∞ Helping people, aversion to.[1]
∞ High places.[1]

∞ Hostages for sexual torture.[1]
∞ House for sexual liaisons.[1]
∞ Lascivious, smutty.[2]
∞ Mangled car.[1]
∞ Manure.[1]
∞ Murder.[1]
∞ Mutilated body.[1]
∞ Nakedness, unashamed.[1]
∞ Obstacles easily dealt with.[2]
∞ Prisoner, being taken.[1]
∞ Pursued.[1]
∞ Sexual captivity.[1]
∞ Teeth fallen out by injury.[2]
∞ Water.[1]

## Generals
∞ Sleeplessness & heavy feeling in limbs.[1]
∞ Drenching perspiration, easily dehydrated; heat intolerance.[1]
∞ Aversion to stuffy rooms.[1]
∞ Desire for mayonnaise and salt.[2]

## Sensations
∞ Floating, after drinking coca cola.[1]
∞ Head as if light.[1]
∞ Flashes of light on closing eyes to fall asleep.[1]

## Locals
∞ Pressing frontal headache, like a weight pushing down, & increased hunger and irritability.[1]
∞ Itching forehead.[2]
∞ Epistaxis, left side, bright fluid blood; easily, which >.[1]
∞ Epistaxis from straining at stool.[2]
∞ Distended veins face, spider naevi.[1]
∞ Speech stammering; from excitement; tripping over words.[1]
∞ Toothache > clenching teeth.[2]
∞ Diarrhoea from eating too many cherries.[2]
∞ Cough as from dust.[2]
∞ Nocturnal cramps backside of thighs [hamstrings].[2]

# SIROCCOPTERYX MOROCCOENSIS

## Systematics
• Scientific name: Siroccopteryx moroccoensis [Mader & Kellner, 1999].
• Class: Pterosaurs ['wing-lizard'].

## Biological Profile

One of the most remarkable groups of Jurassic carnivorous reptiles was that of the flying dragons or pterosaurs. The Jurassic, also known as the 'Age of Reptiles', constitutes the middle period of the Mesozoic era. The Jurassic period is preceded by the Triassic and followed by the Cretaceous. The Triassic is the first period of the Mesozoic era and the Cretaceous is the third and last.

Pterosaurs appeared late in the Triassic and were characteristic and important in the Jurassic, ranging in size from that of a crow to 90 cm across the wings. Their forelimbs were modified into wings, as in the bats of today, and like them they actually flew. The head was relatively large, but very lightly constructed, and set at right angles with the neck, as in birds. The legs, like those of bats, were small and weak, and the tail was very short in some species and very long in others, bearing in one form at least an oar-like expansion at the tip. They were carnivorous animals, feeding in the main on fish, small reptiles and crustaceans. Like most reptiles they probably laid eggs and may have been warm-blooded.

Pterosaur remains were only recently identified in 1999 from the Mid-Cretaceous deposits of the southern border of Morocco. To date, the only pterosaur species named from Morocco is Siroccopteryx moroccoensis.

With an estimated wingspan of nearly 6 m, this anhanguerid [meaning 'old devil'] ranks amongst the largest pterosaurs known. There have been comparisons of this creature to other anhanguerid species known from the Early Cretaceous of Brazil. Only jaw fragments and teeth have been discovered from Morocco and much has yet to be learned about this fascinating and giant flying reptile from prehistory.

## Materia Medica

- No symptoms.

# TYRANNOSAURUS REX

## Systematics

- Scientific name: Tyrannosaurus rex [Osborn, 1905].
- Common name: T-rex.
- Family: Tyrannosauridae.
- Class: Theropods ['beast-footed'].

## Biological Profile

- One of the largest terrestrial carnivores of all time; approximately 4.5 m high, about 12.2 m in length, and roughly 6 tons in weight. Its massive head, measuring around 1.5 m was supported by a short and muscular, S-shaped neck. The forelimbs were short with 2 clawed fingers and were just 90 cm long. In contrast, the hind limbs were huge. The massive tail was long and heavy in order to support the massive torso.

- Range: Western North America. First discovered in Montana in 1902 by Barnum Brown, and described and named in 1905 by Henry Fairfield Osborn, the director of the American Museum of Natural History.
- The theropod [meaning 'beast-footed'] dinosaurs are a diverse group of bipedal saurischian dinosaurs. They include the largest terrestrial carnivores ever to have made the earth tremble. Several characters that typify a theropod: hollow, thin-walled bones are diagnostic of theropod dinosaurs. Other theropod characters include modifications of the hands and feet: 3 main fingers on the hand; the fourth and fifth digits are reduced; and 3 main [weight-bearing] toes on the foot; the first and fifth digits are reduced. Most theropods had sharp, recurved teeth useful for eating flesh, and claws were present on the ends of all of the fingers and toes.
- The name Tyrannosaurus says it all. This group of huge carnivores must have tyrannically ruled the land. Short but deep jaws with banana-sized sharp teeth, long hind limbs, small beady eyes, and tiny forelimbs [arms] typify a tyrannosaur.
- Tyrannosaurs are surprisingly common in many North American fossil beds, especially their large, serrated teeth, which they shed periodically like most archosaurs. The teeth of tyrannosaurids are very interesting – rather than being the flat knifelike blades as in most other carnivorous dinosaurs, they are more like giant spikes than razor-edged blades. With a mouthful of this murderous dentition, tyrannosaurs had a whopping bite, which might have made up for their reduced forelimbs. The bite marks of these teeth are quite recognisable on some dinosaur bones. Some tyrannosaur fossils show evidence of bite marks from other tyrannosaurids, suggesting that there might have been fierce fighting between tyrannosaurs, or even cannibalism. [www.ucmp.berkeley .edu/diapsids/saurischia/tyrannosauridae.html]

## MATERIA MEDICA TYRANNOSAURUS REX

### Sources
1 Clinical observations Mangialavori [Italy].
2 Clinical observations Karl-Josef Müller [Germany].

### Mind
∞ Ailments from reproaches.[1]
∞ Ambition, highly ambitious.[1]
∞ Death, wishes. Suicidal disposition.[1]
∞ Delusion of being in another world.[1,2]
∞ Dictatorial, domineering, in children.[1]
∞ Eating, refuses.[1]
∞ Fear of dark and death.[1,2] Must have light on at night.[2]
∞ Obstinate, headstrong, contrary.[1]
∞ Omnipotence.[1]

## Dreams
∞ Animals, dinosaurs.[1]
∞ Cold, snow-covered landscapes.[2]
∞ Greatness.[1]
∞ Night terrors, awakening from sleep.[2]
∞ Pursued; by police.[1]

## Generals
∞ Epileptiform or febrile paroxysmal convulsions/cramps.[2]
∞ Absences, absent-mindedness, after measles.[2]
∞ Absent-mindedness leads to dangerous situations, e.g. in traffic.[2]
∞ Night blindness; cannot drive a car at night or find his way in the dark.[2]
∞ Growing pains in tibiae.[2]
∞ Carnivorous craving for raw meat and fish; or extreme aversion to fish.[2]

## Case Observations
Very openly violent in reactions but feels bad about it afterwards. Wants to be the chief; can't stand to be in second place. Away from home, he is nice and friendly because he is the 'chief' at school. Great fear of water. Gets cramps when angry. Very self-centred.

Strange relationship with death: the dog dying was the first of the family to go – this is not the same as the fascination with death in snake remedies. This is one of the most important features of this remedy. Massimo has only 4 patients of this remedy. All of them had some features similar to Stramonium. In all snake remedies there is a mechanism that makes them able to overcome this anguish. This interest in uncommon things or 'spirituality' or 'religious affection' is a serious issue for snakes, to cut off the problem of the mystery, which cannot be endured. In this case, this compensation does not work at all. For them, life is a very basic problem.

"I have this anguish of not existing and nothing can be done to help me get rid of this problem." This appears to be the main problem for this remedy. "You can say whatever you want about saints, religion, whatever, but none of these things will help me understand this problem."

His perception of the dog dying is that he is the first of many. Eventually they will all die, one by one. Religion doesn't help him. He needs things that are clear, strong and evident to solve a problem for him. It's interesting what he says about dinosaurs: They were able to survive much longer than human beings, however eventually they were extinguished. Against the inevitability of dying, there is nothing that can be done.

The duality in his physical body is interesting. He considers the upper part of his body is not working at all. He gets worried that if the strong part of his body doesn't work anymore, then he has no weapon.

The issue about dying, being extinguished, etc., is very central to this remedy. As is the sensation that the upper and lower parts of the body vary so very much in their strength. It is duality, but of a different kind to that of the snakes.

Despite the strong aggressivity, very often they are considered nice because they look after the other children at school, etc. In Tyrannosaurus there is a great fear of being unable to control their rage. They have serious problems after these fits of anger. In the sense that when it happens to them, they're really unable to control it and there is an issue that it jumps out in a kind of out-of-proportionate way. The first thing they do is to go to their mother and ask for forgiveness immediately. It is as if in some way they could not allow themselves to have this kind of acting out with the fear that they may be even more rejected, abandoned or not considered. They are not able to integrate their aggressivity. [Extracted from Mangialavori, Tyrannosaurus rex cases; RefWorks]

### General Concept of T-rex

'My general understanding of T-rex is that it is appropriate for boys who have the juxtaposition between their wanting to be strong and powerful, and not wanting to show their vulnerable side. So they use a loud voice, aggression, obstinacy, and become interested in big animals [Like dinosaurs but also other large and powerful animals] to compensate for a feeling of low confidence.

'They can share some of the symptoms of reptiles, in particular the more audacious reptiles like Lachesis and Bothrops. The confusion is that they can also look like a nightshade because of the fears.

'The growing pains appear to be a problem that they have with the idea of ageing, growing old, or making transitions. According to Müller & Massimo, these patients are vulnerable around the idea of getting older, of eventually meeting their mortality. The bone pains are showing that they are in fact growing up, getting older.

'The fear of the dark may also be some kind of holding on to an earlier safer time, a younger more dependent sense of self. So perhaps in some sense, these patients are in fact in a kind of limbo, between not wanting to seem vulnerable, yet they also don't really want to grow up.

'They can also have the fear of persecution – in this boy it comes up around homeless people, in Massimo's cases, it was around policemen getting them. Massimo has seen some of his patients be either afraid of death or suicidal. These patients can be quite aggressive and audacious in clinical practice so they can be mixed up with Stram, Lachesis, Bell, Lyssin, Bothrops, and possibly Alligator [See Todd Rowe's excellent proving].

'The differential for these types of cases can be challenging. I don't want to pigeonhole this remedy for boys only or only children. This is the only experience I've personally had with the Rx and I suspect that there are other cases walking around in need of it. Of course, once we begin to have some females and adults, the understanding of the remedy will mature.'

[Tim Shannon, Tyrannosaurus rex: A Case of Conduct Disorder, Violence and Audacity in a Fearful Boy; RefWorks]

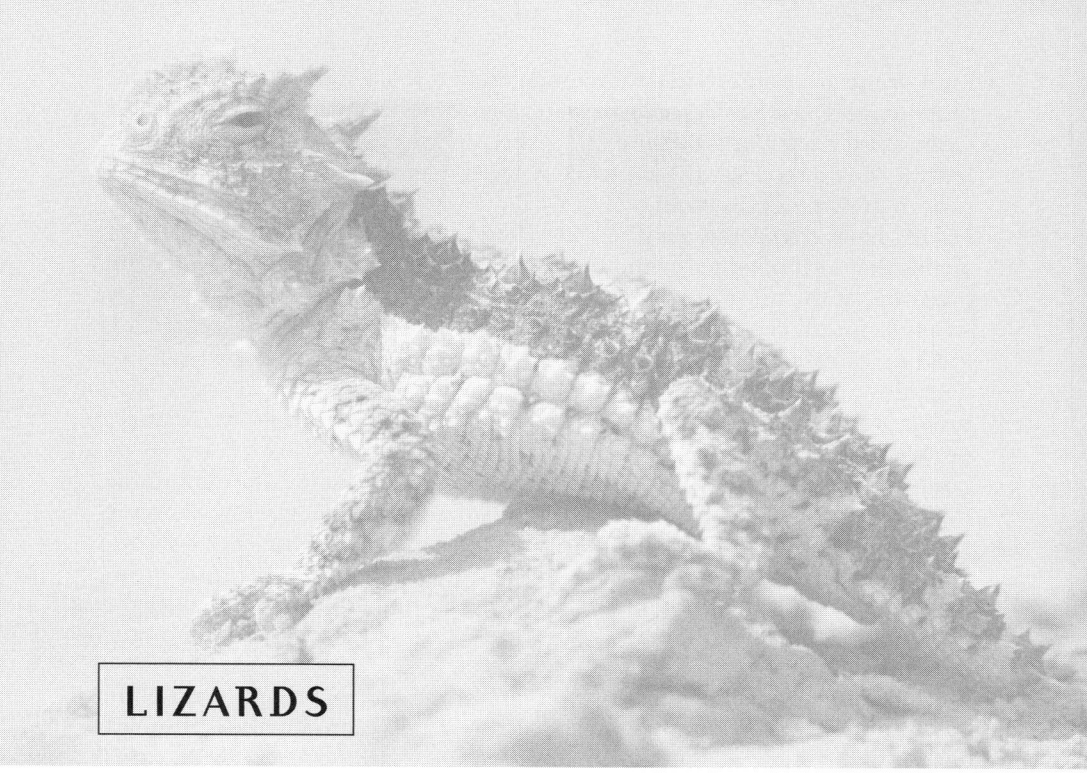

# LIZARDS

## BIOLOGICAL PROFILE

- The largest group of extant reptiles with more than 3000 species, lizards are an extremely diverse group, incl. terrestrial, burrowing, aquatic, arboreal and aerial members. Among the more familiar groups in this varied suborder are the geckos, small, agile, mostly nocturnal forms with adhesive toe pads that enable them to walk upside down and on vertical surfaces; the iguanas, often brightly coloured New World lizards with ornamental crests, frills and throat fans, and a group that includes the remarkable marine iguana of the Galapagos Islands; and chameleons, a group of arboreal lizards, mostly of Africa and Madagascar.
- The great majority of lizards have 4 limbs and relatively short bodies, but in many the limbs are degenerate and a few such as the glass lizards are completely limbless.
- Lizards have radiated extensively into a variety of habitats and reveal an array of functional and behavioural specialisations. Most lizards have movable eyelids, whereas a snake's eyes are permanently covered with a transparent cap. Lizards have *keen vision for daylight* [retinas rich in both cones and rods]; although one group, the nocturnal geckos, has pure rod retinas for night vision.

LIZARDS                                                                      51

- Most lizards have an external ear tympanum that snakes lack. However, as with other reptiles, *hearing does not play an important role* in the lives of most lizards. Geckos are exceptions because the males are strongly vocal [to announce territory and discourage the approach of other males] and they must, of course, hear their own vocalisations.
- Lizards have *excellent vision*; their livelihood depends on it. Mattison [2004] argues that vision, which is the lizard's primary means of detecting prey and predators, is the most important sense in all but a few lizard species.
- As a rule, lizards deposit a moderate number of oval, soft-shelled eggs, hatching in 8 or 10 weeks. In certain families, however, among which are the Iguanidae [iguanids], Lacertidae [wall or true lizards], Anguidae [alligator lizards, glass lizards, and lateral fold lizards] and Scincidae [skinks] are a number of species producing their young alive.
- Lizards possess a variety of protective responses and tactics: fleeing, hiding, freezing, puffing up, hissing, gaping, snapping, biting, crying, charging, shedding tail, squirting blood, and rolling into a ball by biting down on own tail or limb.
- Most species of lizards are diurnal, but some are nocturnal. Nocturnal species include Gekkonidae. Both daily and seasonal cycles of activity are tightly tied to temperature.
- Most lizards, esp. smaller ones, prey on insects and arthropods; some are herbivores, some others are omnivores, while larger lizards eat small mammals, birds and reptiles. Yet again others are dietary specialists, feeding primarily or exclusively on ants, scorpions, snails, tadpoles, termites, mosquito larvae, wasps, fish, or mussels.
- Compared with snakes, a far greater proportion of the lizards are confined to the warmer portions of the globe; only a limited number of species occur in temperate latitudes.
- Lizards can be distinguished from snakes by the presence of 2 pairs of legs, external ear openings and movable eyelids, but these convenient external diagnostic features, while absent in snakes, are also absent in some lizards.

## LISTING LIZARDS

1 **Agamids** – fam. Agamidae, 2–6 subfamilies, 40 genera, about 325 species. Range: Old World.
Includes dragons, bearded dragons, bloodsuckers, tailfins, thorny-tailed agamas, spiny-tailed agamas, frilled lizards, toad-heads, and others.
Typical features: [1] Ranging in type from arboreal tree-dwellers to terrestrial and semi-aquatic types. [2] Agamids have well developed limbs, long tails and often bizarre forms with crest, dewlaps and expandable appendages. [3] Males are usually brightly coloured. [4] Capable of limited change of colours. [5] Oviparous, laying eggs in ground burrows. [6] Cannot cast tail.

2 **Anguids** – fam. Anguidae, 12–14 genera, 90–112 species.
Including slow worms, alligator lizards, glass lizards, galliwasps, California legless lizards, and others. Closest relatives of Heloderma.
Range: Northern Hemisphere.
Typical features: [1] Body covered in body armour consisting of large, nearly non-overlapping scales and underlying osteoderms. [2] Body elongated; tail long. [3] Powerful jaws; notched or forked tongue. [4] Many species have reduced or absent limbs, superficially resembling snakes. [5] Oviparous, except slow worms, which are ovoviviparous. [6] Insectivorous or carnivorous. [7] Can cast tail. [8] Inconspicuous colouration, usually brown, sometimes green or more striking colouration. [9] Slow movements and tendency to utilise leaf litter and other surface cover render anguids fairly inconspicuous.

3 **Beaded lizards** – fam. Helodermatidae, 1 genus, 2 species.
Range: North America, esp. SW United States and Mexico.
Typical features: [1] Venomous stout-bodied lizards with broad head, well developed limbs, and short fat tail. [2] Powerful jaws. [3] Carnivorous. [4] Oviparous.

4 **Chameleons** – fam. Chamaeleonidae, 6 genera, 120–180 species.
Range: Madagascar, Africa, Asia through much of India, the Middle East, and southern Europe. About half the world's chameleons live in Madagascar.
Typical features: [1] Able to change their colour for camouflage and communication. [2] Long, projectile, sticky tongue that can be shot out to an extraordinary length; tongue may be longer than the chameleon's body. [3] Insectivorous. [4] Can rotate and focus their cone-shaped, protruding eyes independently of each other; can look at 2 different objects at the same time and has a full 360-degree view around its body. [5] Body laterally compressed; large head. [6] Arboreal and diurnal. [7] Prehensile tail, can wrap around tree branches while climbing; tail cannot be shed and regrown. [8] Oviparous, with a few ovoviviparous exceptions. [9] Move slowly and methodically. [10] Skeletal structure remarkably flexible; can as easily compress body as expand it.

5 **Flap-foots** – fam. Pygopodidae, 8 genera, about 40 species.
Range: Australia.
Typical features: [1] Related to the geckos. [2] Body unusually long, slender, strongly resembling snakes; essentially legless, with only vestigial remnants of hind legs in the form of small, flattened flaps. [3] Arboreal, terrestrial or burrowing. [4] Feed on small lizards and invertebrates.

6 **Geckos** – fam. Gekkonidae, 5 subfamilies, 97 genera, 600–2000 species and subspecies.
Range: All warmer regions worldwide.
Typical features: [1] Unlike other lizards, geckos have the ability to produce sounds, ranging from soft chirping, clicking or croaking, to loud squeaking, high-pitched calls, or barking, depending on the species. [2] Most geckos have fused

eyelids [like snakes] and they lick them with their protrusible, notched tongue to clean them; they appear never to blink. [3] Mostly nocturnal; narrow, vertical pupils to block out light. [4] Excellent vision; can use colour vision at low light intensities. [5] They all have flattened bodies, short necks and wide flat heads. The toe-like digits of their feet are adhesive due to rows of tiny hooked bristles, which allow them to climb straight up walls and across ceilings. [5] Cast their tail and/or expel a foul-smelling material and faeces onto aggressor when attacked. [6] Can change colour, lightening or darkening their skin colour depending on the time of day, temperature, or background.

7 **Girdled lizards** – fam. Cordylidae, 4 genera, about 70 species.
Range: Africa southeast of the Sahara and in Madagascar.
Typical features: [1] Body with enlarged, girdle-like scales, often spiny. [2] Insectivorous. [3] Ovoviviparous or oviparous. [4] Defend themselves with their spiny tails or wedge themselves into crevices and inflate their bodies. [5] Territorial during the breeding season. [6] Diurnal.

8 **Iguanids** – fam. Iguanidae [including family Phrynosomatidae], 8–11 subfamilies, 54–60 genera, about 550 species. Including iguanas, curlytails, swifts, anoles, collared lizards, chuckwallas, horned lizards, leopard lizards, wood lizards, clubtails, helmeted lizards, basilisks, and others.
Range: New World and on the islands of Fiji and Madagascar.
Typical features: [1] Ranging in type from arboreal tree-dwellers to terrestrial and semi-aquatic types. [2] Limbs well developed. [3] Tongue short and barely protrusible. [4] Most have long tails and display a great variety of crests, dewlaps, and spines. [5] Males are bright and varied in colouration. [6] Most lay eggs in the ground but there are a few who are livebearers. [7] The desert and forest dwellers are mainly herbivores while the smaller iguanids are insectivores or omnivores. [8] Territorial, males defending territory against other males. [9] Omnivorous. [10] Primarily diurnal. [11] Can cast tail.

9 **Monitor lizards** – fam. Varanidae, 1 genus, about 65 species.
Range: Australia, Australasia, Asia, Africa.
Typical features: [1] Large ground-dwelling lizards with well-developed limbs and long whiplike tail. [2] Body elongated, head long with pointed snout; very powerful jaws. [3] Carnivorous; some species are known to eat fruit. [4] Oviparous. [5] High intelligence. Monitor lizards are more closely related to snakes than any other species of lizard, sharing some of the characteristics of snakes – i.e. dropping of lower jaw [in other lizards parts of the lower jaw are fused]; ossified skull; long, deeply slit tongue; capacity to follow olfactory cues.

10 **Skinks** – fam. Scincidae, 3 subfamilies, 130 genera, about 1200 species.
Range: Worldwide.
Typical features: [1] Terrestrials, often burrowing. [2] Mostly insectivorous, occasionally omnivorous. [3] Body elongated and rather circular, with small necks and small pointed heads. [4] Legs short, or even absent in some species;

tails vary from short to long and are generally colourful. [5] Viviparous or oviparous. [6] Can cast tail.

11 **Teiids & Whiptails** – family Teiidae, 9 genera, about 200 species.
Including jungle-runners [or racerunners], false monitors, whiptail lizards, crocodile tegu, caiman lizards, desert tegus, and others.
Range: New World.
Typical features: [1] Ranging in type from arboreal tree-dwellers to desert dwellers. [2] Most have well developed limbs, long tails, large plate-like heads and extensible forked tongues. [3] Carnivorous and insectivorous to partly or mostly herbivorous. [4] Achieve some of the highest body temperatures known in lizards – up to about 40°C in some species. [5] Oviparous. [6] Certain species of whiptails have *all-female or nearly all-female* populations. These lizards reproduce by parthenogenesis. [7] Active diurnal foragers. [8] Can cast tail.

12 **Wall or true lizards** – family Lacertidae, 2 subfamilies, 27–36 genera, about 220 species.
Range: Old World.
Typical features: [1] Distinguished by a collar of large scales on underside of neck. [2] Body slender and elongated with well-defined head above narrow neck; tongue long, extendable, deeply forked; tail long, slender. [3] The structure of their tail supports fast zigzag movements and very accurate jumps that are needed to catch their insect prey. [4] Insectivorous. [5] Oviparous, all but 1 species lay eggs. [6] Diurnal. [7] Cannot change colour rapidly but may change colour over the course of their life. [8] Mostly terrestrial or rock-dwelling. [9] Can cast tail. [10] All use bouts of rapid locomotion to escape predators, to catch prey, and during social interactions.

## Remarkable lizards
A reptilian assemblage with astonishing features, there are lizards that fly, walk over water, bury themselves in sand, squirt blood from their eyes, are vegetarian or on a strict fruit diet, to name a few strange, rare and peculiar lizard manifestations.

- Flying lizards or flying dragons are agamids of the genus Draco, a group widespread in forest areas of SE Asia that has taken adaptation to an arboreal lifestyle to the extreme. They have membranes folded against their flanks, which can be extended to form a pair of broad wings, enabling the lizards to cross open areas between trees in excess of 100 m.
- Thorny devils [Moloch horridus] live in Australian deserts, feeding on termites and ants with their long tongues. Described as 'walking pieces of barbed wire', they have a spiny coat to keep them safe from predators.
- Unique among modern lizards and found only on the Galapagos Islands, marine iguanas [Amblyrhynchus cristatus] live and forage in the sea. These herbivores feed exclusively on algae growing on rocks near the shore. When feeding, they can remain submerged for up to an hour, though dives of 5 to

10 minutes are more common. They look fearsome [Charles Darwin called them 'imps of darkness, sluggish, and sluggish in its movements'] but are quite harmless.

- The short-horned lizard of the southern U.S. and Mexico's Sonora desert, known locally as 'horny toads', uses an unusual defence tactic to repulse predators. A small, flat, round lizard with short, stubby horns on the back of the head, it will squirt blood from ducts in the corners of its eyes to a distance of about 1 meter to keep predators at bay.
- Basilisk lizards, skittish tree-dwelling species found in Central America, have the amazing capacity to scurry across the surfaces of ponds and streams, which has earned them the nickname Jesus Christ lizard. When frightened by a predator's approach it will drop to the water and run across the surface. Smaller basilisks can run about 10–20 meters on the water surface without sinking and the young can usually run farther than older basilisks.
- Burrowing sand lizards occur in various genera. They display sand-burying and sand-swimming behaviour, which allows them to bury themselves in sand and to move 1 or 2 meters under the surface, to avoid predators or for thermo-regulation.
- Whereas nearly all lizards are carnivorous or insectivorous, 2 monitor lizards of the genus Varanus, both native to the Philippines, are adapted for a diet of almost entirely fruit.
- The Australian shingleback skink Tiliqua rugosa is an exception to the polyga-mous rule among lizards – it is monogamous. Slow-moving, blue-tongued and with a short, stumpy tail resembling its blunt head, it is known as 2-headed skink and sleepy lizard in Australia. In the spring the male pairs up with a female, staying with her for up to 8 weeks prior to mating. After mating the partners separate and remain solitary until the following spring, when the relationship is actively re-established by both partners. Pairs have been known to return to each other every year for up to 20 years.

## LIZARDS FROM HEAD TO TAIL

### Diversity of Lizards

'Even the most passive of observers cannot refrain from expressing amazement at the array of varied forms in the suborder of the lizards. Under the head of the Lacertilia we shall consider creatures 7 feet long, with claws as long as those of the leopard – animals strong and active enough to leap at the throat of a young gazelle, tear, dismember and devour the prey; and passing such we stop to realise that tiny, limbless and worm-like, slow-moving things, burrowing their life away deep in the ground where they need no eyes – in fact, have none – are also true lizards. Among these hordes of scaly life we shall find lizards that rush over the ground with such speed they appear as but a streak to the human eye; others having adhesive digits and with equal speed can traverse the smooth face of a precipice or run head downward over a horizontal surface; and yet others that swim with the strength of crocodilians, while a few have parachute-like wings with which they sail from tree to tree. From one family we may abruptly arrive at another where the species are so slow in movements they rely upon a remarkable resemblance to the hues of their arboreal homes for protection, for with these the motions might appeal to us like the slow relaxation of the muscles of some dying creature. Again we come upon lizards without vestiges of limbs, gliding away like serpents, or species with limbs so small they fold these useless members against the side of the body in times of fright, when, with the aid of a sharpened snout, they plow their way, literally swim into the desert sands.' [Ditmars, 1937a]

## Scales & Skin

The outer skin of lizards, like that of snakes, is covered with protective scales that are dry to the touch and differ significantly in appearance and arrangement among species.

'Lizards may be fairly well separated . . . according to the structure of their scales. Some have very coarse, overlapping scales, each terminating in a sharp point and having a strong keel; species thus coated are rough, lusterless and bristling with sharp points. Others have smooth, rounded scales as polished as glass. While a number of lizards have the scales arranged in oblique rows, many display a ringed arrangement on both the body and the tail. A good proportion of the larger [as well as the smaller] lizards have such a fine, granular scalation they appear to be covered merely with a bare, rough skin unless closely examined. Some of the degenerate, worm-like species have lost their scales, in place of which are hardened, polished and movable rings of skin, encircling the body; these are used in precisely the same fashion as the segments of an earthworm – to assist in locomotion.' [suborder Worm Lizards] [Ditmars, 1937a]

## Shedding & Sloughing

'When a lizard "sheds" its skin, it doesn't slough its only covering. These reptiles actually have 3 layers: the epidermis, or outer skin; the dermis, which consists of connective tissues, membranes, blood vessels, nerves and cells that affect colour; and the subcutis, or lower skin, which anchors the skin to the muscles below.

'Shedding, which is more frequent among juveniles than among adults, usually takes place shortly after hatching and at irregular intervals, depending upon temperatures, moisture, food supply, growth, and general health. A lizard often endeavours to speed the process of shedding by pulling the outer skin with its mouth or scratching with its feet and claws. Some lizards [like some frogs] eat the rejected skin as they peel the flakes off their body. . . . Just as some frogs and salamanders will initiate the shedding process by "popping" their eyes to stretch their skin, some lizards will bulge their eyes and loosen the neighbouring skin by contracting muscles and forcing blood into a system of sinuses in their head. Some geckos even rely on their skin-shedding talents to help them escape from predators. Quammen notes that the island-dwelling *Gehyra mutilata* is one of a handful of geckos that engage in "shock-shedding" – casting off their entire skin when handled or grabbed and slipping away all "pink and naked and raw." This unusual defensive behaviour triggers minimal bleeding and apparently causes no injury to the gecko.' [Badger, 2002]

## Shape & Size

'The general form greatly varies. Yet the vast majority of lizards have 4 well-developed limbs. Among several of the families – and these by no means nearly allied – we find startling illustrations of degeneracy; and all along similar lines. In adopting subterraneous habits certain species have ultimately lost their limbs while their eyes have become small and nearly useless. Such degenerative tendencies are always marked with decided elongation of the body – into a snake-like or worm-like form. We find all stages of development. Most striking are those species with the limbs so aborted the creature folds them against the sides of the body and glides like a snake, or where there is but one pair of microscopic limbs, these are of absolutely no use though going through all the motions of walking during the animal's gliding progress. In the degenerate family Amphisbaenidae, not only the limbs and scales have disappeared, but the pectoral and the pelvic arch have been reduced to mere vestiges.' [Ditmars, 1937a]

## Tongue 'n Teeth

'The structure of the tongue varies greatly among lizards. With many of them it is long, black, deeply forked and snake-like; it is darted from the mouth to examine objects in the lizard's path. On others the tongue is flattened yet rather fleshy, and but bluntly nicked at the tip; in combination it is used as an organ of investigation and to pull the food into the animal's mouth.

'A number of lizards have a thick, viscid tongue, employed in the same fashion as that of the toad, namely to lap up small insect prey. The true chameleons have an enormously long tongue – club-shaped at the tip – that is darted at an insect, which sticks fast when squarely hit.

'With the arrangement of the teeth we find an important character bearing on classification. Two phases of development should be thoroughly understood. Some lizards have an *acrodont*, others a *pleurodont* dentition. Acrodont lizards have the teeth set along the edges of the jaws; there are no well-defined alveoli [sockets] or a longitudinal socket groove.

'Pleurodont lizards have the teeth set in a deeply cleft, longitudinal, continuous socket. The teeth of lizards may be conical or flat, straight or recurved, sharply pointed or terminating in queerly serrated fashion that makes each tooth look like a "bit" of some fancy drill. Among the vast aggregation of lacertilians, only 2 are known to be poisonous; these are the species of Heloderma – the Beaded Lizards, inhabiting the deserts of the southwestern portion of the United States, besides the arid regions of southern Mexico and northern Central America.' [Ditmars, 1937a]

## Tail

The lizard's tail performs at least 4 major functions: grasping, balancing, fat storage, and defence.

'For purposes of defence, the tail is an invaluable organ. With it, the larger lizards deal lashing, whip-like blows. Many lizards have a tail of extraordinary length – 4 or 5 times as long as the combined length of the head and body; a number possess a diminutive, stumpy appendage. With the majority of lacertilians the tail is readily discarded, and it is soon reproduced. Let us take one of the extremes of caudal development as an illustration, noting how the brittle appendage may save its owner's life in time of danger.

'Suppose a limbless lizard – a glass "snake" – is pursued by an active, reptile-eating serpent. The former's stiff, undulatory movements are hopelessly slow in comparison with the sinuous glide of the pursuer. In a moment the snake has seized its prey. There is a quick twist and instantly the snake is busily engaged in subduing what appears to be its frenzied victim. Actually, this is what has happened: In that twisting movement the lizard has snapped off its tail. The muscles of the discarded member have been thrown into a state of great excitability – evidently a provision of Nature. Meanwhile, an abbreviated lizard has, under cover of the excitement occasioned by the antics of the tail, glided slyly for a safe retreat. . . .

'A number of the geckos run away from danger with the thick tail well elevated and the animal parts with the caudal member at barely a touch, when the tail jumps and wriggles in a manner sure to attract the attention of the enemy. In this casting off of the tail the organ is not "disjointed" as is often the popular idea. Owing to a curious structure of the caudal vertebrae the break occurs in the middle of a vertebral joint and the broken end of bone immediately begins a reconstructive process, resulting in a new tail. The new member is completed in a few months. It is seldom as long as the original one, nor covered with a normal scalation.' [Ditmars, 1937a]

## Limbs & Locomotion

Lizards exhibit tremendous variation in morphology and behaviour with respect to locomotor function and have served as a model system for testing *maximal sprinting performance*, which may be important for many activities such as escape from predators and feeding. Lizards' legs are mounted sideways: they are better sprinters than distance runners. Lizards bend their trunks laterally with each step of locomotion and, as a result, their locomotion appears to be fundamentally different from mammalian locomotion. The same muscles lizards use to breathe are used to sway their bodies side-to-side.

The majority of lizards are quadrupedal [walking on 4 legs], with powerful limb musculature. They are capable of rapid acceleration and possess *great ability to change direction of motion rapidly*. Racerunners [Cnemidophorus], collared and zebra-tailed lizards can attain speeds of 26–29 km per hour, which, in terms of their own body length, puts them in a class with fast terrestrial mammals. To achieve top speeds, some lizards run on their hind legs alone

'Movement patterns have been used to categorise lizards as sit-and-wait or wide foraging. Sit-and-wait foragers rely primarily on vision to ambush prey [and accordingly have poorly developed chemosensory abilities], and use large sticky tongues coupled with short broad skulls to capture and process prey. In wide foraging, lizards use an oscillating forked tongue to search for prey [with highly developed chemosensory systems] and use their long narrow jaws to capture and process prey.

'During foraging, sit-and-wait lizards remain *motionless* most of the time and then use short bursts of fast locomotion [~10% of activity period] to ambush passing prey. In contrast, wide foraging lizards move slowly most of the time [~10–90% of activity period] over long distances chemically sampling the environment to locate hidden caches of prey.' [McElroy, 2008]

Predator evasion and territorial defence in all lizards involves short bursts of fast locomotion.

In addition to the standard reptilian repertoire of locomotive techniques – walking on 4 legs, swimming, climbing, burrowing – lizards possess 'some other, more unusual skills: gliding from trees, flinging their bodies into the air, "swimming" through sand, running on water and walking upside down across a ceiling. . . . Lizards with 4 legs have mastered the art of *outrunning* most predators, incl. humans, as anyone who has ever chased an anole or skink can attest. Since their very survival may depend on their speed, the swift flitting, dashing, and darting of lizards have attracted human attention. . . . The flying dragon of tropical rain forests spreads its wing-like membranes, "runs forward a short distance, leaps into the void . . . and floats away," Mertens recounts. . . . Equally amazing is the so-called Jesus Christ lizard of Central and South America, a basilisk celebrated for its ability to walk – actually, to skim – across water.' [Badger, 2002]

## Anoxia

Diving and burrowing reptiles are often exposed to oxygen lack for prolonged periods. Crocodiles, lizards and snakes are usually able to survive without oxygen about 45 minutes at 22°C [71.6°F]. The tolerance of turtles to anoxia is remarkable, exceeding that of all other tetrapod vertebrates. Turtles of all families except the Cheloniidae [sea turtles] commonly survive without oxygen at 22°C for about 12 hours; sea turtles are less tolerant, having an average survival time of 2 hours.

## Lizards Loved or Loathed

'In calling the hideous and ill-tempered alligator *el lagarto*, the lizard, I think the Spanish explorers were guilty of a crying injustice to the lizard family, many of the members of which are the *most delightful* little creatures imaginable.

'How often in Italy, seated by some ancient ruin or on a stone wall draped in rose vines, I have watched the merry little lizards, dressed in crimson, orange, or green, darting among the grey stones like flashes of living light, or running along the trailing vines like animated blossoms.

'How often in the warm fragrant silence of the Tuscan hills, have I seen, thrust from the chinks of a pile of crumbling masonry, a pert little head, with a pair of diamond-bright eyes, watching me with intent interest. Friendly, graceful, entirely harmless, these little lizards seem to suit the beauty-loving Italians. I have never seen the smallest or rudest Italian boy throw a stone at one of them or try in any way to hurt them.

'The lizards in our own country are no less friendly and beautiful, but it seems to me our people are less in harmony with nature than some others and cherish more unjust traditions; for certainly among us the lizards are received in less hearty good-fellowship and are very wrongly feared and esteemed harmful. But some people know how to treat my dear lizards with courtesy. A young friend in Florida has made pets of sundry emerald-green lizards. No creatures are more capable of *maintaining an absolute stillness* if they are suited with their circumstances. Like most of the cold-blooded reptiles, they delight in warmth. My young friend often placed a little green lizard in the knot of lace at the throat of her evening dress, where, delighted with the softness and warmth of the lace and its owner's neck, it would lie motionless for an entire evening. It was often mistaken for a piece of jeweler's work in rich green enamel, upon the beauty of which her friends sometimes commented. One of these little lizards would remain for hours, twined bracelet-wise about my young friend's wrist.

'*Inoffensive in disposition and unprovided with weapons of attack* as lizards are, I have often admired nature's protective methods in their behalf. Walking once in a wood in New Jersey, I was surprised to observe a fragment of the bark of a tree some 2 feet from me, run round the tree and appear on the farther side. Here was a little lizard of the exact colour and markings of the bark of the tree that it frequented; it was only by its motion that it could be discovered when it clung against the trunk or branches. When at rest its little, bright, jet-black eyes were the only noticeable part of it. In that same wood I was equally startled by seeing a dead leaf run away from a heap of leaves as I approached and a little twig in my path darted out of danger just as I was about to put my foot upon it. These also were lizards, with their slender bodies dressed in grey and brown, with little markings of black and white, a coat closely simulating the colours of dry and decaying vegetation.

'While capable of lying for hours in entire quiet, still as if fashioned out of gems or metal, the lizard, when it moves, is remarkable for the swiftness of its motions: it darts with the rapidity of an arrow; it seems to have *no hesitancy, no afterthought, no change of mind*; its spring is with the precision of entire certainty. Perhaps its sure-footedness has something to do with this; on wall or wood, tree, stone, grass, who ever saw a lizard slip or lose its footing?' [McNair Wright, 1895]


## BASIC BEHAVIOUR PATTERNS

### Behaviour Patterns Common to both Lizards & Mammals

In order to interact, lizards use static modifiers [body posture] and dynamic modifiers [display movements]. Static modifiers alter the appearance of the displayer, whereas dynamic modifiers alter the appearance of the display. There are 4 main kinds of displays: challenge, submission, courtship, and signature [head bobbing; push-ups; dewlap or throat extension; etc.].

Altogether, more than 25 special forms of basic behaviour patterns are seen in lizards that are also seen in mammals, incl. human beings. The most prominent forms are as follows:

1 Domain – Selection and preparation of homesite.

2 Domain – Establishment of territory.

3 Domain – Use of home range.

4 Showing place preferences.

5 Trail making.

6 Marking of territory.

7 Patrolling territory.

8 Ritualistic display in defence of territory, commonly involving the use of colouration and adornments.

9 Formalised intraspecific fighting in defence of territory.

10 Triumphal display in successful defence.

11 Assumption of distinctive postures and colouration in signaling surrender.

12 Use of defaecation posts.

13 Foraging.

14 Hunting.

15 Homing.

16 Hoarding.

17 Formation of social groups.

18 Establishment of social hierarchy by ritualistic display and other means.

19 Greeting.

20 Grooming.

21 Courtship, with displays using colouration and adornments.

22 Mating.

23 Breeding and, in isolated instances, attending offspring.

24 Flocking.

25 Migration.

[MacLean, 1985]

## Daily Routines

'At present, there is almost no information about brain mechanisms accounting for the highly complicated business of regulating an individual's daily routine and subroutines. . . . Apart from the matter of daily rhythms, there is as yet no information as to whether or not there are particular cerebral structures involved in linking together the daily master routine. . . . In view of his emphasis of treating the mind and body as a whole, Adolf Meyer would have looked kindly upon research concerned with the daily routine.'

[Swiss-born Adolf Meyer, 1866–1950, was the most prominent and influential American psychiatrist of the first half of the 20th century. Particularly after his appointment to Johns Hopkins, as its first professor of psychiatry, he dominated psychiatry in the United States until his retirement in 1941. His focus on collecting detailed case histories on patients is the most prominent of his contributions; along with his insistence that patients could best be understood through consideration of their life situations.]

'Lizards are *ideal subjects for studies on routine*. Every day they engage in no less than 7 sequences of behaviour that occur almost with the regularity of Meyer's clocks at the Hopkins [Johns Hopkins University, Baltimore]. An incapacitating illness is a poignant example of what we forfeit when there is a break in our routine, and we are confined to bed and regulated by the routines of those taking care of us. Psychiatric illness, however, may present quite a different situation, as illustrated by the psychotic person who is perfectly able to ambulate and who has everyone dancing to his or her routines. The over-and-over repetition of disrupting subroutines may be particularly difficult to deal with. Neuroleptic drugs with a rather specific action on the striatal complex have become widely popular as a means of restraining psychotic patients.

'It is pertinent to mention here that patients with Huntington's chorea [characterised by a widespread loss of nerve cells in the corpus striatum] may, early in the disease, lack the initiative to pursue any daily routine, but are grateful for the opportunity to follow a prescribed routine. They may also have difficulty in executing subroutines. Patients who are recovering from Sydenham's chorea may be *obsessed with repeating disrupting subroutines* over and over again, such as counting to one hundred after each brushing of the teeth.' [MacLean, 1985]

Regarding the 'sequences of behaviour' that constitute the daily routine of lizards, MacLean explains in his book *The Triune Brain in Evolution* [1990] what these are. He refers to observations by Greenberg, who found that lizards in a quasi-natural environment will follow the same kind of master routine and engage in the same type of displays as are seen in the field. Their daily master routine is characterised by

1 cautious emergence from a shelter [as though expecting at any moment to be seized by a predator];
2 a period of basking, followed by
3 defaecation in an accustomed place [like many kinds of mammals, lizards have a defaecation post];
4 morning feeding within the territory;
5 a period of afternoon quietude;
6 afternoon feeding farther afield;
7 late afternoon basking; and
8 return to the shelter.

### Lizard's Dilemma – To Be or Not To Be Noticed
'Colour is an important aspect of lizard biology for several reasons. Because lizards are the most visually orientated of the reptiles, patches of bright colour are important in communication between individuals. Colour is also important in helping the lizard to blend into its surroundings and thereby escape the notice of predators. These 2 requirements seem to be at odds with each other, and many species compromise.

'Thus, many lizards have brightly coloured undersides, or patches of bright colour on their flanks and throats. When displaying to one another, these lizards expose their bright flash markings by raising their bodies up in a series of push-ups. Others signal by raising and lowering coloured flaps.

'In the majority of species, it is only the male that is colourful, the females being much duller and well camouflaged. The reason behind this is that females may be more vulnerable when they are carrying the extra burden of a develop-ing clutch of eggs or young, apart from the fact that it is normally the male's job to defend the territory and to attract a mate – the onus of communication at a distance therefore lies with him, whereas all the female has to do is to respond to his signals if she so desires.

'Selection for bright colours can also occur even when these are detrimental – males that are brightest have the best chance of attracting mates and passing on their genes, even though this may make them more vulnerable to predation. Dull males are not likely to be eaten but rarely become fathers. Bright courtship colours are therefore a trade-off between reproductive success and predator avoidance.' [Mattison, 2002]

### Showing One's Colours

'Involuntary changes of the body hues may be observed among several of the [lizard] families. The process is influenced by light, temperature, excitement and the health of the individual. It is a mistake to imagine the colour changes to be strictly in line of protection to the lizard in immediately conforming to the colours of surfaces on which the animal rests. A specimen capable of exhibiting all phases of colouration between a dull brown to an emerald green may for some time rest upon a dark tree trunk and be clad in a suit of conspicuous steel-grey; from this hue it may transform into a livid green; a few minutes later it may jump among the leaves and shrubbery, where it takes on an almost blackish hue. In fiction, theory is an excellent stand-by.

'Who can blame certain romantic authors for elaborating upon such an admirable point as the "power" displayed by a dull brown lizard to jump upon a leaf and transform into a leafy green, thence upon a tree trunk where it immedi-ately turns brown again, and from there, possibly, upon a gorgeous flower where the reptile assumes a hue to match the richly-coloured petals?' [Ditmars, 1937a]

The most conspicuous examples of lizards that vary in hues and pattern are among the Gekkonidae [geckos], Iguanidae [iguanids], Agamidae [agamids] and Chamaeleontidae [chameleons]; others exhibit no trace of this characteristic; among the latter are the members of the Lacertidae [wall lizards], Teiidae [tegus, racerunners and whiptail lizards] and Scincidae [skinks].

'Since most diurnal [day-active] lizards can also identify colours, the bright red, yellow, orange, and even lavender dewlaps of certain anoles – as well as the vivid blue throats, tails, flanks and tongues of other lizards – are readily apparent to rivals, intruders and prospective mates.' [Badger, 2002]

### Colour as Communication

Lizards *communicate through visual displays*, in contrast to acoustically communi-cating animals such as birds, frogs, and primates.

Skin colour and patterns of lizards are esp. important as *communication* cues because, as herpetologist Chris Matheson explains, "lizards are the most visually oriented of the reptiles." Although the brighter, bolder colours of males are often characterised as "nuptial colours" intended to attract the opposite sex, authority Hobart Smith argues that the real function of an anole's bright red [or yellow or purple] dewlap, or the bright blue on the throat or flank of a chuckwalla, is not to attract females "but rather to send other competitors or enemies away." Accordingly, these often-vivid colours and striking patterns require a well-developed sense of vision, rather than the well-developed sense of hearing that frogs and toads exhibit when courting.

'The colours of lizards, particularly those of colour-changing chameleons, anoles, and geckos, are especially attractive to hobbyists and breeders. Of the quick-change artists, chameleons are probably the best known but also among the least understood, since most people believe chameleons alter their colours to blend in with their surroundings. Colour change for chameleons and certain other lizards is *not a disguise*, Martin explains, but rather a way to make the chameleon "more conspicuous" in courtship or in response to threats – the change in colour is essentially a form of *communication*.

'Researchers have identified 8 significant variables that can affect the colour of a lizard. As enumerated by Smith, these include:

1 age or stage of growth;
2 gender;
3 colour of the environment;
4 season of the year;
5 temperature;
6 mood or state of excitement;
7 physical state of health;
8 intensity of light.

'While some changes in colour are voluntary, others are strictly involuntary, as close observation of the sleeping habits of chameleons and anoles reveals. In the morning, for example, when temperatures are still cool, many lizards assume a darker shade of colour to absorb radiant heat. Then, if the temperature becomes too hot, the dark colour "suddenly changes to a quite light one," explains herpetologist Robert Mertens, to avoid "heating beyond the optimum." During courtship, a male chameleon adopts his flashiest colours and bobs his head repeatedly to signal his gender to a prospective mate or to warn off a rival suitor. A startled chameleon may suddenly turn black with anger or exhibit a pattern of spots and stripes – sometimes in less than a minute.

'Anole lizards [mistakenly called "chameleons" in Florida and other Southern states] are famous for their quick transformation from bright green to brown and then back again. Bright green is the "activity colour," explains researcher Hilda Simon, displayed "when the animal feels insecure, endangered, or uncomfortable, as well as during periods of exertion." Brown, the "response colour," signals that the anole is "comparatively calm, tranquil, or sleepy, regardless of the colour of its background." As for camouflage, colour phases "may very well have a protective value," she says, "not so much because of the animal's background, but because of its own condition." . . . Some members of another family, the agamids of Asia and Africa, can change colour as strikingly as chameleons.' [Badger, 2002]

## Eye-catching & Jaw-jawing Messages

'Lizards that signal to rivals with a visual display "shout" to get their point across, UC Davis researchers have found. Male anole lizards signal ownership of their territory by sitting up on a tree trunk, bobbing their heads up and down and extending a colourful throat pouch. They can spot a rival lizard up to 25 meters away, said Terry Ord, a postdoctoral researcher at UC Davis who is working with Judy Stamps, professor of evolution and ecology. The lizards' signals need to be strong enough for a rival to see, but not vivid enough to say "eat me" to a passing predator. But their forest home can be a visually noisy environment, with branches and leaves waving in the breeze and casting patterns of light and shade.

"They have to have a strategy to get their message across," Ord said. Ord videotaped 2 species of anole lizards, Anolis cristatellus and Anolis gundlachi, in the Caribbean National Forest in Puerto Rico. He found that the more "visual noise" in the background, the faster and more exaggerated the movements of the lizards.' [UC Davis, 2007]

Another method of getting your message across is the gaping display of adult male lizards. '. . . Researchers showed that when an adult male lizard gapes his jaws at a rival male during an intense territorial interaction, information is made available to his opponent about how hard he can bite – indeed, the lizard's jaw muscles become clearly visible. Further, some lizards have evolved bright patches that reflect ultraviolet light, which lizards can see, to delineate the jaw muscles. Lappin and colleagues point out that the information about bite force provided by the display does not correspond to body or head size because males of similar size can vary substantially in how hard they can bite.

'The display thus provides unique and honest information about weapon quality, as well as a mechanism for making the decision to fight or to back down. Adult male collared lizards . . . are larger than the females, have hypertrophied jaw muscles, and are highly territorial toward other males. All of this relates to males having evolved the ability to bite with great force, which means that they can seriously wound rivals in fights.

"When you've seen what these lizards can do to each other with their jaws, inflicting deep lacerations and even breaking bones, it makes sense that avoiding fights would be advantageous, even if you are likely to win," Lappin says. When 2 competing males engage in a gaping display, each shows off its weapon while simultaneously affording an opportunity to evaluate its rival's weapon. In animals from insects to humans, such displays likely play an important role in assessing the risks associated with fighting, as well as in reinforcing the experiences of past fights with specific individuals.

"You see the same with humans," Lappin explains. "Think back to the *rivalries of adolescence*. Fights took place in order to establish dominance relationships in the neighbourhood, but the fights themselves were rare. Most of it was *posturing and showing off*, displays per se, that served to advertise physical prowess as well as to reinforce the consequences of previous confrontations." ' [Lappin, 2006]

## Poseurs & Polygamists

'Male lizards "out on quite a display," Carr notes, and, for maximum effect, many adopt "stereotypical" poses or body motions to call attention to themselves. Bobbing the head vigorously up and down is one common male ritual; doing "push-ups" is another. If a female is receptive and stands her ground [some species tread in place], the male will proceed to court her with nudges, licks, or a firm bite on the neck or flank – then slip the base of his tail beneath hers and insert one hemipenis into her cloaca.

'Many males are "polygamists" [Blair calls them "promiscuous"], engaging in copulation with more than one female during the breeding season. Some males simply entice eligible females that wander into range; others [such as chuck-wallas] operate what Mattison calls "a kind of harem system," exercising control over females that populate a specific territory. "Large tyrant males defend large territories [and] patrol their territories daily," observes researcher Bayard Brattstrom; "only the tyrant mates with the females."

'Some Madagascan day geckos actually form permanent relationships and if one partner dies, "the remaining partner will not normally mate with another," Henkel and Schmidt report.

'Roughly one-fifth of species give birth to living young [viviparity], and others produce eggs that hatch just prior to or at the time of laying [ovoviviparity]. Most lizard eggs are leathery or hard-shelled, yet they are also permeable to moisture, without which the embryo will die; accordingly, many females lay their eggs in moist locations, such as leaf litter, rotting wood, damp soil, or sand. . . . Females of some species – esp. geckos – lay their eggs in communal nesting sites, perhaps when conditions are not ideal.

'In about a dozen species of geckos and lacertids, the gender of offspring may be dependent upon the temperature of the nest – as is also the case with croco-dilians, many turtles, and some snakes. Among the temperature-dependent lizards, "females are produced at cooler temperatures and males at warmer ones," Pough and his co-authors report. This is exactly the opposite of the pattern in other reptiles. . . .

'Even more remarkable is the ability of some 30 species of lizards in 6 different families to reproduce asexually [i.e. without the female having her eggs fertilised by a male]. This method of reproduction, called parthenogenesis, produces offspring [usually all female] that are clones of their mother and that share an identical genetic makeup.' [Badger, 2002]

## Surrendering the Behind

Tail-casting lizards are found in the families Anguidae [anguids], Gekkonidae [geckos], Iguanidae [iguanids], Scincidae [skinks], Teiidae [teiids and whiptails] and Lacertidae [wall or true lizards].

Relinquishing part of the body seems a drastic thing to do under any circum-stances. But for many lizards, casting off the tail can mean the difference between life and death. Not all lizards get away but enough escape to make the strategy worthwhile.

Other animals also shed parts of their bodies easily: many salamanders lose their tails, while brittle stars, spiders, crabs, lobsters, octopuses and some insects readily give up limbs. This process of self-amputation is called autotomy and is often followed by regrowth of the shed part.

Autotomy in lizards is enabled by special zones of weakness at regular intervals in the vertebrae below the vent. Essentially, the lizard contracts a muscle to fracture a vertebra rather than break the tail between 2 vertebrae. Sphincter muscles in the tail then contract around the caudal artery to minimise bleeding. The new section will contain cartilage rather than bone, and the skin may be distinctly discoloured compared to the rest of the body.

However, despite the immediate survival benefit, autotomy carries substantial cost, and thus should be avoided except as a last resort. Surrendering expendable body parts imposes multiple longer-term costs and risks, incl. reduced levels of reproductive investment [i.e. reductions in territory size and access to females], inhibited locomotor performance, restricted growth rates, diminished escape capabilities, modified habitat use, *lowered social status*, impaired competitive abilities and reduced survival in natural populations.

If Lizard is your 'power or totem animal . . . detachment is also part of what lizard can teach. They can help us to *become more detached in life* to survive. Sometimes it is necessary to separate ourselves or part of ourselves from others to be able to do the things we most desire to do. The lizard helps us to awaken that ability for objective detachment so that it can occur with the least amount of difficulty. Lizard can show up to help us break from the past. It may even indicate a need to explore new realms and follow your own impulses before you get swallowed in what is not beneficial for you.' [Andrews, 1998]

Given the fact that lizards tend to be *routine-bound in their daily activities* . . . 'Lizard will aid you in becoming more detached from situations in your life. Now and again it is required to be detached, to separate yourself from others, to succeed in what is necessary. Lizard will also show you how to leave the past in the past! To move on and quit being attached to what has been. Lizard is proposing immediate change in one or more areas of your life. You may need to let go of old ideas, patterns, belief systems, habits, actions or lifestyle because the old may threaten you in some way now. It is time to let go. Lizard prompts the need to go within and examine your present reality and then, move with confidence and utmost assuredness into a new chapter of your life.' [Woolcott, 2015]

## No Families

Notably *lacking* in lizards [and other reptiles] is the family-related, behavioural triad consisting of nursing [in conjunction with maternal care], audio-vocal communication for maintaining maternal-offspring contact [also known as the separation call] and play [which may have functioned originally to promote harmony in the nest]. Recent findings suggest that the development of such mammalian family-related behaviour may have depended on the evolution of the thalamocingulate division of the limbic system, a derivative from early mammals, which in turn stem from the mammal-like reptiles [therapsids].

The pivotal role of the forebrain in mammals is supported by its involvement in the regulation of specific behaviours during nursing and maternal care of offspring. For instance, the thalamocingulate division of the forebrain, which has no counterpart in reptiles, is believed to have evolved in parallel with social behaviours related to the development of familial acculturation, which are established to a large extent through audio-vocal communication. The perception of emotional information in species-specific communication sounds of non-human mammals – involved in securing emotional bonding and social interactions – depends at least partially on thalamocingulate neural circuits, both in parents and offspring.

### Benefits & Costs of Social Rank

'Depending on space requirements and the distribution of key resources in the environment, social behaviour among lizards can vary from defence of exclusive territories to the formation of dominance hierarchies. As anyone who has watched large groups of lizards is aware, increases in population density usually lead to more social interaction and heightened aggression, esp. among mates. In captivity, where dispersal is not possible, dominance hierarchies tend to emerge even in species that appear to be strictly territorial in nature. Dominance hierarchies can become established quite quickly among captive lizards, almost always within a day, but sometimes after only a few hours.

'In many lizard species, *dominance hierarchies are characterised by a pecking order*, in which higher ranking individuals dominate those of lower social rank. In other species, a single highly dominant individual tyrannises all others in the local vicinity. In either case, the potential benefits of dominant social status are many. For carnivorous species such as Komodo monitors, Varanus komodoensis, feeding order at carcasses depends on size and social status. Dominant male brown anoles, Anolis sagrei, are far more successful at acquiring and defending preferred perch sites than are subordinate males. Higher ranking spiny-tailed iguanas, Ctenosaura sp., tend to occupy the best rocky crevice retreats, restricting lower ranking males to lower, more marginal areas. Perhaps most importantly, dominant males in virtually all lizard species are much more likely to attract females and mate successfully.

'The benefits of being a dominant lizard do not come without costs, however. Compared to subordinates, dominant males probably consume a great deal more energy, suffer from increased exposure to predators and run a higher risk of serious injury during fights. In male mountain spiny lizards, Sceloporus jarrovi, dominance is associated with higher mortality, probably as a result of the tremendous amount of time and energy expended in aggressive interactions. In order to avoid the costs of escalated interactions with dominant males, subordinate male lizards often conspicuously advertise their low status. For example, subordinate male anoles become darker in the presence of dominants and subordinate male spiny lizards adopt submissive postures, which hide their bright blue belly colours. In bearded dragons, Pogona [= Amphibolurus] barbota, submission is signaled by a distinctive overhand wave. . . .

'The consequences of social subordination in lizards appear to extend far beyond restricted access to preferred sites within enclosures. Among captive 6-lined racerunners, Cnemidophorus sexlineatus, subordinate individuals lose weight over the course of the breeding season and may exhibit other physiological signs of social stress. When male green anoles, Anolis carolinensis are housed in pairs, one male invariably becomes dominant. Levels of *corticosterone, the major steroid hormone associated with stress in lizards*, are much higher in subordinate males, which are also less advanced spermatogenically. Dominant male anoles tend to monopolise positions that afford the best access to heat and light, preventing subordinates from thermoregulating normally and rendering them more vulnerable to a variety of infectious agents.' [Alberts, 1993]

*Body size is the main determinant of male competitive ability and mating success in lizards.*

## Hostility & Dear Enemies

'Aggressive interactions, usually between sexually mature males, occur in most lizards. The associated behaviours include visual displays, posturing, chasing, grappling, and in some instances fighting, with potential for serious injury. Aggressive interactions in territorial species – most Iguania – are usually directed toward establishing and maintaining territorial boundaries.

'At the heart of aggressive interactions between individuals is competition for resources in short supply, incl. females. Aggressive interactions in non-territorial species – most Scleroglossa – also occur over scarce resources, or rather, one particular resource: individual females.

'In both cases, relative body size is among the most important variables determining success in aggressive encounters between males, even though hormone levels and established residency play roles as well. . . .

'Establishment of territorial boundaries lessens the likelihood of fights – which, because they require energy and are always risky, are engaged in only when there is a reasonable chance of winning – especially when potential opponents are familiar with each other: a phenomenon known as "dear enemy recognition." '

[Dear enemy recognition implies reduced aggression toward territorial neighbours relative to strangers. It is a widespread occurrence in many species of lizards, as well as in territorial amphibians, presumably because a stranger represents more of a threat to a resident than a neighbour.]

'In collared lizards and green anoles, for example, males holding adjacent territories seldom interact aggressively, unless an intruder is a stranger. Similarly, territorial male *Platysaurus broadleyi* in South Africa allow neighbour males to approach more closely than unfamiliar males and more readily attack the latter. Members of the opposite sex are not "enemies," thus response to an unfamiliar female is quite different. In *Holbrookia propinqua*, males court unfamiliar females more intensely than resident females, possibly to increase the chance of successful mating or to induce the female into becoming a resident of the male's territory.' [Pianka & Vitt, 2006]

## Cooperation

Most examples of cooperative behaviour in animals involve cooperation between genetically related individuals, which is explained by the theory of 'kin selection'. Researchers have recently described an example of cooperation between genetically similar but unrelated side-blotched lizards [Uta stansburiana], a species of lizard common on the Pacific coast of North America, from Washington to western Texas and NW Mexico. Barry Sinervo, a professor of ecology and evolutionary biology at the University of California, has been studying the side-blotched lizard since 1989, making some fascinating discoveries that show cooperative behaviour in this species.

The side-blotched lizard can be identified by the bluish-black blotch on either side of its chest, located just behind the forelimb. This species of lizard has 3 different colour morphs [a 'morph' is a morphologically distinct subset of a species]. The orange, yellow, and blue colour morphs differ not only in their throat colour, but also in their territorial behaviour and mating strategies. Orange-throated males, 'usurpers' as Sinervo terms them, are very aggressive and mate with multiple females by enlarging their territories, taking over those of other males. Yellow-throated males are 'sneakers' who don't defend territories but resemble females in their colouration, which enables them to sneak behind the backs of territorial males to cuckold them. Blue-throated males are mate guarders; they keep a close eye on their mates and form partnerships in which 2 males co-operate to protect their territories.

The cooperative behaviour of blue-throated males plays out differently depending on the frequency of aggressive orange males in the population. In years when there are few orange males, cooperating blue males both benefit. But when orange males are common, one blue male ends up serving as a buffer for his territorial partner, bearing the brunt of the advances of aggressive orange males. Thus, the behaviour of the blue-throated males oscillates between mutualism and altruism, depending on where the population as a whole is in the rock-paper-scissors cycle. [In the rock-paper-scissors game rock beats scissors, paper beats rock, and scissors beats paper.] In nature, altruism seems contradictory to an animal's goals of survival and passing on its genes, so researchers have been trying to understand why one of the blue males in a partnership will put himself in harm's way to allow the other to reproduce. Even though it may forfeit their own reproductive chances, the fighting blue throats secure the persistence of their genes in future generations by enabling their blue buddies to avoid the aggressors and go on to mate.

Mapping the genomes of these heroic blue throats, Sinervo and his co-workers found that the partners would share not merely the one gene that controlled the colour of their throats, but multiple genes that, they speculate, allowed the 2 lizards, who were not bound by close kinship ties, to mutually recognise the presence of cooperative genes.

## Cooperation, Aggression, or Deception

Male competition in side-blotched lizards drives a cycle of 3 strategies: yellow-throated sneakers beat orange-throated usurpers [deception triumphs over force], blue-throated mate guarders defeat sneakers [cooperation overcomes deception] and usurpers prevail over mate guarders [force trumps cooperation]. Each strategy in this game has a strength and a weakness, which keeps the wheels spinning. The lizard populations go through cycles in which one colour after another increases its numbers at the expense of the others, but none are able to maintain dominance.

The triangle of competing strategies may be far more common than previously recognized, and may even shape the way humans behave, Sinervo suggests. 'The models we propose . . . are a general phenomenon for all animals, humans included. . . . When faced with the task of gathering food or finding mates . . . you either cooperate, or take by force, or take by deception. Those are the 3 ways you can make a living in any social system. It's one of those basic games that structures life.'

Other lizard species are known or expected to have adopted strategies similar to those of side-blotched lizards.

For example, in male European common lizards [Lacerta vivipara] the strategy used to pursue females is revealed by their underside. Males sporting orange bellies are bullies who invade other lizards' territories to mate with any female they can grab hold of. While they're at it somewhere in their sizeable territory, drab yellow-bellied males sneak in and mate with unguarded females. The third side of the triangle, white-bellied males guard their mates closely, and cooperate with other white-bellied lizards to keep the yellows at bay.

Involved in an endless frequency-dependent cycle, one strategy predominates for some time, after which it declines in frequency as the strategy that manages to exploit its weakness increases. Orange aggressors may be dominant for a couple of years, followed by yellow deceivers, succeeded by white cooperators and then back to orange as the cycle starts anew.

## Lizards & Music

'Popular tradition has, from time immemorial, ascribed to music a vague and mystic power over the brute creation. Birds were supposed to hush their own songs in listening to those of the divinities; shepherds drew their flocks around them while they played on the Pandean-pipe; horses thrilled and neighed responsively to martial strains with equal elation to that aroused in their riders; and serpent-charmers are said, even in the present day, to exercise their art under some occult protection derived from cadences which, however, are rather cacophonous than tuneful. . . .

'But it is among reptiles that we should find this influence most strikingly manifested, according to popular opinion – an opinion so widely prevalent, so universally received, that I hesitate in expressing my own incredulity. . . . Snake-charming I think we may dismiss from consideration in this paper. . . .

'With lizards the case wears an aspect of greater probability, since the smaller species, such as some of the Gekkonidae, the Lacertidae and the Iguanidae, certainly betray a sense of musical vibrations. Little geckos and other house-lizards, if they do not exactly "come out to listen," as they are reputed to do, will stop instantly in their flight over walls and floor when a note is struck and remain motionless for some seconds, as though actually listening for its repetition; and I have seen taraguiras in a garden "mesmerised" by a guitar in the same way. But it is to be observed that in neither instance is the mesmerism complete enough to prevent their eluding capture and that if the music be continued, they soon become habituated to it, and resume their wonted movements. I am inclined to attribute the effect to the reception of the air-waves by the general sensibility of the cutaneous surface, the feeling of what is most likely a disagreeable thrill, rather than to any impression on the special sense of hearing.

'Sitting at an open grand piano one day, looking at some manuscript, but not touching the keys, a "legatitia," making his way down the wall, against which the instrument stood, by a series of running crooked jerks, caught my eye, his little sprawling hands and iridescent body sharply defined against the white background. On the farther end of the piano lay a paper of "dulces"; this had attracted a swarm of flies and the flies in their turn attracted the legatitia. Down he came, with abrupt suspicious darts and turns to this side and that, until he stood on the level ground of the piano-top, paused, elevated his tiny bright sharp head, flitted half across it and paused again. Just as he began to run once more, having cautiously brought my hands and feet into position, I struck a tremendous double chord with the hard pedal down. Poor little chap! I thought I had killed him. He was absolutely knocked off his legs and turned over on his back, where he lay feebly kicking. Before I could reach him, however, he had recovered, regained his feet, flashed up the wall and disappeared into a crevice. I expect that that lizard, at any rate, had a very low opinion of music afterwards.

'The true auditory function in all reptiles is dull and imperfect. A snake perceives the shock of approaching footsteps on the earth and evades them or takes instant alarm at the falling of a shadow, whereas the noise of laughter and voices in close proximity to it are often powerless to disturb it. That they are not actually deaf can be demonstrated by experiment as well as dissection. . . . and a huge teguexin lizard of my own communicates a small earthquake to the quiet mound of hay and moss under which he usually lies buried, and waddles forth in response to a certain whistle, shooting out his long red tongue in confident expectation of a dead mouse or bit of raw meat.' [Dickens, 1882]

'In *Music for Chameleons*, New Orleans-born author Truman Capote claims he once watched 3 "green chameleons" race one another across a stately terrace and pause at his hostess' feet. "Chameleons [are] such exceptional creatures," remarked the hostess. "Did you know they are very fond of music?" Capote was skeptical, so his friend sat down at her piano and began playing a Mozart sonata.

"Eventually the chameleons accumulated," Capote recalled; "a dozen, a dozen more, most of them green . . . They skittered across the terrace and scampered into the salon, a sensitive, absorbed audience for the music." Afterwards, when the pianist rose from her bench, "the chameleons scattered like sparks from an exploding star."

How charmingly exotic – but do chameleons really respond to music? In truth, Capote was observing anoles, which many Americans persist in calling "chameleons" because of their similar talent for changing colour. But Capote, one suspects, would not have been pleased with the less elegant-sounding title *Music for Anoles.*' [Badger, 2002]


## LIZARDS & LEPROSY

### The Most Loathsome of Diseases

'A spectre haunted large parts of the Western world in the last decade of the 19th century – the spectre of the most "loathsome" of diseases, leprosy, lapping on European and American shores. At the high point of Western imperialism, great anxiety was felt about the likely importation of the dread disease endemic in the colonies, into "civilised countries."

'The paranoia was the more ironic, because only a few decades earlier endemic leprosy had been viewed as evidence of civilisational backwardness, – implicitly this was a category not applicable to the West. For example in 1862, an authoritative medical journal in England opined that the countries of Asia continued to be infested by leprosy, "to a greater or less extent, generally speaking, in proportion to the physical and moral degradation of their people" [BMJ, 12.6.1862].

'The smugness of the 1860s was rapidly overtaken by panic in 1889, in the wake of the widely publicised Father Damien incident. That European priest had succumbed to leprosy after associating with the lepers in the settlement on the Hawaiian island of Molokai. Thereafter, it became painfully clear to imperialists that physically and morally degraded indigenous peoples could endanger Western well-being.

'In his incisive analysis of lepra-phobia in 19th-century white America, Gussow [1989] argues that one of its inspirations was racism. In a country that was undergoing a demographic transformation by immigration, the entrants were particularly feared and stigmatised by white Americans, as it was the case of the Chinese, who according to the 1882 legislation were prohibited to immigrate into the United States. A particularly emotive allegation in the United States was that germ-laden Chinese "coolie" labour had carried the disease into the pristine Hawaiian Islands, a territory deeply important to American commercial interests.

'Gussow also argues that on the other hand leprosy-endemic Norway, also a source of immigration, did not excite such prejudice: "Norwegian leprosy never generated horror and alarm simply because Norwegians were never perceived as a 'loathsome' people whose germs were considered culturally and biologically anathema to Anglo-Saxon civilisation." . . .

'There were 2 alternatives, either the healthy must evacuate, or the lepers must be put outside the community and be isolated. For the greater good, the leper was duty-bound to endure the disadvantages of isolation.' [Pandya, 2004]

### Unclean Things that Cling to the Ground

The ancient Egyptians disliked geckos and believed that they were a danger to human health. This attitude has continued to the present day as many modern Egyptians also fear geckos, believing them to be capable of poisoning food and *causing skin diseases.* Apparent similarities between the symptoms of dermato-logical problems and characteristics of gecko skin may have led to the association between the reptile and skin disease.

'The gecko's particular ability to lighten and darken their skin colour may have struck the Egyptians as alarmingly similar to pigmentation changes caused by rashes and skin-whitening conditions, such as vitiligo. There is no firm, physical evidence for leprosy in Egypt prior to the Ptolemaic period. It is nevertheless intriguing to note striking similarities between this disease and characteristics of gecko morphology and behaviour. Leprosy is a chronic, contagious, disfiguring disease that attacks the skin, peripheral nerves and mucous membranes. The infection is characterised by a rash of flat, white ulcers that eventually enlarge and become discoloured. Multiple lesions and accompanying nerve damage can cause affected areas [the extremities] to lose sensation. Often, because of the loss of feeling, the fingers and toes become mutilated and fall off. The tendency for geckos to release body parts [tail, skin] when seized by a predator may consequently have given rise to the belief that these reptiles carry leprosy.

'Furthermore, if the humidity level drops while geckos are shedding, the skin can fail to come away from their toes; subsequent infection often causes these to fall off. Leprosy can also affect the facial nerves around the eyes, causing patients to lose the ability to blink. The gecko's apparently similar inability to close their eyes may also have cast suspicion upon them. It is not currently clear whether these associations can account for the ancient dread of geckos, but they are likely to explain why later inhabitants of Egypt, for whom leprosy was a constant fear, saw them as carriers of this disease.' [Evans, 2002]

In the Bible various references are made to the word lizard as being related to Hebrew and Arabic meaning 'hiding' and 'that which clings to the ground'. Leviticus 11:29–30 provides a list of unclean 'creeping things', comprising particularly reptiles: tortoise, great lizard, gecko, chameleon, 'land crocodile' [probably either the desert monitor or the thorny-tailed lizard, both common in Palestine], lizard, and sand lizard. In the Revised Version of the King James Bible it says in the margin that Leviticus 11:30 contains 'words of uncertain meaning, but probably denoting 4 kinds of lizards.'

In Palestine, the gecko is common in houses. It clings with ease to smooth walls that other lizards cannot scale. Although perfectly harmless, it is believed to be poisonous and is much feared. It is called abu-brais, '*father of leprosy*,' either on account of its supposed poisonous qualities or because it has a semi-transparent and sickly appearance, being of a whitish-yellow colour with darker spots. In the eastern Mediterranean, geckos were at one time also associated with the development of leprosy.

In large parts of Asia, similar superstitions are perpetuated, as becomes evident from Jürgen Frembgen's 1996 paper *The Folklore of Geckos*. 'Proverbs, sayings and information provided by numerous informants show that the common small house geckos are regarded as ominous creatures associated with ill fortune. They are also considered highly impure and thought to be carriers of leprosy and other diseases. People are nevertheless rather ambivalent on the question of whether geckos should be killed; in some cases there is evidence of underlying beliefs that link the animals with fertility and well-being. . . . [In India] the Bengalese also say, "If a house-lizard [gecko] utters its peculiar cry 'tuck tu' when a man is speaking of something, then he cries out 'Satyi, satyi' – 'true, true', and it is believed that the thing spoken of will surely happen." . . .

'In Punjab and Uttar Pradesh it is claimed that a gecko dropping on a person will result in serious skin disease unless the person takes a full bath, particularly in "gold water" [hot water in which one or more pieces of gold have been laid]. . . . Geckos as carriers of leprosy and leukoderma [vitiligo]. Geckos have the capacity to change their colour between pale and dark by shifting the melanophores in their skin cells. They shed their skin, so that when one touches them some of the regenerating epidermis is likely to be left on one's hand. The tail also detaches quite easily. These qualities have tended to link the gecko through association – similia similibus evocantur – to certain diseases whose symptoms are the same. In the Punjab leprosy is generally attributed to contact with this animal, or, more especially, with its urine.

'Similar ideas are reflected in the Arabic name for a leper, bas, which derives from bors [gecko]. In Yemen and other Arab countries skin diseases are attributed to a gecko having run over the face of the afflicted person as he or she slept at night. In the region between North India and Afghanistan it is believed that contact with the gecko, or with its excreta, will cause the skin disease known as leukoderma, an acquired type of skin depigmentation characterised by whitish blotches on the face, hands, feet, back, arms, and legs. Leukoderma . . . often appears after inflammations caused by syphilis, psoriasis, leprosy, eczema, neuro-dermatitis, etc.'

Further down to the south, in New Zealand, some Maori tribes thought lizards ['ngarara' in their language] to be the cause of all diseases. In the afflicted part a lizard was supposed to exist; thus, a pain in the chest was due to lizard, and so with pains in the head and elsewhere. They believed that lizards actually existed in those organs and willfully caused these evils. A little green lizard was held especially baneful.

## Lizards for Treating Leprosy

The Scottish physician William Gourlay worked for more than 18 years as a 'Physician to the Factory at Madeira', a Portuguese island off the NW coast of Africa that later came to house a leper asylum. In his *Observations on the Natural History, Climate, and Diseases of Madeira* [1811], Gourlay gives a quite accurate description of leprosy, or 'elephantiasis, or Arabian leprosy' as he terms it.

Stating that it is 'very common among the lower classes of people in Madeira . . . it generally shows itself by tubercles upon the face and upper extremities and sometimes upon the trunk of the body and penis. Ill-conditioned ulcers of the legs also take place, in some instances attended with acute pain; large indolent glandular tumours occupy the upper and anterior part of the thigh. The fingers become contracted and the feet hard and swelled. The fingers also, and toes, are occasionally destroyed by ulccration; the same disposition to irregular tumours and ulceration attacks the throat. . . . In those affected by the disease, previous to the age of puberty, the usual signs that mark this period of life do not appear.

'The beard, the usual sign of virility, is wanting; the hair is deficient on the pubis and scrotum, as well as on the axilla and breast. No desire prevails for the venereal passion: the *voice preserves its puerile tone* and does not acquire the real strength and masculine expression. Even the testicles, not called upon for the exercise of their functions, gradually waste. Young females affected with this disease experience no increase or fulness of the breasts, no growth of the external parts of generation, no appearance of the menses, have no hair on the pubis or axilla and feel no disposition to venery. Even where the disease makes its first attack, at a much later period, the marks of sexual maturity, which are already established, gradually disappear, and are attended with *impotence or very impaired powers of generation*. These circumstances denote that the elephantiasis of Madeira differs from the same complaint in other countries: for almost every writer on the subject has described the unhappy victims of this disease, raging with insatiable irresistible desire for venery.'

Whereas leprosy hitherto was viewed as incurable, Dr. Gourlay occasionally succeeded in affording relief. In some cases he found 'great benefit of the internal administration of the lacerta [agilis] or common lizard.'

There can no certainty about the identity of the lizard species mentioned by Gourlay. Lacerta agilis does not occur on the island of Madeira, nor is it the 'common lizard'. The latter is Lacerta vivipara, a species that might have been present in Madeira. If Gourlay, however, meant to indicate commonly found on the island with the term 'common lizard', it could have been a small number of other Lacerta species, all of them endemic to Madeira.

Since there is no way of knowing whether the beneficial effects were specific for one particular species, we assume they were generic, particularly since they are in line with the use of other lizards – geckos – in Arab countries as effective agents for extracting urine or foreign bodies, as well as with the use of lizards in an ointment against 'evil patches on every limb' in ancient Egypt.

'As a medicine,' Gourlay surmises, 'this reptile acts as a powerful stimulant on the living solid, opening the several excretions and producing large evacuations, particularly by the skin and urine, which are at the same time not attended with any debilitating effect. By this mode of operation, it will be found to have the certain influence of arresting the progress of the worst symptoms of elephantiasis, if not the whole, and in many cases to have surprisingly restored parts, which for years had been morbidly enlarged, to their natural size and even sensibility; though for that period they had continued in a torpid state. Its operation also seems to vary somewhat in different cues; at times the different secretions seem increased by it all at once, viz. the perspiration, urine, and saliva; at other times, merely an increase of saliva takes place.

'Diarrhoea was not an uncommon effect of its operation, but as noticed and what would hardly be supposed, these evacuations produced no proportionate degree of debility. On the contrary, in every case, the appetite for food and the natural strength and vigour continued unimpaired. One effect of its administration was at times to occasion vertigo or giddiness, but this symptom seemed merely a transient attack and was never attended with any bad consequence. On what peculiar principle the active operation of this remedy depends, admits much conjecture, the viper, a reptile of the same structure, was considered by the ancients an infallible cure for leprosy, the active powers of which were supposed to reside in its volatile saline parts.

'The form of administering this remedy was that of pills of an ordinary size, [or about 5 or 6 grains each], into which it was made up with a little flour. In order to do it, the head, tail and legs were previously cut off, the skin removed, and the intestines taken out; of these pills, from 6 to 12 or more were given daily.

'. . . we are convinced that this reptile possesses considerable efficacy in the cure of elephantiasis. It has also been administered with advantage in herpes, chronic rheumatism, dropsy, and scrofula.'

### A Dose of Lizard

For centuries lizards have been used as medicine for everything from leprosy to syphilis. In various cultures they were believed to restore old men and to make young men great lovers, lizards being killed for medicine *for men who need help being men.*

Hahnemann had this to say about the practice in his *Organon:* 'Did not the renowned *excitantia* and *aphrodisiaca*, ambergris, lacerta scincus, cantharides tincture, truffles, cardamoms, cinnamon and vanilla invariably bring about complete impotence when used for the purpose of restoring the gradually declining sexual power [which always depended on an unobserved chronic miasm]?'

Although mixing up the species, Hahnemann appears to have been more positive about the lizard as medicine in his Lesser Writings, 1829: 'The lizard, which was first employed in America and subsequently also in Europe, according to reports with extremely happy effects, in inveterate syphilis with nodes, pains in the bones, ulcers and slow fevers, besides other diseases, is the *lacerta agilis*, L., a large [greenish coloured] species; the smaller varieties also are useful, though in a less degree. They reside in old walls and prey upon spiders, flies, ants, earthworms, crickets and locusts.'

Hahnemann's allusion to America relates to Dr. José Flores [ca. 1730–1795], a Mexican physician who published a treatise in 1781 claiming to have discovered that the raw flesh of lizards of the Amatitlán region of Guatemala cured cancer, syphilis, 'hydrophobia' [rabies] and 'all the varieties of cutaneous disease'. Based on Flores's description, arboreal alligator lizards of the genus Abronia appear to have been the species preferred for the treatment. As the following descriptions, comments and opinions demonstrate, the alleged medicinal properties of a specific New World lizard turned into generic medicinal properties of Old World lizards, coinciding partly with the traditional employment of Old World lizards and accounting for the muddled materia medica on these animals. [Note that the old term 'cancer' often was applied for canker sores or inveterate phagedenic ulcers!]

- 'Grey Lizard [Lacerta agilis] is one of the anti-cancerous remedies, the virtues of which have been the more exalted on account of its singularity. J. Flores, of the University of Guatimala [sic], in Mexico was the first who published on the subject in 1781, his memoir being reprinted the year following, at Madrid. His recipe ran thus – the heads and tails of lizards to be cut off, and after stripping off their skins and entrails, to be bolted forthwith, "tout palpitans." One, 2, or 3 were thus to be devoured daily. Cataplasms were applied to the cancers.

'The use of this specific was said to be followed with febrile heat, anxiety, sweats, profuse alvine and renal discharges – convulsions, etc. The grey lizard was so celebrated by the Spanish physicians that Daubenton and Mauduyt, 2 celebrated naturalists, were requested by the Royal Academy to ascertain its species. The case of a wench at Cadiz was much spoken of, who got cured in the space of 20 days of an ulcered cancer of the breast, by gobbling a lizard every morning. Theses were published on the virtues of the lizard in Sicily and Germany by Grass and Römer. It appears that the French Doctors were not so successful in their experiments. M. Bayle directed a man affected with a cancerous tumour of the face to take the remedy – 50 grey lizards were swallowed in the space of 15 days! "This remedy so vaunted produced no physiologic nor therapeutic effect." ' [Johnson & Johnson, 1834]

- 'As somewhat connected with the class of remedies we are at present enumerating, in its mode of action, [which has been compared to that of Mercury] may be mentioned a medicine of the animal kingdom, employed as a specific against this disease [cancer]. We have the account of it in the Transactions of the Royal Society of Medicine at Paris, being the translation of a Spanish Memoir on the subject. In the province of Guatimala [sic] in New Spain, we are informed that the use of the small Green Lizard is common in the cure of Cancer and attended with the greatest success in the ulcerated stage.

  'Two or 3 of these animals are directed to be swallowed daily, on an empty stomach, being first prepared by skinning them and cutting off their heads and tails. Their operation is attended with strong symptoms of fever, viz. great heat, sweating, and salivation; but the success is very sudden, generally in the course of 3 or 4 days a cure is affected. This practice is said to have been very common among the Indians in South America. It was attempted by the Spanish physicians with the Lizard of their own country; the circumstance of its being exhibited newly killed, preventing any being procured from America: But experience has shown the same inefficacy of it in Europe, as that of many other boasted Indian specifics; and this remedy has the farther objection to it, in being highly disagreeable to the patient, though this last circumstance might be somewhat removed by forming it into pills.' [Nisbet, 1795]

- 'The Scink [Scincus officinalis; Lacerta scincus L.] [now Scincus scincus, sandfish skink] was long regarded as a most useful and valuable remedy. In the Materia Medica it was said to be stimulant, restorative and anti-syphilitic, but esp. serviceable in restoring the powers of the body when they had been exhausted by voluptuous indulgences. It entered into the composition of several complicated formulae.

  'The common Lizard [Lacerta agilis] has been proposed as a substitute for the Scink. A species of Anolis [Anolis bullaris Cuv., green lizard] [now Anolis carolensis, green anole] and an Iguana [Iguana delicatissima; I. nudicollis]

[Lesser Antillian iguana, a mainly grey lizard, the juveniles of which are bright green] have also been mentioned for the same purpose.

'Very recently Dr. Gosse, of Geneva, has advocated the therapeutic properties of the Scinks. He maintains that the ancients were justified in employing them and that these animals possess powerful stimulant and sudorific properties, which might be usefully employed in various diseases. [Moquin-Tandon, 1861]

- 'The Officinal Scink has been long celebrated as a medicine among eastern nations, and once obtained a place in the British pharmacopoeias. It is a small animal, seldom exceeding 6 inches in length, and is of a pale yellowish grey colour. . . . This species of Scink is found in Nubia, Abyssinia and Egypt, from whence it used formerly to be brought to Europe by way of Venice and Marseilles. In its manners it is perfectly harmless; and so active in its motions that it hides itself in the sand in an instant. . . . The Scink is one of those medicines that we owe to the superstition of former ages. . . .

'The virtues for which its flesh has been extolled are extremely numerous; but it has been principally recommended as a restorative and as a remedy in elephantiasis, lepra, and other cutaneous diseases. In consequence of its reputed alexipharmic powers it entered as an ingredient into the old compound preparations, which went under the names of Theriaca Andromachi and Confectio Damocratis.

' "For a long time," says Mr. Griffith, "the Scink has been regarded as a remedy against certain maladies. Before this it was extolled by Pliny as a specific for the wounds caused by poisoned arrows; subsequently it has been vaunted as an aphrodisiac and quackery or ignorance has placed it in the rank of those medicaments which merit the distinguished honour of being employed to reanimate the exhausted powers and to *rekindle the fires of love*, when exhausted by the frosts of age or at the expense of debauchery. Its flesh has been administered as depurative, excitant, anthelmintic, analeptic, anticancerous, sialagogue and antispasmodic. 'Notwithstanding this confused mass of medical properties, thus put together without discrimination, as if to form the vademecum of some empiric, now appears completely ridiculous, yet even at the present day, in many countries, fables are still published respecting the success of this remedy. In spite, however, of the discredit into which it has fallen among the faculty in general, it does not appear to be totally devoid of efficacy in some complaints." [Stephenson, 1832]

### Lizards & Salmonella

Recent epidemiological studies have shown that geckos carry salmonella. Salmonella has been isolated from the blood and faeces of many reptile species. Exposure to this bacterium can cause an infection of the intestinal tract called 'salmonellosis', resulting in severe nausea, diarrhoea, fever and vomiting approximately 12 to 48 hours after exposure. Although most often contracted through ingesting contaminated foods of animal origin [e.g. meat, eggs, etc.], salmonella may also be passed on by handling animals carrying the bacteria. Outbreaks of salmonellosis have been linked to the presence of geckos and other lizards in homes and public water supplies. Compared to other lizards, geckos appear to pose a greater threat to human health. They are usually prevalent within the urban environment, congregating in large numbers in homes and other buildings. Moreover, their climbing skill gives them access to any surface, so that they through faecal deposition can contaminate food and water storage areas that other reptiles are incapable of reaching.

## Lizards & Lyme Disease

In parts of Asia, Europe, Africa, and the southern and western United States, lizards are frequently parasitised by species of Ixodes, a genus of ticks often infested by the Lyme disease spirochete Borrelia burgdorferi.

Studies indicate that lizards may act as barriers to the acquisition, maintenance, and/or transmission of B. burgdorferi, which has been suggested as a contributing factor to low Lyme disease prevalence in the western United States and Europe. Such barriers have been documented for the western fence lizard [Sceloporus occidentalis] and the southern alligator lizard [Elgaria multicarinata], and are likely to exist in the sand lizard [Lacerta agilis] and common wall lizard [Podarcis muralis] of Europe.

*See* Materia Medica Sceloporus occidentalis below.


## LIZARD SAYINGS & PROVERBS

- Whom a serpent has bitten a lizard alarms. [Africa]
- Better be the head of a lizard than the tail of a dragon. [Italy]
- The lizard that jumped from the high iroko tree said he would praise himself if no one else did. [Nigeria]
- The smaller the lizard the greater the hope of becoming a crocodile. [Africa]
- He who is bitten by a snake fears a lizard. [Uganda]
- A lizard that fell from the top of a tree wastes its time looking back to where it fell from; if there was anything good the lizard deserved, it could not have missed it while it was there on top of the tree. [Nigeria]
- It is difficult to throw a stone at a lizard that is clinging to a pot. [Ashanti]
- If the lizard were good to eat, it would not be so common. [Haiti]
- The lizard says that he knows the condition of his underbelly. The reason he has it pressed against the ground. [Igbo]
- The lizard would like to stand erect, but his tail will not permit him. [Igbo]
- A grasshopper that sleeps about will be soon awake in a lizard's mouth. [Africa]
- A lizard can't be a snake even without its limbs. [Africa]
- A lizard longs to sit down but its tail doesn't let it. [Africa]
- He who brings firewood infected with maggots in his house should not complain when lizards start visiting him. [Africa]
- In the absence of water lizards can claim to be crocodiles. [Africa]
- No matter how much you feed a lizard it cannot become a crocodile. [Africa]
- A lounging lizard catches no crickets. [Nigeria]
- I am the Lizard king. I can do anything. [Jim Morrison]

- Precisely the least, the softest, lightest, a lizard's rustling, a breath, a flash, a moment – a little makes the way of the best happiness. [Nietzsche]
- The long days seduce all thought away, and we lie like the lizards in the sun, postponing our lives indefinitely. [Elizabeth Smart]
- I suspect that the principal function of human reason is to rationalize what your lizard brain demands of you. [Dave Hickey]
- When you are in a creative or appreciative zone, you literally have no access to your inner lizard, to that fear-based, non-creative, shrieking little beasty who's so afraid you're going to be a bag lady. [Martha Beck]

## LIZARDS IN THE MATERIA MEDICA

In sharp contrast to the division Snakes of the reptilian materia medica, which is well-developed and adequately trustworthy, the section lizards is sadly deficient at best and badly defective at worst.

That Heloderma horridum and Heloderma suspectum are mixed up frequently in the literature is rather understandable, given their close overall similarity. It is quite another matter with the lizards lumped together under the catch-all name *Lacerta*.

Allen is the main authority on Lacerta, faithfully reproduced by Clarke. In Allen's Encyclopedia, Vol. 5 p. 432 and Vol. 10 p. 570, 3 sources are given for the symptoms listed under Lacerta:

1 an anonymous, unspecified reference to Stapf's Archiv für die homöopathische Heilkunst, 1834;
2 ingestion of 4 lizards, cut into pieces, over the course of one day by the Sicilian physician Filippo Baldini [not Baldelli as Clarke calls him], 1790s;
3 fatal bite in a 13-year old girl by a 'large green spotted lizard', in Georgetown, Maine, 1836.

Both Allen and Clarke give Lacerta agilis as the specific name of the lizard concerned and 'green lizard' as its common name. The large green spotted lizard, Clarke explains, 'is probably an American variety of *Lacerta*.'

Three things are wrong. Firstly, Lacerta agilis is neither green nor 'widely diffused throughout Europe', as Allen states, being absent from most of southern Europe. Secondly, Baldini used green lizards [most likely Lacerta *viridis*] for his self-experimentation and for the treatment of patients. Thirdly, Lacerta is a group of lizards restricted to the Old World and unknown in North America.

The culprit of the fatal case in Maine remains a mystery. The uppermost northeastern state of the U.S., Maine harbours no venomous reptiles, let alone green ones, with the exception of Crotalus horridus, the timber rattlesnake. The latter, apart from not being green, is unlikely to be mistaken for a lizard. Both the green iguana and the snapping turtle can deliver a nasty bite, but the former does not live in Maine and the latter is neither green nor a lizard. However dubious the cause, the symptoms have been included with Lacerta agilis. Here is the case in full:

*Bitten by a lizard [?]*

'To the Editor of the Boston Medical and Surgical Journal.

'Dear Sir, As I have not opportunity to examine the classification of venomous reptiles of the United States, I have copied from my diary the following singular case of the bite of the large green spotted lizard, so called. The case involves a question for the naturalist, rather than the physician. It is therefore submitted to your decision, whether its publication in your Journal may not elicit some new light of a scientific, if not practical nature. As the symptoms are entirely abnormal, partially tinctured as they were with those of a tetanic character. I shall give them precisely as they were noted at the time and leave others to their own pathological inferences.

'On the 31st of Aug., 1836, I was called to a little girl, 13 years of age, the daughter of Capt. Joseph G. Rowe, of Georgetown, about 9 miles from my residence in Boothbay, Maine. Thirteen days previous to my visit, this little girl, as she was gathering an armful of sticks, felt something pricking severely the inside of the sole of the left foot. On looking down she discovered a large, green spotted lizard fastened to her naked foot, which she extracted with a fold of her gown and with it that portion of skin on which it had seized. The next day she complained of numbness in the foot, as though it had been deprived of sensation by cording the ankle and that occasional "prickling" that occurs on the return of circulation.

'The numbness continued extending upward – the whole limb became severely swollen, and the most excruciating pain on the slightest motion followed; and over the direction of the lymphatics, I observed the inflammatory blush. The muscles of the neck and jaw of that side were rigid and tender to the touch; much difficulty of swallowing; occasional delirium, particularly the first week, and a wonderfully increased mental acumen during her intervals of reason. The whole left side continued paralysed and the pain unabated. A short time before death, the limb became spotted. She lingered along in great agony until the 21st day of the bite, when death terminated her sufferings.

'Owing to my distance from the patient, I had not opportunity for an autopsy, or to examine whether a filament of the internal plantar nerve might not have been wounded; but there were so many symptoms of the introduction of a morbid septic poison into the system that I carefully recorded them at the time, more particularly as these symptoms, it is well known, bear a close analogy to tetanus. I have excluded the treatment in this case; 1st, owing to the time that elapsed previous to my visit; 2d, because the sole object of this communication is to ascertain, through your Journal, whether the lizard tribe are venomous [which has been doubted], and whether in tetanus, the paralysis, great tumefaction, and spotted livid appearance, before, and gangrenous, after death, are symptoms that ever occur.

Yours, with much respect,
Boothbay, Me., Dec. 28, 1839. Sidney B. Cushman.'

| Homeopathic name | Common name | Abbreviation | Symptoms |
|---|---|---|---|
| Anguis fragilis | Slow-worm | Anguis-fr. | + |
| Askalabotes laevis[1] | Smooth gecko | Ask. | – |
| Basiliscus basiliscus | Common basilisk | Basl-bs. | – |
| Basiliscus vittatus | Brown basilisk | Basl-vt. | – |
| Chamaeleo chamaeleon | Common chameleon | Chamel-ch. | – |
| Chamaeleo dilepis | Flap-necked chameleon | Chamel-dil. | ++ |
| Chamaeleo zeylanicus | Indian chameleon | Chamel-zl. | – |
| Chlamydosaurus kingii | Frill-necked lizard | Chlams-k. | – |
| Elgaria coerulea | Northern alligator lizard | Elga-c. | – |
| Elgaria kingii | Madrean alligator lizard | Elga-k. | – |
| Furcifer oustaleti | Giant Madagascar chameleon | Furc-ou. | + |
| Heloderma horridum | Mexican beaded lizard | Helo-h. | + |
| Heloderma suspectum | Gila monster | Helo-s. | +++ |
| Hemidactylus sp. | House lizard [gecko] | Hemid-fl. | – |
| Iguana iguana | Green iguana | Igu-ig. | – |
| Lacerta agilis | Sand lizard | Lacer. | + |
| Lacerta muralis | Common wall lizard | Lacer-mr. | – |
| Lacerta vivipara | Viviparous lizard | Lacer-viv. | – |
| Pogona vitticeps | Central bearded dragon | Pogon-v. | – |
| Sceloporus occidentalis | Western fence lizard | Scelop-oc. | – |
| Varanus komodoensis | Komodo dragon | Varan-ko. | – |

1  During his residence in Suriname, South America, in the early 1830s, Hering proposed the use of a lizard believed to be venomous by the local population. He gave it the name Askalabotes laevis, sometimes spelled Askalabotes laevigatus, mixing some of the then current scientific names – Ascalabotes surinamensis, Gecko laevis, Thecadactylus laevis – for a lizard now known as Thecadactylus rapicauda, the smooth or turnip-tailed gecko. A large nocturnal lizard, often found clinging to walls [both indoors and outdoors] or tree trunks, the smooth gecko is mistakenly held to be venomous throughout much of its native range [Central America, Caribbean, Amazon]; like other geckos, they were assumed to climb on a person's body and inject venom with their webbed feet. Smooth geckos in addition are in the habit of resting under some object or inside a crevice in a coiled position possibly mimicking [and looking quite like] a small viper. It would seem that Hering accepted the supposedly venomous nature of this harmless gecko as true. Although he enters it in his *Analytical Repertory of the Symptoms of the Mind,* as Askalabotes laevis, abbreviation Askal. [Ask. in modern repertories], marking it as 'somewhat proved', no symptoms of it could be found.

## Lizard Family – a Concept

There is a distinct connection between the Lizard family and Strontium and the entire 5th row of the periodic table. Strontium's dreams of lizards point the way to that connection. Rajan Sankaran's Strontium carb. proving revealed the issues of dependence and independence, lack of self-confidence, a strong need for help, guidance, support and direction. Yet also there is the polarity of resisting and resenting help that is offered and willfully wanting to do things for himself. All of these issues and themes are basic to the Lizard family too, with the general animal features blended in.

All Lizards feel weak, helpless and dependent, without their own mind, necessitating reliance on others for help and guidance. Some of the words used are insecure, dumb, average, stupid, nothing special, unattractive with many flaws, having no talents or creative abilities, fragile with a fear of being judged and criticised. Inability to concentrate or think properly, confusion, all of which resulting in inability to make one's own decisions. Additionally, the animal issues of attractiveness come out as the feelings of being ugly, disfigured and disgusting and are related to the need to attract guidance.

All animals experience the world as a hazardous place, where they must compete for survival. The world is full of evil demons, snakes, accidents and competitive, selfish people, who just want to win and get more than you. In such a world he will be targeted, beaten up, picked on, hunted, raped, and killed. He feels others will specifically go after him by plotting how to hit his most painful spot.

What differentiates Lizards from other animals is their survival strategy. For safety, stability and security Lizards rely on guidance, help, support from those around them such as their family, social group or other close-knit group. They take care of them, provide a shoulder to lean on and are generally the backbone to keep them standing upright and strong. In this competitive world, he needs a place where there is no hierarchy, everyone is the same, and where there is emotional support, confidence, respect, honesty, reliability, common interests and values. In times of need, he will have someone to hold his hand and guide his every step, to show him the basics giving him the clues and discipline he needs so he can figure out things. He needs someone to tell him exactly what to do and he can rely on their support to make decisions. He can be confident and carefree when there is someone older and experienced to depend on and help with decisions.

In the midst of this dependence, Lizard wants attention to feel important, special, loved, respected and independent. He wants to be acknowledged as a special case as if he is a celebrity or movie star, where he gets recognition and can be the centre of attention and get more attention than anyone else. For the Lizard family, attractiveness also has to do with the need to attract guidance as well as feeling independent. He becomes preoccupied with appearance and wants to be lean, clean, strong, beautiful and alluring. Being attractive, he will draw more attention to himself and therefore feel confidence, strong and independent.

On the other hand, being attractive means that others will lust after him and then he will get extra advantages, favours, benefits, help and guidance. When he accepts these perks, he feels dependent and therefore must do exactly what they want him to do. He has the upper hand, all the power and control. Everything is dictated by that person and he will make all the decisions. Beliefs are imposed by those who are opinionated, close-minded and think they are always right. He cannot be himself. He is trapped, becoming the slave of a domineering person who is abusive. A nurturer becomes an abuser. Yet if he doesn't follow the guidance, he will lose the support for survival.

He feels forced, controlled, suffocated, trapped, attacked, encompassed. As a result he feels dirty, unworthy, ashamed, filthy, and disgustingly helpless, weak, restricted with no way out. He wants to stand up to their power by going against their wishes, fighting back. He wants to retaliate, have revenge in a vindictive and spiteful way. 'You did it to me and I will do it to you.' He hopes they feel the same pain or worse, so they feel all the pain and suffering that he had to endure.

Additionally, he feels ugly and unattractive, scarred, disfigured as if he lost an arm. By losing his attractiveness and appeal, those he trusted for guidance will betray him, cheat him and leave him. He will lose his survival advantages, favours and help. He will be all alone, left to fend for himself in dangerous situations. That also makes him resentful and bitter, ready to seek revenge. He will target and plot to make those who betrayed him pay by making them suffer in any way possible.

For whatever reason, once he would retaliate, he would be kicked out and be completely separated from the group, disowned, disgraced, rejected, becoming an outcast, as if he was not from the same lineage. He would have the freedom to think on his own, make his own decisions and not have beliefs imposed; however, he is weak and confused, being unable to think straight. He can't think or make decisions. He needs the group and their guidance and support for his very survival. Therefore, he wants to take revenge and retaliate but he can't because he is far too vulnerable and helpless. [Divya Chhabra]

*Chameleon*
The outstanding characteristics of Chameleon patients are the same as the animal; the ability to change its colours to blend into the background. The particular way Chameleon expresses the Lizard themes of seeking guidance is to change himself to be accepted, please others, conform and to fit in the close-knit group from which he gets support, guidance and help. He puts up a façade, is not genuine, not himself. He is a fake. He will not show his real feelings or express his real thoughts and is constantly on guard never to reveal anything about his real self. He becomes like a cookie-cutter, being the same, looking the same way with the same interests and the same ideas. This is all essential because even in one's own family, people are selfish and only work for their own satisfaction through ulterior motives, evil intentions, and deceptions. People can't be trusted; they hide things about themselves. They always have something planned in the back of their mind. If one's true colours showed, he would be rejected out from the group. Alone, he would not be able to survive.

## LIZARD THEMES

*According to Divya Chhabra [India]:*

1 Importance. Attention. Appreciation. To be liked. Best. Win. Ambitious. Independent.
Wants attention, importance, to be the best [like other competitive animals].
2 Love for excess money, fame. Worldly possessions. Selfish. Greed, unsatisfied, wanting more. Playful, jovial, fun loving. Travel.
3 Feels weak, helpless, dependent & needs family for guidance.
4 Issues with right and wrong. Duty and responsibility. Fairness, honesty and trust.
5 Feels wronged, harmed, hurt, mistreated, cheated, taken advantage of by the very people they are dependent upon.
6 Feels neglected, left out, excluded.
7 Wants to retaliate, speak out, take revenge [snakes, reptiles] but can't for fear of bad opinion of others, non-acceptance & being left alone without support.
8 Feels split between desire to retaliate & guilt & fear of losing support if they do.
9 Not expressing [keeping quiet] & lack of independence makes them feel locked up, curbed, closed in like a caged animal & they long for freedom & independence ['doing things my way'; 'doing whatever I want']. Social pleasures.

# ANGUIS FRAGILIS

### Systematics
- Scientific name: Anguis fragilis [L., 1758].
- Common names: Slow-worm. Blindworm.
- Family: Anguidae.

### Biological Profile
- Semi-fossorial [burrowing], cool-temperate, legless lizard, 30–50 cm long, smooth-skinned with shiny [glassy], non-overlapping scales. Males vary in colour from grey to light brown or bronze with a pale belly and may have blue spots dorsally. Females typically browner than males and have darker brown flanks, a dark belly and a thin dark stripe running along the back.
- Head small, elongated, somewhat angular and conical. Mouth of almost equal length with head. Eyes lateral, oval, distinct, though not prominent. Neck short, at times observably smaller than head.
- Body, from the neck, gradually swells to the middle, then gradually declines in thickness to the cloaca, and from thence becomes smaller and smaller to the extremity of the tail, which ends a little short of a minute point.
- Range: NW Asia and most of Europe; absent from far north, Ireland and southern Spain.

- Habitat: Humid environments, incl. grassy meadows, gardens, farmland, woodland margins and open fields, where their main prey – slugs, snails, spiders, insects and worms – can be found.
- Highly elusive, usually remaining unnoticed, spending much of its time hiding beneath rocks, logs, sheet metal, or in self-made burrows.
- Mostly active during twilight or after rainfall.
- *Low body temperature* [means range from 22.1 to 26.4°C – 71.8–79.5°F], compared with many other lizards.
- Hibernates from October to February/March under piles of leaves, within tree roots and in crevices of banks.
- Hibernates both communally and solitarily. Sometimes shares hibernating sites with other reptiles. May burrow in soft substrates so that just its head is visible.
- Ovoviviparous; 6–12 live young per brood.
- Males will fight each other for possession of females.
- Females may pair with several males throughout breeding season.
- Sheds tail readily.
- Individuals of both sexes are often *scarred*: females, because they get gripped around the head and neck by males during mating, and males, because they bite one another vigorously when fighting.
- Specific name refers to the *extreme fragility* of the tail, which is shed readily and from the slightest cause.
- Slow-worms *stiffen their body when touched or handled*, which gives the impression that the tail breaks or snaps off. Formerly it was believed that this lizard *would break in several pieces*.

## Behaviour & Temperament

'As far as the character of the slow-worm is concerned it may challenge comparison with almost any animal and is certainly more docile than most other reptiles. Though extremely timid at first, it rapidly becomes familiar with its owner and will feed from the hand after a short time in the vivarium.

'But – and this is a point that many observers appear to have overlooked – slow-worms have their individual idiosyncrasies like other creatures, and some of them will exhibit a great tendency to bite. Even when they do, the small size of the teeth renders the bite perfectly harmless, the only result being a series of small depressions on the skin showing the marks of the teeth. This exhibition of temper is generally seen in old females before the young are born, and I have had several such in my cages that would attempt to bite on every opportunity.

'The great majority, however, never attempt any such thing so long as they are handled carefully, being *quiet and docile* to a degree. They are extremely clean and take to life in a vivarium well, and therefore make most interesting pets. One cannot help being struck with their patience and curiosity. Time after time will they raise themselves up on to the tail to examine the side of the cage, until they may be said to stand on the tip of that organ, or very nearly so. In fact, the total sum of the characteristics of the slow-worm, or blind-worm, forms an entire negation of those implied by the popular names, since the creature is neither slow, blind, deaf, nor a worm.' [Leighton, 1903]

## Slugging Slugs

'Slow-worms will eat worms in captivity, and insects, and possibly many other invertebrate creatures, but the result of much watching of them in nature has been to convince me that their one aim in life as far as food is concerned is to find good fat slugs, not too large. The number of these that a slow-worm will eat during an hour or so about sunset, when they feed most, is simply astonishing. I can vouch for a meal that consisted of 17 slugs, the slow-worm being a large male 16 inches long. But the usual number taken seems to be from 4 to 10. Doubtless they feed during the night also, but not during the heat of the sun. In other words, when the slugs emerge from beneath stones and debris, then comes the slow-worm also.

'Very interesting to watch is the slow-worm feeding. The whole process is carried out very *methodically and deliberately*, and with evident satisfaction. The slug is seldom taken except when moving, and, as far as I have seen, never when dead. The slow-worm either gradually approaches or allows the slug to approach until the latter is within reaching distance, then poises its head in a delicate curve over the body of the slug and with a quick movement – the only sign of haste in the whole business – seizes the mollusk by the middle. There is then a momentary pause as if to make sure that the grip is satisfactory, during which the reptile remains motionless while the slug exudes frothy bubbles. A sudden wide gape of the jaws and mouth – as far as the fixed jaws allow of distension – and the slug disappears head-first down the throat of the slow-worm, as if it were the direction of least resistance. Then follows much gaping and licking of jaws on the part of the slow-worm, and should another slug come into range the process is immediately repeated. The slug never takes the slightest notice of the slow-worm until it is seized, indeed they will frequently crawl all over the creature that a few minutes later feeds upon them. I have found that the larger slugs are refused and so also are the brightly coloured ones; probably the latter are flavoured in a manner disagreeable to the slow-worm.

'Slow-worms should never be allowed to be short of water. They drink frequently and some are very fond of lying in a shallow bath, while others do not seem to care about it. They will also take milk.' [Leighton, 1903]

## Meet the Slow-worm

'First let us briefly review her many wrong names, "blind-worm," "slow-worm," "deaf-adder," "brittle-snake," and endeavour to account for them. Of her name "snake" [Anguis], from its external aspect, enough has already been said. The "brittleness" shared in common with several of her foreign relatives, known as "glass snakes," proceeds from a power of *contracting the muscles into rigidity when molested*: that is, when, on finding themselves in a helpless condition, slow-worms grasp firmly whatever they can attach themselves to.

'In fact, this little lizard only displays constricting powers as far as it is able; for it really does constrict the fingers that detain it, with a force as great for its size as its cousin Anaconda uses in killing its prey. Were the giant constrictors to entwine us with proportionate power, they would gain the day. In the case of Anguis fragilis, we are the masters; and were we to attempt violently to unwind one from our fingers, it would break 'in halves' in its resistance, or rather in its redoubled efforts to cling the tighter and so save itself.

'In handling the little reptile, you will feel it pressing the tip of its tail against whatever part comes in contact with it, as a hold, a fulcrum, and motive power. Upon a smooth surface it would be entirely helpless without this assistant to progression, its scales being too even and polished to afford hold of any kind. You will see it sweeping its long tail this way and that, in search of some hold or obstacle against which to push itself forward; and failing this, the point is pressed close to the table or floor as may be. When in any unaccustomed position, as, for instance, when held in the hand, you will see the tail instantly twining itself about the fingers for safety, the creature trusting itself entirely to its aid and *being helpless when its movements are fettered* in any way.

'Seeing her so wonderfully energetic and by no means "slow," either in action or intelligence, the next thing was to ascertain whether Lizzie was "deaf" in addition to her other pseudo-failings; but by the various tests used to exercise her aural faculties, I am inclined to think her powers of hearing served her almost better than those of sight. When permitted to ramble among the plants and over the table, the sound much more than the sight of her box and its contents attracted her. Never averse to go home and retreat into her moss, the rustling of this or the scraping and rubbing the sides of the box – any noise with it with which she was familiar, would cause her to turn towards it, when the sight of it alone failed to entice her.

'After a time she turned her head, if even from across the room I made a sudden and sharp noise to attract her attention, such as the tapping of a spoon against a cup, or the peculiar talk I indulged in for educational purposes. She undoubtedly became familiar with certain sounds, which were repeated till she did look round. Not – as I am bound to confess – that it was a strikingly intelligent look! rather the contrary, I fear: still, as the object was to test her powers of hearing, the result was satisfactory. The origin of this reputed deafness is difficult to conjecture. In the way of external ears, those of the slow-worm are less distinct than those of lizards generally, but more so than in snakes, which have no visible aural apertures; whereas in the slow-worms they can be discerned if sought for, though they are very small and indistinct.

'Of the 6 or 7 that have been in my keeping at one time or another, not one has, under any provocation, attempted to bite me. They were handled continually, twirled about and tied into knots [with gentle treatment, of course], but not one of them ever broke itself in "halves" or opened its mouth with malice intent. Lizzie sometimes in winding about my fingers got herself into very pretty knots, and in such tied-up fashion when placed on the table she would remain motionless for a time and then begin to move away. Curious was the effect at this juncture. The knot was not loosened at all; but as the little reptile began to move, the knot passed downwards and she crawled out of it, while its form remained the same to the very end of the tail.

'Its quality of "slowness" is only another name for caution. Quick and active it can be; but in retreating down among the moss or hay, or whatever you provide in its cage, then you see the *perfection of slowness*. Not a blade stirs, not a sound is heard, and one may repeat here that the manner of progression in Anguis fragilis is not the least of all the ophidian wonders we have witnessed. In the earth it can burrow itself to the depth of several feet. In soft rubbish it simply vanishes slowly; its hard, polished scales permitting it, as it were, to slide down into and among the hay with that gently gliding motion that enables us to perceive how very well it does manage without the ancestral limbs. . . .

'Imagine that poor little shred of life passing the night in frantic efforts to burrow into the carpet and retire below according to custom! Whenever held or touched, their first impulse was to conceal themselves beneath, and they would dive and butt with impetuous agitation in their endeavours to *push themselves out of sight.*' [Hopley, 1882]

## MATERIA MEDICA ANGUIS FRAGILIS

### Sources
1 Clinical observations Karl-Josef Müller [Germany]; in: Wismut Materia Medica Müller 2.0, 2009.

### Symptoms
∞ Fear of going blind.
∞ Fear of losing limb[s]; obsessed with amputation, guilt feelings.
∞ Fear of snakes and other reptiles.
∞ Colour blindness for red and green.
∞ Loss of orientation in dark; eyes as if closed up.
∞ Insomnia, awake 'whole nights'.
∞ Use of words related to 'cutting off'. Dreams of cutting hair.
∞ Cold sensitive; coldness begins in hands.
∞ Coldness through and through [cf. *Heloderma*].
∞ Sluggish in morning, can't hurry.
∞ Backache as if broken [*fragilis*, fragile].

# BASILISCUS BASILISCUS

### Systematics
• Scientific name: Basiliscus basiliscus [L., 1758].
• Synonyms: Lacerta basiliscus [L., 1758]. Basiliscus americanus [Laurenti, 1768]. Iguana basiliscus [Latreille, 1802]. Thysanodactylus bilineatus [Gray, 1845].
• Common names: Common basilisk. Jesus Christ lizard
• Family: Corytophanidae.

### Biological Profile
• Large lizard whose tail generally comprises 70–75% of total body length; total length to 80 cm. Generally brown or olive in colour but can range from bright

green to olive-brown and bronze. Dark cross bands and cream to yellow lip and lateral stripes. Males larger than females.
- Has long digits with sharp claws for climbing.
- Males have sail-like crests supported by elongate neural spines incl. a rounded or pointed head, dorsal and caudal crest.
- Tail can be used as a whip when threatened.
- Extremely swift and agile.
- Range: SE Nicaragua, Costa Rica, Panama, NW Ecuador, Colombia, Venezuela.
- Habitat: Lowland dry and moist forests, often adjacent to rivers and other waterways.
- Males display size-related hierarchal dominance in which larger males often attack smaller males and prevent them from breeding. Because of this, many male basilisks do not enter the breeding cycle until 3 or 4 years of age.
- Preys on arthropods, small lizards, snakes, birds, mammals, fishes, freshwater shrimps, and occasionally frogs; will also feed on flowers and fruits.
- Male courtship behaviour includes head-bobbing, which is typical of many iguanid lizards.
- Oviparous; 2–18 eggs per clutch. Female lays the eggs in a hole and covers them up. No parental care is given after that.
- Named after the Greek 'basiliskos', meaning small king, in reference to the expanded parietal blade symbolic of a crown.
- Two recognized subspecies [basiliscus and barbouri].

## Crossing the Water

The Jesus Christ lizard swims well and sometimes dives and hides in the water. Usually it runs away on its hind legs when disturbed, crossing water as readily as it crosses dry land. It manages to do this by trapping pockets of air beneath its long toes and fringes of skin, and using its long tail for balance. It may also launch itself directly from its perch onto the surface of the water and run. Juveniles are more apt to run across water than adults. Running instead of swimming minimizes the time of exposure to aquatic predators.

'Common basilisks are diurnal, spending most of their time foraging, basking, and resting along waterways. At night, they sleep in perches up to 20 m high. When disturbed or in the pursuit of prey, common basilisks will exhibit the behaviour that earned them the nickname "Jesus Christ Lizard". Using erect bipedal motion, basilisks are able to run across the surface of water. Smaller individuals are more adept at this sprinting and may reach 20 or more meters on the surface. Larger lizards may sink and resort to swimming [or even diving] after just a few meters. Large feet and flattened toe pads also aid common basilisks in this behaviour. The hind feet have large rolled-up scales that are pushed up when the lizard begins to cross the water. Male basilisks are territorial and will display head bobbing as a territorial threat.' [animaldiversity.org]

## Materia Medica
- No symptoms.

# BASILISCUS VITTATUS

## Systematics
- Scientific name: Basiliscus vittatus [Wiegmann, 1828].
- Synonyms: Corythaeolus vittatus [Kaup, 1828]. Oedicoryphus vittatus [Wagler, 1830]. Cristasaurus mitrella [Gray, 1852].
- Common names: Striped basilisk. Brown basilisk.
- Family: Corytophanidae.

## Biological Profile
- Smallest of the 4 Basiliscus species, with average length of 16–20 inch [41–51 cm]. Males larger than females. Males have a very large crest on back of head.
- Displays a checkerboard body pattern of black, white and brown, along with yellow and black stripes that extend from just behind the eye all the way down both sides to the vent.
- Tail can be used as a whip when threatened.
- Range: From central Mexico south to northern Colombia. Widely distributed throughout southern Florida after an initial introduction to Miami-Dade County in 1976.
- Habitat: Near inland streams in a variety of forests, lowland dry to wet rain-forest.
- Excellent swimmer and climber; able to run on water.
- Diurnal. Commonly seen basking on sunny, hot rocks.
- Sleeps until daybreak in suspended vine thickets, on twigs or branches over-hanging rivers, within thick underbrush, in palm fronds, etc.
- Very territorial; small home range up to 20 square meters [215 square foot].
- Swift, agile runner relying on lightning fast bursts of speed to attack and surprise its prey.
- Preys on flying insects, grasshoppers, scorpions, freshwater shrimp, and small lizards or snakes; will eat fruit.
- Oviparous; 2–12 eggs per clutch. Female lays the eggs in a hole and covers them up. No parental care is given after that.
- Named after Latin 'vittatus' for ribbon, or decorated by a ribbon, referring to the parietal blade of male vittatus, which is shaped like a thin ribbon.

## Stressed into Submission
'The average time that it takes for a striped basilisk to sexually mature can be as early as 10 months of age and as late as 15 months. While they are sexually mature at a young age, they normally are still not at adult size yet. Males of this species develop more slowly than the females. It's important to note that females of both striped and green basilisks are incredibly food aggressive. This means that if you are housing multiple young females together with one young male, he will develop slowly and may even get stressed into submission by the females. To prevent this, I recommend housing juvenile basilisks separately so that the

males may grow at a healthy pace and become established before introducing them to the females. This is esp. recommended when working with B. vittatus, because *striped basilisk males are incredibly submissive* and will prefer to hide than compete with females for food.' [Chermel, 2018]

## Materia Medica
• No symptoms.

# CHAMAELEO CHAMAELEON

## Systematics
• Scientific name: Chamaeleo chamaeleon [L., 1758].
• Synonyms: Lacerta chamaeleon [L., 1758]. Chamaeleon vulgaris [Daudin, 1802].
• Common names: Common chameleon. Mediterranean chameleon.
• Family: Chamaeleonidae.

## Biological Profile
• Slow moving, arboreal lizard, greenish or brown with paler markings, with disproportionately large, helmet-like head, high thin body and dorsal crest. Yes independently movable, stereoscopic. Long, rapidly extrudable tongue. Prehensile tail and special leg adaptations for grasping vegetation. Able to change skin colouration.
• Like other chameleon species exhibits a distinct locomotion in which they *slowly* rock back and forth between each step taken.
• Range: S Europe, N Africa, W Asia to Indian Subcontinent.
• Habitat: Semi-desert scrubland, coastal scrubland, crop plantations, forested areas up to 2600 m elevations.
• Solitary, territorial, aggressive.
• Intolerant of cohabitation and disturbance.
• Field experiments show that juveniles actively avoid the presence of adults by concealment or flight. Adults readily attack and consume juveniles, regardless of their own mass.
• Preys on insects, young birds, small reptiles.
• Oviparous; up to 60 eggs per clutch.
• The common English name 'chameleon' comes from Greeks words meaning 'on the ground', also 'dwarf', and 'lion'; chameleons are therefore 'ground-lions' or 'dwarf-lions'.
• Four recognized subspecies [chamaeleon, musae, orientalis, recticrista].

## Slow to Flee
Some lizards are swift and lithe, others are *slow and deliberate*. Chameleons belong to the *slowest extreme* of the latter category. In her book on snake-catcher Ionides and his African assistant Rashidi, Margaret Lane recounts the capturing of a giant chameleon in Tanzania.

'Few Africans will touch these harmless creatures. We would often be sitting indoors in the afternoon, snake-catching over for the day, when word would come that someone had spotted a chameleon, and we would walk out with military speed to some nearby tree to find the reptile calm and contemplative above us. Their appearance alone is responsible for their evil reputation, for they move with a dreamlike slowness and have no defence but a hard and toothless bite.

'Once disturbed they will begin a stately climb to a safer position, opening their mouths in a roaring hiss and swiveling their strange eyes backward towards the pursuer. It was touching to see the confident lack of haste with which they went up hand over hand, coiling their tail at each step at the bending branch as Ionides carefully pulled it within reach. He taught me the way to take them, in a firm grip along the ridge of the back, using both hands and snatching the animal off the branch by surprise.

'They *go flat at once*, like an empty pouch, all the breath knocked out of them, and twist, slowly as ever, reaching for one's wrists with corkscrew tail and with leathery palms wide open. Their claws are sharp and long and *their grip powerful*; it is unwise to let them get a hold, for they can break the skin, and Rashidi's technique, which never fails to deceive, is to grasp the 2 hind feet and give them to each other, when they clasp together in a slow-motion handshake and give no further trouble.

'Their reactions are so slow that it is a miracle they have not been extermi-nated, esp. among people like the Makua tribe, who will eat anything; only the spell of their appearance saves them, the *magical stare*, the fluted pie-crust frill along the back, the *menacing lack of haste* with which they place one careful hand before the other, opening their pointed mouths in a breathy roar. Their rage on finding themselves captured was slow to manifest, but very serious; they would gradually change their tint from bright to dark, turning an angry slate-colour as they twanged the wires of their cage, for days refusing our offerings of cock-roaches.' [Lane, 1963]

## Quick to Anger

'The "reptilian vicar of Bray," as the late Mr. Grant Allen termed this lizard, has got an unjust reputation for capacity of colour change, mainly due to a well-known ballad, where these changes lead to misunderstanding on the part of some who have not been present to witness the whole series.

'As a matter of fact the chameleon does change its colour, and incidentally and at the same time, unlike the leopard, its spots. But these changes are not precisely what they are in popular imagination, which will accordingly be disappointed when the chameleons at the Zoo can begot to "perform." Popular imagination in this, as in other matters, has raced well ahead of the facts and has assigned to the chameleon the entire chromatic scale. Its actual performance falls far short of this, and is limited to greens, yellows, browns, greys and almost blacks. Some colours are beyond their powers. Nor can they entirely blanch or blacken.

'The faculty of colour change, though characteristic enough of these singular lizards, is by no means confined to them; it is a common attribute of many lizards, some of which even excel the chameleon in their variety and rapidity of change. The chameleon, however, is a fairly quick-change artist. Apparently, rage is the most potent factor in inducing alterations and a chameleon, when pinched gently, becomes spotty with wrath. Sunshine blackens them and death leaves them black or pale straw colour. In fact, anger, heat, cold and death would seem to be the main factors in turning their coats.

'That chameleons are lizards is probably known to most, but in almost every feature they differ from the more typical and nimbler, scaled, creatures that are called by that name. To watch a chameleon in the Reptile House side by side with a lacerta for example, will bring out so long a series of differences that it seems almost necessary to establish another order for these divergent creatures. Their prehensile tail is unique among limbed reptiles and its very prehensility is remarkable, for it only works downwards: the toes are bound together in 3s and 2s, 3 on one side of hand and foot, and 2 on the other. This is suggestive of a bird, and esp. of the woodpeckers, where, however, there are but 4 toes altogether, grouped in 2s.

'The independently moving eyes above the grinning mouth are weird in the extreme and not reptile-like; they are indeed like nothing except a human being with an inordinate squint and like the eyes of such a being they move independently. Then too the tongue, nearly as long as the body of its possessor when fully extruded, is an extraordinary organ, unparalleled in the reptilian series and only partially paralleled by the ant-bear, the woodpecker and the echidna.

'The chameleon when it detects its prey, an insect for choice, literally "gives tongue" to the extent of 6 inches or so. To watch a chameleon shows that profound mental differences accompany these structural differences from the remaining crowd of lizards. Its movements are characterised by an almost *judicial deliberation*. It is *elephantine in its slowness*. The reptile is in fact not by any means unlike in these particulars to its fellow-dweller upon tree-tops – the American sloth. Finally, the lean and really emaciated form of the chameleon mark it out as something greatly different from the ordinary run of lizards, who are plump in comparison. This leanness, however, has its uses.

'The chameleon has, somewhat rashly for so small a creature, an *ungovernable temper*; it literally *swells with anger*, grunts, bites and flashes changes of colour. If all this fails and the enemy is not to be daunted by bluff, the chameleon relies upon its scragginess in this way. Its lean sides, like those of a tiger, can by contraction of the muscles lying between the ribs become still more attenuated. This accomplished, the chameleon prudently, but in another sense to the usual one, turns its back upon its foe and remains perfectly quiet. The leanness reduces its dimensions to those of a straight line, which has no breadth, and seen in profile, the chameleon escapes unwelcome attention.' [Beddard, 1905]

### Prone to Quarrel

Although male chameleons display mate-guarding, long-term interactions do not occur; the male abandons the female when she is no longer receptive, demonstrating that their relationship is transient rather than long-term.

Like most other species of chameleon, common chameleons generally are *intolerant and aggressive towards each other*. Males of the common chameleon engage in similar fighting as most other species of chameleon do. A typical chameleon confrontation goes like this:

'On first interaction, the body changes to a lighter colour, with blotches disappearing and spots intensifying; the gular region is expanded and the back arched, giving a general impression of increased size as males approach each other; the tail and body are lifted off the perch and the tail is moved around. As long as both chameleons assume the expanded display posture, the interaction escalates, with lunges being made at the throat and bites inflicted on the gular region until one of the lizards loses, possibly with serious injuries. If a male assumes a submissive posture, however, stretching his body out longitudinally, the winning chameleon ceases to attack.' [Pianka & Vitt, 2006]

Richard Robert Madden [1798–1886] believed that the chameleon's green colour was connected to both its gall bladder and its fiery, irascible, choleric nature, bringing to mind such phrases as *stirring one's bile, rousing one's choler, and galling, all denoting the lizard's crankiness*. 'Dr. Madden, in whose observations we may place much reliance, states that he paid much attention to this animal when he was in Egypt. He says: "Of all the irascible little animals in the world, there are none so choleric as the chameleon. I trained 2 large ones to fight and could at any time, by knocking their tails against one another, ensure a combat, during which their change of colour was most conspicuous. This change is only effected by paroxysms of rage, when the dark green gall of the animal is transmitted into blood and is visible enough under its pellucid skin. The gall, as it enters and leaves the circulation, affords the 3 various shades of green that are observable in its colour."' [Kitto, 1841]

## Mating

Males actively follow females closely as a typical mate guarding behaviour during the mating season. Guarding behaviour results in territorial behaviour, with 'stable' as well as 'mobile' territories. In 'stable' territories, males defended non-overlapping areas where the home range of one female or more was included. Intrusion by a solitary intruder in stable territories evokes aggression and chasing by the male guarding the territory and the female. A female may accept or reject the courting male. If she rejects him, she might run away or she might face the male and hiss at him with an open mouth. She might even attack and bite him. These bites can kill. Females that are not sexually receptive assume a spotted colouration and a more aggressive than usual attitude if approached by a male. The spots may be yellow on green or tan on grey-green.

## The Outcome of Proceeding Slowly

According to African traditions, human mortality is the result of the dim-witted chameleon's laziness and slowness. It was one of the first living creatures, appearing before the Earth had completely emerged from the primal waters. It had learned to walk in the mud by adopting its deliberate and apparently lazy gait. One day the Creator decided to inform mankind that when they died, they would live again, entrusting the chameleon to deliver the message. The chameleon went on his way, but lingered and dawdled, so that the Creator, annoyed with the delay, altered his mind and sent the lizard with another message that mankind would die. The swift lizard arrived ahead of the chameleon, announcing that man must die. By the time the chameleon arrived with his message, man had already accepted the lizard's message and that's why man distrusts the chameleon and despises the lizard.

## Seven Distinctive Attributes

'In the legends of the Kaydara, the chameleon is endowed with 7 qualities, as many symbols as are revealed to the initiate.

'1  It changes colour whenever it wishes. On the positive side this is to be sociable, tactful and able to engage in pleasant conversation with anybody and to adapt oneself to any circumstance and to any social environment. Negatively it is to be hypocritical, changeable, swayed by sordid interest and base intrigue. It is also to lack originality and individuality. It is to spend one's life in the anteroom courting the mighty.

'2  Coiled in its belly is a long, sticky tongue, which enables it to take its prey from a distance without having to pounce upon it. If it misses its prey, it simply retracts its tongue. This is carefully concealed greed, persuasive talk that deprives the hearer of all means of resisting its argument. It is the art of escaping from every dilemma, of deceiving with sweet talk, the ability to lie and wait patiently in ambush, the better to surprise one's victim.

'3  It steps carefully, one foot after the other, unhurriedly. The wise man is circumspect and never rushes headlong into anything. He balances its importance and its risks without a spark of generosity and without taking the slightest risk. He spies out the land and makes sure before advancing a step or venturing advice or making a decision.

'4  It does not need to turn round to see what lies about it. Slightly bending its head, it lets its eye revolve in its socket and sweep the horizon. It is the crafty watcher, impervious to external influence as it gathers in every scrap of information.

'5  Its body is slender-flanked, soft-skinned but lithe and dexterous.

'6  It has a spiny ridge along its back. In a positive sense, this may be taken as an assurance against any surprise; negatively, as empty vainglory.

'7  It has a prehensile tail. Hypocrite and coward, it steals others' goods behind their backs and without the least appearance of ill intent. This is a trap set to obtain an advantage in a manner that could not be foreseen.' [Chevalier & Gheerbrant, 1994]

## Blending In vs Standing Out

Changing colour constitutes undoubtedly the chameleon's best-known quality. This is universally interpreted as mastery of camouflage and disguise, a superior quality of blending in with one's surroundings so as to become invisible. However, camouflage is now known to be only half the story of the chameleon's outstanding peculiarity. The other half is about communication, *showing one's colours*, saying it with colour. New research indicates that some of the chameleon's colour changes evolved for the purpose of *attracting attention* instead of avoiding it. Rather than allowing them to fit in with more colourful surroundings, chameleons appear to have such a wide-ranging colour palette in order to produce more conspicuous social signals. Rather than changing colour to look like something they're not, chameleons actually *change colour to reveal their true feelings and inner stirrings*. Changes in colour, it has been observed, occur most rapidly and dramatically when chameleons are interacting with each other.

These modern findings substantiate the general concept of the lizard's dilemma of to be or not to be noticed, of which the chameleon is conceivably the optimum case in point. It has earned it a place in literature and language as the embodiment of blending in. For example, the Australian novelist Max Rittenberg depicted the 'chameleon mind' thus:

'Many men are chameleons. They take their mental colour from the surroundings of the moment. They are swayed by every fresh change of circumstance, influenced by every strong mind with whom they come in contact. If such a man goes on from year to year in the same groove of work, the chameleon mind may not be apparent on the surface; but if by any chance he is suddenly jolted from his accustomed groove, the mental instability becomes plain to read.' [Rittenberg, 1913]

The Urban Dictionary, a Web-based dictionary of slang words and phrases, presents 5 definitions of human chameleonism, termed social chameleon:

1 A person that has the ability to be social with anyone and any setting and still fit in.
2 Someone who changes the way they interact with people depending on who they're with.
3 One who has such wide interests they can relate to anyone.
4 A social behaviour exhibited by those who were or are shy. This usually stems from a sheltered upbringing or inferiority complex. He grew up away from others, so having no social skills of his own, he became bit of a social chameleon; learning what was right by observing those around him.
5 One who pretends to be your friend until the more popular people show up and then acts differently.

### Social Chameleons

'Everyone wants to make a good impression, but for some people it is almost a way of life. Such social chameleons, who in every situation strive to make the best impression they can, do so at a psychological cost, new research suggests.

'Those who always try "to be the right person in the right place at the right time," according to Mark Snyder, a social psychologist at the University of Minnesota, become extraordinarily attuned to the ways others react to them. They continually monitor their social performance, skillfully adjusting it when they detect that they are not having the desired effect. . . .

'Social chameleons, for whom Dr. Snyder uses the rather infelicitous term, "high self-monitors," display these key traits: They pay careful attention to social cues, scrutinizing others with keenness so as to know what is expected of them before making a response. In order to get along and to be liked, they try to be as others expect them to be. For example, they try to make people they dislike think they are friendly with them. They use their social abilities to mould their appearance as disparate situations demand, so that, as some put it, "With different people I act like a very different person."

'Those low on the self-monitor scale, would be unlikely to espouse ideas they do not believe, while those high in self-monitoring would do so if it were expedient. Certain professions, by their very nature, seem to draw people who are adept at impression management. "Professional actors, as well as many of the more mercurial trial lawyers, are among the best at it," Dr. Snyder said. "So too are many successful salespeople, diplomats and politicians."

'Such people can swing with ease from bubbly sociability to reserved withdrawal, or even from conformity to non-conformity, as the situation demands, Dr. Snyder said. And while these same abilities make them skilled at lying, they are just as likely to apply them in smoothing social interactions.' [Goleman, 1985]

### Chameleons in the Making

'To success-hungry people who work in challenging, rapidly changing, highly unpredictable environments where worry awaits and humiliation and betrayal stalk the unwary and insecure, the world seems dangerous and hostile, populated with predators who seek to pull them down. Losing is always a terrifying possibility. Feeling beleaguered, they fall victim to loneliness and a sense of helplessness. They believe themselves the prey of enemies out to abuse, cheat, and defeat them, and feeling endangered they can become disabled by anxiety. To prevent this calamity, some of them [even figuratively] take refuge in chameleonism.

'Human chameleons, like their reptilian counterparts, ward off danger by assuming a protective colouration whenever danger arises. Not willing to run away, not wanting to put up their fists [even figuratively], reluctant to give in, chameleons take cover. *Deception is their game.* They pretend to be what they are not. They spread smoke to hide their actions, skillfully arrange mirrors to confuse the enemy and don masks to conceal their true faces, hiding their real intentions and designs from envious competitors and implacable enemies.

'Although chameleonism begins as a deliberate attempt to fend off competitors and to guard self-esteem, in time and with practice it becomes automatic, a mostly unconscious way of ensuring personal safety. When it works properly, chameleonism helps win over needed clients and friends, and protects self-regard from the appraisals and actions of fierce rivals. With training it becomes a tool in the struggle for success, an invaluable aid in the struggle to keep from falling behind in a ferociously competitive world.

'In general, chameleons try to please whomever they are with – adversaries, neutrals, and friends alike – hoping in this way to blend inconspicuously in the group. . . . Another way of looking at chameleons is to think of them as salesmen whose principal item of sale is themselves.

'Chameleons are skilled at sensing changes in their environment and quickly adjust their behaviour to suit the expectations of others. Impression management is their forte. Seeking to blend safely into hazardous surroundings, they behave congenially, ingratiating themselves with superiors and doing as little as possible to arouse suspicion or attack. . . .

'Chameleonism is more than a habitual response to danger, more than the concealment of one's true identity. . . . It is a trait to which the individual can become strongly attached, one not easily abandoned . . . Moreover, chameleonism has several advantages. For example, chameleons can move easily in out of relationships as their situation requires, without emotional turmoil and regret. . . . Being a successful chameleon is not easy. It takes concentration and luck, because a chameleon's path is strewn with mines. One misstep and all is over. Chameleons are always at risk. They cannot afford to lower their guard, even for a second. . . . Chameleonism well done is difficult to discern. Even chameleons are often deceived by their own façades: they begin by fooling others and end up fooling themselves. . . . As Nietzsche wrote, "Whenever a man strives long and persistently to appear someone else, he ends up finding it difficult to be himself again." . . .

'On the positive side, chameleons possess qualities that commend them to other people. They are bright, often charming and resourceful, since they like to enjoy themselves, fun to be with. . . . Finally, chameleonism is riddled with contradictions. On the one hand, chameleons want to be inconspicuously embedded within their milieu; they seek to *mask their superiority under the pretense of ordinariness*. On the other, chameleons are convinced of their own personal superiority and want it publicly acknowledged. . . . In sum, chameleons are beset by contrieties, *torn by inner conflicts and pulled in opposite directions*. They treasure independence but want to blend into the group; they cultivate self-detachment but seek to convey an impression of genial collegiality; they present an inviting façade but at heart want to keep people at a distance; they pretend to be part of the group but are reluctant to establish enduring relationships with anyone. In fact, they want to go their own way. They view dependency as a weakness and avoid true intimacy as a trap.' [Rosen, 2001]

## Materia Medica
- No symptoms.

# CHAMAELEO DILEPIS

## Systematics
- Scientific name: Chamaeleo dilepis [Leach, 1819].
- Synonyms: Chamaeleo bilobus [Kuhl, 1820]. Chamaeleo planiceps [Merrem, 1820].

- Common name: Flap-necked chameleon.
- Family: Chamaeleonidae.

## Biological Profile

- Semi-arboreal chameleon with a flattened head with a low casque. Females up to 36 cm in length, larger than males. Males have a short, backward-pointing spur on hind legs.
- Occipital flaps protruding over neck, hence the common name, can be raised to deter predators or rivals.
- Basic colouration light green, brown and yellow with a light or dark stripe on flank extending from axillae to rear legs. A second, smaller and less pronounced stripe may extend from head to shoulder. Many small spots decorate body. Normally dark, these spots may take on a bright yellow or orange colour when sexually receptive, gravid or excited. Large brown or grey splotches may appear on body.
- Range: Central and southern Africa.
- Habitat: Savannah woodland, scrubby and forested habitats.
- Generally considered to be wanderers, esp. males, probably looking for prey and/or mates. Often seen on the ground, crossing roads.
- Preys on arthropods, esp. orthopterans [grasshoppers, crickets, locusts, katydids] and coleopterans [beetles].
- Oviparous; up to 60 eggs per clutch.
- Eggs are laid in a tunnel 15–30 cm deep, excavated in damp soil. After egg laying, females are emaciated and generally vulnerable to a wide variety of predators.
- Young are fully capable of foraging minutes after hatching.
- Eight recognized subspecies [dilepis, idjwiensis, isabellinus, martensi, petersii, quilensis, roperi, ruspolii] of which C. dilepis dilepis was used for the homeopathic proving.

## Bloating Allows Floating

'Another adaptive feature is that of its lungs, which have branches spreading through the body that allow the body to blow up to a large size on inflation. This happens when attacked, or when it lets go of a branch it can fall to the ground, bouncing without being hurt. The same thing happens rapidly if it falls into the water, allowing it to float or swim to the shore.' [Moore]

## Aggressive Displays

'When a chameleon is annoyed or attacked, it will turn a blotchy-black, blow itself up, dilate its throat, open its mouth displaying the red inside, hiss and suddenly lunge forward. This ferocious behaviour is more for show and is intended to frighten or surprise the attacker, thus giving the chameleon a chance to take cover in the nearest vegetation.

'*Chamaeleo dilepis dilepis* are considered to be solitary creatures and resent competition for food. When 2 of these animals meet there is typically a show of aggression and a fight may ensue, with both of them turning black and attacking with open mouths and biting or pushing with the head. The battle typically ends suddenly with one giving way and being rapidly pursued by the other.

'They are generally considered to be non-social creatures but may be found in discrete colonies, spacing themselves out by this sort of aggressive displays.' [Moore]


## MATERIA MEDICA CHAMAELEO DILEPIS DILEPIS

### Sources
1  Proving Liesl Pistorius and Debora Moore [South Africa], 24 provers [9 females, 15 males], 30c; 2006.

### Mind
∞ Disconnected and disoriented, on waking; impressions rushing in and retreating; cannot integrate visual and auditory input, staring at things and words just passing by; taking a long time to process any sensory input. As if body and mind do not work sharply together.
∞ Disconnected, disorientated, scattered, incompetent.
∞ Dullness, unable to think long.
∞ Forgetful, esp. in morning after waking.
∞ Sensation as if everything is moving past very smoothly, as if being on another plane or dimension [but also semi-here].
∞ Getting bored very quickly and switching off concentration.
∞ Delusion being restricted, controlled, imprisoned by expectations.
∞ Feeling of procrastination midday. Unable to complete tasks, & mild irritation, > sleep.
∞ Poor self-image; feels fat, disgusting, repulsive.
∞ Destructive and full of self-hatred.
∞ Emotional blankness; struggling to pretend being happy.
∞ Emotional coldness, and even hardness.
∞ Extreme irritability on waking.
∞ Anxiety > warm food.
∞ Anxiety on waking > sunlight.
∞ Excessive sensitivity to noise; sounds are overwhelming, intensified, seem very loud.
∞ Despair, as if looking into a black hole; as if being a fully functioning empty shell.
∞ Delusion being paralyzed.

### Dreams
∞ Bombs exploding.
∞ Changing backgrounds and blending in.
∞ Cheating.
∞ Disease.
∞ Embarrassment – toilets, disgust.

∞ Helpless feeling.
∞ Helplessness.
∞ Old friends.
∞ Paralysis.
∞ Reckless driving.
∞ Sports.
∞ Strangers.
∞ Travelling, exploring new places.
∞ Water, oceans, seaside, lakes, rivers.

## Generals
∞ Tiredness [19 pr.], on waking; throughout body; drained and sleepy; cold and weak.
∞ Physical and mental exhaustion accompanied by feeling of light-headedness.
∞ Restless sleep > lying on back or left side.
∞ Waking in morning < – anxious; depressed; disoriented; irritable; worried; tired eyes; stuffy nose.
∞ Thirst for cold water when light-headed/dizzy or from dryness mouth/throat.
∞ Movement alterations – Leaning against walls when standing. Walking funny, falling forwards with small paces; not well coordinated. Frequent tripping, left foot especially seems to stick to ground every so often.
∞ Dryness mouth, lips, tongue [like cardboard], skin.
∞ Coldness, spreading up legs.
∞ Coldness worse on right side.
∞ Very cold, as if in the bones, < cold; must sit in the sun to get warm.
∞ Coldness makes lethargic.
∞ Appetite increased or ravenous after eating.
∞ Craving for chocolate [2 pr.]; eggs; fatty food [butter; cheese sauce; cream; peanuts; pizza; pork] [3 pr.]; fruit/fruit juice [3 pr.]; salty; sour [citrus; sauerkraut; yoghurt]; sweets [3 pr.].
∞ Aversion to coffee; eggs; vegetables.

## Sensations
∞ Floating or as if falling into space.
∞ Head congested as if brain were swollen.
∞ Tight band around head.
∞ Iron vice around head, squeezing it.
∞ Head as if quivering or shaking internally around the eyes.
∞ Back of eyes as if pierced by a needle, during headache with photophobia.
∞ Eyes as if dried up.
∞ Eyes as if filled with water and wanting to bulge.
∞ Tired, fixed feeling in facial muscles, as from a mask.
∞ Numbness tip of tongue after eating.
∞ Teeth as if cracking from cold water.
∞ Throat as if a tube, hollow, enlarged.
∞ Lump in anterior throat.

- ∞ Butterflies in stomach, > coffee.
- ∞ Needles inside chest.
- ∞ Chest as if a hollow tube.
- ∞ Cold feeling in chest, like alcohol evaporating, spreading to beneath ribs.
- ∞ Palpitations as if blood is thick and sluggish.
- ∞ Chest as if pulsating with hard heartbeat, < lying on left side. Blood as if hot.
- ∞ Cardiac region as if full, making breathing difficult.
- ∞ Blood as if thick and getting stuck in aorta, building up, then suddenly forcing through.
- ∞ Fullness in heart region, making breathing difficult.
- ∞ Lower mid-back as if broken.
- ∞ Back muscles as if strained, causing stiffness, > cold application.
- ∞ Pins and needles sensation from base of spine, radiating up and out.
- ∞ Left arm as if lame.
- ∞ Legs like jelly.
- ∞ Feet as if broken.
- ∞ Feet as if sticking to the ground when walking, causing stumbling.

## Locals
- ∞ Dizziness on rising, > cold water on face.
- ∞ Occipital headache, < coffee, fizzy drinks, > cold ice application, heat of sun, warm food.
- ∞ Headache behind eyes < quick movements of eyes or head, shaking head.
- ∞ Dull ache behind eyes > drinking water.
- ∞ Right-sided headache & numbness of right side of tongue.
- ∞ Headache centred in right eyeball.
- ∞ Eyes watery and light sensitive; margins red.
- ∞ Excessive watering eyes > fresh cold air.
- ∞ Increased salivation from salty or strong-smelling foods, > cold water.
- ∞ Nausea from looking at rich food.
- ∞ Nausea from smell of tobacco.
- ∞ Heart complaints & numbness right arm.
- ∞ Stiffness of neck in morning > cold application.
- ∞ Legs heavy, weak, tired.


# CHAMAELEO ZEYLANICUS

## Systematics
- Scientific name: Chamaeleo zeylanicus [Laurenti, 1768].
- Synonyms: Chamaeleo zebra [Bory de St. Vincent, 1823]. Chamaeleo coromandelicus [Fitzinger, 1843]. Chamaeleon calcaratus [Werner, 1911].
- Common name: Indian chameleon.
- Family: Chamaeleonidae.

## Biological Profile

- Arboreal chameleon. Body colouration pale green, dark green or yellowish-brown, with dark spots and streaks. Body dorso-laterally flat with a distinct low, serrated crest or ridge on the dorsal [spinal] aspect. Male larger than female. Length up to 43 cm.
- Range: Sri Lanka, India, Pakistan.
- Habitat: Forest, shrubland, inland wetlands.
- Solitary, territorial, aggressive.
- Hisses loudly with laterally flattened body and displays a deep green colour with black blotches and spots.
- Female intolerant of close approach of other chameleons of either sex except for suitor males during a period of a few days when they are ready to mate.
- Male display directed only to other males competing or thought to be competing to court a female. Such male display includes close approach, pausing to inflate and hiss, and attacks on the flanks.
- Mainly insectivorous, also preys on small amphibians, skinks and geckos.
- Oviparous; 10–31 eggs per clutch.

## Post-Mating Male Avoidance Behaviour

'The post-mating male avoidance behaviour of the female is highly pronounced. Trench, who had also noticed this, stated: after mating the female "showed rage if the male came near her, rocking her body to and fro and gaping at him with faint hissings. He on the other hand would fly in ludicrous terror falling head long from his perch if she came near, as though paralysed."' [Singh, 1984]

## Materia Medica

- No symptoms.

# CHLAMYDOSAURUS KINGII

## Systematics

- Scientific name: Chlamydosaurus kingii [Gray, 1825].
- Common names: Frill-necked lizard. Frilled lizard. Frilled dragon.
- Family: Agamidae.

## Biological Profile

- Semi-arboreal lizard, grey and brown in colour, to 1 m long [incl. about 60 cm tail].
- Range: Australia and New Guinea.
- Habitat: Savanna woodland areas, sometimes found in tropical and temperate forests.
- Preys on arthropods in trees and ants, termites and small vertebrates on the ground.
- Oviparous; 7–8 eggs per clutch.
- Diurnal, spending most of its time on trunks of trees and lower branches.

- Name derived from the skin frill around its neck, which is normally folded down, but is flared out when frightened or agitated.

## Behaviour & Temperament

'Both males and females use the neck frill when frightened and as a defensive measure. If the frill does not frighten their predator, they begin to run away on all 4 limbs and then *accelerate* and begin to run on their hind legs. Australians have given the Frill-necked Lizard the nickname of "bicycle lizard" due to this behaviour. They will run to a tree, climb, and use camouflage to hide.

'Frill-neck lizards certainly do their best to look like a scary dragon when they feel threatened but *looks is all there is to it*. They are perfectly harmless. Frill-neck lizards rely on camouflage for their safety, so their mostly grey and brown colours match those of their surroundings. Lizards from different regions will have different colours. The only brightly coloured body part is the actual frill around their neck, which often contains bright red and orange scales. . . . Whether in the tree or on the ground, a frill-neck lizard with its frill folded around the shoulders, lying down and perfectly still, blends in very well with its surroundings and is hard to spot.

'If you do spot a Frilled Lizard on a tree it's still near impossible to take a photo: as you approach the tree the lizard moves around the trunk to the other side. And as you go around to the other side the lizard does the same, always remaining exactly on the opposite side, while both of you try to sneak a look at the other.

'The story is a different one if a frilled lizard is on the ground. Again, first it tries to be "invisible." Once a frill-neck lizard realises that its cover is blown it changes its strategy: The lizard opens its mouth to expose the strong teeth, which also opens the impressive orange frill, making the lizard look twice as big. In addition it rears up on the hind legs, hisses, thrashes its tail on the ground, and it might even jump towards an attacker hoping to scare them off. . . . But if our Frilly Lizard realises that the attacker is not impressed it turns and runs for the nearest tree for safety, using the hind legs only. That's when the "attacker" doubles over laughing . . . They look so funny when they run . . . [Outback Australia Travel Guide]

## Jolly & Comical

'Another oriental lizard is named "the frilled," because he wears a large quilled collar, or ruff, all around his neck; upon his head is a crest deeply indented, and down his back from head to tail-tip a full ruffle like a cloak close folded, or a court train. In fact, whenever I have seen a frilled lizard, I have had a laugh, not only at its truly pert and comic appearance, but because he seems such a jolly little caricature of stately Queen Bess in her head tire, ruff, farthingale, and court train. Then, too, other ideas come to heighten my mirth over a frilled lizard.

'You must know that lizards' tails are very brittle and not infrequently break off; when this happens the organ grows again just as a crab's claw does. I wonder if the tail of the frilled lizard is apt to break off and how long it takes such a cumbersome appendage to grow. Then, again, here is my other little joke over him: all lizards, as they grow cast their skins; toads and frogs do this also, and crabs cast their shells. The process is far from unusual, but the lizards like the toads swallow their worn-out garments, and how can my frilled lizard swallow such an amount of frilling and furbelow and flouncing! I should say be must choke!

'It would be as bad as being obliged to eat a birthday cake, candles, wreaths of flowers and all. But when I stand before a frilled lizard and laugh at all these queer notions concerning him, what does he do but bob and move his head and neck, until all his ruffles quiver and curl in a most threatening way, as if he meant to alarm me by his ferocious appearance. But he is really a timid creature and would rather fly than fight. If you persecute him and drive him into a corner he will now and then turn at bay, and bite with some sharp little teeth that he has.' [McNair Wright, 1895]

## Putting on Frills

'There are few subjects in Natural History more interesting than the power that many animals possess of suddenly altering their appearance, to the end either of terrifying an enemy or conciliating the fair sex of their own species. In many, perhaps in most cases, the attitude assumed is the same or nearly so, for it must be borne in mind that the creature is in all probability usually quite unconscious of any deliberate intention to produce an effect, and is merely instinctively employing the natural means of expressing emotion, which is an attribute if its particular species.

'Ruffs and frills about the neck are naturally particularly well calculated to produce a striking alteration in appearance when suddenly expanded, and it is therefore not surprising to find many animals decorated with these, and these of the most diverse classes.

'Among the beasts, we have the mane in the lion and the peruke of some baboons; and these serve a double purpose, as they not only increase the apparent size of the animal when bristled up but are apt to baulk an adversary of a throat-hold with the fangs. Very possibly the beard of man has the same significance, for primitive man certainly did not fight according to Queensberry rules, but in all probability flew at his enemy's throat like a modern monkey. Of course, all races of men have not beards, but neither have all animals frills, in spite of the manifest advantages of the decoration; natural selection has to work on the variations which come ready to hand and cannot produce a structure just because it would be useful.

'Reptiles are particularly addicted to endeavouring to *make themselves as horrible as possible to the eye when enraged*, but only a few species have a neck decoration to exhibit on such occasions. The flat, horizontal expansion forming the hood of the cobras is well known, and many lizards and snakes can expand their throats vertically, but the Frilled Lizard of Australia alone rejoices in a perfect Elizabethan ruff for use as a war-mask.

'When not in use, this remarkable appendage lies folded along the sides of the neck, but if the reptile be alarmed, it is widely spread, and the mouth being opened at the same time, produces a *tout ensemble* so uncanny that, as Mr. Saville-Kent tells us, it will deter a dog, which will fearlessly tackle the larger and really more formidable monitor lizards. It is not only that the ruff increases the apparent size of the creature, but it is also very brilliantly coloured in red and yellow, while the inside of the mouth is altogether of the latter colour.

'It is just as well for the lizard that it is able thus to impose on enemies, for it is by no means a powerfully-armed reptile and is far more given to making these grimaces than actually fighting.

'A parallel case is found among birds in the so-called Painted Snipe [Rostratula sp.] of the Old World tropics. This bird, a highly coloured sandpiper rather than a snipe, seems to have no idea of really fighting, but attempts to terrify an enemy by the display of its beautifully-spotted quills, which are concealed in repose, accompanying the exhibition by a formidable-sounding hiss. This has been actually seen to frighten some small creatures and no doubt disconcerts larger ones long enough to allow the painted fraud to escape attacks to which it would otherwise fall a victim, for it has not the swift dodging flight of the true snipes.

'Another member of the sandpiper family, and that a British bird, the Ruff [Philomachus pugnax], has a ruff very similar in outline to that of the frilled lizard. In the ordinary way it lies close to the bud's neck, but when courting or fighting it is spread out widely. The individual with the speckled ruff is just assuming the courting attitude, as is shown by the downward-pointing bill; for when paying his addresses to his consort the reeve, the Ruff affects the greatest humility, and crouches down even to the ground when at full show. When fighting, however, he assumes much the same position, except that he does not crouch so much, and points his bill forward. His aim is then to seize his foe with his bill and, with a spring, to slap him with his wing, for the contests of Ruffs are mere boxing matches, and the vanquished is merely driven off the field, not hurt. The frill can here be of no advantage to the fighting birds, as it merely gives a better hold for the bill, and it cannot be needed as a shield, as the Ruff's bill is too blunt and weak to do any damage, the real weapon being the wing.

'Similarly, it may be noted that the hackled ruff of the common rooster is such a convenient handle for opponents that cock-fighters used to cut it off when preparing their birds for the pit.

'It would seem, then, that frills in some birds are essentially of use in courtship, and they are certainly widely distributed in the class, though only sporadically as a rule. . . . Thus, until it is more definitely proved that hen-birds really do select their mates according to beauty, the question must remain open whether, even among the birds, the beautiful plumes and attitudes we admire so much are not really in many cases simply the further development of the goblin war equipment of their coarser relatives, the reptiles.' [Finn, 1905]

## Materia Medica
• No symptoms.

# ELGARIA COERULEA

### Systematics
- Scientific name: Elgaria coerulea [Wiegmann, 1828].
- Synonyms: Gerrhonotus coeruleus [Wiegmann, 1828]. Gerrhonotus burnetti [Stejneger, 1893]. Gerrhonotus coeruleus utahensis [Woodbury, 1945].
- Common name: Northern alligator lizard.
- Family: Anguidae.

### Biological Profile
- Medium-sized, smooth, shiny terrestrial lizard with broad head, long body, small limbs, and extremely long tail. Body colour grey, olive and rust, to greenish or bluish dorsally with heavy blotching or barring in a dusky colour. Underside light grey with dark shadows around edges of each scale. Back and belly armoured with large, stiff, rectangular, scales reinforced with bony plates. Fold of skin along each side of body to expand for breathing or to make room for food and eggs. Length: 32 cm.
- Range: Canada [S British Columbia], USA [Washington, Oregon, Utah, Idaho, Montana, northern and central California].
- Habitat: Grassy, bushy, or rocky openings within forested areas. Also found in areas of low to moderate development, incl. in rock retaining walls, woody debris, rock piles, and near the bases of newly emerging buildings.
- Secretive. Often heard rustling through leaf litter before it is seen.
- Capable climber.
- Primarily diurnal and crepuscular.
- Hibernates during cold months of winter.
- Preys on crickets, spiders, mealworms, ticks, moths, snails, small lizards. Stealthily stalks its prey and pounces from a short distance.
- Mating 'love bite': Male grasps neck of female in his jaws and holding her thus, manipulates posterior portion of body to bring the genital orifices into contact.
- Viviparous; 2–15 live young per brood.
- Four recognized subspecies [coerulea, palmeri, principis, shastensis].

### Materia Medica
- No symptoms.

# ELGARIA KINGII

### Systematics
- Scientific name: Elgaria kingii [Gray, 1838].
- Synonyms: Gerrhonotus kingii [O'Shaughnessy, 1873]. Gerrhonotus multi-fasciatus [Duméril & Bibron, 1839].
- Common name: Madrean alligator lizard.
- Family: Anguidae.

## Biological Profile

- Medium-sized, smooth, shiny terrestrial lizard with broad head, long body, small limbs, and extremely long tail. Base colouration tan or grey. Dark brown to red-brown crossbars with dark posterior edges dorsally. Crisp black and white markings on the lips. Back and belly armoured with large, stiff, rectangular, scales reinforced with bony plates. Fold of skin along each side of body to expand for breathing or to make room for food and eggs. Length: 32 cm.
- Range: SW USA [Arizona, New Mexico], NW Mexico.
- Habitat: Broadleaf riparian corridors, semidesert grassland, interior chaparral, woodlands, and montane conifer forest.
- Frequents moist areas, often in association with loose ground cover such as fallen leaves, pine needles, and other dead plant material.
- Secretive. Often heard rustling through leaf litter before it is seen.
- Capable climber.
- Primarily diurnal and crepuscular.
- Hibernates during cold months of winter and late fall.
- Difficult to capture; quickly slides and zigzags through ground cover.
- Writhes, expels faeces, and often bites when captured.
- Preys on a variety of insects, incl. grasshoppers, caterpillars, and moths. Also feeds on scorpions. Stealthily stalks its prey and pounces from a short distance.
- Mating 'love bite': Male grasps neck of female in his jaws and holding her thus, manipulates posterior portion of body to bring the genital orifices into contact.
- Female capable of storing sperm. Embryonic development arrested during cold winter months.
- Oviparous; up to 15 eggs per clutch. Female may stay with the eggs to tend to them.
- Three recognized subspecies [kingii, nobilis, ferruginea].

## Materia Medica

- No symptoms.

# FURCIFER OUSTALETI

## Systematics

- Scientific name: Furcifer oustaleti [Mocquard, 1894].
- Synonym: Chamaeleon oustaleti [Mocquard, 1894].
- Common names: Giant Madagascar chameleon. Oustalet's chameleon.
- Family: Chamaeleonidae.

## Biological Profile

- Large chameleon to 60–70 cm in total length with characteristic dorsal crest, which extends to the vent and consists of 45 or more short, triangular spines with regular spacing between them. Females reach half the size of males. Colouration primarily grey, tan and brown with broad, vertical russet or deep brown bands of varying intensity. Females tend to be slightly more colourful

than males; gravid females often assume a golden hue with dull-red bands and spots.
- Range: Madagascar. Introduced to Florida, USA.
- Habitat: Inhabits both warm and humid coastal lowlands but seems to prefer drier forests. Most common in disturbed areas, it even occurs in parks and gardens.
- Oviparous; up to 60 eggs per clutch.
- Mostly insectivorous, but may feed on small vertebrates and fruits.
- Moderately aggressive toward con-specifics; docile to aggressive toward keepers.

## Thoroughly Solitary

The electronic magazine Chameleons! Online E-Zine provides information about chameleon husbandry and the thoroughly solitary nature of these lizards:

'Despite the fact that chameleons are beautiful animals and people are drawn to them, they become extremely stressed by exposure to people and other animals. Minimising this exposure must be a priority. Specifically, these animals should not be purchased with the intention of being handled more often than for the occasional health check. They do best as display animals in a low traffic area of your home where other animals will not be bothering them, and children will not be interacting with them unsupervised.

'Chameleons are not social animals; they are actually quite solitary. Keeping multiple chameleons, even those of the same sex, in a single enclosure is extremely stressful for them. A cage for multiple chameleons would need to be excessively large and complicated in design to ensure the animals' complete ability to *avoid each other*. . . .

'One of the common major mistakes that beginners make is to house chameleons together.

'Chameleons are not community animals the way we humans think of communities. Although we cannot know what goes on inside of a chameleon's head, decades of keeping chameleons has shown us that chameleons not only do not get lonely, but that they do very well living life without ever seeing another chameleon. In fact, the long-term evidence shows that they live longer lives in better health if they *interact with each other as little as possible*.

'In captivity, the results of co-habitation usually end up with a stunted, poor health, or dead chameleon. The reason why there is any debate at all about this issue is the combination of a strong innate desire in human beings to group animals together and the fact that health issues related to co-habitation usually manifest themselves over time and indirectly. This makes the official cause of death something other than co-habitation. . . .

'There is virtually no scientific evidence that a solitary-living animal such as a chameleon forms any sort of affectionate bond with another chameleon, much less with a member of a large, strange primate species such as Homo sapiens. Neither is there evidence that early handling will make an animal less aggressive. Certainly, hand feeding a chameleon will teach him to associate you with food and might even cause him to approach you when the cage door opens. But it does not facilitate the formation of a "bond" and it likely does not reduce the stress of handling.' [www.chameleonnews.com]

## MATERIA MEDICA FURCIFER OUSTALETI

### Sources
1 Clinical observations Karl-Josef Müller [Germany], in Wissmuth Materia Medica Müller 2.0, 2009.

### Symptoms
Two things are typical for *Furcifer*: swelling and immobility [motionlessness, absence of movement]. When suffering of pollinosis [hay fever], the patient has the sensation as if his eyes were coming out of his head, whilst moving the eyes is impeded by conjunctival swelling [chemosis].

As a child *Furcifer* had the febrile dream his tongue continued to swell, growing too large for his mouth. Although he is athletic and keen on sports, he can also remain for hours in one spot. He dreams of wanting to run away, yet being unable to do so; movement is difficult and he doesn't know how to use his legs properly. The warmer the weather, the more sluggish and worn-out he becomes. Coldness refreshes him.

Tight clothing [cf. *snake remedies*] causes choking and he gets the feeling he cannot move well any longer. If his suppressed anger comes out, he feels as if his thyroid were distending and rage boiling in his belly. He is afraid to go to sleep lest he would not wake again. Sleeping could mean dying; the infinity of death frightens him.

Becoming a paleontologist was Furcifer's childhood dream; he is fascinated by dinosaurs and fossils [cf. *Tyrannosaurus*]. What captivates him particularly about chameleons is that they can move their eyes in opposite directions simultaneously.

# HELODERMA – HORRIDUM & SUSPECTUM

### Biological Profile
- 'The 2 species in this family, the Gila monster and the Mexican beaded lizard, are both large, heavy-bodied lizards coated with small, rounded bumps that look like the beadwork on clothing. The bumps, which are actually pebble-like scales, cover the tops of the arms, legs, head, and tail, as well as the back and sides of the body. The generic name Heloderma means 'studded skin', from the Ancient Greek words *hêlos*, the head of a nail or stud, and *derma*, meaning skin. Its specific name, *horridum*, is Latin for rough or rude.

  'These lizards have rather short, but strong arms and legs and long, thin claws. The tail may be thin or thick, depending on how well fed the individual is. This is because these lizards store fat in their tails.

'Beaded lizards have slightly longer tails than Gila monsters. An average beaded tail is at least two-thirds the length of the entire body, but the typical Gila tail is about half the total body length. Unlike many other lizards, these 2 species also have thick, forked tongues. Members of the same species can look very different from one another. Some adults are brightly patterned, while others are faded and dull. The patterns may be made up of spots, blotches, circles, bands, or squiggles on a background of pink, orange, yellow, dark gray, or black. Juveniles are usually banded.

'Gila monsters and Mexican beaded lizards are the only 2 venomous lizards in the world. Unlike venomous snakes that deliver venom from the upper jaw and through grooves in just the 2 fangs, these lizards store their venom in the lower jaw and deliver it through grooves in numerous teeth.

'The beaded lizard is larger than the Gila monster but has duller colouration, being black with yellowish bands of differing width, depending on the subspecies. A specialised predator that feeds primarily upon eggs, the primary use of its venom is still a source of debate among scientists. However, this venom has been found to contain several enzymes useful for manufacturing drugs in the treatment of diabetes, and research on the pharmacological use of its venom is ongoing.

'Because the Helodermatids have remained relatively unchanged morphologically, they are occasionally regarded as living fossils.' [Wikipedia]

- Unlike most other lizards, helodermatids *cannot run swiftly*. A painful venomous bite is an important feature of their ability to avoid predators.
- Males vie for access to females by performing spectacular combat rituals, reminiscent of the entwining combat dances of viperid snakes. Both Gila monster and beaded lizard males engage in hours of snorting, head pressing, and body twisting, all aimed at claiming access to a breeding female. Their low metabolic rates, ability to eat large meals and to store energy as fat in their sausage-shaped tails enable helodermatid lizards to offset the energy costs of searching for a widely distributed food source and to subsist long periods without feeding. These traits make frequent foraging unnecessary and contribute to their ability to feed almost solely on the contents of vertebrate eggs and young in their nests, a specialised feeding niche shown by few other lizards. The ecology, physiology and behaviour of the Helodermatidae has helped us refine our thinking about reptilian life in the slow lane, and as ancient members of the clade from which snakes likely arose, they are putting a new spin on what it means to be a lizard.

## Monster Paradox, like Strolling Snakes

The specific epithets *horridum* [meaning 'rough' but suggesting 'the horrible one'] and *suspectum* [the suspect] appear to indicate a sinister side of the helodermatid lizards.

'As they do with venomous snakes, humans have historically regarded helodermatid lizards as loathsome and dangerous, reminding us of the dark side that lurks in the shadows, both in nature and in our imaginations. But, because they are *lizards*, the archetypal feature of snakes that lies embedded in the human psyche does not fully extend to *Heloderma*. They don't slither; they walk. Even though bumpy lizards are venomous, most people do not perceive the same sinister threat from them as they do from snakes.

'Nonetheless, the development of our knowledge about helodermatid lizards mirrors our discovery and gradual understanding of *all things sinister and misunderstood*. First there are fantastic tales of pain, horror, and death, accompanied by fear and repugnance. Size and dangerousness are often exaggerated. There is fierce debate. Facts may be ignored. As we learn more, fear is replaced with respect – a respect that, in the case of *Heloderma*, has blossomed into full-blown fascination. No other species of lizards have spawned as much folklore, wonder, and myth as those of the Helodermatidae. And new discoveries about this small but remarkable family of lizards are even more intriguing than the folklore.

'Helodermatid lizards present a number of paradoxes. They are venomous, yet they don't appear to use their venom for subduing prey, as do nearly all other venomous reptiles. They are at once cryptic and aposematic. Their mottled patterns of yellow/orange and black mingle with the broken shadows and textures of their desert and tropical dry forest habitats. But approach more closely and the cryptic pattern is transformed into a bright, bold *beware*: a wide-open mouth – soaked in venom – hisses a warning that a very nasty bite awaits those who advance further. The bite is delivered with a *lockjaw tenacity* that surely qualifies *Heloderma* as the pit bull of the lizard world.

'*Tenacity* is also reflected in their evolutionary history – they are survivors. . . . Gila Monsters and Mexican Beaded Lizards present a textbook example of reptilian *life in the slow lane*. Their keen chemosensory abilities and excellent memories allow them to forage on vertebrate eggs and nestlings, a feeding niche shared by very few other lizards. . . . The low-energy lifestyle of helodermatid lizards stands in stark contrast to their remarkable capability for aerobic activity and endurance. They cannot quickly sprint to escape danger, as can most other lizards, but they can walk for hours at speeds much greater than their normal foraging pace in nature. *Heloderma* has among the *highest aerobic capacities* of any lizard measured. Endurance and high aerobic capacities seem puzzling traits for slow-moving lizards like *Heloderma*, until one considers behaviours other than foraging.' [Beck 2005]

## Economic with Energy

'Lizards that forage widely, such as the monitors, are generally more active and have higher resting metabolic rates than sit-and-wait predators. Monstersaurs [Gila monster and beaded lizard] buck the trend: Even though they do forage over wide ranges, their overall activity levels and their resting metabolic rates are remarkably low. Rather than being steady performers, they are like athletes who perform superbly in bursts, then spend the rest of their time on the bench.

'Even in the spring and summer, when monstersaurs are most active, they spend more than 90% of their time hidden in shelters. And over an entire year they spend far less energy in activity than most sit-and-wait predators do. Such apparent sloth is the result of extreme seasonal fluctuations in the monstersaurs' environment. Food, when available, needs to be *gorged on, stored as fat, and used slowly*. Compared with monitors, monstersaurs can feed only infrequently, but when they do, they *can eat meals that put supersizing to shame. . . .* Of course, monstersaurs don't use up all that energy right away; they store it in their sausage-like tails and within their body cavities. Because the capacity to store energy is directly proportional to body mass, the larger the lizard, the longer it can subsist between meals. Gila monsters and beaded lizards, 2 of the largest lizard species in the New World, therefore have impressive abilities to store energy.

'But if monstersaurs are good savers of energy, they're even better at spending it very, very slowly. At rest, Gila monsters and beaded lizards have among the lowest metabolic rates ever measured in lizards – far lower than the rates in monitor lizards. Furthermore, because monstersaurs spend so much time at rest – much of it in shelters where reduced temperatures confer even greater energy savings -the stored energy is used frugally. Monstersaurs are ectotherms [or, as they are sometimes erroneously known, cold-blooded animals], lacking internal mechanisms to regulate their body temperatures. With each drop in body temperature of 18 degrees Fahrenheit [10 degrees Celsius], their metabolic rates decrease 3-fold.

'The resulting energy conservation makes frequent foraging unnecessary and enables the monstersaurs to occupy a feeding niche exploited by few other lizards. Indeed, their frugal lifestyle is causing herpetologists to rethink what they know about lizards. Contrary to the received wisdom, predators that search widely can have low rates of overall activity – provided they have the right combination of high storage capacity, large meals, and low metabolic rates.

'Nothing about the foregoing should be taken to imply that monstersaurs are always sluggish. On the contrary, they have striking aerobic capacities. On a treadmill, beaded lizards can walk at half a mile per hour for hours. Both monstersaur species display some of the highest capacities for sustained aerobic activity of any lizard ever measured, right up there with their monitor cousins. Large capacities for aerobic activity have traditionally been interpreted as adaptations to the needs of foraging. But why would inactive lizards have such *remarkable endurance*? For monstersaurs, endurance may fit into a different context: competition for mates.' [Beck, 2004]

### Gripped by Pain
Although not highly toxic to man, Heloderma venom is principally a neurotoxin that causes respiratory failure.

'Perhaps the most frequent comment on bites by these lizards relates to the *force of their jaws and their tenacity*. Their bite has been described as "forceful," "bulldog-grip," "crunching," "crushing," "firm," "grasping," "good mouthful," "seizing," and "tenacious hold." The length of time that they hold on, or the time it takes to remove them from the bite site varies, but probably it is less than most of the stories in the literature would indicate. Some appear only to "nip," while others have been reported to hold on for 10 to 15 minutes. In any event, if the animal chooses to hold fast, it will do so with great vigour and mechanical means may be necessary to free it from the bitten part.

'If envenomation has taken place, pain about the wound area will usually be present within the first 5 minutes following the bite. If considerable venom is involved, the pain will be more severe and may appear within the first 30 seconds of the bite. The pain is usually described as "burning," "intense," "excruciating," or "violent." Although it is usually confined to the injured area during the first 5 minutes, it may spread to involve the entire part, hand, or foot within 10 minutes. It can radiate up the arm, where it may be described as "shooting," "stabbing," or "burning." Radiating pain is common in the more severe envenomations but infrequently extends beyond the involved extremity.

'Oedema is also one of the important presenting signs. It usually appears later than in rattlesnake bites and it progresses more slowly. In one case the oedema was quite marked and eventually extended up the arm and into the axilla. As in rattlesnake bites, the oedema appears to be soft.

'*Weakness, faintness, or dizziness* [related to primary hypotension] are common complaints following Gila monster bites. Most patients complain of some weakness within the first 15 to 30 minutes following the bite. Weakness may persist for several days. . . . Pulse was usually increased and tended to be thready in some cases.

'Cyanosis or bluish discolouration around the wound was seen in several of our cases and has been reported by others. It is certainly not as evident as that seen following rattlesnake bites. Increased perspiration appears to be another common complaint following envenomation, although in our own patients it appeared less frequently than in those reported in the literature. It is a less frequent complaint than weakness, fatigue, or dizziness. When it does occur, it is first seen within 30 minutes of the bite and may persist for several hours. In 2 patients that I treated, skin temperature was decreased during the first 2 hours following envenomation.

'Shannon notes tinnitus in 2 cases following bites by helodermatids. The only time I inquired of this symptom in a patient he reported that he had had some bilateral ringing, lasting for approximately 4 hours after the bite. Muscle fasciculations appear to be rare. Numbness of the affected part has been reported. . . . Headaches are rare and reliable evidence of respiratory depression is lacking.

'Other reported manifestations include chills and fever, "lumps on the tongue," "bulging eyes," slight dysphonia, and "seeing blinding lights."' [Russell, 1980]

## Chemistry of Venom
'In the 1980s, researchers discovered in the venom of helodermatid lizards some remarkable biologically active peptides that have strong physiological effects in mammals, incl. humans. Most of these compounds are similar in structure and action to vasoactive intestinal peptide [VIP], a mammalian hormone secreted by nerves throughout the gastrointestinal tract and other tissues. VIP is a powerful relaxant of smooth muscle and plays a role in the secretion of water and

electrolytes by the small and large intestines. One of the VIP-like peptides discovered in *Heloderma* venom, named *helospectin*, binds to VIP receptors in a number of human tissues in the gut, brain, lungs, and even the genitalia. In these tissues, helospectin may play a role in regulating secretory activities and local blood flow.

'Helospectin has been immunohistochemically located in the corpus cavernosum of the penis, the clitoris, and the human vagina, where it may play a role in the regulation of local blood flow and lubrication. Helodermin, another peptide discovered in the venom of *Heloderma* [and similar to helospectin] also binds to receptors in several human tissues including breast cancer cells. It has even been shown to inhibit growth and multiplication of lung cancer cells. These bioactive peptides from *Heloderma* venom are, in a sense, part of our physiology!

'So it is a funny coincidence that ancient Mexican cultures thought extracts of *H. horridum* might "awaken the sexual appetite better than any known medicament" and that Boocock noted the effects of Gila Monster venom on erection and sexual performance [although he also noted dozens of other effects not unexpected in a person his age in the United States during the late 19th century].

'The powerful vasodilatory effects of some *Heloderma* venom constituents have not escaped the attention of modern researchers in pharmacology. Helospectin has been shown to relax tissue preparations of the corpus cavernosa, which mediates penile erection, to relax the vaginal wall of rabbits and to possibly play a role in the female sexual response. In the human bronchi, helospectin also produces a potent relaxation response, which may open the airways of the lungs.

'We do not know why peptides from lizard venom reside in the most intimate places of our anatomy, or why they mimic our hormones. It is doubtful that extracts of *Heloderma* venom will become the next Viagra. . . . And there are even more promising modern uses for constituents of *Heloderma* venom. The best known is Exendin-4, found naturally only in Gila Monster venom. Exendin-4 mimics another mammalian hormone, glucagon-like peptide, which mediates insulin release and glucose uptake from the blood after a meal.' [Beck, 2005]

### Dogged Persistence

Heloderms present a stubborn perseverance that can be best defined with the ambiguous term '*doggedness*'. They are dogged in the sense that their bite will be generally compared with that of a bulldog [although pit bull would be fitting even better] and that they use their highly developed sense of smell to track down their prospective meals [eggs, nestling birds, baby animals], suggestive of bloodhounds.

Heloderms are equally dogged in the other meaning of the word: obstinate, stubborn, tenacious. Reluctant to bite unprovoked, Heloderma's mild and non-combative disposition will undergo a sudden reversal when injured or teased, or if escape is not feasible. Then, when it does grab hold, it has no intention of letting go, hanging on with unyielding resolve. Under Heloderma suspectum we will come across reports on the lizard's 'tenacity of life'. Massimo Mangialavori has found that *patients requiring Heloderma as a remedy are very obstinate people, esp. when engaged in conflicts.*

The last word is for Roger Caras, who allotted them a whole chapter in his book *Dangerous to Man* [1977]: 'Heloderms are not a cross between a lizard and an alligator, but have a respectable lineage as pure, albeit rather singular, lizards. As far as is known, the Gila monster possesses no magical powers and is quite killable, although it is tenacious of life. All in all, these animals are just about what a sensible person might expect them to be; they are all lizard, not terribly bright, not at all affectionate, very poor pets, very intent on minding their own business, but different in that they are [1] large, as North American lizards go, and [2] venomous.'

# HELODERMA HORRIDUM

## Systematics
- Scientific name: Heloderma horridum [Wiegmann, 1829].
- Synonyms: Trachyderma horridum [Wiegmann, 1829]. Heloderma hernandesii [Wiegmann, 1834].
- Common names: Beaded lizard. Mexican beaded lizard.
- Family: Helodermatidae.

## Biological Profile
- Less colourful than its cousin, the Gila monster, but larger and more arboreal, the Mexican beaded lizard has black or pale yellow bands or is all black, depending on the subspecies. Average length 60 cm, maximum 90 cm.
- Range: Coastal regions of Mexico through Guatemala.
- Habitat: Primarily tropical deciduous forest and thorn scrub forest, but also found in pine-oak forest, with elevations from sea level to 1500 meters. In the wild, the animals are only active from April to mid-November, spending about an hour per day above the ground.
- Skin comprised of bead-like small, bead-like and non-overlapping scales. Except for the underside of the animal, the majority of its scales are underlaid with bony osteoderms.
- Short tail, used to store fat so the animal can survive during months of aestivation [sleeping throughout summer]. Unlike many other lizards, this tail does not autotomise and cannot grow back if broken.
- Like snakes, H. horridum has a forked black tongue that it uses to smell, with the help of a Jacobson's organ; it sticks its tongue out to gather scents and touches it to the opening of the organ when the tongue is retracted.
- Sexual maturity is reached at 6 to 8 years of age and mating takes place between September and October.
- Males engage in ritual combat that often lasts several hours; the victor mates with the female.
- Young lizards are seldom seen. It is believed they spend much of their early life underground, emerging at 2 to 3 years of age after gaining considerable size.

- Specialised vertebrate nest predator feeding primarily on bird and reptile eggs; will climb deciduous trees in search of prey when encountered above ground. It will occasionally prey upon small birds, mammals, frogs, lizards and insects. Captive specimens, both wild-caught and captive-born, will often refuse any food, *except for eggs*.
- Oviparous; 2–30 eggs per clutch.
- Four recognized subspecies [horridum, alvarezi, exasperatum, charlesbogerti].

### Venom

A short-tempered lizard, it will turn and open its mouth in a threatening manner when molested.

'Its venom is a weak haemotoxin and although human deaths are rare, it can cause respiratory failure. It consists of a number of components, including L-amino acid oxidase, hyaluronidase, phospholipase A, serotonin, and highly active kallikreins that release vasoactive kinins. The venom contains no enzymes that significantly affect coagulation. Almost all documented bites [8 in the past 100 years] have resulted from prodding captive animals with a finger or bare foot.

'While invertebrates are essentially immune to the effects of this venom, effects on vertebrates are more severe and varied. In mammals such as rats, major effects include a rapid reduction in carotid blood flow followed by a marked fall in blood pressure, respiratory irregularities, tachycardia and other cardiac anomalies, as well as hypothermia, edema, and internal hemorrhage in the gastrointestinal tract, lungs, eyes, liver, and kidneys. In humans, the effects of bites are associated with excruciating pain that may extend well beyond the area bitten and persist up to 24 hours. Other common effects of bites on humans include local oedema, weakness, sweating, and a rapid fall in blood pressure. Beaded lizards are immune to the effects of their own venom.

'The compounds which have been studied in its saliva have pharmacological properties relating to diabetes, Alzheimer's disease and even HIV. This hormone was named exendin-3 and is marketed by Amylin Pharmaceuticals as the drug Exenatide. One study done in 1996 revealed that it binds to cell receptors from breast cancer cells and may stop the growth of lung cancer cells.' [Wikipedia]

### Scuffling for Love

Combat in H. horridum more closely resembles fighting in monitor lizards, *Varanus*, than in H. suspectum.

'Male beaded lizards have even more spectacular combat rituals [than Gila monsters]. The 2 challengers begin by pressing against each other, first side-to-side, then belly-to-belly, gradually creating a lizard arch with only snouts and tails contacting the ground. Larger size and a stronger, longer tail may give one lizard an edge. A bout ends when one male topples the arch and forces the other onto his back; the 2 competitors repeat the contest until one lizard gives up. Beaded lizards have been observed to continue wrestling for more than 15 hours.

'Ritualised battles are all about dominance. For both species, remaining on top and forcing the opponent to the ground appear to be the primary objectives.

Consistent losers retreat from the fight, while the winner gets access to a shelter housing a female. The exhausting contests test the limits of endurance, giving obvious advantages to the animal with the higher aerobic capacity.' [Beck, 2004]

## MATERIA MEDICA HELODERMA HORRIDUM

### Sources
1 Clinical observations Karl-Josef Müller [Germany], in Wissmut Materia Medica Müller 2.0, 2009.
2 Synthesis Treasure Edition 2009.
3 Degroote, Dream Repertory.
4 Effects of bite; envenomation.

### Mind
∞ Inability to speak/Loss of speech, due to migraine or more chronically, due to failure dealing with conflicts.[1]
∞ Knows what she wants to say, but can't express it and instead utters inarticulate sounds [cf. *Bothrops*].[1]
∞ Personal history of feelings of helplessness and abuse [cf. *Cenchris*] induced by alcoholic father; hoped he would drink himself to oblivion, unable to speak and walk.[1]
∞ Longing for harmony; not wanting to cause anyone grief.[1]
∞ Fear of lizards. Dreams of walking through a scenery filled with lizards.[1]
∞ Concentration difficult.[2]

### Dreams
∞ Basket filled with chocolate eggs.[3]
∞ Crocodiles in pits.[3]
∞ Fighting insects by cutting them in two.[3]
∞ Helped, being.[3]
∞ Helping people.[3]
∞ Sea being frozen.[1]
∞ Sinking into mud.[3]
∞ Suicide as the only way to escape trouble.[3]
∞ Suicide attempt by holding breath.[3]
∞ Taking care of a little child.[3]

### Generals
∞ Paralysis agitans.[2]
∞ Before menses < [cf. *snake remedies*] – swollen, tender breasts; water retention; headache; spontaneous bruising.[1]
∞ Icy coldness, coldness through and through [*Anguis fragilis*], even near a source of warmth or under a thick blanket in the night.[1]
∞ Despite coldness, loves ice cream and views of glaciers and snow-covered mountains.[1]

∞ Snow air <.[1]

∞ Craving for eggs.[1]

## Locals
∞ Pressure in eyes and on eyelids.[1]

∞ Breath cold, as if frozen.[1]

∞ Constipation.[1]

∞ Respiration: Asphyxia during anaesthesia.[2]

### Envenomation by the Mexican Beaded Lizard: A Case Report
'Envenomations by venomous lizards are rare. A single report of envenomation by a Mexican beaded lizard [Heloderma horridum] has been published. Further, anaphylaxis secondary to lizard envenomation has only been reported with the Gila monster. We report an envenomation that resulted in both systemic toxicity and anaphylaxis.

'Case Report: A 40-year-old male was bitten on his hand by a captive Mexican beaded lizard. The patient experienced severe local pain, dizziness, vomiting and diaphoresis. Upon arrival to the hospital, he was lethargic, vomiting and in severe pain with marked swelling of his hand, lips and tongue. His blood pressure was 110/63 mm/Hg with a pulse of 60 beats/minute. The patient's oxygen saturation decreased to 55% and he required oxygen, although cyanosis was not observed. He was treated with normal saline, diphenhydramine, methylprednisolone, famotidine, ondansetron, morphine and hydromorphone.

'The patient was admitted to intensive care where he continued to complain of severe pain requiring morphine. Local X-ray revealed only soft tissue swelling. . . . Over the next 8 hours, the patient's symptoms gradually improved. He had persistent local swelling at the bite site along with erythematous streaking up the forearm. He had an uneventful hospital course until his eventual discharge the following day.

'Conclusion: Significant envenomations by members of the Helodermatidae family are rare. Systemic toxicity usually resolves within 1 to 2 days with supportive care. Prior envenomations may predispose patients to anaphylactic reactions.' [Cantrell, 2003]

# HELODERMA SUSPECTUM

## Systematics
- Scientific name: Heloderma suspectum [Cope, 1869].
- Common names: Gila monster. Reticulate Gila monster.
- Family: Helodermatidae.

## Biological Profile
- Only venomous lizard native to the United States, and 1 of only 2 known species of venomous lizards in North America, the other being its close relative the Mexican beaded lizard, Heloderma horridum.

- Robust lizard with large head and heavy tail. Body covered with beadlike scales. Markings consist of a pattern of black bands or reticulations on a peach, orange, yellow or pink background. Usually 3 to 5 black bands on the tail. Snout and sides of face black. Average length 30 cm, maximum 50 cm.
- Range: Arizona, New Mexico, Utah, Nevada, northern Mexico, and extreme corner of southeast California.
- Habitat: Arid areas, most commonly mountain foothills dominated by saguaros and palo verde trees.
- Skin has a 'beadwork' appearance made up of individual rounded, raised scales. Embedded within the scales are osteoderms or small boney plates. Although such protective 'bony skin' appears to have been fairly common in dinosaurs, the Gila monster [as well as the Mexican beaded lizard] are among the few living reptiles with such extensive use of this type of armour.
- Has very good hearing and can detect very minor sounds in its vicinity. It is believed that Gila monsters can locate their prey, e.g. young mice, rats, rabbits or birds by their sensitive sense of hearing.
- Capable of storing fat in its tail against lean times when food is scarce.
- Prefers a body temperature around 30°C [86°F], which is a fairly low for a diurnal desert lizard. The body temperatures of winter-dormant animals may drop below 10°C [50°F].
- Comes out at night or early morning hours during the dry season [spring and early summer] in search of small rodents and bird eggs; later in the summer it may be active on warm nights or after a thunderstorm. During the heat of the day it stays under brush or rocks.
- Despite the arid climate prevalent in its range, favours areas of high humidity and spends the vast majority of its time in fairly moist underground retreats. When kept in dry zoo exhibits, Gilas will soak in water bowls for hours on end.
- May enter a burrow and eat the nestlings of whatever it finds living there, to next assume the ready-made burrow as its home.
- Returns year after year to the same foraging and overwintering areas, sometimes re-using the same shelters.
- Oviparous; 2–12 eggs per clutch.
- The species name *suspectum* was coined in 1869 by renowned herpetologist and paleontologist Edward Drinker Cope – upon noting the Gila's grooved teeth, he 'suspected' that it was venomous. Common name derived from Arizona's Gila River basin, where the species was first discovered.
- Two recognized subspecies [cinctum and suspectum].

## Slowly Forwards, Retreating Backwards

'Gila monsters are the slowest of lizards and their pace can be described as only a purposeful waddle under normal conditions and a hurried amble when pressed. The alternate movement of the feet give the animal a peculiar rolling gait, each foreleg moving in synchrony with the opposite rear leg.

'Like crocodiles, the Gila monster holds its belly above the ground when traveling, as well as the heavy tail. If surprised or controlled, the Gila monster's usual response, when not totally ignoring the intrusion, is to *retreat backwards*, using the same alternate pattern of steps. Should escape appear unlikely, the Gila monster backs into a rock or other hard surface and curls into a semi-circle where it holds its ground huffing and hissing with mouth agape. The Gila monster may lunge at an adversary who gets too close, but it does not "jump up or spring" as some writers would have you believe. . . .

'Gila monsters have good daytime vision and *amazingly keen hearing*, as anyone who has ever attempted to sneak up on a basking animal can attest. The animal can also sense an oncoming intruder by detecting minute vibrations in the ground – a good thing given that the Gila monster is a slow traveller and incapable of high speed sprints. The average foraging mode is only 13 feet [4 m] a minute or 0,15 miles [240 m] per hour, with maximum bursts of about 50 feet [15 m] per minute. But while the lizard does not move forward with speed, it is neither as awkward nor as sluggish as it first appears. The Gila monster can spin around and face an attacker with lightning suddenness. More than one handler of a Gila monster has been surprised by the animal's agility and quickness, particularly if one of the clawed feet obtains a grip on an article of clothing or other surface.' [Brown & Carmony, 1999]

## Diet

'The Gila monster feeds primarily on bird and reptile eggs, and occasionally upon small birds, mammals, frogs, lizards, insects, and carrion. The Gila monster eats infrequently [only 5 to 10 times a year in the wild], but when it does feed, it may eat up to one-third of its body mass. It uses its *extremely acute sense of smell* to locate prey, esp. eggs. Its sense of smell is so keen that it can locate and dig up chicken eggs buried 15 cm [5.9 inch] deep and accurately follow a trail made by rolling an egg.

'Prey may be *crushed to death* if large or eaten alive if small, swallowed head-first and helped down by muscular contractions and neck flexing. Unusually, after food has been swallowed, the Gila monster immediately resumes tongue flicking and search behaviour, probably as a result of a history of finding clumped prey such as eggs and babies in nests. Gila monsters are able to climb trees and cacti in search of eggs.' [Wikipedia]

'Gila monsters are adapted to eating large meals infrequently. In fact, an adult male Gila can consume its entire yearly energy budget in 3 or 4 meals! This is because of the large meals they can consume as well as their limited food require-ments. This allows them to consume most of their food during the limited Spring activity period. Their food requirements are reduced by a low metabolic rate, as well as the relatively cool body temperatures they maintain for most of the year. . . . Gila monsters also have unique physiology to assist them in storing food for their long periods of inactivity. Immediately after eating, large quanti-ties of a hormone-like molecule called exendin-4 circulate in the Gila's blood. With this unique mechanism of metabolic control, the act of eating primes the organism to receive the incoming nutrients, by, for example, stimulating insulin secretion. A synthetic version of this protein is currently being developed as a treatment for human diabetes.' [www.docseward.com]

## Behaviour & Temperament

Not an aggressive lizard, but ready to defend itself when provoked. If approached too closely, it will turn toward the intruder with its mouth open. If it bites, it hangs on tenaciously and must be pried off. Its venom glands and grooved teeth are on its bottom jaw.

'One of the reasons Gila monsters are so poorly understood is the fact that most of their life is spent underground and out of sight. Although Gilas can be seen throughout the year, even basking at the entrance of their shelters on unseasonably warm winter days, most of their aboveground activity occurs during a 3 month period of time in the Spring. Their reproduction, feeding, and even metabolic controls are uniquely adapted to this short activity period.

'After a winter of hibernation, Gilas emerge in the spring to feed and mate. After this 90-day peak activity period they rarely come to the surface. In fact, even during this spring activity period they are active for only brief periods of time. Consequently, more than 99% of the Gila monster's life is spent inactive and underground.

'Adult Gilas are predominately diurnal, not nocturnal as previously thought. To avoid the extreme heat of the desert, most of their activity occurs in the morning and the late afternoon. Sometimes they are seen out after dark during the summer monsoon season, esp. in the southern part of their range.' [www.docseward.com]

## Pre-Monstrual Bickering

Gila monster wrestling matches have been observed repeatedly near shelters where males pair with females in the spring, when both sexes are primed for mating. In such a bout, one male climbs on top of his adversary and tries to remain there, while his opponent twists around in an effort to reverse their positions.

The lizards use intricate techniques equivalent to those of Olympic wrestlers, incl. Dorsal Straddle, Body Twist, Neck Arch, Head Raise, and Roll. Daniel Beck [2005] informs us that captive female Gila monsters also 'exhibit aggressive behaviours toward other Gila monsters. Especially during the weeks preceding and following oviposition, females become quite defensive and frequently hiss, chase, and bite other lizards [males or females] that approach. Some of these fights may even resemble male combat.'

## Persistent Determination

'Popular accounts are rife with examples of the supposed power and endurance of the Gila monster. Fights have been staged between Gila monsters and a 12-year-old alligator, a wildcat, a red coachwhip [viz. fast-moving, thin-bodied snake preying on lizards and rodents], a copperhead, and several varieties of rattle-snakes. In all of these accounts the Gila monster emerges triumphant, or at the very least, giving as good as he got. The only reptile known to best a Gila monster in combat is its ancient adversary, the desert tortoise.

'There is some justification for the animal's reputation as a *combatant*. Gila monsters are immune to their own poison and appear to be resistant to rattlesnake venom. Their hides are protected by an armour-like covering that only the sharpest and strongest of teeth can penetrate. Moreover, the Gila monster is capable of sustaining a higher level of activity for a longer period of time than any other lizard yet studied. . . .

'The Gila monster's tenacity of life is also legendary. Taxidermists and animal collectors have reported the lizard to be *nearly indestructible*, after attempting to club them to death, suffocate them, drown them, and even inject them with alcohol. Even today, rural residents of Sonora are said to assure the death of a Gila monster that they have killed by hanging it by the neck with a wire noose, lest the animal recover and seek revenge on its tormenter. This "refusal to die" is of course due to the reptile's low metabolic rate and primitive nervous system that allows the muscles to twitch long after the animal is clinically dead. . . .

'Gila monsters appear to be almost incapable of drowning. A Phoenix undertaker reported many years ago that he "kept one under water for 10 hours, taking him out at the end of that time still alive and in fighting condition." . . . This amazing ability has been attributed to the lizard going into a state of suspended animation or torpor for hours at a time.' [Brown & Carmony, 1999]

### Difference with Heloderma horridum

'It appears that the Arizona Gila monster, inured to xeric conditions and exposed to the hot, bright desert sun, is quite responsive in its actions when met in the wild. Its movements when disturbed may be quite rapid forward or back and alarming, as it throws its mouth open with a loud hissing sound to warn would-be captors or enemies. On the other hand, the Mexican Gila monster [H. horridum] seems to be much more docile in nature, often assuming a "play-opossum" attitude to some extent.' ['play-opossum' = to feign death]

'However, if held, its long, lithe body is very powerful as it tries to escape by twisting and turning. If one does not have a good hold it is best to drop the creature and then start over. Probably these very habits may account for the single case of Gila monster [H. horridum] bite in Mexico as compared with numerous bite accounts in our country.' [Bücherl & Buckley, 1968]

### Effects of bite

Hans-Joachim Schwandt on his website www.heloderma.net observes the following frequency of symptoms occurring in 17 cases of Gila monster bite:

Pain [14 cases];
local oedema, swelling [14];
weakness, faintness, dizziness [11];
nausea [11];
hypotension [8];
sweating [8];
tachycardia [6];
vomiting [6];
leukocytosis [5];
hypersensitivity around bite [4];
reduced blood potassium levels [3];

reduced platelets [3];
bluish discolouration around bite [2];
cardiac abnormalities [2];
swollen or painful lymph glands [2];
lethargy [2];
anaphylaxis [1–2];
diarrhoea [1];
tinnitus [1];
exophthalmia or peri-orbital haemorrhage [1];
hypothermia [1];
miosis [1].
*See* also above, Gripped by Pain.

## Personal Accounts of Bites

In the November 1882 issue of the *American Naturalist*, Dr. Shufeldt gave the following account of a painful experience with a Gila monster:

'On the 18th, in company of Prof. Gill of the [Smithsonian] Institution, I examined for the first time Dr. Burr's specimens of the Heloderm, then in a cage in the Herpetological Room. It was in capital health and at first I handled it with great care, holding it in my left hand, examining special parts with my right. At the close of this examination I was about to return the fellow to his temporary quarters when my left hand slipped slightly and the now highly indignant Heloderma made a dart forward, and seized my right thumb in his mouth, inflicting a severe lacerated wound, sinking the teeth in his upper maxilla to the very bone.

'He loosened his hold immediately and I replaced him in his cage with far greater haste perhaps than I removed him from it. By suction with my mouth I drew out a little blood from the wound, but the bleeding soon ceased entirely, to be followed in a few moments by very *severe shooting pains up my arm* and down the corresponding side.

'The severity of these pains was so unexpected that added to the nervous shock already experienced and to a rapid swelling of the part that now set in, it caused me to become so faint as to fall and Dr. Gill's study was reached with no little difficulty. The action of the skin was greatly increased, and the perspiration flowed profusely. A small quantity of whiskey was administered. This is about a fair statement of the immediate symptoms: the same night the pain allowed of no rest, although the hand was kept in ice and laudanum, but the swelling was confined to this member alone, not passing beyond the wrist.

'Next morning this was considerably reduced, and further reduction was assisted by the use of a lead water wash. In a few days the wound healed kindly and in all probability will leave no scar; all other symptoms subsided without treatment beyond the wearing, for about 48 hours, so much of a kid glove as covered the parts involved. After the bite our specimen was dull and sluggish, simulating the torpidity of the venomous serpent after it has inflicted its deadly wound, but it soon resumed its usual action and appearance, crawling in rather an awkward manner about its cage."

U.S. biologist Ernest R. Tinkham [1904–1987] was bitten on the left index finger on July 6, 1948.

'My bite had occurred at 10:50 a.m. At 11:05 I felt a twinge of pain in the middle of my forearm. I hastily applied a handkerchief tourniquet there. . . . By 11:20 I started to feel ill. I tried another doctor and succeeded in reaching him. Suddenly a wave of sickness struck me. My legs grew weak and blinding lights flashed before my eyes. I lay back on the couch as nausea seized me. I threw up – the vomitus was yellow.

'Entering the hospital I vomited again. A doctor gave me a shot of tetanus in my left shoulder and one of Demerol in my right. My hand was now so puffed I could not bend my fingers and the swelling had advanced far up my arm. Most of it had taken place since cessation of the ice-water bath when I was taken from the house. Equipment was brought next to my bed and soon a saline solution slowly filtered into the vein of my right arm to replace the body fluid loss by my *vomiting every 10 minutes*, which condition endured for 4 hours.

'I was very weak and breathing heavily, but I do not remember having any speech difficulties and I could think coherently. . . . A long series of penicillin shots – 1 every 3 hours – was started at this time. By now I *could not tolerate the slightest touch* to my left arm. . . .

'After 4 hours in the hospital, my vomiting cycle lengthened from 10 to 15 minutes, then to every 20 minutes and finally every half hour or so. The last spell came at 8:30 that evening. By midnight, after taking little sips of water now and then, I drank half a gallon in 3 hours to relieve my *extreme thirst*. After that I fell into a sleep induced by sedatives. . . .

'On Saturday – I had entered the hospital Tuesday – I was released. It took a month for my hand and arm to recover, although my fingers still were sore to the touch. Hot baths of Epsom salts took away most of this soreness. By mid-August of that year much of the arm's *sensitivity to sunlight* had disappeared and I considered myself fully recovered.' [Tinkham, 1957]

## Diabetes type 2 Drug

'In 2005 the U.S. Food and Drug Administration approved the drug exenatide [marketed as Byetta] for the management of type 2 diabetes. It is a synthetic version of a protein, exendin-4, derived from the Gila monster's saliva. In a 3-year study with people with type 2 diabetes, exenatide led to healthy sustained glucose levels and progressive weight loss. The effectiveness is due to the fact that the lizard hormone is about 50 percent identical to glucagon-like peptide-1 analog [GLP-1], a hormone in the human digestive tract that increases the production of insulin when blood sugar levels are high. The lizard hormone remains effective much longer than the human hormone, helping diabetics keep their blood sugar levels from getting too high. Exenatide also slows the emptying of the stomach and causes a decrease in appetite, contributing to weight loss.' [Wikipedia]

# MATERIA MEDICA HELODERMA SUSPECTUM

## Sources
1 Self-experimentation Boocock [USA], 6x and 30x, 1892–93.
2 Clinical observations Boocock, Johnson, and Case [USA], 1890s.
3 Proving Todd Rowe [USA], 11 provers, 30c; 1996.
4 Clinical observations Römer [Germany], 14 cases, 1960s.
5 Clinical observations Mangialavori [Italy].
6 Degroote, Dream Repertory.
7 Synthesis Treasure Edition 2009.

## Mistaken Identity
Boocock calls the lizard and thus the remedy 'Heloderma horridus'; erroneously since Boericke & Tafel produced it from the venom/saliva of a specimen from Arizona, where Heloderma suspectum is endemic.

H. horridum can be excluded with certainty as the source of the remedy [and the proving] for the simple reason that this species is not found in the U.S., but much further south in Mexico.

The mix-up is due to misidentification some decades earlier. In *Amphibians and Reptiles from New Mexico* [2005], Degenhardt et al. explain how this came about: 'During the U.S. and Mexican boundary survey of 1855, 3 specimens of *Heloderma suspectum* were collected by Arthur Scott at Sierra de la Unión in Sonora, Mexico. These specimens were deposited at the Smithsonian Institution and Baird [1859] misidentified them as *Heloderma horridum* following an earlier description by Wiegmann [1829]. He illustrated one of these specimens for the Boundary Survey that actually became the first illustration of *Heloderma suspectum*. Cope [1869] noticed differences between these specimens and *Heloderma horridum*, and designated these 3 specimens, USNM 2971, as syntypes. In 1869, Cope formally described *Heloderma suspectum* in a publication of the Academy of Natural Sciences of Philadelphia.'

Any lingering doubt ought to be put aside by Anshutz, who writes in *New, Old and Forgotten Remedies*: 'The provings and the clinical cases that follow were from the virus of the Gila monster obtained by Dr. Charles D. Belden, Arizona, in 1890. . . . A supply of this poison was sent to Dr. Robert Boocock at his request for proving and he made 3 different trials of it.' As if this shed too much light on the question, Anshutz confuses matters again by including it in the remedy section 'Heloderma horridus' in his book.

## Mind
∞ No inclination for exertion in any way.[1]
∞ Aversion to household duties. Indolence, aversion to work.[5]
∞ Laziness, thinks work will harm him.[7]
∞ Difficulty in remembering the spelling of simple words while writing.[1]
∞ When excited could not get hold of the right words and dropped some when speaking from a want of flexibility or a catch in the tongue.[1]
∞ Mistakes in spelling and talking, omitting words.[5]

∞ Fear heart will stop beating, causing restlessness at night.[1]
∞ Depressed; feels blue.[1]
∞ Disinclined to talk.[2]
∞ Communicative.[7]
∞ Very irritable; easily provoked.[2]
∞ Easily startled from sounds, with trembling; startled from sound of bell ringing.[1]
∞ Sensitive to noise.[3]
∞ Fear of cats; of lizards.[5]
∞ Fear of lions, even of picture of lions.[6]
∞ Slowness. Slow learning to talk.[5]
∞ Childish behaviour. Forsaken feeling. Jealousy. Obstinate, headstrong.[5]
∞ Mentally restless; not able to confine mind to one object.[2]
∞ Difficulty concentrating on one subject.[7]
∞ Racing thoughts [4 pr.], < waking [3], cannot control thoughts.
∞ Rushed [4 pr.].[3]
∞ Busy [4 pr.]. Industrious [4 pr.].[3]
∞ Restless [3]. Feels manic [3 pr.].[3]
∞ Restlessness driving out of bed.[6]
∞ Hurry, as if from imperative duties.[6]
∞ Wants to be let alone [3 pr.].[3]
∞ Desire for company; when alone <.[6]
∞ Lack of self-confidence, feels oneself a failure.[6]
∞ Lack of self-confidence alternating with confidence.[6]
∞ Postponing due to lack of self-confidence.[6]
∞ Defiant.[6]
∞ Loss of ambition in evening.[7]
∞ Expansive.[7]
∞ Delusion being possessed.[7]
∞ Tranquility during conflicts.[7]

## Dreams
∞ Animals with tails [6 pr.].[3]
∞ Attending cases of malignant diphtheria.[2]
∞ Choking, difficult breathing.[3]
∞ Construction [4 pr.].[3]
∞ Dead people and graveyards.[2]
∞ Drowning in a sea of tears.[3]
∞ Falling into a bomb crater.[6]
∞ Fast motion [3 pr.].[3,6]
∞ Feasting/celebrating, family.[6]
∞ Foreign country.[6]
∞ Hearing telephone bell ring.[2]
∞ Helped, being.[6]
∞ Laughed at / mocked, being, over misfortune.[6]
∞ Lizards.[6]
∞ Ocean and water.[3]

∞ People fighting, surrounded by.[3]
∞ Poisoned, being.[6]
∞ Poisoning.[3]
∞ Rain.[3]
∞ Resignation, handing in.[6]
∞ Robot killing other robots.[6]
∞ Scorpions [3 pr.].[3,6]
∞ Speech, making a, eloquent; lecture.[6]
∞ Speeding on dry, dusty roads [4 pr.].[3]
∞ Standing in water.[3]
∞ Tortured, being.[6]
∞ Urinating in bed.[2]
∞ Violence/poisoning [5 pr.].[3]
∞ Water/underwater [5 pr.].[3]

## Generals
∞ Moving quickly = dizziness and weakness.[2]
∞ Great thirst.[2]
∞ Dryness, parched sensation – lips, throat.[1]
∞ Wakened out of sleep by pains [abdomen, right lung, lumbar region] and/or trembling [arms and thighs].[2]
∞ Wakened out of sleep by shocks through head.[7]
∞ Wakes at 3 a.m.[6]
∞ Sleeps with head against head of bed.[6]
∞ Stretching > pains in muscles and limbs.[1]
∞ Moving does not < pains.[1]
∞ Left side more affected.[4]
∞ Allergy to Primula [4 cases], strawberries [3 cases], coldness [2 cases].[4]
∞ Aggravation at night [4 cases], cold air [4 cases], cold drinks [2 cases].[4]
∞ Hot weather >.[6]
∞ Desire for eggs[5]; meat and coffee[3].
∞ Aversion to eggs; meat; sweets.[3]
∞ Desire for crunchy food, cornflakes.[6]
∞ Trembling limbs that can be suppressed by will-power.[7]
∞ Weakness < slight exertion.[7]

## Coldness
∞ Coldness, objective and subjective, partial or general; tongue, breath, dorsal region, limbs, etc.[1,2]
∞ Arctic coldness.[1]
∞ Internal coldness, from the heart; as if being frozen to death internally.[1]
∞ Arctic coldness throughout body except head and face, with great tiredness and aching in bones; feels as if frosty winds were blowing through holes in his garments and freezing his flesh.[1]
∞ Coldness from within outward; as if filled with a deathly coldness; > eating hot sour pickles.[2]

∞ Coldness > hot food.[2]
∞ Cold waves ascend from feet or go downward from base of brain.[2]
∞ Coldness = trembling.[1,2]
∞ Cold pressure within skull.[1]
∞ Cold band around head.[1]
∞ Cold, crawling feeling from temple down right cheek.[1]
∞ Cold feeling in genitals, as if frozen.[1]
∞ Right lung as if cold.[1]
∞ Coldness and trembling around heart.[1]
∞ Coldness in and around heart.[2]
∞ Heart as if cold.[6]
∞ Feeling as if a cake of ice were on back, & hands blue with cold and feet like lumps of ice.[1]
∞ Right biceps as if cold.[2]
∞ Tingling and burning of feet as if recovering from being frozen.[1]
∞ Cold rings around body, beginning between scapulae.[1]

'Quite a number of those who read the proving of Heloderma shrugged their shoulders and cried, "too sensational." Among them was a young clerk in the employ of Boericke and Tafel. He laughed at the whole thing and in a spirit of bravado took 6 doses of the 6th dil. On the second night he awoke with a cold sensation creeping down his body and legs, and found himself in a very cold and clammy sweat. This lasted all the remainder of the night and he was unable to go to sleep again; by morning the disagreeable experience began to pass off and he felt no more of it.' [Hom. Rec., Oct. 1895]

## Sensations
∞ Sensation as if would fall on right side; desire to bear to the right side and could not walk straight because of this; had repeatedly to stop or step to the left to get a straight course. When bending forward, inclination to fall forward or backward.[2]
∞ Heat on vertex.[1]
∞ Brain as if scalded.[1]
∞ Brain as if numb.[7]
∞ Skull as if too full; pressure in head and scalp.[1]
∞ Band around head.[1]
∞ Constriction head, band or hoop, < cold.[7]
∞ Scalp as if drawn tight over skull.[1]
∞ Headache as if top of head would come off.[7]
∞ Occiput as if stiff.[7]
∞ When looking at stars or distant lights there always appeared a cluster of lights below to the right of the main one. Comet-like tail to stars appearing on upper left side.[2]
∞ Wax as if running out of ears.[1]
∞ Left cheek as if pricked with points of ice.[1]
∞ Facial muscles as if drawn tight over bones.[1]

∞ Molars as if elongated, painful when chewing food.[2]
∞ Waist band as if too tight.[2]
∞ Bowels as if filled with pins, awakening from sleep.[2]
∞ Testicles as if swollen and painful.[1]
∞ Lungs as if stiff and difficult to inflate.[1]
∞ Lungs and heart as if stiff, as if they were tied or unable to move.[1]
∞ Twitches about heart as if blood had difficulty in entering or leaving heart.[2]
∞ Boiling heat beneath left scapula.[6]
∞ Numb feeling down right leg.[1]
∞ Numb feeling down left leg.[2]
∞ Tight band around left ankle, as if it would cut foot off.[1]
∞ As if walking on sponge and feet as if swollen; a springiness and sense of looseness in stepping, which requires caution, as if he were not sure of his steps.[1]
∞ As if stepping on wool.[7]

## Locals
∞ Dizziness & inclination to fall backwards.[1]
∞ Dizziness followed by perspiration.[7]
∞ Dizziness < rapid motion of head.[7]
∞ Intense pain over left eyebrow, through eye to base of brain and down back.[1]
∞ Pain in head and back of neck going down back and right leg.[1]
∞ Pain occiput and cervical region/nape of neck on coughing.[6]
∞ Headache over right temporal bone, as if a tumour were forming and pressing within the skull, affecting entire right side of head and producing numbness down left side of body.[2]
∞ Bores head in pillow.[7]
∞ Weight on eyelids, difficult to keep them open.[1]
∞ Pain beginning in right ear, extending round back of head to left ear.[2]
∞ Nasal congestion [6 pr.], < eating [1 pr.].[3]
∞ Pain abdomen on drawing in abdomen.[6]
∞ Urine profuse and pale during night.[2]
∞ Urine greenish-yellow.[1]
∞ Urine thick like milk after standing a short time.[2]
∞ Urine foetid with odour of decaying fruit.[1]
∞ Urinary incontinence when laughing.[6]
∞ Heartbeat felt all over body; body throbs, he can feel and hear it, as if it were some labouring engine; slow laboured thumping of heart.[2]
∞ Trembling of arms; difficulty in holding hand steady when reading and writing.[2]
∞ Hands and feet blue with cold; cold as ice.[2]
∞ Formication lower limbs at night in bed.[5]
∞ Twitching as if foot would spring when walking, making him walk as if he had the 'cock's gait'.[2]
∞ When walking lifts feet higher than usual and puts down heel hard.[1]
∞ Cracks, fissures < cold weather.[5]

## Clinical Observations & Confirmations

'In Heloderma we see this feeling that you are not receiving what you deserve from your environment. . . . In Massimo's experience, his cases of Heloderma have a very good structure to support what happens. Even if they complain about this feeling of not being recognized and not getting enough, all the patients so far that Massimo has had are very strong, very tough people. They are capable to do more or less what they want and to do this in their own proper way.

'The anger in Heloderma is often acted in a very aggressive nature, but not with common aggressive tools [fits of violence for example]. But in a more precise and extremely efficient way, they try to find out the weak point of their enemy. The aggression is more or less a kind of apparently passive aggression. "I can stay here for as long as I need to and if you don't come to me there is no way we can have a communication."

'The eroticisation you don't find in these cases. It's more evident [eventually] that they don't give too much importance to a communication based on feelings. Often they look like pretty cold people. Whenever you have to do with remedies where the feeling of coldness is so deeply rooted, they often lack the feeling or even the possibility of a 'warm' relationship with another person. They even don't consider that this may be possible. There is a deep sense of distance that is not possible to overcome.

'What seems to be specific to Heloderma suspectum is the characteristic kind of stubbornness with which this remedy expresses itself. Those patients whom I have successfully treated with this remedy are often described by their family and friends as very obstinate people, esp. when engaged in conflicts or in their most destructive strategies. They are described as apparently lazy people who even find it a chore to talk. In actual fact I find them to be restrained and careful in their behaviour, as well as verbally, giving the impression that the whole world should turn around them and adapt to their rhythms. They present themselves as being apparently passive, but stubbornly flaunt theirs as being the only possible way.

'This aspect does not seem to me to be so typical of the other remedies in this family. The other reptiles attain their objectives using a wide variety of strategies, first and foremost among which is their highly effective charm, easily able to penetrate their victims' defences.' [Massimo Mangialavori, RefWorks]

## Themes of Proving

'The central idea of this remedy is expressed in the following: I am busy [industrious], centered [balanced] and speeding in my space but don't bother me or I will get irritable and lunge. This idea was well expressed in the dream of prover #3 who dreamt that she was possessed by a scorpion and had to keep attacking others who would get into her space but when left alone she felt centered and at peace.

'The idea of centeredness vs. being out of balance [expressed on the physical level of vertigo] seemed to come up repeatedly during the proving. A number of the provers described feelings of peace and contentment by the end of the proving relating to feeling as if they were coming into greater balance.

'Three of the provers felt more social by the end of the proving. Prover number 5 in particular noted a significant change from isolation and being a loner to greater socialness and calmness. For several provers, this also took the form of connecting more to deceased relatives. Prover number one described feeling as if she was much closer to her patients after the remedy and could see more clearly. The animal is known for its solitary habits.

'Another theme was that of increased energy. This took on many forms, which ranged from apprehensiveness and anxiety to mania. Key words that provers used to describe this state included anxiety, busy, industrious, working constantly, rushed, not able to shut off the flow of ideas, insomnia and agitation.

'The theme of aggression was also present. For the most part this took the form of irritability and the need to protect one's space. However, a number of provers had violent dreams and one prover described aggressive feelings of wanting to punch others in the jaw. The aggression and irritability seemed to be without remorse or much emotion. In general the provers noted a lack of maternal feeling with this proving.

'Animal themes were present throughout the proving. By the end of the exit group proving, participants predicted that the remedy was an animal, which had a tail, was involved in some type of construction [burrowing] and had the potential to be aggressive. The colours red, white, black and yellow also came out, which match the colours of the lizard. The craving for eggs is also interesting in that this is the one of the primary foods that the lizard eats. Reptilian themes were also present involving a lack of maternal feeling, striking out and aggression.

'The physical center of the remedy seems to revolve around the upper respiratory system, nervous system and gastrointestinal system. Many of the participants developed upper respiratory symptoms. One participant also experience a cured symptom of chronic severe stabbing stomach pain. Symptoms also were generally worse in the morning. Chilliness was noted by several participants [the leading keynote of this remedy prior to the proving]. One prover had a dream of being in snow and woke up with intense shivering.' [Todd Rowe, 1997]

# CASE

An auburn haired woman, 55 years of age, had numbness in the feet 2 years ago. It has gradually extended upward until it now includes the lower part of the abdomen.

Tingling, creeping sensation on legs as if from insects; < lying in bed at night; < exposure to cold air; < touch; cannot endure to place bare feet together. Legs insensible to an electric battery. Legs wasting away, skin very dry and inelastic. Ankles turn easily when trying to walk.

Numbness of arms from hands to elbows.

Forgetfulness. Melancholy with weeping; < stormy weather; < thinking of her ailments, cheered by company.

Pain in forehead in morning, < turning eyes. Tongue dry and cracked in morning. Swallowing difficult.

Empty eructations, especially before breakfast. Empty, gone sensation in stomach.

Dislikes sweet things and < from taking them.

Sensation of constriction about whole abdomen. Constipation from torpor of rectum. Haemorrhoids and itching of anus. Burning in urethra during and after micturition. Burning and dryness of vagina.

Palpitation and dyspnoea from slight exertion.

Drawing sensation in extremities.

Yellow skin.

April 11, 1895. Heloderma horridus 4 powders, one every 4 hours.

April 23, 1895. Decidedly more cheerful and memory is better. Bowels more active. Legs more reliable, with the numbness and tingling. No medicine.

April 26, 1895. Alarmed because palms and soles are swollen and itching. No medicine.

May 22, 1895. She gained rapidly in both flesh and strength, until a week ago. Heloderma one powder.

Soon after this an itching eruption came all over her, which subsided without any further medication. She was restored to a fair degree of health so that she has taken care of her house and family up to the present time.

[Summarised from a case by Dr. Erastus E. Case, in Anshutz. Note that the remedy is *not* H. horridus, but Heloderma suspectum.]

# HEMIDACTYLUS FLAVIVIRIDUS

## Systematics
- Scientific name: Hemidactylus flaviviridus [Rüppel, 1835].
- Synonyms: Boltalia sublevis [Gray, 1842]. Hemidactylus bengaliensis [Anderson, 1871].
- Common names: Yellow-belly gecko. Indian house gecko. Indian leaf-toed gecko.
- Family: Gekkonidae.

## Biological Profile
- Medium to large gecko, dorsoventrally flattened, with total length of about 18 cm. Limbs somewhat short and thick. Dorsal colouration yellowish-grey, pale yellow or yellowish-green, unmarked or with rather feeble dark wavy transverse bands; underside pale to bright yellow.
- The structure of its tail is adapted for autotomy at every joint.
- Range: Egypt, Kuwait, Saudi Arabia, Oman, Iraq, Iran, Afghanistan, Nepal; Pakistan, India, Socotra Island [Yemen]; N Somalia, Sudan, Ethiopia, Eritrea.

- Lives in close association with humans and human-made structures both in urban and rural areas.
- Nocturnal.
- Largely insectivorous, but will also consume spiders and other invertebrates as well as any animal it can overcome, incl. other geckos and smaller snakes.
- Occasionally shows cannibalism.
- Larger prey is battered to death, to a manageable softness and eaten.
- Strongly territorial. Can be quite vocal at night, making a series of crisp, rapid chirps.
- May make a squeaking noise when captured.
- Oviparous.

### Darting Forward Without a Warning Shadow

'The skill and agility that the house-gecko shows in hunting its prey is remarkable. When it observes an insect fluttering about, it hastens to the spot, slows down its pace on nearer approach and finally sits 'crouched', ready to pounce upon the unsuspecting creature in an unguarded moment. Now and again, it steals a step or 2 nearer. Its remarkably depressed body lies so flat against the wall that there is hardly a warning shadow; its attitude is of complete attention. All of a sudden it darts forwards, snaps at the insect and holds it struggling in its mouth. Lizards do not wait for their prey to die but start swallowing them as soon as they catch them. If the prey is large, the lizard might strike it right and left against the wall before beginning its meal; but it rarely loses its fatal grip on the insect.

'How far the house-lizard [H. flaviviridis] exerts a sense of selection amongst the creatures that it preys upon, is not definitely known, but some observations show that it generally excludes dangerous insects from its menu. It appears, for instance, to refrain from attacking wasps.

'Like many other reptiles, house-geckos have remarkable powers of going without food. Unless properly kept, they may refuse food in captivity. According to Baini Prashad [1916], "they are very shy, and not at all sociable in captivity." . . . These creatures have a nervous temperament and resent much tampering. They can fast a great deal. I have known them fast as long as 5 or 6 months and ultimately die of starvation.

'Besides gnats and mosquitoes, the house-gecko controls the numbers of such other harmful insects as the house-flies, crickets, cockroaches, etc. When this lizard is absent or rare in a particular locality, the noxious insects are apt to multiply so much that human habitation becomes extremely inconvenient, if not altogether impossible.

'Although it might be widely known that the house-gecko hardly ever ventures abroad from its own locality, most persons do not know that even in the same house, it remains true to its own accustomed site and does not migrate to another part, unless compelled to do so. One gecko might stick to a place behind a bookshelf, another remain in a particular crevice in a wall, a third inhabit the cellar, and so on; all being true to their own sites.' [Mahendra, 1936]

## House Geckos

House geckos resemble each other very closely in habits.

Greyish to pinkish-brown in colour with uniform to marbled patterning, H. frenatus can be distinguished from other common 'house geckos' by its tail, which is oval in cross-section and possesses a row of tiny spikes on either side. It has large toe pads and the bulging, lidless eyes that are typical of nocturnal geckos.

Native to south and south-east Asia, but spread around the world by ships, Hemidactylus frenatus has now a worldwide distribution in tropical and subtropical regions, and is known as the Pacific house gecko, the Asian house gecko, or simply, the house lizard.

A member of a quartet of small, prolific, aggressive and nocturnal aggressive lizards, these geckos can be seen climbing walls of houses and other buildings in search of insects attracted to porch lights. Like many geckos, this species can lose its tail when alarmed.

And like all geckos, its call or chirp rather resembles the sound "gecko, gecko." However, this is an interpretation and the sound may also be described as "tchak tchak tchak" [often sounded 3 times in sequence]. Its vocal repertoire consists of 3 functionally, physically distinct calls that are important in its social behaviour. The multiple chirp call is the most common and is closely associated with agonistic behaviour and territorial defence. Call frequency varies directly with the air temperature and has been observed to reach a peak in the early morning hours. The 'churr' call is heard less frequently, occurring solely during aggressive encounters between males, and is thought to function as intimidation.

Males will strongly defend a good feeding territory. Battles between males during the spring breeding season can be quite dramatic, beginning with the twitching of tails and lots of 'churring' as they advance to the fray. Once engaged, physical damage may be done to opponents, but rarely do they kill.

Females normally lay 2 eggs at a time. Eggs are hard-shelled, like those of birds, and slightly sticky, so that they can be attached to a suitable surface in a safe place. The calcium needed to produce the shells is obtained from the diet and stored until needed in a pair of pouches in the throat. Due to their thin and semi-transparent skin, both these calcium deposits and developing eggs can often be seen in living specimens. Females frequently lay collectively in secure places; large numbers of eggs, as well as remains of previous clutches, will often be found together.

Depicted in the pet trade as 'a well-adapted escape artist, managing to get out of the smallest spaces and taking advantage of any loss of concentration . . . it is next to impossible to handle this species.'

## Geckos in Indian folklore

'Geckos are regarded as highly poisonous, so that physical contact is – with few exceptions – considered quite dangerous for the health. It is commonly believed that any contact with the animal requires a thorough washing, though Khush-want Singh, the famous Indian writer, says that "it [is] not the sort of dirt which [can] be wiped off or wiped clean." . . . Writing on Hindu beliefs, S.S. Mehta remarks, "If [a gecko] happens to fall on the body of a human being, the person is believed to suffer from illness in a short time; and if, while the person is asleep it creeps over the body, he or she is believed to meet death in a few days."

'The Bengalis say, "If a lizard falls on the body or passes urine or ordure thereon, then it beckons illness. Sprinkling the body with Ganges water averts the evil." In Peshawar I was told that a gecko falling directly on the face will cause one to become an albino, while in Punjab and Uttar Pradesh it is claimed that a gecko dropping on a person will result in serious skin disease unless the person takes a full bath, particularly in "gold water" [hot water in which one or more pieces of gold have been laid]. The faith in gold water stems from the belief that the yellow colour of the metal can absorb and neutralise the yellow substance of the gecko. A similar notion is reflected in the Arab belief that storing yellow saffron in the kitchen keeps geckos away.

'In Uttar Pradesh Muslims and Hindus alike generally believe that a gecko falling on the right shoulder is a good omen, while one falling on the left shoulder is a bad omen. One woman from Peshawar told me that if a gecko falls on a man's head, then that man will become king.

'Among North Indian Hindus there is an oral tradition that the god Siva, described in Hindu texts as a carrier of disease, dispensed poison to every living creature. Only the gecko, the last to arrive, received none. Siva himself thus prepared a strong poison with a grater and gave it to the gecko, which licked it up and has been deadly poisonous ever since. Eating one, it is believed, can lead to vomiting, serious illness, or even death.

'Similar beliefs are widespread in the Arab world, where the little lizard is called *bors sum*, "poisonous gecko." Popular oral traditions perpetuate such beliefs.' [Frembgen, 1996]

Geckos of the genus Hemidactylus generally have rather small teeth and weak jaws, and are therefore not capable of causing severe human injury through biting. Bites usually just cause teeth marks, minor scrapes or, at worst, some puncture marks without any other symptoms. This is contrary to the common belief in the region that the house lizard is capable of delivering a life-threatening bite. Additionally, geckos, like other reptiles, do not carry the rabies virus, and are therefore not a cause for serious concern.

## Leaving its Taint Wherever it Passes

No other group of lizards is probably surrounded by so much superstitious fear as geckos. From ancient belief to popular view to 'scientific' conclusion, geckos have been disliked and mistrusted for their unusual abilities to meander upside-down across ceilings and to move on smooth surfaces such as glass. Add the gecko's vocalisation, bulging eyes, sticky feet, nocturnal habits, slow colour change, dropping down on sleepers, the haunts where it hangs out, and we start getting the picture why the gecko in Charles F. Partington's authoritative British Cyclopedia of Arts and Sciences, published in 1836, is portrayed as follows:

'The appearance of these animals is peculiarly loathsome; they not only in-habit places which are dark and obscure, but those which are rank and offensive; and as they bear no inconsiderable resemblance to toads and salamanders, they have had the stigma set upon them of being venomous. That it poisons by stinging or biting, or any other species of offensive apparatus, or instrument, of attack, is not true, and cannot be true, of any species of gecko; for none of them possesses a sting of any description, and the teeth in all are so very minute that they are incapable of penetrating the skin of any animal of moderate size.

'That some of them discharge a poisonous liquor is, however, well understood, but this liquor is discharged from pores in the feet; it is of so very virulent a nature as to inflame or even blister the skin when they run across it; and it is particularly dangerous to those who have eaten any provisions over which these animals have passed. . . . This circumstance, together with the toad-like aspect and clumsy gait of these creatures, is in all probability the reason why they are looked upon with so much aversion by most people; and this is, no doubt, also further increased by the foul places in which they reside, and their nocturnal habits.

. . . [Spiders and insects] 'constitute the principal food of the geckos, which seek after them with go much assiduity that in many places where the habits of the people are slovenly, they are encouraged for the purpose of keeping the houses as clear of the others as possible, though, according to our notions of domestic cleanliness, the cure would be considered as even worse than the disease. . . . There is great difficulty in expelling the house gecko . . . but its croaking and its crawling are equally offensive during the night; and when it does come into contact, there is nothing but to submit, and let it run across, for any attempt to seize it with the hand is attended with very painful consequences, as, when alarmed, it sheds its poison more copiously than when left alone. . . .

'Nor is the very offensive danger of this loathsome reptile directed against the skin alone, for it prowls about wherever the people deposit their food and is said to be especially fond of salt meat. It is not the quantity that it eats which is the offensive part of the matter, for its powers of mastication are but limited, but it paddles over everything, leaving the taint of its feet wherever it passes; so that, unless the people have made certain that no house gecko could pass over any provisions that may have remained in the house during the night, they have no security that those provisions shall not be poisoned; and thus, whether the fact is so or not, the uncertainty of this species of feeling is equally bad; because they who live in constant apprehension of any disease, be it what it may, always run a risk of some mated; or other arising from their own apprehensions.'

### Materia Medica
• Introduced as a homeopathic remedy by Divya Chhabra [India] under the name 'common house lizard'.

# IGUANA IGUANA

### Systematics
• Scientific name: Iguana iguana [L., 1758].

- Synonyms: Lacerta igvana [L., 1758]. Iguana minima [Laurenti, 1768]. Iguana tuberculate [Laurenti, 1768]. Iguana coerulea [Daudin, 1802]. Iguana viridis [Spix, 1825].
- Common names: Green iguana. Common iguana.
- Family: Iguanidae.

## Biological Profile
- Diurnal lizard, to 1.5–2 m in length from head to tail. Weight 4–8 kg.
- Range: Central and South America.
- Habitat: Arboreal, living high in the tree canopy. Juveniles establish areas lower in the canopies while older mature iguanas reside higher up. The tree dwelling habit allows them to bask in the sun, rarely coming down except when females dig burrows to lay eggs.
- Row of spines from just behind head to tail. Powerful jaws and strong whip-like tail, used to deliver painful bites and strikes, respectively. Can cast and regenerate tail.
- Agile climber; can fall up to 15 m and land unhurt, using hind leg claws to clasp leaves and branches to break fall.
- Often found near water; excellent swimmer, will dive beneath the water to avoid predators.
- Prefers to stay on the ground for greater warmth during cold, wet weather.
- Superb eyesight, sharp colour vision, but poor vision in low-light conditions.
- Males have highly developed femoral pores on underside of thighs that secrete a scent; females have similar but smaller femoral pores. Dominant males mark rocks, branches, and females with a waxy pheromone-containing substance secreted from their femoral pores.
- When threatened will extend and display the dewlap under its neck, stiffen and puff up its body, hiss, and bob its head at the aggressor. Can lash with its tail, bite and use its claws in defence.
- Herbivorous, predominantly feeding on green leafy plants, flowers and fruits. Juveniles, with higher need for protein, are likely to eat eggs and insects.
- Feeling water, being in moist, wet places, or having water run over hind legs and tail triggers defecation in iguanas.
- Oviparous; 20–70 eggs per clutch.
- No parental care, apart from defending the nesting burrow during excavation.
- Juveniles stay in familial groups for the first year of their lives. Males in these groups often use their own bodies to shield and protect females from predators and it appears to be the only species of reptile that does this.
- Among the most popular reptile pets in the United States.

## Colour Alteration
'Although called green iguanas, these animals are actually variable in colour. The adults become more uniform in colour with age, whereas the young may appear more blotchy or banded between green and brown. Colour of an individual may also vary based upon its mood, temperature, health, or social status. Such colour alteration may aide these animals in thermoregulation. In the morning, while

body temperature is low, skin colour will be darker, helping the lizard to absorb heat from sunlight.

'However, as the hot mid-day sun radiates upon them, these animals become lighter or paler, helping to reflect the sunrays and minimizing the heat absorbed. Active dominant iguanas usually have a darker colour than lower-ranked iguanas living the same environment. Most colour variation seen in this species is exhibited by males and may be attributed in part to sex steroids. Six to 8 weeks prior to and during courtship, males may acquire a bright orange or gold hue, although colouration is still related to dominance status. Mature females, for the most part, retain their green colouring.' [Animal Diversity Web]

## Behaviour & Temperament

'In the wild, most disputes between iguanas take place over basking sites. There is usually adequate food for these herbivorous lizards, but good perches are limited. Basking is important for increasing body temperature and aiding digestion.

'During the breeding season, males become territorial and display head bobbing, dewlap extension, and colour changes. They will bite at each other. Injuries in the wild are rare, as there is ample space for males to retreat when threatened. However, in captivity where space is limited, injuries are more common. Females may also display some of these behaviours when nesting sites are limited.

'Green iguanas may travel considerable distances in several cases. Females migrate to the same nesting site for several years in a row, then travel back to their home territory once their eggs are laid. Hatchlings may disperse over large distances as well.

'When frightened, an iguana will usually freeze or hide. If caught, twisting and rotating around or tail whipping may occur. Like many other lizards, iguanas can autotomatise, or drop off part of their tail. This gives them a chance to escape before their predator figures out what is going on. A new tail will sprout from the autotomatised spot and regrow within a year, though not to the length it was before.

'These animals are known to use visual signals, such as head bobbing and dewlap extension, as means of communicating with rivals. In extreme cases, physical contact is involved in altercations. In addition, males scent mark females as well as branches. Hissing, which is a form of auditory communication, sometimes occurs.

'One of the best methods for iguanas to avoid predation is their cryptic colouration. Because they look like so much of their green environment, they can remain immobile when a predator has been spotted and remain unnoticed themselves. Young iguanas may be found in small groups and use the "selfish-herd" or "more eyes are better" strategy to avoid predators. Iguanas prefer to bask in tree limbs that overhang water so when threatened by a predator they can dive into the water and swim swiftly away. In addition to these strategies for avoiding predation, green iguanas are able to shed a large portion of their tail, thus distracting predators and allowing the "rest" of the animal to escape.' [Animal Diversity Web]

## Amusing, Brash, Aggressive

At the conclusion of the 1980s Los Angeles denizen Henry Schiff renamed himself 'Henry Lizardlover' because he 'decided to go all the way to having a house full of lizards by collecting iguanas, to keep in my home as pets.' When he was growing up, other kids called him Lizard Boy because he liked to catch them. Since the 1980s he likes to keep them, maintaining 'a group averaging 30 to 50 iguanas' in his house ['plenty of room']. Lizards became more and more of a fascination for him, resulting in a 'total commitment to them'. As time went on, he 'was living and breathing lizards,' incorporating them in all his activities. Lizards became a major part of his life, one favourite pet iguana, named Hasbro, sharing his bed at night for over 14 years and others accompanying him wherever he would go.

Raising hundreds of iguanas throughout the years granted Henry Lizardlover 'a rare opportunity for a broad view into their behaviour' . . . and 'to recognise truly human-like character in them.' The author of *The Iguana Owner's Manual*, 1993, 'the first book that honestly reveals who the lizard is and what's on his mind,' the iguana aficionado maintains a website, where he portrays iguanas thus:

'There is generally a very classic difference in personality between the male and female iguana. The female is clearly more timid, shy, sensitive-scared, inde-pendent, and less adventurous, usually. The male is generally the opposite. The male's *bold assertiveness and sense for adventure* is not without various drawbacks or even serious potential problems. Each male iguana will manifest his charac-teristics differently, which determines whether he will be a heavenly thrill or a pet out of hell.

'The more dominant male is bold, arrogant and more active. The male has a passion for adventure, he wants to cruise throughout the house or yard and challenge, conquer, possess, mate or whatever to satisfy his big male ego. He is definitely the most interesting and fun to watch but will require more patience to supervise the trooper that he is. Guaranteed to intrigue, fascinate and amuse anyone, anywhere, anytime.

'Example: Hasbro, "the perfect pet": This *prince of primal power* walks around the house like he owns the place. Then bobs his head every 2 or 3 feet and also when he succeeds to climb on to something like a chair, table or me. He will bob and shake his head as a "Hey, I'm the king, I'm the Master, My territory" as I offer him food and whenever I come into his view. Just like a gorilla that pounds his chest. He is a macho man and commands respect as he maintains his pompous attitude anywhere I take him.

'This dominator will want to watch and stand guard over his territory during the day. Many other male iguanas just want to relax and enjoy living in a safe environment, but a dominant male tends to have a serious mission and to be on a fulltime guard for competition. Some males will only become warriors if another male comes into their territory, but the dominant male will be active on a mission to search out and destroy other males.'

Regarding the matter of aggression in iguanas, Henry warns that male iguanas in breeding season *attack mood and mode* 'can inflict truly serious and multiple, deep flesh wounds if given the opportunity.' Attacks come fast and powerful, 'their sensitivity and paranoia toward male iguana competition is brought to a fever pitch, they seek out other males, will travel to other territory to do battle. They get completely charged up and crazed about male iguana competition, and when only humans are all they see, then humans are male iguanas to them.'

We are informed 'not to confront him or [to] get in his attack range while he is showing any signs of aggressive body language. In most cases, the mood only lasts about 2 to 4 months, then the mood subsides, and the iguana gets back to his normal non-aggressive sweet lovable self. . . . Placing the iguana in a completely strange and new environment such as another room of the house or another house or place altogether, which takes him out of his area of familiarity, will be a shock and tends to intimidate him, makes him feel less confident, which often cancels his aggression right away.'

## Circling to a Clash

Interactions among males of some large-bodied iguanas can be quite impressive. 'Male green iguanas [*Iguana iguana*] initially display at each other with a series of rapid head bobs. Once sex is established based on response to this signal, a male struts in a circle around the challenging male with his large dewlap fully erected and body expanded to give the impression of maximum size. The males may hiss, lash their tails, and continue to bob their heads. As males circle, the diameter of the circle of interaction becomes smaller and smaller and the interaction intensifies proportionally, with pushing and leaning now being interspersed with head bobs and possibly tail twitching. If the interaction continues to escalate, which becomes more likely the more similar in size the 2 males are, one male will attempt to mount the other and bite it on top of its neck or back. If this male succeeds in inflicting a bite, it pulls back, causing the opponent to rapidly flee. The defeated male usually darkens in colour. If the mounting male is thwarted before biting, the escalating interaction is repeated until one male wins.' [Pianka & Vitt, 2006]

## Dominators & the Dominated

'Our own research on green iguanas, Iguana iguana, at the San Diego Zoo has taught us much about how dominance hierarchies are established and maintained in this species. Among adult green iguanas inhabiting a large outdoor exhibit, we found that *high social rank was associated with elevated levels of testosterone*, highly developed jaw musculature and a greater incidence of head-bob display.

'Dominant males won more aggressive encounters and spent more time patrolling a centrally located rock where most of the females preferred to bask. In addition, top-ranking males possessed greatly enlarged femoral glands compared to subordinate males. Presumably, dominant males that produce more secretions can scent mark their home ranges more effectively and as a result may be better able to attract females and defend them from rival males.

'Among juvenile male green iguanas, dominance relationships are established surprisingly early in development. We investigated the effect of limited resources on the establishment of dominance hierarchies by housing a group of 10-day-old hatchlings such that the available heat resources were restricted to only 10% of the perches in the enclosure. A second group was housed in a similar enclosure, but with the available heat spread out more evenly over 50% of the perch sites. In the group with limited heat resources, a dominance hierarchy developed among the males within the first month of life.

'Approximately a third of the males *monopolised* all of the heated perches, denying access to the remaining individuals. By the end of the study, the socially dominant males had grown significantly larger than their subordinate counterparts. In the group without limited heat resources, all males grew at approximately the same rate. Interestingly, hatchling females were not excluded from heat resources by either males or by each other and their growth rates remained unaffected by the distribution of heat resources within the enclosure.

'It appears that the presence of dominant adults can profoundly affect the growth and health of juvenile green iguanas. For one year, a group of juvenile males at the zoo was exposed to the sight of an adult female, a second group was exposed to both the sight and smell of an adult female, a third group was exposed to the sight of an adult male, and a 4th group was exposed to both the sight and smell of an adult male. Juvenile males continuously exposed to chemical and visual signals from adult males showed signs of chronic stress, incl. reduced growth rates, lower testosterone levels, higher corticosterone levels, and fewer head-bob displays. Although the sight of an adult male alone was sufficient to induce some of these effects, visual and chemical signals appeared to act in concert to influence the behaviour and physiology of juveniles.' [Alberts, 1993]

### Third Eye
'Green iguanas have a white photo-sensory organ on the top of their heads called the parietal eye [also called third eye, pineal eye or pineal gland], in contrast to most other lizards, which have lost it. This "eye" does not function the same way as a normal eye does, as it has only a rudimentary retina and lens and cannot form images. It is, however, sensitive to changes in light and dark and can detect movement. This helps the iguana when being stalked by predators from above.' [Wikipedia]

### Guts to Grow
Baby green iguanas spend the first 3 months of their lives feeding and sunning on the lower 30 feet of vegetation. Older iguanas sun above them. While they are at these lower levels, the younger iguanas consume greenery that has been inoculated with the faeces of the older iguanas in the upper story. During these months, the younger iguanas develop the same intestinal flora as the adults. The bacteria help digest the low-quality and hard to process vegetarian only diet the young lizards consume throughout the rest of their lives. Baby iguanas kept in

captivity [and not allowed to consume inoculated leaves] do not develop the intestinal flora and grow more slowly than their wild brethren. After 3 months, the now-larger-grown baby green iguanas move to higher perches in the vegetation.

### The Iguana's Fundamental Nature

Henry Lizardlover raises and loves iguanas since 1982. In his *Iguana Owner's Manual* he elaborates in-depth on the fundamental nature of this reptile, 'faithfully embracing the spirit of iguana.' While conceding that 'every iguana is an individual, similar yet different,' he condenses its essence simply as coming down to 'an emotional child [and always will be]'.

'When people get an iguana,' the *Manual* clarifies, 'they usually assume it will react in a similar manner as other pets [cats, dogs, birds] whereas if you show it kindness [petting and handling] it will like you. Cats, dogs, and even birds . . . begin the pet owner relationship in a rather neutral and receptive mode, being "neutral," neither considering you an enemy [to be feared] or friend and simply await the treatment you give them and act accordingly. . . .

'The iguana . . . is not always starting from this neutral and receptive attitude; he usually is in a position of fear, he is scared, scared, scared, usually. The iguana is not viewing his new owner with a "fair" or unbiased viewpoint; he starts off convinced that people will harm him. That means that an iguana is much more sensitive and more worried about his safety than a dog or cat would be. . . . Essentially, the iguana is quite the "same" as other earth creatures. He wants to breathe, eat his veggies, get some sun, have a safe place to sleep and live another day in the busy jungle. He clings to life and is *very, very afraid of being hurt.* . . .

'Once the iguana establishes an inner feeling of confidence, safety and security, the rest comes easy. . . . The iguana has the potential to live comfortably with friendly animals and humans when given the opportunity in the right situation. He is however basically a very *sensitive creature that can be easily overwhelmed and live in fear or madness*. If he does not surrender [let go] of the fear and develop an attitude in some degree of trust [faith in his safety], he will most certainly be a miserable unhappy pet. . . .

'It is clear that the iguana is very aware and perceptive of everything in his environment. . . . He is always watching and evaluating every detail in the environment. . . . He will notice changes and be very careful and suspicious. . . . The iguana's ability to recognise friendly or safe creatures is the most important thing. . . . The iguana is very able to differentiate new things or new animals and adjust if necessary as long as no harm comes to him. . . .

'He is a passive observer . . . always very alert, very aware. Even during sleep he is somewhat alert to the noise of approaching creatures. . . . He knows where his personal resting place is located in the house. He will develop regular routines and be very predictable. . . . He will behave so reasonably and sane that you think he is a person that only looks like a lizard.' [Lizardlover, 1993]

### Materia Medica

• No symptoms.

# LACERTA AGILIS

## Systematics
- Scientific name: Lacerta agilis [L., 1758].
- Synonyms: Lacerta stirpium [Ménètries]. Lacerta paradoxa [Bedriaga, 1886].
- Common name: Sand lizard.
- Family: Lacertidae.

## Biological Profile
- Fast-moving, terrestrial lizard to 25 cm long. Colouration varies between subspecies and populations; back and sides grey-brown or brownish and flanks sometimes strewn with dark patches with light centres. Belly whitish-grey with small blackish speckles. Individuals may show various patterns of broken stripes and spots. Males show a vivid grass green colouration along the flanks in the mating season.
- Range: Europe [but absent from most of SW Europe] and Asia into Mongolia.
- Habitat: Sandy habitats, coastal dunes, heathlands. Hibernates in winter.
- Accomplished burrower in order to create a safe refuge and also to bury eggs at sun exposed bare batches of sand. Begins its excavation with shovel-like movements of the head and then follows up with one forearm at a time, making surprisingly rapid progress.
- Insectivorous [incl. spiders and other arthropods]. Active forager. Cannibalism does occur.
- Oviparous; 4–18 eggs per clutch.
- Ten recognized subspecies [agilis, argus, boemica, bosnica, brevicaudata, chersonensis, exigua, grusinica, ioriensis, mzymtensis].

## Behaviour & Temperament
'Male sand lizards emerge from their hibernation burrows in late February to mid-March and are joined by the females around 2 weeks later. The largest males are the last of the males to emerge and smaller males are often displaced from territories as a result. Cooler air temperatures at this time of year necessitate basking for longer periods. This combined with the comparative lack of ground cover in early spring causes the lizards to be particularly vulnerable to predation at this time. The majority of the lizard's time at this time of the year is spent basking or in refuge. Hunting sorties at this time are short-lived and seldom successful, although opportunities to grab passing food when basking are quickly taken advantage of.

'As the year and heat levels progress, less time is spent basking and by early April most mature males having sloughed adopt their gaudy breeding attire. It is at this point that sand lizards are easily one of the most colourful of British fauna. Mid-April finds male sand lizards especially preoccupied with mating and feeding. Note that mating precludes feeding in that last sentence. The author grew up on the southern heaths of England and spent many happy hours watching sand lizards. Some males visibly lost condition due to the vigour and stress of breeding and would undoubtedly have benefited from a good feed.

'Male sand lizards whilst preoccupied with patrolling, displaying to rival males and looking for females have in the past chased one another across the author's walking boots on more than one occasion. Male sand lizards often meet during the breeding season whilst patrolling overlapping routes. On such occasions, a series of warning displays are observed. Rising up on the forelimbs whilst sometimes arching the back and almost always puffing out the neck all combine to make the animal appear larger and more intimidating. Often the mouth gapes wide open and the tail almost always twitches from side to side. Invariably the situation progresses no further other than one animal vacating and the "victor" either viewing the departure or following this up by pursuing the retreating animal for a distance [often across the observer's walking boots!].

'On occasion the situation can progress to violence. If the threat display is not heeded and a closer approach is made [i.e. to within a few centimeters] then surprisingly loud hissing is employed, no doubt brought about by sudden expulsion of air from the lungs. Lunging and butting the head and neck region of the opponent then follows, until one or other of the combatants succeeds in grasping the head, neck or base of tail of the other in his jaws and then tossing the animal to one side. On every occasion the animal, which was thrown to one side, wandered rather drunkenly off. On 3 separate occasions however the author has witnessed evenly matched males combating which resulted in a grappling stalemate for about 15 seconds or more, and on at least 2 occasions visible war wounds on both combatants. On 1 or 2 occasions, female sand lizards were in the vicinity and appeared to pay absolutely no attention to the proceedings whatsoever.' [West Glamorgan Amphibian and Reptile Group; www.swwarg.co.uk]

## MATERIA MEDICA LACERTA AGILIS

### Sources
1 Clinical observations Mangialavori [Italy].

### Symptoms
∞ Busy.
∞ Fear of reptiles.
∞ Before menses <.
∞ Constipation < before menses.
∞ Heat soles of feet, uncovers them.

All other symptoms listed in repertories for Lacerta agilis are *misapplied*.

1 Three symptoms come from Stapf's Archiv, 1834, but are unspecified as to the species of lizard: Large vesicles under the tongue. Moist, white eruption in several parts of the body, especially on the inner canthus of the eye. Ulcerated places on the female genitals.
2 Then there are effects observed by Baldini on himself from swallowing 4 *green lizards* [Lacerta *viridis*] one shortly after the other [minus their heads, tails and

entrails]. Small wonder this resulted in an upset stomach. Baldini held a thermometer against the pit of his stomach in order to measure differences in temperature in addition to counting his pulse.

Baldini's symptoms included – [After the first lizard] Violent eructations and some distress in the stomach. Temperature rising from 26° to 32°C. Pulse from 70 rising to 80. [After the second lizard] Immediately, nausea and a feeling of weight in the stomach. Temperature 34°C, falling to 26°C after one hour. Pulse 80, falling to 66 in one hour. [Two more lizards later] Great nausea, violent pressure in stomach. Temperature 6°C up, pulse 8 beats up. After one hour pain in intestines, relieved by frequently drinking water and vinegar. Constant accumulation of saliva in the mouth. Heavy sweating the subsequent night, after which all symptoms disappeared.

His suffering notwithstanding, can this be called a proving? In case we want to include Baldini's symptoms, they should be listed under *Lacerta viridis*, European green lizard.

3 The final source of the Lacerta agilis supposed materia medica is even more doubtful. It concerns the bite by a so-called 'large, green spotted lizard' in Maine, USA, and the consequent death of the victim, a 13-year old girl, 3 weeks after the bite. While the culprit is anybody's guess, one thing is certain: it could not have been the European sand lizard, Lacerta agilis.

The unfortunate girl suffered the following symptoms [Allen's Encyclopedia, Vol. 10 p. 570]:

'Numbness of the foot, as though it had been deprived of sensation by cording the ankle, and that occasional prickling that occurs on the return of circulation; numbness continued spreading upward; the whole limb became severely swollen, with most excruciating pain on the slightest motion. Inflammatory blush over the direction of the lymphatics [second day]. The muscles of the neck and jaw of that side were rigid and tender to touch. Much difficulty in swallowing. Occasional delirium, particularly the first week. Wonderfully increased mental acumen during her intervals of reason. Whole left side paralysed. The limbs were spotted a short time before death, which occurred on the 21st day.'

Mind, Industrious [mania for work], a symptom credited to Boericke appears to be a misinterpretation of 'Increased mental acumen' [Boericke, p. 323].

# LACERTA MURALIS

## Systematics
- Scientific name: Lacerta muralis [Laurenti, 1768].
- Synonyms: Seps muralis [Laurenti, 1768]. Lacertus terrestris [Garsault, 1764]. Lacerta muralis [Duméril & Bibron, 1839].
- Common name: Common wall lizard.
- Family: Lacertidae.

## Biological Profile

- Small, slender terrestrial lizard with elongated, pointed head and very long tail [2/3 of overall length]. Body colouration generally brownish or greyish; may occasionally be tinged with green. Pattern highly variable: prominent black spots, mottling or stripes. Belly with reddish, pink, or orangish rectangular scales. Dark brown stripe on flanks that continues from ear opening to eyes. Up to 20 cm in overall length.
- Range: Europe, except for northern parts. Northern Africa. Introduced in Canada [British Columbia], USA and England.
- Habitat: Rocky environments, incl. boulders, rocks, walls, and urban settings. Has established strong populations in human settlements and big cities.
- Well adapted to cool temperature climates.
- Diurnal.
- Extremely fast moving, lively and agile.
- Territorial, aggressive.
- Insectivorous.
- Oviparous; 2–10 eggs per clutch.
- Thirteen recognized subspecies [albanica, appenninica, baldasseronii, beccarii, breviceps, brongniardii, colosii, maculiventris, marcuccii, muralis, nigroventris, sammichelii, tinettoi].

## Testosterone

- Increasing levels of testosterone in males bolster conspicuous colouration, stimulate territoriality and trigger antagonistic interactions among rivals. By defending a territory a male gets exclusive access to females, since females never copulate with non-territorial males.
- 'Chemosensory tests showed that female conspecifics tongue flick at a higher rate and more quickly towards the secretion of males with experimentally increased testosterone levels than towards the secretion of control males, suggesting that females can discriminate between males with dissimilar testosterone levels based on chemical cues of secretion alone.' [Baeckens, 2016]

## Materia Medica

- No symptoms.

# LACERTA VIVIPARA

## Systematics

- Scientific name: Zootoca vivipara [Lichtenstein, 1823].
- Synonyms: Lacerta vivipara [Jacquin, 1787]. Lacertus cinereus [Lacépède, 1788].
- Common names: Viviparous lizard. Common lizard.
- Family: Lacertidae.

## Biological Profile

- Fast-moving, terrestrial lizard to 20 cm long, with short limbs and a rather round head. Colouration very variable. Dorsal colouration grey brown to dark brown, often with a darker streak that may run the entire length of the spine. A continuous dark band bordered by light yellow or white spots is often seen on either side of the body. Belly egg yolk yellow to orange spotted with black in males, yellowish-grey in females. Throat white, sometimes blue.
- Range: Europe and Asia; lives farther north than any other reptile species.
- Habitat: Lives at high elevations in the southern parts of its distribution range, occurring as high as 3,000 m in the Alps, living in damp places or near water, incl. meadows, swamps, by brooks and in damp forests. In northern part of range, also found in lowlands, where it occurs in drier environments, incl. open woodland, meadows, moorland, heathland, fens, dunes, rocks, roadsides, hedgerows and gardens.
- Hibernates in winter.
- Insectivorous.
- Ovoviviparous; 3–11 live young per litter.
- Oviparous in the extreme southwest portion of its range.
- Four recognized subspecies [louislantzi, pannonica, vivipara, carniolica].

## Quicksilvery Quick

'It is generally conceded that the specific name Agilis, given to the sand lizard, is a rather unfair inference that it is the more active of the 2. Nimble it undoubtedly is; but *in alertness, swiftness and agility, the little Vivipara can scarcely find a rival.* Supple as if they were boneless, if you do succeed in catching one, to retain it in your hand without risk of injury is almost impossible. Secure, as one thinks, in the tightly closed hand, it finds escape where least expected. If its head be thumbwards, it will turn in some marvellous fashion and make instantaneous exit at the 4th finger, or between the fingers, however close together.

'As well try to manage and restrain a stream of quicksilver. And the Viviparas are *more shy of being touched* than the sand lizards, which will remain in the hand in seeming enjoyment as long as you please to keep them there. One of my 5 Viviparas, more elusive than the rest and much disliking to be handled, would watch me through the glass, and if she saw me coming would disappear among the moss, when to find her was impossible, unless spray by spray were taken out; so swiftly did she flit among it, without disturbing a feather.

'Sometimes you might discern one bright eye on the lookout for the enemy; eye and owner vanishing utterly at a hand ever so cautiously approaching. I half suspected sometimes as much frolic as fear in this game of hide-and-seek. Her bird-like look and her manner of eyeing one with her head on one side gained for her the name of "Birdie." Many physiological features in both lizards, esp. in the smaller species, disclose their relationship to birds. . . .

'And as regards intelligence, the lizards rank much higher than the Batrachians [amphibians], esp. the newts. Their manner of watching and of hiding, even of biting, as an instinct of self-preservation, and afterwards ceasing to do this, as if having gained experience, indicates something nearer to reason than frogs and salamanders ever display. To hurry-skurry away and hide is the only impulse of the latter, who on no provocation attempt to bite. Nor must it be forgotten that the little Vivipara bit and hung on to my finger with its tiny jaws as persistently as its larger relative, until it ceased to be alarmed at humanity generally.' [Hopley, 1888]

## Desperate Haste

'Reptiles are frequently described as being sluggish and slow of movement. This is certainly not true of many lizards and is very wide of the mark in the case of the viviparous lizard. A more difficult creature to catch it would be hard to mention. The pace at which one of these creatures will cross a piece of open ground to the nearest cover is simply astonishing and almost defies capture by the hand.

'The observer sees the lizard *first here, then there, and then not at all*, and it is a hundred to one against finding it, unless it has sought the shelter of an isolated tuft of grass, from which it may be dislodged. Even then it is very difficult to see the little creature amongst the roots and just as it is exposed and you are about to grasp it, like a flash it darts out and away to another more secure hiding-place. As to attempting to see the individual movements of the limbs it is a sheer impossibility. In fact, all the movements of this lizard are rapid. Feeding is carried out in *desperate haste*, as well as locomotion.

'During the hot summer months they may be seen sunning themselves in the open, esp. the gravid females, at which time, of course, their movements are more deliberate and less speedy, and therefore they are at this period more easily captured.

'J.A. thus describes some habits of this lizard [Newcastle Weekly Chronicle, 1881]: "Some years ago I remember being on a bird-nesting excursion in Belford Cragg. Seeing a bird flying about with food in its mouth, I concealed myself up the branches of a tall, thick holly-bush, and there waited quietly to see where the bird would go to feed its young. I had not sat more than a few minutes, when a small lizard crept out from the side of a stone and laid itself quietly down to bask in the sun's rays. It was presently joined by a second, and then a third, fourth and fifth. I watched the motions of these little creatures for nearly an hour, and so interesting and amusing were they that I forgot to observe what became of the bird with the 'bait' in its mouth.

'Sometimes they would lie motionless, separated from each other by a few yards; then suddenly one would dart swiftly towards his neighbour, who, in turn, with equal agility, would avoid the attack; then a general darting to and fro, helter-skelter, would occur amongst the lot. Suddenly there was a pause, and all would lie still; then one would dart at some insect, secure it, and resume his vigils; then in a moment all was commotion again, a general darting here and there in all directions.

'Could not I secure one of these little lizards, thought I. But how was it to be done? The slightest movement on my part alarmed the whole and they were all out of sight in an instant. In a short time they would return and resume their manoeuvres. I thought the best way to secure one was to overturn the stones under which they had taken shelter. Accordingly I began to turn over first one stone and then another, and after seeking for a considerable time, and turning over several stones under which I felt sure one at least had taken shelter, I was compelled to give up the search in despair, without getting a glimpse of the animals again.

'Such is the capacity of the lizard for keeping out of sight that it is next to impossible to capture it when once it gets among rough stones, grass, or heath; and the rapidity with which it darts about on a surface of loose sand can only be likened to the movements of a dragon-fly on a pool of water."' [Leighton, 1903]

### Materia Medica
- No symptoms.

# POGONA VITTICEPS

### Systematics
- Scientific name: Pogona vitticeps [Ahl, 1926].
- Synonyms: Amphibolurus vitticeps [Ahl, 1926].
- Common names: Central bearded dragon. Inland bearded dragon.
- Family: Agamidae.

### Biological Profile
- Bulky, diurnal lizard up to 60 cm in length, with broad, triangular head, round bodies, stout legs, and robust tails, ranging in colour from dull brown to tan with red or gold highlights.
- Range: Eastern and central Australia.
- Habitat: Great deserts of the interior to the woodlands of the eastern coast.
- Omnivorous; feeding on plant matter [including greens, fruits, flowers], insects, and the occasional small rodent or lizard.
- The social behaviour of bearded dragons includes a full set of body movements, which represents their language. They have actions for dominance, appeasement, playfulness, and competition. When threatened, bearded dragons make a hissing sound similar to a cat.
- Oviparous, up to 24 eggs per clutch.
- Females are known to store sperm and are able to lay many clutches of fertile eggs from one mating.
- Very popular in the pet trade because of their manageable size and pleasant temperament. With their array of social behaviours and inquisitive nature, bearded dragons quickly become endearing to their keepers.

### Behaviour & Temperament
'When intimidated, they flatten their bodies and stand erect with mouth agape. The light-coloured mouth lining, spines bordering the lower jaw and puffed-out blackish beard give a formidable appearance. This defensive display has earned these lizards the common name of "bearded dragon".

'Aggressiveness is shown through body movements when approaching other members of the group. The tip of the tail is slightly curved at the end and the head is bobbed in a rapid motion. Submission is demonstrated by rotating the arms in a full circular motion, which looks like waving. Ritualistic sparring matches take place in which both are in flat postures, with beards and tails up and outward; they circle each other, biting at one another's tail, but usually no damage is done.

'Their ability to change shades from light to dark helps them to regulate body temperature. Colour changes can also depend on emotional state, as well as be used for concealment when threatened. When injured, sick, or dying its back becomes black and its legs pale yellow. Australian desert lizards often make their escape by rising on their hind legs and running bi-pedally. They cannot run as fast as quadrapedally, but it is thought to be a matter of temperature control. They lift their bodies from the hot ground to counter-balance the heat they generate in running. This reduces the amount of heat they take in from the ground and increases the cooling airflow over their bodies.' [website Oakland Zoo]

### Bobbing & Waving

'Beards are not limited to males; the females will show off their beards as well, in a very interactive communication. Indeed, bearded dragons are *very social* animals. They have a rich gestural language, bobbing their heads at one another, gaping their mouths, flattening their bodies and tilting as they circle one another ["see how big I am!"], swishing their tails, using their tongue to check each other or their environment out, etc.

'They even have a variety of submissive gestures. For instance, both sexes will raise one arm and hold it stationary or slowly wave it in circles, evidently to signal "hey, its ME, stop harassing me, I'm harmless!" They rapidly establish a hierarchy and *adapt to their caretakers*, so the more extreme aggressive gestures become rare in captivity [unless you give them new territory to conquer]. They are very curious, and love being let out to investigate.

'Some dragons can recognise humans' clumsy attempts at their body language. My male adolescents become excited if I extend my hand with fingers held together and pointed, to mimic a dragonhead, and then "bob" my mock dragon-head. They will often bob right back. However, they will become quiet and assume a satisfied "I am dominant" pose if I then circle my thumb at them to mimic submission.

'I initially suspected that my dragons responded to my signals only because I had trained them. I tested this hypothesis during a visit to the San Diego Zoo, which has a large outdoor habitat for bearded dragons. During my visit, several dragons were sunning themselves and ignoring human gawkers. After surreptitiously assuring myself that no one was looking, I began a "bobbing" display with my hand. Instantly, dragonheads turned toward me. The closest dragon ran a few steps toward me and bobbed his head. I bobbed in return. He advanced and bobbed more emphatically. I bobbed back. He ran closer and bobbed with such amplitude that his chin hit the ground. I pointed my hand somewhat downward and slowly moved my thumb in a circle. He bobbed once [which I translated as a "So, there!" gesture], turned sideways to me and raised his head in the "I am supreme!" gesture. I concluded that I can speak dragon! Well, at least in pidgin form.

'One of the joys of caring for this species is its *mellow but interactive nature*. Beardeds appear to communicate with us, at least in broad terms. Long, piercing stares are apparently designed to transmit the mental message "feed me crickets . . . crickets . . . crickets. . . ." Although they will interact with you, they show their full social repertoire only to one another, an argument for keeping more than one dragon. If your dragon has a buddy, you will be able to enjoy a full behavioural series as they set up and maintain a dominance hierarchy. You will see "lizard stacks" as they pile up on one another beneath their basking light. If you have a male and female, you will see mating displays [and mating]. Some- times however, interactions become aggressive and such individuals require separate quarters. If you have 2 dragons together and one stops eating, likely he has been intimidated and will require special feeding or even different quarters. Do not house dragons together if they differ dramatically in size. One could furnish lunch for the other.' [Tosney, 2004]

## Materia Medica
- No symptoms.

# SCELOPORUS OCCIDENTALIS

## Systematics
- Scientific name: Sceloporus occidentalis [Baird & Girard, 1842].
- Common names: Western fence lizard. Pacific blue-bellied lizard.
- Family: Phrynosomatidae [formerly included in Iguanidae].

## Biological Profile
- Medium-sized lizard to 21 cm long with overlapping, pointed ['spiny'] scales on back and limbs. Total length comprised of a tail that is approximately 1.5 times the snout-vent length. Will readily lose its tail.
- Dorsal ground colouration usually some shade of grey, tan or brown; some individuals are black. Can lighten or darken the ground colour to some degree. Ground colour broken by a series of wavy dark transverse lines or blotches. Females and juveniles often a lighter colour than males. Males have blue patches on underarms, throats and underside of abdomen.
- Range: W USA, NW Mexico.
- Occupies a variety of habitats that usually have a vertical component; avoids dense, moist forests and low flat desert valleys. Most often found in open areas on rocks, logs, and trees.
- Preys on beetles, flies, caterpillars, ants, other insects, and spiders.
- Both males and females defend their hibernation area, food supplies and home range throughout the year; re-establishing home territory in the same area year

after year during the spring [after hibernation]. Seasonal home range is generally much less than 0.01 ha. Both genders will establish dominance over their territory from other lizards by posturing and posting chemical cues or scent marks.

- Inactive during cold weather.
- Oviparous; 3–17 eggs per clutch.
- In times of stress, such as food and water shortages, western fence lizards secrete *glucocorticoids*. These hormones help it to survive by affecting the catabolism of fats and metabolic rate.
- Five recognized subspecies [biseriatus, bocourtii, longipes, occidentalis, taylori].

## Mating & Breeding

'During the breeding season males will sit atop their territory to both fend off other males and to attract females. The lizards begin to mate their second year, the males will do what looks like a rhythmic set of pushups to attract mates. Females are usually closer to the ground and harder to spot than males. Once ready to mate she will appear and the male will vertically flatten his body to display his brilliant blue colours.

'He then holds the female's neck in his jaws while mating commences. If the female changes her mind during copulation she turns on her back and kicks the male off with all 4 legs. During mating the normally tan to brown dorsal scales on the male will turn a brilliant blue. At present it is unknown if the couple is monogamous during the breeding season.

'To assure species success the female will have 2 to 3 clutches per breeding season. She will expend more energy in the present season in case of her death before the next. Her first clutch will have the largest egg size and the final the smallest. To compensate for the difference in egg size the female will expend more energy on the care of the last clutch than the first, to maximize offspring survival. Once the eggs are laid they can range in size from 6 to 14 millimeters, she buries them under shallow moderately moist soil. If consistent with similar species of reptiles the female will bury and *care for the eggs* without assistance from the male. The eggs usually hatch after 2 months in late April to June or July. Clutch sizes can range from 3 to 17 and appear to increase with higher latitudes; larger females typically have more offspring. After a couple of months the infants emerge at around 26 mm in snout-vent length. Most of their growth will occur during their first year of life.' [Bailey, 2001]

## Lyme Disease

When Lyme-disease carrying ticks bite western fence lizards, the lizard's blood produces a chemical that disinfects both the lizard and the tick. Something in the reptile's blood appears to destroy the spirochetes. Test tube experiments found that Lyme disease bacteria bathed in western fence lizard's blood died within 1 hour, while control samples grown in mouse blood lasted 3 days.

'Ticks harbouring the Lyme disease bacterium can be cleansed of the infection when they feed on the blood of the common western fence lizard, UC Berkeley researchers have discovered.

'The scientists . . . speculate the new finding may help explain why Lyme disease is less common in California but epidemic in some northeastern states, where lizards are rare. "Lizards are doing humanity a great service here," says Robert Lane, professor of insect biology at UC Berkeley and principal investigator on the tick project. "The lizard's blood contains a substance – probably a heat-sensitive protein – that kills the Lyme disease spirochete, a kind of bacterium."

'Even better news, the newly discovered protein apparently leaches into the mid-gut of infected nymphal ticks as the tick feeds and destroys spirochetes stored there, permanently cleansing the ticks before they mature to adults. Nymphal ticks feed abundantly on the lizards, and in some habitats in Northern California, lizards are more numerous than rodents. Unlike wood rats and some other wild rodents, western fence lizards [Sceloporus occidentalis] produce the newly discovered "spirochete-killing factor," not yet identified.

'In California, the western black-legged tick is the primary carrier of Borrelia burgdorferi, the bacterium causing Lyme disease. The nymphal tick is an immature stage about the size of a poppy seed. These tiny ticks can do big damage, causing most cases of Lyme disease in the state, where the disease occurs in people who frequent tick-infested areas during the spring and summer.' [Scalise, 1998]

### Materia Medica
- No symptoms.

# VARANUS KOMODOENSIS

### Systematics
- Scientific name: Varanus komodoensis [Ouwens, 1912].
- Common names: Komodo dragon. Komodo monitor. Ora.
- Family: Varanidae.

### Biological Profile
- Largest and heaviest extant lizard, with the smallest range of any large carnivore, males reaching an average length of 3 m, and weighing up to 150 kg.
- Body stout and flattened, with a thick tail that accounts for half of its length. Legs short and squat; feet ending in long, powerful claws. Skin very leathery, grey-brown in colour with red circles spotted here and there. Juveniles have vertical bands of green and black around their neck, which disappear with age.
- Range: Komodo Island, and several other small, adjacent Indonesian islands in the Lesser Sundas, incl. Padar, Flores, Gili Motang, and Rinca.
- Habitat: Mostly open savannahs, occasionally rainforests.
- Carnivorous glutton that will eat most anything, preying mainly upon pigs, deer, goats, and monkeys. Will feed also on carrion and have been known to

attack and kill humans. Can locate a dead or dying animal from a range of up to 9 km, and actively seek it out.

- Oviparous, 2–30 eggs per clutch.
- Mature adults often form pair bonds, a feature rare in lizards.
- Komodo monitors have 2 main activity ranges. A foraging area, which includes a core area where the most foraging activity [and territoriality] is observed, and a scavenging area, which is much larger and much less defended [if at all]. The scavenging areas of many monitors overlap each other and for the most part, confrontations are neutral.
- Adults have no natural enemies; eggs may be dug up and eaten by feral dogs and pigs, while birds and adult komodos eat young dragons.

### Family Varanidae

The Komodo dragon is the largest member of a group of some 65 species of monitor lizards known to exist today across Africa, Asia, and Australasia. About two-thirds of the species are found in Australia and Australasia.

Comprising a single genus, Varanus, the Varanidae family is part of the infra-order Anguimorpha, which also includes alligator lizards, galliwasps, legless lizards, knobby lizards, and the extinct mosasaurs, as well as the Gila monster and Mexican beaded lizard.

'Monitor lizards tend to be robust, diurnal lizards, with elongate necks and non-autotomous tails. They have long, forked tongues, which are used for chemoreception, and their hemipenes are unusually ornate, with paired apical horns. Unlike lizards in all other families, except Lanthanotidae [Lanthanotus genus], varanids have 9 cervical vertebrae, while all other lizards have 8 or less. Notably, some authors consider Lanthanotidae to be a subfamily [Lanthanotinae] of Varanidae. Monitor lizards differ greatly from other lizards in possessing a relatively high metabolic rate for reptiles and several sensory adaptations that benefit the hunting of live prey.

'Recent research indicates that the varanid lizards, including the Komodo dragon, may have very weak venom. Monitor lizards typically are diurnal and almost all monitor lizards are carnivorous; however, they have diverse feeding behaviours, with not all species fully carnivorous predators. Diets of various species of monitor lizards include fruit, invertebrates, mammals, birds, fish, and carrion.

'The genus name Varanus is derived from the Arabic word *waral*, which is translated to English as "monitor." It has been suggested that the occasional habit of varanids to stand on their 2 hind legs and to appear to "monitor" their surroundings led to the original Arabic name. According to legend, these lizards were supposed to warn people that crocodiles were nearby.' [Wikipedia]

Monitor lizards exhibit an extraordinary degree of intelligence and retain what they have learned for long periods.

### Varanid Behaviour

'Monitor lizards adopt characteristic defensive postures, flattening themselves from side to side and extending their gular pouches, presumably to make themselves appear as large as possible. Often they hiss loudly and flick their tongues.

Big species lash their tails like whips with considerable accuracy. Some species stand erect on their hind legs during such displays.

'Male monitor lizards engage in ritualised combat, fighting over females. Larger species wrestle in an upright posture, using their tails for support, grabbing each other with their forelegs and attempting to throw their opponent to the ground. Blood is sometimes drawn in such battles. Smaller species grapple with each other while lying horizontally, legs wrapped around each other as they roll over and over on the ground. The victor then courts the female, first flicking his tongue all over her and then, if she concurs, climbing on top of her and mating by curling the base of his tail beneath hers and inserting 1 of his 2 hemipenis into her cloaca. . . .

'Varanids differ from other lizards in several ways: they have more aerobic capacity and a greater metabolic scope; most range over larger areas; and they appear to be much more intelligent than most lizards. . . .

'After following Komodos in the field using radiotelemetry for over a year, Auffenberg summed up their ambush technique thus: "when these animals decide to attack, nothing can stop them." He followed one lizard for 81 days, during which time it made only 2 verified kills. Auffenberg himself was attacked by a "maverick" *V. komodoensis,* from which he barely escaped by climbing a tree. Juvenile Komodos are highly arboreal, which may protect them from being eaten by their larger, less agile brethren.

Because of their size, large monitor lizards retain body heat in their nocturnal retreats and can emerge the next morning with body temperatures well above ambient air temperatures.' [Painka & Vitt, 2006]

## Medicinal & Other Uses of Monitor Lizards

'A bewildering array of tonics, medicines and potions are made from various parts of the monitor lizards' anatomies. The fat is used to treat deteriorating eyesight and for a variety of other ailments [particularly arthritis, rheumatism, piles and muscular pains]. It is also used as a sexual lubricant. Dried gall bladders are particularly therapeutic, curing heart problems, impotency and liver failure as well as a number of more serious complaints. In North Africa dried heads of monitor lizards are sold to be pulverised and used for the treatment of various external and internal afflictions.

'Amnesiacs in Sri Lanka sometimes prepare a meal of monitor lizard tongues, which is said to restore the memory to its full capacity. Krishnan [1992] reports that a man who had sustained a serious thigh wound as the result of an encounter with a wild boar was treated by his friends in the following manner: thin slices of fresh, Bengal monitor flesh were inserted into the deep wound, which was then bandaged up. The man later claimed that the wound had healed completely within 10 days and exhibited a "surprisingly small" scar.

'As far as I am aware none of the monitors' therapeutic properties have yet been subjected to serious scrutiny. In Sri Lanka it was also believed that a mixture of water monitor fat and flesh and human blood and hair makes a very strong poison when boiled, and that a drop is sufficient to cause the instant death of an enemy. Water monitors were also said to be instrumental in the preparation of the Singalese assassins' most favoured poison, kabara-tel. The raw ingredients [fresh snake venom, arsenic and various herbs] were mixed with water in a human skull and placed on a fire, at 3 corners of which bound water monitors were strategically placed and beaten, so that their hisses would hasten the boiling process and add to the strength of the concoction. The froth from the lizards' lips was added at the last minute, and when an oily scum rose to the surface the dreadful potion was complete. . . .

'A number of cultures were said to allow monitor lizards to feed on their deceased relatives and thus eliminated the need to dispose of corpses by burying or burning them. In the Mergui Archipelago corpses were left on exposed platforms in the forest whilst on Bali the bodies were covered with wicker baskets that kept dogs and monkeys out and allowed the lizards to feed in peace. Such free and nutritious meals attracted large numbers of water monitors, Anderson reports that up to 15 specimens were seen "engaged in a ghastly meal of this kind." . . .

'By far the most conspicuous use of monitor lizards is for their skins. Traditionally used for drumheads and shields, monitor skins are in great demand in the richer parts of the world to make watchstraps, shoes, wallets, handbags and other leather goods. The exquisite patterns of the lizards combined with the durability of their hides make them the most popular family of lizards in the skin trade. Most are caught in the poorer countries of central Africa and SE Asia and are sold in Europe, North America and Japan. . . . Not all monitor lizards are exploited for their skins, in fact the brunt of the trade is borne by just 5 or 6 species.

'A few large monitors will eat people when given the opportunity, but most have to be content with buried corpses that they locate by smell and exhume. In many parts of the world graveyards have to be heavily protected against monitor lizards by packing the ground with clay or coral, or by enclosing the area within a strong fence. Only a few, very large, komodo dragons are capable of catching and consuming a healthy adult, but small children could potentially fall victim to a number of species. Monitors have an unfavourable reputation for stealing animals [usually young chickens] from man in most parts of the world and for this reason are often killed when encountered by farmers. In some cultures monitor lizards are tolerated rather than encouraged. Local customs often forbid the killing of monitor lizards for any reason, but their antisocial behaviour does not necessarily go unpunished.' [Bennett, 1995]

### Almost Alone on an Island
'Komodo is an Indonesian island of approximately 390 km and home to over 2,000 people who are mostly descendants of former convicts once exiled to the island.

'Komodo is part of the Lesser Sunda chain of islands and Komodo National Park. The island is especially known for its native Komodo Dragon – the world's largest living lizard.

'For centuries, local tradition required feeding the dragons by leaving deer parts after a hunt or sacrificing goats. This practice maintained a friendly relationship with the dragons, which can live for more than 50 years and recognise individual humans. Also, taboos strictly forbid hurting the komodos. This is the most likely explanation why they have survived here while becoming extinct elsewhere.

'In 1995 a conservation project led by a US environment protection group began to create a more natural habitat for the komodos, prohibiting the traditional feeding and deer hunting practice by humans. While the deer population consequently stabilised and now provides the komodos with a more natural hunting environment, the komodos often prefer to seek easier prey in the vicinity of human settlements, entering villages and hiding under stilt houses while waiting for the opportunity to snap passing goats or chicken. At the same time, the komodos have become more aggressive towards humans than ever before, sometimes resulting in deadly attacks. Nevertheless, the komodos remain a primary attraction of the island and a major financial contributor to a local tourism industry.

'Komodo Island is known not only for its heritage of convicts and fearsome lizards but also for its rich marine life and exceptional dive locations.' [www.komodo.asia]

### Venom rather than Bacteria

Komodo dragons have around 60 long, highly serrated teeth, which are frequently replaced during its lifetime. These teeth create deep lacerations in prey for entry of the venom, enabling dragons to bite and then release prey, leaving it to bleed to death from the horrific wounds inflicted. A 2009 study by Fry and co-workers has shown that the effectiveness of the komodo dragon bite is a combination of the highly specialised teeth and venom.

The komodo must rely on its venom in enhancing the effects of the deep lacerations induced by its powerful bite for predation since its skull is poorly adapted to resist the erratic forces generated in a sustained bite and hold attack on large prey. Sit-and-wait ambushers or stealthily following well-marked hunting paths, komodos typically use their tooth/venom killing apparatus, causing massive injury, to incapacitate large prey with minimal risk to themselves. While knocking large prey off their feet, it goes straight for the neck in smaller prey, demonstrating a straightforward strategy of battering and ripping apart.

This crash-grip-and-rip technique is the consequence of the structure of the komodo's skull and jaws, as Fry explains. 'Further, its skull is least well adapted to resist torsion. In contrast, the Varanus komodoensis skull is best adapted to resist forces generated in *pulling* on a prey item [or a prey item pulling back]. These results are consistent with observational data showing that V. komodoensis opens wounds by biting and simultaneously pulling on prey by using post-cranial musculature, thereby supplementing relatively weak jaw adductors by recruiting postcranial musculature. Our findings are also in accord with the view that the killing technique of V. komodoensis is broadly similar to that of some sharks and Smilodon fatalis [saber cat].'

The study dismisses the widely accepted theory that prey die from septicaemia caused by pathogenic bacteria living in the dragon's mouth. 'Although wild-caught individuals have been shown to harbour a variety of oral bacteria, no single pathogen was found to be present in all V. komodoensis studied. Moreover, the bacterial species identified were unremarkable in being similar to those identified in the oral cavities of other reptiles or being typical gut contents of the mammalian species on which they prey. . . . Variability in bacterial load within and among individuals . . . makes it exceedingly unlikely that toxic bacteria could reliably induce sepsis in prey animals to the extent that this would become an evolutionarily successful mechanism on which V. komodoensis could rely on for prey capture.'

The effects of venom were tested by Fry's team and found to be similar to that of helodermatid lizards [Heloderma suspectum and H. horridum] and snakes that cause a *severe loss in blood pressure by widening blood vessels*, thereby inducing shock in a victim. These findings may explain the observations that komodo dragon prey become still and unusually quiet soon after being bitten. Bitten prey bleeds profusely, consistent with the team's discovery that the venom was also rich in toxins that prolong bleeding.

Fry's team investigated the biochemical composition and toxicological properties of the dragon's venom and found it to be a mixture of proteins as complex as that of snakes. The properties were defined as coagulopathic, hypotensive, haemorrhagic, and shock-inducing. [Fry, 2009]

### A Full Meal

Solitary animals, most of the social interactions of komodo dragons take place when breeding and feeding. Once a prey has been killed and more individuals show up, a pecking order develops with size dictating who eats first and who eats most, large males having first choice, followed by smaller males and females, and finally the tiniest. No time and very little of the prey is wasted, komodos packing away up to 80% of their body weight in one sitting.

'The muscles of the komodo's jaws and throat allow it to swallow huge chunks of meat with astonishing rapidity. Several movable joints, such as the intra-mandibular hinge, open the lower jaw unusually wide. The stomach expands easily, enabling an adult to consume up to 80% of its own body weight in a single meal, which most likely explains some exaggerated claims for immense weights in captured individuals. Komodos can throw up the contents of their stomachs when threatened to reduce their weight in order to flee.

'Large mammalian carnivores, such as lions, tend to leave 25 to 30% of their kill unconsumed, declining the intestines, hide, skeleton and hooves. Komodos eat much more efficiently, forsaking only about 12% of the prey. They eat bones, hooves and swaths of hide. They also eat intestines, but only after swinging them vigorously to scatter their contents. This behaviour removes faeces from the meal. Because large komodos cannibalise young ones, the young often roll in faecal material, thereby assuming a scent that the large dragons avoid.' [Smithsonian National Zoological Park]

### Meeting at the Dinner Table

According to Janine Benyus, 'mealtimes are the only times when the normally solitary monitors see one another. . . . You'd see males lavishing females with attention while sniping at one another with deadly accuracy. . . . [Monitors] tend to do all their social business here; establishing rank, courting, and even copulating take place around the dinner table!'

With the increasing numbers of monitors joining in, the chances of discord and hostility also increase, making rules of engagement imperative. Order is maintained by proper social conduct including appeasement and deference.

'If a monitor wants to partake of a kill . . . it must shrug off its reluctance and stand shoulder to shoulder with other monitors, even ones much larger than itself. Like dogs and wolves, monitors have a clear-cut ranking system [usually based on size], and small monitors are therefore well-versed in how to appease the larger lizards. Before daring to come near, they traverse the outskirts of the circle with a stately *ritualised walk* that shows that they mean no harm and know their place. With a slow, stiff-legged, stereotyped gait, they throw their body from side to side with exaggerated undulations. They compress their torso laterally, arch their spinal column, and hold their tail up off the ground and straight out behind them. With neck arched and throat inflated, they lower or even cock their head as if tipping their hat to the dominant. Because it's important to hide weaponry, they keep their mouth closed and dare not hiss.

'These appeasement gestures communicate humbleness and the promise that the smaller monitors will wait until the larger one has had its fill of the choicest meat. When the subordinates finally enter the circle, they are *nervously attentive to the dominant's wishes*. The slightest move will cause them to bow out of the way and let the dominant pass. Monitors may perform these same appeasement gestures when confronted by humans.

'When komodo monitors are attacked or handled roughly, they may become so afraid that they *disgorge* their stomach or intestinal contents. This happens most often in the few days after a big meal, when they need a way to slim down before fighting or fleeing.' [Benyus, 1997]

## Materia Medica
• No symptoms.

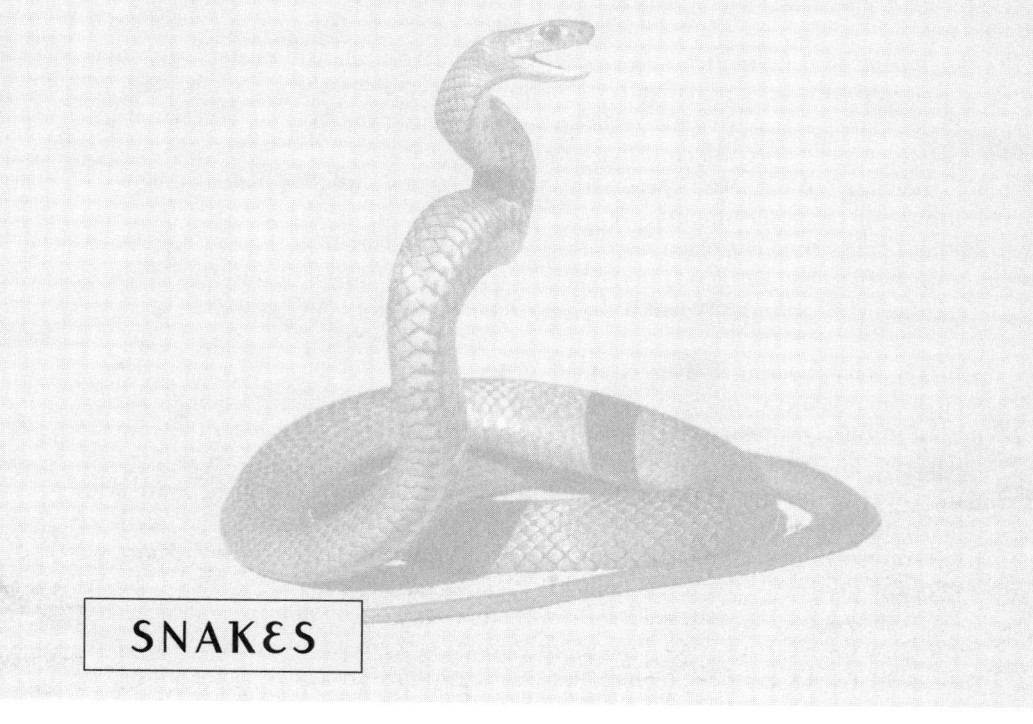

## SNAKES

### BIOLOGICAL PROFILE

- Snakes are entirely limbless and lack both pectoral and pelvic girdles; the latter persists as a vestige in pythons and boas.
- The numerous vertebrae of snakes, shorter and wider than those of legged vertebrates, permit quick lateral undulations through grass and over rough terrain. The ribs increase rigidity of the vertebral column, providing more resistance to lateral stresses. The elevation of the neural spine gives the numerous muscles more leverage.
- In addition to the highly kinetic skull that enables snakes to swallow prey several times their own diameter, snakes differ from lizards in having no movable eyelids and no external ears. Snake eyes are permanently covered with upper and lower transparent eyelids fused together.
- All vipers have a pair of teeth, modified as fangs, on the maxillary bones. The fangs lie in a membranous sheath when the mouth is closed. When a viper strikes, a special muscle and bone lever system erects the fangs as the mouth opens. The fangs are driven into the prey by the thrust, and venom is injected into the wound through a canal in the fangs. A viper immediately releases its prey after the bite and follows it until it is paralysed or dies. Then the snake swallows it whole.
- Most snakes are oviparous species that lay their shelled, elliptical eggs beneath rotten logs, under rocks, or in holes dug in the ground. Most of the remainder,

including all the American pit vipers except the tropical bushmaster, are ovovi-viparous, with eggs that hatch on laying. Very few snakes are viviparous; in these snakes a primitive placenta forms, permitting the exchange of materials between the embryonic and maternal bloodstream.

- Snakes are able to store sperm and can lay several clutches of fertile eggs at long intervals after one mating.
- The 4 traits that are often used to distinguish snakes from lizards are: a tail shorter than the elongated body, lack of external ears, lack of movable eyelids, and a forked tongue. Worm lizards possess all these 4 traits as well.

## Solitary, Non-social & Non-territorial

Snakes are not social animals. They are almost unique in the vertebrate kingdom in not showing any regular form of grouping, and of being essentially non-territorial. Snakes have home ranges but not territories, in contrast to lizards, which are highly territorial. Territoriality implies that an organism will guard and defend its home range against other members of its species. Snakes don't defend their home ranges. Only in times of breeding interactions may occur to determine dominance amongst snakes.

As solitary animals, *snakes associate with others only incidentally*, when necessary for mutual preservation, e.g. joining with others to keep warm in winter. Despite the use of the term 'social' for snakes hibernating in groups or aggregating for purposes other than hibernation or mating, these are not really social activities, as Mattison [2002] points out, 'because the groups may contain snakes of various ages, sexes and species and may occur at almost any time of the year: they do not show any consistent patterns. There appear to be few if any interactions between the individuals of such aggregations although they must obviously tolerate one another at close quarters.'

## Sense Organs

Most snakes have relatively poor vision, the tree-living snakes of the tropical forest being a conspicuous exception. Arboreal snakes possess excellent binocular vision, which they use to track prey through the branches where scent trails would be difficult to follow.

Snakes are deaf in a technical sense, i.e. they lack the ability to detect high frequencies of sound conveyed through the air. They do hear or more correctly feel low frequencies and have a tremendous ability to detect the *most subtle of vibrations* transmitted through sand, leaf-litter, dried grasses and to a lesser degree hard ground.

Most snakes employ the chemical senses rather than vision or vibration detection to hunt their prey. In addition to the usual olfactory areas in the nose, which are not well developed, snakes have a pair of pit-like Jacobson's organs in the roof of the mouth. The forked tongue, flicked through the air, picks up *scent particles*; the tongue is then withdrawn and sampled molecules are delivered to Jacobson's organs. Information is transmitted to the brain, where scents are identified.

Since snakes have no tactile appendages such as limbs, the sense of touch is not so important to them as it is to many other kinds of animals. Despite being sheathed with scales that might be expected to dull their sensitivity, they are *apparently responsive to the slightest external contact*. Dropping particles of sand on rattlesnakes or brushing them with feathers show them to be sensitive even to these light contacts.

## Thermoregulation Through Colour

'Colour also plays a part in heat absorption. It is well known that black objects absorb heat much better than light coloured ones and so snakes living in cooler climates have a tendency to be black or dark in colour. In Australia, for instance, 2 of the most characteristic southern genera, the copperheads, *Austrelaps*, and the tiger snakes, *Notechis*, both of which are represented on Tasmania, have darker than average species, often black, in the southern portions of their ranges.

'This difference is not restricted to entire species, however; sometimes individuals from temperate parts of the range are darker in colour than those from warmer areas, where a species has a wide range. For instances, black examples of the common garter snake, *Thamnophis sirtalis*, are found in isolated colonies towards the northern limits of the species' range, in Canada and northern USA, and European adders, *Vipera berus*, have a similar tendency to be darker in the more northern parts of the species' range, especially in Scandinavia and northern Britain.

'There is growing evidence that snakes living in areas with distinct warm and cool seasons may even change colour slightly in order to improve heat absorption during cool weather and also to prevent overheating during hot weather. So far, only Australian snakes belonging to the Elapidae have been shown to do this, but it is possible that snakes in other parts of the world have evolved similar mechanisms.

'Female Madagascan tree boas, *Sanzinia madagascariensis*, take on a darker, more subdued colouration during pregnancy – again, this is almost certainly due to the need to improve heat absorption, in this instance because the growing embryos will develop more quickly if the female keeps her body warmer and so speed up pregnancy.

'Still on the subject of colour, an unusually high number of snakes have black heads. It seems possible, or even likely, that these snakes expose their heads while keeping the rest of their bodies under cover. The dark pigmentation will help the head to absorb heat, which can then be shunted, via the blood, to the rest of the body. The advantages of this system would be that the brain and the sense organs, practically restricted to the head, would be the first parts of the body to begin operating efficiently, so the snake could be alert to danger before it took the risk of exposing itself completely. Black-headed species are found in many parts of the world.

'Conversely, snakes living under hot conditions are often pale in colour in order to reflect heat [although this may also result from camouflage]. Because they move about in close contact with the substrate, which is often extremely hot, their undersides are also pale in colour and this may also help to prevent them from overheating, allowing them to remain active longer than they would if they had dark undersides.' [Mattison, 2002]

## Parental Care

There is little to no parental care in snakes. Some snake species may engage in guarding their eggs, while the females of a small number of rattlesnake species typically remain with their young after giving birth until they shed and disperse. Female bushmasters brood their eggs until hatching, similar as female ball pythons and other python species, which remain coiled around their clutch for 2 months and refuse to feed during nest attendance.

The myth of mother snakes swallowing their own young to protect them probably started because some snakes will eat the young of other snakes, even their own species, although, usually not their own brood.

## Limbless Locomotion

'John Ruskin remarked "that no scientific book tells us why the reptile is a *serpent*, i.e. serpentine in its motions, and why it cannot go straight." . . . Now, may not the fact that snakes have acquired these ever-varying sinuations arise from their sensitiveness to the slightest, and what would be to other creatures almost impalpable, obstructions in their path? – mere inequalities which in their lazy nature it is easier, they know not why, to circumvent than to surmount; because they can go straight, and do go straight when the way is plain.

'. . . Even in intermediate ages, when travellers and naturalists began to confront fiction with fact, even in the days of Buffon and Lacépède, a serpent was regarded as a living allegory rather than a zoological reality by many intelligent, albeit unscientific persons. Of such was Chateaubriand, in *Genius of Christianity*, whose contemplation of the serpent partook of religious awe. "Everything is mysterious, secret, astonishing in this incomprehensible reptile. His movements differ from those of all other animals. It is impossible to say where his locomotive principle lies, for he has neither fins, nor feet, nor wings; and yet he flits like a shadow, he vanishes as if by magic, he reappears, and is gone again like a light azure vapour on the gleams of a sabre in the dark. Now he curls himself into a circle, and projects a tongue of fire; now standing erect upon the extremity of his tail he moves as if by enchantment. He rolls himself into a ball, rises and falls like a spiral line, gives to his rings the undulations of a wave, twines round the branches of trees, glides under the grass of the meadow, or skims along the surface of the water," and so forth.' [Catherine C. Hopley, Snakes: Curiosities and Wonders of Serpent Life; 1882]

Snakes move through their environment by one or several different means of locomotion: [1] lateral undulation or serpentine movement, is the most frequent gait encountered in snakes; this movement requires a minimum of 3 contact-points. The second method of locomotion is variously known as [2] rectilinear, caterpillar movement, or creeping, and is seen most in large snakes, which have a proportionately greater bulk to move across the ground. The third type is called [3] concertina progression, because the snake moves like a concertina. Requiring a rough surface, this type of movement is almost as common as lateral undulation and some snakes use the 2 in combination. Although it is available to most snakes, few use [4] sidewinding effectively. It has the advantage of speed over flat terrains. A speedy journey over hot sandy unobstructed surfaces ensures a greater chance of survival since overheating can kill a snake in a few minutes. [Russell, 1980]

## Snakes in Motion

'That rivulet of smooth silver – how does it flow, think you? It literally rows on the earth, with every scale for an oar; it bites the dust with the ridges of its body. Watch it when it moves slowly; a wave, but without wind! a current, but with no fall! all the body moving at the same instant, yet some of it to one side, some to another, and some forward, and the rest of the coil backwards, but all with the same calm will and equal way – no contraction, no extension; one soundless, causeless march of sequent rings, a spectral procession of spotted dust, with dissolution in its fangs, dislocation in its coils. Startle it: the winding stream will become a twisted arrow; the wave of poisoned life will lash through the grass like a cast lance. . . . I cannot understand this swift forward motion of serpents. The seizure of prey by the constrictor, though invisibly swift, is quite simple in mechanism; it is simply the return to its coil of an opened watch-spring and is just as instantaneous. But the steady and continuous motion, without a visible fulcrum [for the whole body moves at the same instant, and I have often seen even small snakes glide as fast as I could walk], seems to involve a vibration of the scales quite too rapid to be conceived.' [John Ruskin, The Queen of the Air; 1869]

## The Silent Might of Motionlessness

'He had seen it lying extended, apparently asleep, on the floor of its box, when a rat, which had been placed with it, ran over it, but not quite over it, for, quick as lightning, it had wound itself round the rat's body, coil over coil, like hand grasping hand in squeezing a lemon, until the bones of the constricted animal cracked audibly; then it was dropped, dead and crushed and limp, on to the floor; and the serpent, having revenged the indignity, resumed its interrupted repose. With this lightning-like deadly quickness of motion and the melting mazy evolutions at the other times, he also contrasted its statue-like immobility, when, with head raised high and projecting forwards, it would actually remain for hours at a stretch, its brilliant eyes fixed on some object that had alarmed it or excited its curiosity.

'This power of continuing motionless, with the lifted head projecting forwards, for an indefinite time, is one of the most wonderful of the serpent's muscular feats, and is of the highest importance to the animal both when fascinating its victim and when mimicking some inanimate object, as, for instance, the stem and bud of an aquatic plant; here it is only referred to on account of the effect it produces on the human mind, as enhancing the serpent's strangeness. In this attitude, with the round, unwinking eyes fixed on the beholder's face, the effect may be very curious and uncanny. Ernest Glanville, a South African writer, thus describes his own experience. When a boy he frequently went out into the bush in quest of game, and on one of these solitary excursions he sat down to rest in the shade of a willow on the bank of a shallow stream; sitting there, with cheek resting on his hand, he fell into a boyish reverie. After some time he became aware in a vague way that on the white sandy bottom of the stream there was stretched a long black line that had not been there at first. He continued for some time regarding it without recognising what it was; but all at once, with an inward shock, became fully conscious that he was looking at a large snake.

'Presently, without apparent motion, so softly and silently was it done, the snake reared its head above the surface and held it there, erect and still, with gleaming eyes fixed on me in question of what I was. It flashed upon me then that it would be a good opportunity to test the power of the human eye on a snake, and I set myself the task of looking it down. It was a foolish effort. The bronze head and sinewy neck, about which the water flowed without a ripple, were as if carved in stone, and the cruel unwinking eyes, with the light coming and going in them, appeared to glow the brighter the longer I looked. Gradually there came over me a sensation of sickening fear, which, if I had yielded to it, would have left me powerless to move, but with a cry I leapt up, and, seizing a fallen willow branch, attacked the reptile with a species of fury. . . . Probably the idea of the Icanti originated in a similar experience of some native.

'The Icanti, it must be explained, is a powerful and malignant being that takes the form of a great serpent, and lies at night in some deep dark pool; and should a man incautiously approach and look down into the water he would be held there by the power of the great gleaming eyes, and finally drawn down against his will, powerless and speechless, to disappear forever in the black depths.

'Not less strange than this statue-like immobility of the serpent, the effect of which is increased and made more mysterious by the flickering lambent tongue, suddenly appearing at intervals like lightning playing on the edge of an un-moving cloud, is that kind of progressive motion so even and slow as to be scarcely perceptible.' [W.H. Hudson, 1919]

### Life Persistence

'It is popularly supposed that snakes – rattlers included – are highly tenacious of life. This belief is no doubt founded on the persistence of reflex body movements that continue long after a snake has been fatally injured, or even decapitated. Probably the earliest statement as to the persistence of life in the rattlesnake was made in 1615 when it was reported that the head, if cut off, would live for 10 days or more.

'Although this is an exaggeration, it is true that there is a surprisingly long continuance of body movement in a decapitated snake, and that it is dangerous to handle the head of a venomous snake for some time after it has been separated from the body. Serious accidents have resulted from picking up severed snake heads of fatally injured snakes, and I wish to voice a warning against any care-lessness in this respect.

'Despite their seemingly strong hold on life, as indicated by the perseverance of movement in decapitation tests, rattlers are relatively frail creatures and are easily killed. And though they can be dangerous as long as capacity for movement continues, their backbones are both delicate and vulnerable, so that a smart blow of no great force will produce a fatal injury, although it first it will seem to interfere only with locomotion.' [Klauber, 1982]

## Defensive Behaviour

Most snakes will try to stay camouflaged. They can be very difficult to detect, even though they can be very abundant. When they are detected they may

[1] flee;
[2] 'freeze', remain motionless;
[3] musk, or excrete unpleasantly smelling substances;
[4] gape, or display inside of mouth;
[5] rattle or vibrate tail, or rasp specialised scales on flanks;
[6] hiss, or emit bubbling or popping sound from cloaca;
[7] try to appear larger;
[8] bluff, intimidate;
[9] play dead;
[10] spit;
[11] strike, as a last resort.

Most venomous snakes are *more bluff than bite*; life does not permit a small and fragile species to deliberately seek confrontation with bigger animals that can kill them with 1 footstep. In fact, the Creator has very effectively designed snakes to actively avoid violent confrontations with behaviours and physical traits designed to warn, scare, bluff, hide and evade.

## Feigning Death

An interesting defensive strategy is that of death feigning or thanatosis. Death feigning is not rare in the animal kingdom. Beetles do it, as well as crickets, sandhoppers, spiders, frogs, fish, birds [chickens, vultures, partridges, babblers], mammals [squirrels, foxes, possums], lizards, and snakes. So famous is the possum for pretending to be dead when threatened that the Americans use the phrase 'playing possum' for the strategy, which in a wider sense includes pretending to be injured, unconscious, asleep, or otherwise vulnerable, often to lure an opponent into a vulnerable position himself. Pasteur classified playing dead as a form of self-mimesis, a form of camouflage or mimicry in which the 'mimic' imitates itself in a dead state, such that its pursuer no longer takes notice of it. Death feigning has been acquired in at least 3 and possibly 4 snake lineages: the hognose [Heterodon spp.], the European grass snake [Natrix natrix], the African spitting cobra [Hemachatus haemachatus], and possibly the Egyptian cobra [Naja haje]. The hognose, otherwise known as 'puff adder', 'blow snake' and 'spread adder,' is a big bluffer and the 'possum' among North-American snakes. It is absolutely harmless in spite of its warlike posturing and hissings and can under no conditions be induced to bite.

Anthony [2008] regards hognose snakes as 'possibly nature's greatest Shakespearean actors. Diurnal toad hunters preferring sandy areas where they can turn out prey with their shovel-like snouts, 3 species of *Heterodon* tour an impressive stage show throughout North America. The eastern form, *H. platyrhinos*, has the most polished act. When threatened, the snake hisses loudly, thrashes mightily, and spreads the forepart of its body like a cobra. It may then move on to a savage display of striking – with mouth closed – or proceed directly to the finale: death feigning.'

If necessary, the snake may follow up by vomiting, smearing its own waste over its body, or going into a squirming fit. As a last resort, it will roll onto its back, open its mouth with its tongue dragging, and play dead. If the attacker turns the snake onto its belly, it will promptly roll onto its back again as if it can play dead only when it is upside down. The belly of the western hognose is heavily marked with black. Scientists have guessed that exposing this dark belly when playing dead makes the snake look as if it is not only dead but also decomposed. Once the attacker leaves, the snake turns over and scoots away.

## More Ballet than Battle

Combat behaviour exists in many animal species. It is also common in many snake species. The reasons for the combats can be territories, food sources or breeding mates. Two different kinds of combat behaviour exist, the ritualised combat and the escalated combat. In the escalated combat the participants try to harm or even kill the rival, while the ritualised combat prevents severe damage. The ritualised combat is very common in animals with dangerous 'weapons' like ungulates with horns, and venomous snakes.

Combat behaviour occurs between young, females and animals of both sexes for different resources, but in most cases it is a ritualised combat of sexual mature males for receptive females. While it is said that in love and war everything is allowed, for the combat dances of snakes' strict rules appear to be in play. More ballet than battle, as is evidenced by the following firsthand observation of a performance:

'On a recent Sunday morning, we'd walked for only a few minutes when we suddenly stopped. Two rattlesnakes blocked our way. By detouring slightly, we could have passed them, but in the time it took us to debate a strategy, [better to sneak slowly or whiz by?] we became entranced. The snakes were engaged in some sort of ritual. We quickly sensed we were witnessing something extraordinary, a spectacle none of us had ever encountered.

'The snakes, each about 3 feet long, rose up, perpendicular to the ground. With a foot between them, they held their position, then, as if on cue, pulled farther back, where they remained immobile for a beat. Then they slammed together. They wriggled on the ground, wrestling in the dust, then disengaged. Once again, they faced each other, their linear bodies extended straight up. Separately, but as precisely as synchronised swimmers, they carved a slalom pattern in the air. Advancing and retreating, a crescendo of activity followed by a period of rest, the serpentine ballet was so exquisitely choreographed that "Bolero" might have been playing.

'As we watched, we assigned meaning to the snakes' darts and feints. We crafted a narrative. The broader snake was a male. The other, a female. They were mating, we decided. The sensuality of their instinctual movements, the way they teased each other and collided with what seemed to be passion wasn't that different from human sexuality. How interesting, we thought, that this simpler species flirted, that they were as playful and seductive as if they were a man and a woman in Eden.

'Interesting, but wrong. "What you saw was a combat dance," Russ Smith, curator of reptiles at the Los Angeles Zoo, tells me. "It was 2 males in a territorial spat, or they were struggling to decide who would get to breed a female in the area. In most cases, it's a prelude to mating. It's a competition thing in which the stronger male wins out. The weaker one isn't hurt, other than his pride." [Mimi Avins, 2002]

## Winners Take it All, Losers Take the Fall

Analysing data for 374 species of snakes from 8 families, Richard Shine found that species in which rival males did not engage in physical combat during the mating season generally had females larger than males, whereas males grew at least as large as females – and often larger – in most species of snakes in which male-male combat had been reported.

'Because of their elongate shape, male snakes are apparently unable to forcibly inseminate females, so that selection for large body size to facilitate forcible insemination [a possible selection pressure on male lizards] does not apply to snakes. Instead, selection should favour male abilities to locate receptive females and induce them to copulate. Although these abilities might depend on body size [e.g. if larger males are more mobile, face greater energetic costs in loco-motion, or are less vulnerable to predators during mate-searching movements] male body size is likely to be especially important in taxa that show male-male combat during the mating season. This kind of behaviour has now been recorded for 100 species of snakes [23 boid species from 10 genera; 31 colubrids from 17 genera, 29 elapids from 14 genera and 40 viperids from 10 genera]. Large males are more likely to engage in combat and more likely to win combat bouts, and thereby obtain matings. Hence, straightforward Darwinian theory predicts that male-male combat should impose a selection pressure for large body size in adult males.' [Shine, 1994]

Large males tend to be more successful than small ones. Winners are awarded with copulation; losers loose more than their pride. Winners take it all, losers take the fall. According to Natalie Angier [1995] the dance determines the dunce:

'They are gentlemen jousters, and they keep their venomous fangs tucked away, struggling for hours and often ending their encounter in a draw. But woe to the snake that cannot stand its ground. Among copperheads, a trounced male ends up so demoralised that for days afterward even far punier males, which normally would be loath to pick a fight, will take on the loser and defeat it. Behind the pitiable behaviour of the defeated is a change in hormone levels, notably a rise in the stress hormone, cortisol, and a tumble in the testosterone concentrations that lend male snakes their randy aggression. On occasion, a female copperhead will take advantage of the loser syndrome. Approaching a potential mate, she will mimic another male, rearing up as though ready for battle. Should the mock display terrify the suitor, she will take it as evidence that the male is a loser and reject him as unfit for paternity. Females mate almost exclusively with winners.'

# FROM FALSE NOTION TO DEVOTION

## 1 SNAKE LEGENDS

### Snakes Chase People

If a crowd of 500 adults is asked how many been chased by snakes, at least 200 will raise their hand, U.S. professional herpetologist Terry Vandeventer has found.

Kenneth Vinton in *The Jungle Whispers* tells the story of how a ranking officer and his wife accidentally ran over a bushmaster [Lachesis] on a dirt road in Panama. The angered snake chased the vehicle, striking at its tires, at speeds exceeding 20 miles per hour for over 1 mile. [cited by Greg Bedayn, Lachesis: Metaphor and myth as medicine; RefWorks].

European settlers told tales of black mambas chasing down riders on horseback or dropping through chimneys to wipe out whole families. The Africans claim a mamba will stick its tail in its mouth and chase you as a rolling hoop.

Stories of snakes giving chase are told worldwide, and widely believed. Here is an exciting one quoted by Fayrer [*Thanatophidia of India*, 1874], citing the Rev. Dr. Mason, who heard from 'an intelligent Burman . . . that a friend of his one day stumbled upon a nest of these serpents, and immediately retreated, but the old female gave chase. The man fled with all speed over hill and dale, dingle and glade, and terror seemed to add wings to his flight, till reaching a small river he plunged in, hoping he had then escaped this fiery enemy; but lo! on reaching the opposite bank, up reared the furious Hamadryad, its dilated eyes glistening with rage, ready to bury its fangs in his trembling body. In utter despair he bethought himself of his turban, and in a moment dashed it upon the serpent, which darted upon it like lightning, and for some moments wreaked its vengeance in furious bites; after which it returned quietly to its former haunts.'

See Toxicophis pugnax, Calling the bluff.

### Snakes Retaliate, Take Revenge & Are Unrelenting

In India there are legends about female snakes taking revenge on people who kill their mates, esp. during the act of mating. Such mortified females are said never to forget the grievance, singling the killer out to strike back. Similar beliefs exist in other cultures, the glamour of pervasive myth accrediting snakes with such enduring affection for each other that if one were killed, its spouse will track the slayer unrelentingly until it can avenge its companion's death.

The myth that snakes travel in pairs and wreak vengeance on anyone who may injure their mates is also often attributed to rattlesnakes.

In Syrian belief the serpent extracts revenge independent of a harm-doer's repent; killing or wounding a snake causes its entire clan of kindred critter to pursue the murderer and his kin till their vengeance is satisfied.

Mantravadis [charm makers] in southern India possess the power of neutralising the effects of snake poison by repeating mantras and performing certain rites. It is believed that there are revengeful snakes, which, after they have bitten someone, coil themselves round the branches of a tree, and render the efforts of the mantravadi ineffective. In such a case the mantravadi, through the aid of mantras, sends ants and other insects to harass the snake, which comes down from the tree, and sucks the poison from the punctures that it has made.

Conversely, snake-like behaviour likewise induces vengeance, as Shakespeare lets King Lear declare of his daughter: 'Struck me with her tongue, most serpent-like, upon the very heart: All the stored vengeances of heaven fall on her ungrateful top!'

See Naja, The Cobra's Revenge.

## Snakes Don't Tolerate Disrespect
Snakes are extremely popular objects of veneration in south India, where they are worshipped as the source of happiness, wealth and fame. It is believed that when they are angered by disrespect, they curse people, resulting in sickness, death and the loss of property. Snakes are also believed to be spirits of the dead. Therefore, most homes have their own snake shrines in a corner of the garden, often under a neem tree [Azadirachta indica]. This is usually a stone with a snake carved on it.

## Snakes More Shrewd & Crafty than Any Other Wild Animal [Genesis 3:1]
Cast as a character in innumerable myths and legends, subject of extensive taboos, the snake is generally thought to be imbued with supernatural powers, usually evil. Especially in Western religion, the snake is regarded as a vile creature of sly deception and destructive forces.

The loathsome, detestable, abominable, villainous, sneaky snake enticed Eve to eat of the forbidden fruit. Accursed, blighted, banned, curse-laden, the snake is doomed and damned in biblical hyperbole 'upon your belly shall you go, and dust shall you eat all of the days of your life. And I will put enmity between you and the woman, and between your offspring and her offspring; he will crush your head, and you will bite his heel.' [Genesis 3:14–15]

## Snakes Charm, Fascinate, Hypnotise Prey with their Unblinking Eyes
They exert some mysterious influence over bird or beast at a distance of many feet. Frozen in fear, prey is deprived of power to escape and haplessly succumbs.

'A very intelligent Hindu told Torrens how he had seen the way in which the Hamadryad [king cobra] procures the snakes that form its favourite food. The Hindu in question happened to be on the flat roof of his house, when a young Hamadryad appeared quite close to him. The snake raised its head, expanded its neck, and emitted a shrill hissing noise. Thereupon a dozen snakes came crawling up from all directions and assembled round the Hamadryad, when the latter made a dart at one of them and hastened to devour it.' [Calmette, 1908]

Because snakes detect the slightest movement, the safest strategy is to 'freeze', to stay still and motionless. In addition, fear often paralyzes and victims may be spellbound by the sudden and near appearance of an enemy.

Prolonged, uninterrupted staring is disconcerting. Such an unrelieved, unblinking gaze has been the *reptilian stare*. Since snakes are one of man's archetypes of evil, it is implied by association that a human being with a reptilian stare is a conscienceless individual with a fundamentally evil nature.

### Mother Snakes Swallow their Young when Confronted with Danger

As Klauber noted, this is a myth 'whose denial brings out the greatest flood of indignant eyewitness protestations.' Despite countless hours of observation, this behaviour has never been documented. Swallowing young would be counter-productive rather than serve the purpose of a protective strategy in snakes because anything that enters the esophagus soon arrives in the stomach where it is promptly digested. Although thousands of dissections have been performed on female snakes, none have revealed a stomach full of baby snakes belonging to the same species.

### Miscellaneous Beliefs

The rattlesnake acquires a new thimble to its rattle for every man it kills.

Those who recover from snakebite are subject to a recurrence of the symptoms at the same time of each year as long as the aggressor lives.

Snakes like milk. Venomous snakes are milked for their venom, but milk is not a natural food of any snake.

Rattlesnakes will refuse to bite an unfaithful wife. Unfortunate women under suspicion would seem to be in a very awkward predicament if submitted to such an ordeal, whichever way the augury may point.

## 2 HELPLESS TO BREAK THE SPELL

Hering lists for Lachesis the symptom: 'Sensation as if in the hands of a stronger power, as if charmed, and as if she could not break the spell.' Naturalists have claimed, *and* disputed, that snakes possess the power of fascination. In the 1850s, T.B. Thorpe, a close observer of the animal worlds, was fully convinced of the existence of such a power and gave the following captivating description of it:

'The rattlesnake has certainly an eye of command as had Napoleon; and the power of the reptile's gaze is not only acknowledged by the humbler class of animals, but man, with all his superior powers, has felt a thrill of helplessness pass through his soul as he beheld that mysterious eye glaring full upon him. Approach a rattlesnake, and with the first convenient thing dash out his brains; but dare not to make a close examination of the death-dealing object before you. If its spiral motions once find a response in the music tune-markings of your own mind; if you look into those strange orbs that seem to be the openings into another world; if that forked tongue plays into your presence until you find it as vivid as the lightning's flash; and, meanwhile, the hum of those rattles begins to confuse your absorbed senses, you will be conscious of some terrible danger; that you stand upon some dread precipice; that your blood is starting back from your heart; and you can only break through the charm with an effort that requires the whole of your resolution.' [cited in Hartwig, 1877]

It is believed in various cultures that certain human beings can establish a telepathic power over snakes, which, if it is true, would imply an interesting reversal of the above notion that it is snakes who possess a hypnotic power. The contrary may be true: snakes are good hypnotic subjects, at the mercy of the stronger psychic powers of man. [Wilson, 2006]

## 3  FANG CLUB MEMBERS TAKING ON THE SERPENT

### Taking on the Snake Nature
Mrs. Martha Learn established in 1896 a business for the buying and selling of venomous snakes. Whilst it was at the time 'strikingly unusual for a woman to engage in business because she loves snakes', Mrs. Learn's chief qualification and best asset at the opening of this business was her absolute lack of fear. In her childhood she played with mice, birds, spiders, and snakes. Mrs. Learn believed that her mastery over snakes and ferocious animals was through her power of concentration. She impressed the animal intelligence with her poise and courage, overcoming all resistance on their part. She has had continually to guard against taking on something of the snake nature because of her close association with snakes, that she finds herself 'crawling within herself,' or feeling that she is not welcome, and quickly assuming the defensive attitude, 'coiling to strike,' when there is actually no provocation for such feeling. [The American Magazine, July-December 1921]

### Love of Desolate Places
American herpetologist of Polish descent Joe Slowinski was entranced by the strength and strange beauty of snakes from his earliest childhood on, which caused his father to say: 'Joe always thought of himself as a critter, not a person.' Slowinski's experiences in Costa Rica, studying coral snakes, 'awakened in him a lifelong wanderlust – the passionate love of desolate places that field herpetologists share with religious mystics and soldiers of fortune,' writes his biographer Jamie James. James carries on with a sweeping characterisation: 'When asked to describe Joe, his friends always come up with the word "macho.' His father said he was "masculine almost to a fault."'' Slowinski died at the age of 38 from the bite by a many-banded krait in the jungle of northern Burma in 2001.

### Outcast. Don't Tread On Me
'Like every outcast, the snake has always attracted passionate admirers, particularly among outsiders, those who flout the social order. In the American Revolution, the native rattlesnake was a defiant symbol of resistance. One of the most

popular American flags before the adoption of Old Glory [the current U.S. flag] was the Gadsden flag, with the image of a coiled timber rattlesnake and the legend *Don't Tread On Me*. Ben Franklin [an outlaw at least in the eyes of the British] opposed the bald eagle as the new nation's symbol, calling it "a bird of bad moral character" and proposed in its place the rattlesnake. In a letter to the *Pennsylvania Journal*, published in 1775, Franklin wrote: "She never begins an attack, nor, when once engaged, ever surrenders. She is therefore an emblem of magnanimity and true courage."' [James, 2008]

## Stoic & Fearless
Described as 'his own man in a world of courage, cunning, and solitude', Snake Man C.J.P. Ionides [1901–1968], shed in snake fashion skins of identity almost from birth. Though sixth generation English, he was tagged as 'the Greek', as 'Ironhides' for his stoic composure under the brutal canings at public school, and as 'Iodine' in Africa. From being an ivory poacher, a game hunter and a game warden, he turned into a wild life conservationist, collecting poisonous snakes for zoos and museums, as well as for the preparation of antivenom serums. A devoted, almost fanatical herpetologist, he felt more at home among animals than among men, whom he called 'the least interesting of all animals'. 'Behind the slightly raffish, egocentric cast of Ionides' character lies solid achievement as a naturalist. No less than 4 separate species of snake bear his Latinized name as their discoverer. . . . More memorable than any of "the suborder Serpentes" is C.J.P. Ionides himself, utterly fearless, wily as Ulysses, not wholly admirable and yet strangely endearing, a kind of outcast hero with the rare courage to be his remarkable self.' [Life of a Non-Pukka Sahib; Time Magazine, April 21, 1961]
In Peter Hathaway Capstick's book *The African Adventurers*, Charles Pitman, game warden of Uganda, portrays his friend the Snake Man thus: 'Rebellious by nature . . . with a permanently soured outlook on life and in particular towards authority; he was a self-avowed rebel and it was not his wont to suffer fools gladly. Intolerant of those who did not share his passion for snakes, his life is a refreshing rarity in an over-orthodox world from which he will be greatly missed.'

## Unappreciated & Misunderstood
Chris Wemmer, a Research Associate at the National Zoological Park in Washington, D.C., believes that herpetologists are often emotionally immature, although committed and creative. He suggests that snake scientists tend to feel unappreciated and misunderstood, much like the animals they study.

## Thrill & Attention Seeking
Jackie Bibby, alias 'The Texas Snake Man', knows snakes. He is especially familiar with rattlesnakes. Bibby has shared a bathtub, sleeping bag and sack with rattlesnakes and holds records for all. He spent 45 minutes in a bathtub with 87 rattlesnakes. His testimonial on ESPN Guinness Chat: 'I've been involved in handling rattlesnakes as a hobby and as a sport for 40 years. I'm a thrill-seeker, so that's how I got started. It developed from there. The answer to why I like to

sit in a tub with rattlesnakes is to prove that I can. Why do we do anything that presses the envelope? I'm an egomaniac with an inferiority complex, so I like attention.'

## Rush to Breakthroughs

Dr. Brian Fry, a herpetologist from the University of Melbourne, Australia, has hunted down and collected venom from snakes that feature in the top-10 of lethal snakes. 'Working with some of these snakes is the biggest adrenaline rush you could ever do,' Fry said in an interview The New York Times of April 5, 2005. 'I used to do extreme ski jumping and big wave surfing, but none of that can touch working with these animals.' His goal is to decipher the evolution of snake venoms. Reconstructing their history will help lead to medical breakthroughs, Fry believes. In February 2005, Fry and his colleagues filed a patent for a molecule found in the venom of the inland taipan [Oxyuranus microlepidotus] that may help treat congestive heart failure.

## Defiant, Argumentative, Aggressive

Herpetologists James B. Murphy and Winston Card assembled with a generous dash of humour a profile of the snake scientist, based upon the behaviour of men in herpetology. Among the exhibited characteristics they recognise in the first place the inclination of young herpetologists to continually defend their interest in snakes as 'being acceptable in polite society'. This defensiveness prompts the development of 'argumentative, antisocial and aggressive patterns in response to criticism.' Among the other habits and traits the authors describe as being typical of herpetologists are limited friendships; 'vigorous heterosexual behaviour with little evidence of success in the game of love'; trend toward permanent facial hair; 'dining habits tend to reflect a high degree of carnivory with food consumed in impressive quantities'; penchant for motorcycles. 'There are 2 distinct modes of dress. One group, certainly in the minority, dresses in sartorial splendor with nicely pressed and laundered clothes. The second group appears to have found mismatched clothing at a garage sale. These items seem to be infrequently washed and never ironed.' In summary, 'generally highly focused, somewhat aggressive individuals who enjoy and nurture live animals but may not be as considerate toward their fellow man.' [J.B. Murphy, 1998]

## Snakes in the Grass, Cunning & Vindictive

Mr. Higgins dealt in the 1860–70s with venomous snakes in Colombia and with their kind in human form, the so-called Curers or snake charmers. Intimately familiar with the habits and peculiarities of venomous snakes, Curers cured snakebites, 'boasting of never losing a case,' although, in Higgins's view, 'they necessarily cling to many "hocus pocus" manipulations and performances.'

Higgins saw them clearly as akin to the serpents they brought under their spell: 'The Curers are generally men void of all principle; shrewd; cunning; ever ready to profit by any circumstance that can be turned to their advantage, and as they have to do with a people always inclined to superstitious belief; who attribute everything to "La Suerte" [luck, chance, fatality]; as an inevitable result, these men are in a position to make themselves masters of any and every situation. They never forget an insult or injury given [except in a fellow-curer or "brujo"], and will wait patiently for years with the hope that sooner or later they shall be called upon to cure a snake-bite in their enemy, and if death is not imminent they soon make it so by the administration or application of poisons they keep on hand, and their long-treasured insult is revenged by death.'

## Supernatural Compassion & Care
If Grace Olive Wiley [1884–1948] 'had wished to make a mystery out of her amazing ability' to calm down dangerous snakes by petting and caressing them . . . 'she could have made a fortune by posing as a woman with supernatural power.' [Compare delusion being under superhuman control.]

She studied entomology at the University of Kansas and during field trips to collect insects it was a great joke among Grace's fellow students that she was terrified of even harmless garter snakes. Later, however, after her marriage failed, Grace turned with a passionate interest to the creatures she had so long feared. 'Somehow they know very, very soon that I am friendly and like them,' she wrote. 'They appear to listen intently when I stand quietly at their open door and talk to them in a low, soothing voice. In some unknown manner my idea of sympathy is conveyed to them. What a powerful thing it must be, when even the world's most deadly reptiles respond to kindness.'

Mrs. Wiley's special ability was to demonstrate that even the most feared of deadly snakes will not seek to harm a person at any opportunity, out of sheer cunning and malice [as is popularly believed]. She died of heart failure 90 minutes after an Indian cobra bit her in the hand.

## The Nature of Snakes
John Ruskin, the 19th-century British artist and social thinker, supplied the 'names of the snake tribe in the great languages' in relation to the perceived nature of snakes:

- Ophis [Greek] – 'the seeing'. Meaning especially one that sees all round it.
- Dracon [Greek], Drachen [German] – 'the beholding'. Meaning one that looks well into a thing, or person.
- Anguis [Latin] – 'the strangling'.
- Serpens [Latin] – 'the winding'.
- Coluber [Latin], Couleuvre [French] – 'the coiling'.
- Adder [Saxon] – 'the groveling'. Meaning to cringe; to lie or creep in a prostrate position, as in subservience or humility.
- Snake [Saxon], Schlange [German] – 'the crawling' [with sense of dragging, and of smoothness].

Lord Bacon, in his book *Of the Proficience and Advancement of Learning, Divine and Humane*, to the King, 1605, writes "It is not possible to join Serpentine Wisdom with the Columbine Innocency, except men know exactly all the conditions of the Serpent; his Baseness and going upon his Belly, his Volubility and Lubricity, his Envy and Sting; for without this, Virtue lyeth unfenced.'

## Speaking with New Tongues

Churches that practice snake handling have dotted the Appalachians in eastern North America for over 100 years. 'A typical snake-handling meeting usually consists of songs of worship and preaching. The front of the church, beyond the altar, is the designated area for handling snakes. Many participants bring their own boxes containing rattlers, copperheads or cobras. The snakes are symbolic of Satan [Genesis 3:15; Luke 10:19]. One demonstrates his power and authority over the enemy by picking up snakes. As the service progresses and the anointing flows, those receiving the unction open the box lids and lift the snakes high into the air. Some practitioners hold several snakes at a time, allowing them to slither and wrap themselves around their bodies. Usually the snake-handling members slip into altered states of consciousness during such episodes. Their eyes roll back, and they twirl or dance in the Spirit and speak in tongues. However, not all are expected to handle snakes; only the anointed. . . .

'When a person is bitten in a religious ceremony, it can signify 1 of 5 things: That the person has sin in his/her life. If discovered to be the case, the faithful members shun the sinners. That the person handled the snake without being under "the anointing" of the Holy Ghost. Since God promises no protection to the unanointed, snakes are prone to bite them. That the person lacks the faith to handle the serpent. Handling snakes without faith is presumption. That God is testing the handlers to see if they will deny the faith when they are bitten. That God is a healer. One of the ways to know this is for him to heal the victim of a venomous snakebite. In each case, the embedded poisonous fangs reveal something about the handler or God. . . . Snake-handling churches embrace the Oneness Pentecostal doctrines, including baptism in the name of Jesus, baptism for remission of sins, the giving of the Holy Ghost subsequent to baptism, and speaking in tongues as the evidence of salvation. Additionally they call upon their members to practice holiness in dress and demeanor. Women cannot wear slacks or cut their hair. Members greet each other of the same sex with a "holy kiss." They rarely go to doctors or take medicine.' [geocities.com/alanstreett/snakehan.html]

There were approximately 2,500 snake-handlers in America in the early 1940s. When deaths from snakebites became prevalent, nearly all states in the southern mountains enacted laws prohibiting the handling of serpents as part of religious worship. The laws are violated constantly.

## Reptile Rapture – Dancing with Snakes Following Signs

'A visitor at a snake-handling church might witness these kinds of events: The congregation typically meets on a Saturday evening in a small, one-room, frame church. Accompanied by guitar, piano, and drum music, the minister leads the faithful in inspired hymns. Soon the room is flooded with rhythmically moving bodies.

'Participants move to a large unobstructed area at the front of the room, where they sway, dance, stamp their feet, and clap hands while singing and volunteering praises to the Lord: "Hallelujah!," "Praise Jesus!," "God is Real!," "Amen!"

'Others counter by raising Bibles, many openly testifying their faith. Some brandish tambourines. The preacher expounds on evil, on the devil's influences [alcohol, smoking, and promiscuity]. His compelling, sensational, fire-and-brimstone delivery solicits vociferous praises to Jesus. The sermon intensifies as he proclaims every word in the Bible is true. The pace quickens; several more communicants move to the front, where they are "getting the spirit" [anointing], "talking in tongues" [glossolalia], crying, shouting, praying. The air is heavy with terrific energy, undeniable devotion, and honest faith.

'Dancing about singly or with others, many demonstrate quick, violent, spastic motions. Worshipers thrust their hands upward while tossing their heads backward, praising the Lord. Oppressive heat emanates from the mass of reeling bodies; all are sweating. A tiny elderly woman in a simple cotton dress falls to the floor, writhing uncontrollably, still chanting and uttering unrecognisable words. This ecstatic seizure attracts others who pray over her. Contagiously, others are overcome, and the frenzy continues for more than half an hour.

'A parishioner occasionally gives a contemptuous kick at one of several flat wooden boxes that lie to one side, almost unnoticed. They contain the snakes. The buzzing of the aroused rattlesnakes cannot be heard through the overpowering music and incantations. Eventually the preacher throws open a box, reaches in among the knot of serpents, and quickly pulls out a timber rattlesnake, *Crotalus horridus horridus*, with a sweeping motion. . . . Participants react with the foreseen response, still more delirium. Grabbing the first snake is considered a supreme test of faith, because the first touch to the aroused snake is most likely to elicit a bite.

'The minister passes the snake to a nearby dancing worshiper who holds it overhead and takes out 2 more magnificent timber rattlesnakes. . . . Soon a dozen others are handling rattlesnakes and copperheads, while chanting, swooning, swirling, and continuing the jerking motions. The music is thunderous, overpowering. One woman in a trance-like state, her head pitching from side to side while rolling back and forth, has a half-dozen snakes stretched between and around her hands. She is at a moment of extreme ecstasy. She is fully anointed, receiving a blessing from the Holy Ghost for her devotion. . . . After 30 minutes of near hysteria, the ceremony reaches a crescendo.

'The music subsides, the snakes are returned to the boxes, and the minister continues his impassioned sermon; people volunteer their faith while continuing their reeling motions at a slower pace. Within minutes the tempo of the music builds, and the congregation quickly becomes embroiled in renewed celebration. Snakes again are taken from their boxes and passed among the invigorated, nearly delirious assemblage. After 15 minutes or so the frenzy subsides, and the snake are again returned to the boxes. The minister calls those in need of healing to come forward. Using his palms he grasps the head of a sufferer, and she immediately falls limp into a trance. Staring deeply into her eyes he commands her to have faith in God's power; only with total faith can a miracle happen. She writhes uncontrollably, shaking [almost vibrating], while babbling and sobbing. A group gathers, pressing in, praying and continuing the rhythmical swaying. . . . The service ends much more abruptly than it started, with emotional kissing and hugging.

'Several phenomena are revealed here that are difficult to explain. . . . The intense spiritualness and pervasive supernatural aura produced by the emotionally consumed participants introduce a unique variable. Although many people do not accept that the state of emotional holiness can interfere with normal physical reaction to a rattlesnake bite, this theory requires much more study. An aroused endocrine-immune response or other physiological preparedness to stress deserves serious consideration, and *a form of holistic medicine* cannot be ruled out.' [Rubio, 1998] [emphasis added; Like Cures Like?]

Practitioners of religious serpent handling call themselves *sign-followers* after the text in Mark 16:17–18: 'And these signs shall follow them that believe.' Snake remedies have a penchant for following, too, it appears, considering that Lachesis has the delusion of hearing [commanding] voices that he must follow. Likewise, Crotalus cascavella, in her magnetic state, hears a strange voice and follows it. Elaps and Crotalus horridus appear also in the delusion rubric Hearing voices.

## 5 SERPENT WORSHIP

- The snake has been variously adored as a regenerative power, as a god of evil, as a god of good, as Christ [by the Gnostics], as a phallic deity, as a solar deity, and as a god of death. It has also served as the symbol of Satan and many deities, including Apollo and the Egyptian god Ra.
- The snake's image is ambivalent rather than negative. Even in societies where it represents a destructive or evil power, the snake is given noble or beneficial roles, usually as guardian of a treasure or of vital elements [water, earth, fertility, fecundity, health, knowledge].
- Shakespeare's understanding of the serpent's opposing qualities of curse and grace, the power both to harm and to heal, is demonstrated in a scene from his play King Richard II, where Mowbray says: 'I am disgraced, impeached and baffled here, Pierced to the soul with slander's venom'd spear, The which no balm can cure but his heart-blood Which breathed this poison.' An old English belief claims something similar: 'The beautous adder has a sting, Yet bears a balm too.' The serpent is the cure for what it causes.
- Snake worship in ancient cultures may have arisen out of fear. It is an inherent human tendency to respect power, which the snake symbolises.
- In certain mystical traditions of India, the serpent represents the supreme power in the human body, the energy of Kundalini coiled [and fast asleep] at the base of the spine. Those who have awakened this power, both in Hindu and Buddhist portrayals, are pictured with a cobra rising along the spine and spreading her protective hood over their heads.

- The aborigines of Australia worship a rainbow serpent named Kurrichalpongo. They believe that it created the world and its eggs hatched the mountains and the trees.
- Quetzalcoatl, in Mexican myths, is the feather-clad serpent, half bird, half snake, of Aztec ancestry. It represents the universe, heaven and earth together, thus the forces of nature, both good and bad.
- 'One of the best-known attributes of the serpent is wisdom. The Hebrew tradition of the fall speaks of that animal as the subtlest of the beasts of the field; and the founder of Christianity tells his disciples to be as wise as serpents, though as harmless as doves. Among the ancients the serpent was consulted as an oracle, and Maury points out that it played an important part in the life of several celebrated Greek diviners in connection with the knowledge of the language of birds, which many of the ancients believed to be the souls of the dead. The serpent was associated with Apollo and Athena, the Grecian deities of wisdom, as well as with the Egyptian Kneph, the ram-headed god from whom the Gnostics are sometimes said to have derived their idea of the Sophia. This personification of divine wisdom is undoubtedly represented on Gnostic gems under the form of the serpent. In Hindu mythology there is the same association between the animal and the idea of wisdom.' [Wake, 1888]

## SNAKE SLANG – IMAGERY & METAPHORS

### Mad as an Adder
According to *A Dictionary of Common Fallacies,* Lewis Carroll [author of Alice in Wonderland, 1865] with his penchant for linguistic games presumably knew perfectly well that his 'Mad Hatter' meant 'a venomous adder', but since his readers may have been misled by Tenniel's drawings, it should be pointed out that 'mad' meant 'venomous' and 'hatter' is a corruption of 'adder' or viper, so that the phrase 'mad as an atter' originally meant 'as venomous as a viper'. Support for the 'adder' theory comes from Eliezer Edward's Dictionary of Curious, Quaint, and Out-of-the-Way Matters [1881]: 'In the Anglo-Saxon the word "mad" was used as a synonym for violent, furious, angry, or venomous. In some parts of England and in the United States particularly, it is still used in this sense. "Atter" was the Anglo-Saxon name for an adder, or viper. The proverbial saying has therefore probably no reference to hat-makers, but merely means as venomous as an adder. The Germans call the viper "Natter".' [www.snopes.com]

### Mean as a Rattler
'The rattlesnake's association with danger and its perceived dominant position among the animal world have made it a logical eye-catching symbol. Many more subtle, underlying attributes have been suggested as rationales of its success as a symbol. Some of these include the following: rattlesnakes lie in wait, always at the ready; their fangs are hidden until action is needed; having no eyelids, they are constantly awake and aware; they rattle to warn of their possible response; and when aroused, they fight with viciousness and tenacity. . . . Politicians,

ministers, and other orators are not averse to referencing rattlesnakes for effect in their speeches. Usually they are referenced in a negative connotation, such as "mean as a rattler," "sneaky as an old rattlesnake," or "dangerous as a rattlesnake." During World War II several American forces included rattlesnakes in the design of their group insignia. It was not uncommon during that era for impressionist paintings of them to personalise fighter planes and boats. A potent air-to-air missile called "Sidewinder" was a lethal weapon during the Vietnam War because of its position on the helicopter and its accuracy.' [Rubio, 1998]

## Quick as a Cobra

The cobra is associated with speed: fast cars; racing motorcycles; strategic military offensives; anti-armour and close support/attack stealth helicopters; all-terrain armoured vehicles; very fast and aerobatic model airplanes; the fastest fighting gear, gloves and kicks, 'deadly speed beyond the human eye'; health insurance; British government committee convened to co-ordinate action in cases of national emergency.

Amongst its many facets, the cobra incorporated into the Pharaoh's headdress symbolised the swift and invincible striking force of the king against his political enemies.

## Slippery as a Snake

Denoting a lurking danger, someone who betrays you even though you have trusted them is said to be a snake in the grass. The expression is equally used for [1] a shady, conniving person who could strike at any time without warning; [2] a deceitful or treacherous person; [3] someone who watches an auction but doesn't bid until the last minute.

'A snake in the bush' for the Japanese means to reap ill fortune from an unnecessary act, e.g. poking a bamboo bush may flush out a snake.

## Speaking with a Forked Tongue – Viper's Tongue

To make false promises or to speak in a way that is dishonest. To say one thing and mean another or, in more general terms, to act in a duplicitous manner. To lie; to be 2-faced.

In the common language, 'viper's tongue' was the expression that described that of slanderers, hypocrites, traitors, and liars. Because the tip of snakes' tongues ends in a fork, medieval artists exaggerated the natural form and made the point into a dart, an arrow, or a javelin. Like these weapons, an evil word also strikes and wounds, and sometimes kills.


## VENOMOUS PHENOMENA

### Snake Venoms General

- Snakes attempt to regulate the amount of venom injected relative to the size of their prey, an ability that is believed to be underdeveloped in juvenile snakes. It is thought that the size of a human being confuses the sensory input of the snake, often resulting in a dry bite. Presumably venom is biologically expensive, a commodity that a snake would be reluctant to dispense needlessly. A strike with injection of a minimal quantity of venom would be as effective in temporarily warding off most larger animals as a large supply of venom.

- Venomous snakes are dangerous if not treated with respect.
- Snake venoms are traditionally divided into 3 or 4 types: neurotoxic, haemotoxic, myotoxic, cytotoxic.

The neurotoxic type acts mainly on the nervous systems, affecting the optic nerves [causing blindness] or the phrenic nerve of the diaphragm [causing paralysis of respiration].

The haemotoxic type breaks down red blood corpuscles and blood vessels and produces extensive haemorrhaging of blood into tissue spaces.

The myotoxic type ranges from mild muscle pain and muscular weakness to serious rhabdomyolysis and myoglobinuria.

Cytotoxic venom destroys cells – usually causing massive necrosis or death of large parts of tissue.

Most snake venoms are complex mixtures of various fractions that attack different organs in specific ways; they seldom can be assigned categorically to one or the other of the traditional types. Consequently there may be considerable overlap of clinical features caused by venoms of different species. However, a basic division in neurotoxic and haemotoxic may still be useful for the general purpose of differential diagnosis.

## Neurotoxins – Paresis & Paralysis
Neurotoxins are produced by snakes in the families Elapidae and Hydrophiidae [sea snakes] and by some pit vipers [Crotalinae].

Pharmacologically divided in pre-synaptic [or beta-] neurotoxins and post-synaptic [or alpha-] neurotoxins, these toxins interfere with the pre-synaptic release or the post-synaptic binding of acetylcholine. The net result is the same: no activity of acetylcholine mediated nerve function.

Pre-synaptic neurotoxins are found in Bungarus [krait], Oxyuranus [taipan], Notechis [tiger snake], and some pit vipers [e.g. Crotalus cascavella].

Post-synaptic neurotoxins are particularly found in Naja [cobra], Ophiophagus [king cobra], and Dendroaspis [mamba].

The elapid genus Micrurus [Elaps in homeopathy] produces both pre- and post-synaptic neurotoxins.

Neurotoxins have a high preponderance for the peripheral nervous system because most do not or only minimally cross the blood brain barrier due to the molecular size of snake venom neurotoxins. Following envenomation, the *cranial nerves are usually affected first*, which results in ptosis, ophthalmoplegia [paralysis or weakness of one or more of the muscles that control eye movement], dysarthria, dysphagia, and drooling. This progresses to weakness of limb muscles, paralysis of the respiratory muscles, and ultimately death if prompt treatment is not initiated. Descending paralysis is typical of snakebite neurotoxicity.

*Signs and symptoms of neurotoxic snakebites include:*
- Drowsiness.
- Headache.
- Ptosis; heavy eyelids, external ophthalmoplegia [paralysis or weakness of extra-ocular muscles that control eye movement].
- Blurred vision or difficulty seeing.
- Pupils dilated and fixed.
- Paralysis of facial muscles and other muscles innervated by cranial nerves.
- Inability to open the mouth and protrude the tongue.
- Drooling.
- Abnormalities of taste and smell, transient or permanent, sometimes leaving the victim with permanent complete anosmia.
- Difficulty speaking or swallowing.
- 'Broken neck sign' – weakness/paralysis of cervical flexor muscles.
- Aphonia.
- Respiratory arrest or dyspnoea.
- Convulsions or epileptiform seizures.
- Sudden loss of consciousness.
- Flaccid paralysis.
- Limb weakness – usually ataxic gait first, then inability to walk, then stand or even sit up.
- Paraesthesias.

## Neurotoxins – Sequelae
Most victims of neurotoxic snakebites who have been suffering systemic effects take several weeks before they feel completely well again. They often complain of lethargy, weakness, night sweats, weight loss and/or feeling 'generally run down'.

## Neurotoxins – Sleeping into Aggravation
A classic snake symptom in the homeopathic materia medica, sleeping into aggravation is a typically neurotoxic manifestation. One man bitten by a tiger snake puts the following words to it: 'Approximately 10 minutes after the bite speech was difficult and breathing was almost impossible as the lungs could be felt slowly paralysing. I believe it was only by being sufficiently conscious to inhale deeply at regular intervals and so fully inflate the lungs that it was possible to continue breathing. I feel certain that, should one go to sleep under such circumstances, it would be very difficult to avoid suffocation. Throughout the effects I would have had no difficulty in going to sleep, but this was purposely avoided.' [Sutherland 1983]

## Neurotoxins – Broken Neck
In dissecting a rat that had been killed by the bite of a cobra, Francis T. Buckland got some of the cobra's venom in a little crack under the nail of his left thumb. Shortly after, he noticed the neurotoxic venom taking effect, a characteristic manifestation of which is the 'broken neck sign', flaccid paralysis of the cervical

flexor muscles: 'I had not walked a hundred yards, before all of a sudden I felt just *as if somebody had come behind me and struck me a severe blow on the head and neck*, and at the same time I experienced a most acute pain and sense of oppression at the chest, as if a hot iron had been run in and a hundred-weight had been put on the top of it.' Buckland next loses consciousness temporarily and becomes ataxic: 'I then forgot everything for several minutes, and my friend tells me I rolled about as if very faint and weak. He also informs me that the first thing I did was to fall against him, asking if I looked seedy. He most wisely answered: "No, you look very well." I don't think he thought so, for his own face was as white as a ghost; I recollect this much. He tells me my face was a greenish-yellow colour. After walking or rather staggering along for some minutes, I gradually recovered my senses.' [Buckland, 1858]

The *'broken neck sign'* is deemed characteristic of envenomation by Crotalus cascavella, sea snakes, and elapid snakes in general. Clinically, the sign is a *feature of poliomyelitis and post-diphtheritic paralysis*.

It is interesting that neurotoxic snakes [elapids and sea snakes] appear to seek the nape of the neck, whilst the haemotoxic pit vipers clearly go for the throat.

Bungarus fasciatus has frontal or left temporal headache extending to the cervical region with pain in the neck. Elaps has sensation of weight in right parietal region and pain that penetrates to nape of neck. Elaps has additionally a sensation as if the cerebellum were settling downwards, causing pressing pain in nape of neck.

Crotalus cascavella has pulling pain on sides of neck in turning head. Buckland's experience is included in the materia medica of Naja as Sensation as if someone were coming up from behind and dealing a severe blow to one's neck and head.

Streamlined for rapidity, elapids deliver their venom with break-neck speed. Although not an elapid, a bite by the cascabel [C. cascavella] is held over much of its range in South America to 'break a man's neck, regardless of the part of the body bitten. This is probably due to some selective action of the venom, which causes complete paralysis of the neck. The man's head may, if he be held in a sitting position, slump forward on his chest, roll from side to side, or backward, in such a loosely connected way that the native cannot explain the condition as other than a broken neck.' [March, cited in Ditmars, 1937b]

### Neurotoxins – Losing Control over Everything – Locked in, Buried alive

We cannot imagine what it is to lose control over everything, what it is to be totally aware of your surroundings while at the same time being *completely unable to communicate anything* of what you feel, think, want, or need; thus becoming a silent and unresponsive witness to everything that is happening. Locked-in syndrome is the medical term for this horrific condition, which has been described as 'the closest thing to being buried alive'. The French call it 'maladie de l'emmuré vivant', 'walled-in alive disease', and in German it is sometimes called 'Eingeschlossensein', 'being locked in'.

Merck Manual gives the details: 'Locked-in syndrome is a state of wakefulness and awareness with quadriplegia and paralysis of the lower cranial nerves, resulting in inability to show facial expression, move, speak, or communicate, except by coded eye movements. . . . Patients have intact cognitive function and are awake, with eye opening and normal sleep-wake cycles. They can hear and see. However, they cannot move their lower face, chew, swallow, speak, breathe, move their limbs, or move their eyes laterally. Vertical eye movement is possible; patients can open and close their eyes or blink a specific number of times to answer questions.'

Locked-in syndrome may result from traumatic brain injury, diseases of the circulatory system, diseases that destroy the myelin sheath surrounding nerve cells, or medication overdose. Basically, anything that causes localised damage within the brain stem can produce the syndrome.

The brain stem is the smallest region in the human brain and resembles the entire brain of present-day reptiles. For this reason, it is often called the 'reptilian brain'. It is 'preverbal' [before speech], but controls life functions such as autonomic brain, breathing, heart rate and the fight or flight mechanism. Lacking language, its impulses are instinctual and ritualistic. It is concerned with fundamental needs such as survival, physical maintenance, hoarding, dominance, preening and mating. It is also found in lower life forms such as lizards, crocodiles and birds.

The bite of a neurotoxic snake may cause symptoms very similar to those of locked-in syndrome or related conditions. Florida snake handler Albert Killian expresses it thus: 'The worst thing about a neurotoxic bite is when you go into respiratory failure and go into paralysis, your brain is completely awake. If someone lifts your eyelids, you can see them.'

A man bitten on the right index finger by the South African cape cobra [Naja nivea] developed within 4 hours complete flaccid paralysis. He later said that at this stage he had been able to hear and understand everything but could not move.

Elapids, including mambas, coral snakes and cobras, are typically neurotoxic. Envenomation may mimic brain death, as the following case of a cobra bite shows. 'Snake bite mimicking brain death. A 6-year-old girl woke up with pain and increasing swelling over the left hand and difficulty in breathing. On examination, she had swelling of the left forearm and hand, flaccid quadriparesis and was in respiratory failure requiring mechanical ventilation. Two clean puncture wounds were identified on the left thumb. A provisional diagnosis of snakebite with severe envenomation was made and she was given anti snake venom therapy. Over a period of about 4 hours her weakness progressed. She became areflexic, developed internal and external ophthalmoplegia and loss of other brain stem reflexes mimicking brain death. Mechanical ventilation was continued despite features suggestive of brain stem dysfunction. About 36 hours after ventilation she showed a flicker of movement of her fingers and gradually the power improved. She was weaned off the ventilator and extubated after 5 days. External ophthalmoplegia is an established association with cobra envenomation, but this combination of internal and external ophthalmoplegia can mimic brain death and pose a dilemma to the caregivers regarding continuation of therapy, . . . thus prompting many a pediatrician to consider withdrawing ventilatory support, which would be disastrous.' [John et al., 2008]

## Neurotoxins – Locked in or Locked out

Brian Fry, the Melbourne-based herpetologist, says that one of the classic reactions to elapid venom is hypoxia: 'There's a sense of disconnection, of sensory disruption – a floaty feeling.'

The possibility of getting disconnected or separated from the body, as if being locked *out* from it, makes one wonder whether humans live within their body or *through* it.

Brian Fry's experience after the bite by a neurotoxic Australian elapid, the Pilbara death adder [Acanthophis wellsi] provides an interesting answer to that question: 'Initially, I was just a bit dizzy and uncoordinated. Which was pretty much my default state anyway, being naturally blond, having bad balance from childhood spinal meningitis and easily distracted by passing squirrels. But these effects became more and more severe until breathing became a struggle. My diaphragm muscle was being paralysed by the neurotoxins.

'As I became progressively more paralysed and my breathing became more laboured and inefficient, the most delicious sensation crept over me, like a technicoloured chemical cloud. Blue gave way to black; my pupils became dilated and fixed. The lights became very bright and the colours very vivid in a way quite like being on psychedelic mushrooms. I was unable to open my eyelids or move my eyes, so my vision was limited to the times the doctor manually opened my eyelids to look at the pupils. The medical staff had no idea I was conscious and could hear everything they were saying. I just had no way of letting them know I was in there.

'But I didn't care. The neurotoxins were now having an extremely potent narcotic effect. Life was beautiful. It was like breathing the most potent dental gas [viz. nitrous oxide, laughing gas], times a thousand. Once I lost my ability to move at all and was put on artificial respiration, the sensation kicked up another gear and I was floating high the world without a single care. True, I was locked inside my body, completely cut off from the outside world – the most primordial of fears. Strangely, I did not mind. This was entirely to do with the fact that I was having the most amazing party-for-one inside my immobile shell. Time warped. For aeons I drifted contentedly through the universe, exploring far-off lands and distant galaxies. This was a classic dissociative *out-of-body-experience;* a psychedelic state of mind that is reached by *disconnecting the mind from the body,* either by dissociative drugs like ketamine or, as it turns out, the neuro-toxicity of certain toxins. Unlike a bad mushroom trip, however, I did not wonder if it would ever end.

'Fortunately and unfortunately at the same time, the antivenom did its job and my Rastafarian world faded all too soon back to the *much more mundane reality.* The days, months, years and centuries I had been travelling turned out to be contained within the eight hours I was fully paralysed: a most interesting form of time travel.' [Fry, 2015]

## Haemotoxins – Cardiovascular Assault & Clotting Crisis

Haemotoxins are produced by most pit vipers [fam. Viperidae, subfamily Crotalinae] and all true vipers [fam. Viperidae, subfamily Viperinae].

In this group the following enzymes and polypeptides are included:

- Procoagulant enzymes stimulate blood clotting but result in incoagulable blood. Venoms such as Russell's viper venom contain several different procoagulants, which activate different steps of the clotting cascade. The result is formation of fibrin in the blood stream. Most of this is immediately broken down by the body's own fibrinolytic system. Eventually, and sometimes within 30 minutes of the bite, the levels of clotting factors have been so depleted ["consumption coagulopathy"] that the blood will not clot.
- Haemorrhagins [zinc metalloproteinases] damage the endothelial lining of blood vessel walls causing spontaneous systemic haemorrhage.
- Haemolytic and myolytic phospholipases A 2 damage cell membranes, endothelium, skeletal muscle, nerve and red blood cells.

## Haemotoxins – Signs & Symptoms

- Cardiovascular – Visual disturbances, dizziness, faintness, collapse, shock, hypotension, cardiac arrhythmias, pulmonary oedema, conjunctival oedema.
- Bleeding and clotting disorders – Bleeding from recent wounds and from old partly healed wounds. Spontaneous systemic bleeding from gums, epistaxis, bleeding into the tears, haemoptysis, haematemesis, rectal bleeding or melaena, haematuria, vaginal bleeding, bleeding into the skin [petechiae, purpura, ecchymoses] and mucosae [e.g. conjunctivae], intracranial haemorrhage [meningism from subarachnoid haemorrhage, lateralizing signs and/or coma from cerebral haemorrhage].
- Renal – Lower back pain, haematuria, haemoglobinuria, myoglobinuria, oliguria/anuria, symptoms and signs of uraemia [acidotic breathing, hiccough, nausea, pleuritic chest pain, foetor, drowsiness, muscle twitching].

## Haemotoxins – Stroke

On October 2018, a systematic search was conducted using PubMed and Google Scholar to review case reports about stroke caused by snake envenomation from January 1995 to October 2018. 83 cases were identified, of which in 58 cases the snake species had also been identified.

Ischemic strokes were 77.1% of the cases while ICH were 20.5%. The most common species were Russell's vipers [*Daboia*] with higher incidence of ischemic stroke than intracranial haemorrhage [ICH]. *Bothrops* species were the second most common venoms to be reported with significantly more propensity towards ICH than ischemic stroke. There were single reports of bite by horned viper [*Cerastes cerastes*] and *Pseudonaja textilis* with ICH; *Cerastes* and *Deinagkistrodon* envenomation were associated with large infarcts. The venom of Bothrops species contains metalloproteinases, a type of haemotoxin that can cause haemolysis, thrombocytopenia, disseminated intravascular coagulation. Among Bothrops, ICH was frequently reported with the species *jararacussu*, *atrox*, *marajoensis* and infarcts were reported for the species *lanceolatus*. Most of the patients bitten were young and had no co-morbidity of or risk factors for either haemorrhagic or ischemic stroke, except 2% who had a history of diabetes mellitus or hypertension. [Al-Sadawi, 2019]

## Cytotoxins – Swelling & Tissue Death
Cytolytic or necrotic toxins [proteolytic enzymes and phospholipases A], polypeptide toxins and other factors increase permeability resulting in local swelling. They may also destroy cell membranes and tissues.

Snakes with predominantly cytotoxic venom are found amongst the true vipers [Bitis arietans, Bitis gabonica, Vipera spp.] and the spitting cobras [Naja nigricollis].

## Myotoxins – Muscle Pain & Muscle Destruction
Myotoxic snake venom contains peptides that destroy the protein in the muscle fibres that have a high oxidative capacity, resulting in muscle destruction [myolysis, rhabdomyolysis]. The broken-down protein from the muscle fibres then enters the blood stream through to the kidneys. The kidneys overwork trying to filter out all the excess body tissue often resulting in kidney failure and the urine turning very dark in colour.

The following reptiles produce myotoxic venoms: Australian death adders [Acanthophis], tiger snakes [Notechis], taipans [Oxyuranus], and black snakes [Pseudechis], true vipers [Daboia russelii], and particularly sea snakes; also venomous lizards [Heloderma].

Although less prevalent in pit viper envenomation, rhabdomyolysis, myoglobinuria, and acute renal failure may complicate bites by Crotalus cascavella, Crotalus horridus, Lachesis spp., and Bothrops spp.

## Myotoxins – Signs & Symptoms
• Muscle tenderness.
• Weakness.
• Swollen tongue sensation.
• Dryness of throat with sense of thirst.
• Stiffness of jaw, neck, trunk and limbs muscles.
• Pain when moving muscles.
• Muscular spasms and convulsions.
• Ptosis.
• Difficulty breathing.
• Blackish-brown urine.
• Renal failure.

## Myotoxins – Rhabdomyolysis
The symptoms caused by this group of snakes [and Heloderma] can be compared with other causes of rhabdomyolysis, defined as destruction or disintegration of striated/skeletal muscles with leakage of muscle intracellular contents into circulation and extracellular fluid.

Rhabdomyolysis has a classic triad of symptoms: muscle pain, weakness and dark urine [myoglobinuria]. General manifestations consist of fever, tachycardia, nausea, vomiting and malaise. Concomitant large releases of potassium from muscles may cause cardiac arrhythmias.

Causes of rhabdomyolysis, and thus possible spheres of action of myotoxic snakes, include:

- Trauma and compression – Crush injuries. Prolonged immobilisation. Physical torture. Struggle against restraints. Deep burns; electrical burns.
- Occlusion of vessels – Thrombo-embolism. Prolonged use of tourniquet use.
- Excessive muscle activities – Overexertion such as long-distance running. Status epilepticus. Delirium tremens. Amphetamine overdose. Exercise in extreme heat.
- Hyperthermia – Malignant hyperthermia. Heat stroke.
- Drugs – Alcohol. Cocaine. Cyclosporine. Ecstasy. Heroin. LSD. Methadone. Morphine. PCP [angel dust]. Solvents [toluene]. Strychnine.
- Medications – Diazepam. Haloperidol. Ibuprofen. Lithium. Lovastatin. Salicylates. Thiazide diuretics.
- Infections – Legionella. Streptococcus. Falciparum malaria. HIV. Salmonella. Tetanus. Influenza. Herpes virus infection [herpes simplex virus, Epstein-Barr virus, cytomegalovirus].
- Endocrine disorders – Hypothyroidism. Thyroid storm. Ketoacidosis. Hyperaldosteronism.
- Animal venoms – Insects [wasps, bees, hornets]. Spiders [brown recluse, black widows].

[www.aic.cuhk.edu.hk/web8/rhabdomyolysis.htm]

## Cardiotoxins – Heart & Circulation

- The neurotoxins and cardiotoxins of Elapid and Hydrophid venom are of small molecular size and carry strong positive charge, which is reflected in their low antigenicity and rapid lethal absorption. The lethal potency of cobra venom cardiotoxin is 1/20 of its neurotoxin. The primary action of cardiotoxin is directly on cell membrane, causing many effects on the skeletal, cardiac, smooth muscles, nerves and neuromuscular junctions, thus contributing to circulatory and respiratory paralysis and cardiac asystole. The pharmacological action of cardiotoxin has been shown to be due to an irreversible depolarization of the cell membrane transport mechanism and asystolic cardiac arrest possibly due to release of Ca++ from the surface membrane of the myocardium.

    Many types of snakes are attributed to be causing cardiovascular symptoms and ECG changes. Patients envenomed by Burmese Russell's viper may bleed into anterior pituitary gland [Sheehan's Syndrome]. Hypotension and shock are common in patients bitten by North American rattlesnakes, Bothrops, Daboia and Viper species. Direct myocardial involvement is suggested by an abnormal ECG in cardiac arrhythmia. In European viper bite, ECG changes include flattening or inversion of T-wave, ST-elevation, second degree heart block, brady- or tachyarrythmias, atrial fibrillation and myocardial infarction.

Myocardial infarction and circulatory collapse may be due to DIC and/or direct myocardial toxicity. ECG abnormalities have been reported as unusual but important observations. Sinus bradycardia, ST-T changes, various degrees of AV block and evidence of hyperkalemia have been described, esp. in envenomation by Viperidae, Australian Elapids and Atractaspididae [burrowing asps]. Similar changes have been seen in viperine bites. [Virmani, 2002]

- Viperine snake bite occurred in 93% and elapid snake bite in 7% of 30 cases. Cardiotoxicity was seen in only 25% of patients with viperine bite. 70% of patients had haemorrhagic manifestations and 30% had cardiotoxicity. The disturbance in heart rate was seen in 47%, rhythm disturbance in 6.7%, tachycardia in 36.7% and bradycardia in 10% of cases. Hypertension was found in 6.7%, hypotension in 16.7%. Thirty per cent of patients had gallop rhythm and it persisted in 16.6% of patients till discharge. One patient had evidence of pulmonary oedema and 1 had basal congestion. Cardiomegaly on chest X-ray was found in 1 patient and elevated SGOT titres were found in 10%. Common electrocardiographic changes were sinus tachycardia, sinus arrhythmia [6.6%], sinus bradycardia [10%], tall T-wave in V2 [3.3%], pattern suggestive of acute anterior wall infarction with reciprocal changes [3.3%], myocardial ischemia [10%], non-specific ST-T changes [16.7%] and atrioventricular block [3.3%]. The mortality rate was 10% and all these patients had bleeding manifestations and abnormal electrocardiograms. [Nayak, 1990]

- Envenoming by a number of species of snake may affect the *myocardium* or cause electrocardiographic changes; several different mechanisms have been proposed. In a prospective study of snake bite in Papua New Guinea, electrocardiographic changes were observed in 36 of 69 patients [52%] envenomed by the taipan [*Oxyuranus scutellatus*], 2 of 6 [33%] envenomed by death adders [*Acanthophis* sp.] and 1 envenomed by the brown snake [*Pseudonaja textilis*]. Septal T-wave inversion and bradycardias, incl. atrioventricular block, were the commonest abnormalities. There was no haemodynamic deterioration. [Lalloo, 1997]

- Tachycardia was noticed in 20 [40%] of 50 cases while bradycardia was present only in 5 [10%] cases; 5 [10%] patients presented with palpitations and 4 [8%] patients had breathlessness. Among all cases commonest ECG changes noticed was sinus tachycardia [19], followed by ST segment depression in 12 patients, sinus bradycardia in 5, ventricular ectopics in 4, T-wave inversions in 2 and tall T-waves in 2 patients. [Anitha, 2017]

- The commonest manifestation in 31 cases of vasculotoxic snake bite was tachycardia [16.67%] and hypotension [14.29%]. On admission, ECG manifestations were 39.1% in poisonous [41 neurotoxic and 31 vasculotoxic] bites were sinus tachycardia [17.8%], sinus bradycardia [9.5%], nonspecific ST-T changes [5.9%], AV block [3.5%] and sinus arrhythmia [2.3%] of all cases. In symptomatic cases mortality was 19% with no mortality seen in non-poisonous snake bite. There was significant difference between outcome of abnormal ECG group and normal ECG group patients. [Singh, 2019]

# FOR GOODNESS SNAKES – VENOMS AS MEDICINES

## Polio & Other Neurological Syndromes

The Thailand cobra [Naja kaouthia] is armed with venom that paralyses nerves and muscles and eventually causes respiratory arrest. For more than 20 years, BioTherapeutics, Inc. in conjunction with Esperanza Peptide Ltd and funded through The Esperanza Research Foundation, in the USA, has been conducting clinical trials of Immunokine, a drug derived from alpha-cobratoxin from Thailand cobra venom, on people with multiple sclerosis.

Immunokine seems to prevent immune cells from attacking and destroying the myelin sheath that protects nerve cells. The drug is reported by the manufacturer to reverse chronic fatigue [improve stamina]; alleviate some types of pain; improve coordination/dexterity; usually improve balance; improve walking; help vision; may help incontinence. What it can't do is cure ['wears off in 24 hours']; help spasticity; reverse optic neuritis; prevent relapses [though minor]; protect from viral infections [but general health is better].

Other potential uses of modified alpha-cobratoxin include amyotrophic lateral sclerosis, Huntington's chorea, diabetic neuropathy, Guillain-Barré syndrome, and post-polio syndrome.

## MS & ALS

In the 1970s, there was particular interest, accompanied by a great deal of public controversy, in the purported effectiveness of a modified snake venom mixture. Based on observations that certain snake venoms block the action of poliovirus on the anterior horn cells, patients were treated with inactivated venom from the cobra [Naja kaouthia] and many-banded krait [Bungarus multicinctus]. Significant benefit was purported to be observed. After an average treatment of 14 months, 52 out of 113 ALS patients were reported as stabilised and 13 as improved. During the later 1970s, many ALS patients went to Florida for treatment with snake venom. [Motor Neurone Disease – Bob Broedel's ALS Digest]

## Breast Cancer

Venom of the southern copperhead [Agkistrodon contortrix contortrix] yields the disintegrin contortrostatin [CN]. Disintegrins are soluble peptides found in snake venom that promote bleeding in envenomation by binding to receptors on platelets. These same receptors are abundant on cancer cells. Contortrostatin is under investigation for treatment of breast cancer, extrapolated from the finding that the copperhead peptide, when injected in mice implanted with human cancer cells, reduced the growth rate of the tumour cells for up to 60–70%, and decreased metastasis to the lungs for 90%. The major limitation to the use of disintegrins as anticancer medications is trying to get them selective to the cancer cells without binding in appreciable levels to platelets. Francis Markland, Ph.D., professor of biochemistry and molecular biology at the University of Southern California Keck School of Medicine, has extensively researched contortrostatin, reporting that it 'appears to inhibit the ability of breast cancer cells to adhere to and invade normal cells in the surrounding tissue.' CN also seems to restrict new blood vessel development in tumours, thus starving them of the nutrients they need to grow.

## Vascular Disease

'Ancrod [current brand name: Viprinex] is a fibrinogen-reducing agent derived from the venom of the Malayan pit viper. The defribrinogenation of blood results in an anticoagulant effect. Ancrod is prepared from the crude venom of the Malayan pit viper [Agkistrodon rhodostoma, also termed Calloselasma rhodostoma] and belongs to the group of proteolytic enzymes. Ancrod may also be found in the venoms of many poisonous snakes [crotalids, elapids and viperids] in general, but the Malayan pit viper is most suitable due to a high concentration of ancrod in its venom.' [Wikipedia]

Ancrod has been used in Europe and Canada since the 1970s as reperfusion therapy for clinical conditions such as peripheral vascular disease, deep vein thrombosis, and central retinal venous thrombosis. At present, ancrod is being marketed only in Canada. Viprinex has been evaluated as treatment beginning within 3 or 6 hours of onset of acute ischaemic stroke [reduced or blocked blood flow to a brain area due to a blood clot] with inconsistent results.

## Blood Pressure

The toxic effects of venom from the Brazilian pit viper Bothrops jararaca have been found to be due to a sudden, massive drop in blood pressure. The venom was shown to contain peptides that inhibit ACE [angiotensin converting enzyme], the enzyme that is responsible for converting the inactive peptide angiotensin I into the active and powerful vasoconstrictor angiotensin II. This formed the basis for developing captopril, the prototype of an anti-hypertensive class of drugs called ACE inhibitors. Since then ACE inhibitors have been discovered in the venom of numerous snake species. The effect of some components of certain snake venoms is comparable to an overdose of captopril, with serious hypotension as a consequence.

## Blood Clotting

A blood-clotting protein in coastal taipan venom [Oxyuranus scutellatus], termed Factor X [Factor Ten], has been identified by Queensland University of Technology PhD researcher Liam St Pierre to rapidly stop excessive bleeding during vascular surgery and major trauma.

## Diuresis

Dendroaspis natriuretic peptide [DNP], recently isolated from the venom of the green mamba [Dendroaspis angusticeps] has been established as a potent natriuretic and diuretic peptide that may play a physiological role in the regulation of sodium excretion. DNP possesses cardiac unloading actions but with significant hypotensive properties. Additional natriuretic peptides have been isolated and characterised, particularly from the venom of the snakes Micrurus corallinus, and Bothrops jararaca.

## Topical Analgesic in Rheumatic & Neuralgic Pains

An over-the-counter ointment named Viprosal has been available in Russia and Eastern Europe for the relief of pain. The ointment is a mixture of Vipera berus venom, salicylic acid, camphor, and turpentine oil. It is touted to stimulate re-absorption and repair of scar tissue, as well as used to treat nerve and rheumatic pains.

## Pain Management

'In the early part of the last century, cobra venoms were established products mainly for the treatment of severe pain, but also for rheumatism, trigeminal neuralgia, asthma, ocular therapy, and neuroses. Cobra venom has been widely used for decades in China for the treatment of rheumatoid arthritis and cancer. Prior to use, it is partially denatured by heating. This process will inactivate many of the venom enzymes, although the neurotoxins can retain their toxicity. Such modified venoms proved to be 80% effective in the clinic for the treatment of headache and arthritis pain. One feature of this venom product is its slow onset of analgesic activity. In the United States, 2 cobra venom products, Cobroxin and Nyloxin, were marketed up to 1972 for the treatment of pain and arthritis. With the new FDA drug registration requirements in that year, these products were abandoned over production issues and in favour of newer drugs.' [Paul F. Reid, 2007]

As over-the-counter pain relievers, both Cobroxin and Nylotoxin are available as an oral spray for treating migraine headaches, neck aches, shoulder pain, cramps, lower back pain and neuralgia. They also come in a topical gel for treating joint pain and pain associated with repetitive stress and arthritis.

'A myriad of different toxins and derivatives obtained from various groups of animals have been described as able to relieve pain through activation or blockage of different molecular targets. Among snakes, there are the cobrotoxin and cobratoxin, isolated from the venom of *Naja atra* and *Naja kaouthia*, respectively, which present high affinity to different subunits of nicotinic acetylcholine receptors and exert antinociception. Also, another example is crotalphine, isolated from the venom of *Crotalus durissus terrificus*. This toxin induces antinociception through an *opioid-like activity* without causing some of the typical side effects induced by the use of opioids, such as tolerance or withdrawal symptoms. Likewise, the neurotoxin hannalgesin, isolated from *Ophiophagus hannah*, and the venom of *Micrurus lemniscatus* also exert antinociception via activation of the opioid pathway. In addition, toxins isolated from the venom of the black mamba [Dendroaspis polylepis] causes strong pain relief by blocking acid-sensing ion channels.' [Freitas, 2017]

## Straightening Out Wrinkles

Pentapharm, a Swiss pharmaceutical company, developed a synthetic peptide that mimics the neurological effects of a polypeptide [termed waglerin 1] found in the venom of Wagler's temple viper [Tropidolaemus wagleri]. The product is called Syn-Ake and is now used in several anti-ageing cosmetic products sold in the U.S. and Europe. A Botox alternative, Syn-Ake relaxes/paralyses muscles that cause facial creases such as expression lines by blocking nerve signals that tell muscles to contract.

### Superior to Snake Oil: Lethal Snake Delight

- Bill Haast, director of Miami Serpentarium Laboratories, made a mark in 1949 in polio research when he discovered that cobra venom affects the same nerve endings as the poliovirus. Asked about the effects of neurotoxic snakebites in an interview with Anne Goodwin Sides in 1997, he said: 'Krait venom [Bungarus candidus] usually makes you stop breathing – it paralyses your diaphragm. In fact, I've never heard of another krait bite victim surviving. But it also stimulates the nervous system. My sensitivity – touch and sight – was exaggerated by maybe a hundred times. There was nothing horrible about it. It was all just beautiful texture and tapestry and colours. This was before LSD, but that's probably similar to what I was feeling.'
- After a bite by a king cobra, Ophiophagus hannah, Bob Hughes, an avid snake collector from New York, experienced something similar in 1988, at least initially: 'At first, it was like a nice mild hallucinogenic, a warm euphoric rush that flowed through my body with mescaline-like trails across my vision. I actually enjoyed it for a few minutes. *La La* land. Then, suddenly I couldn't see in colour anymore. Everything became black and white and, whoa, I started to panic. Then came the pain. God, the pain. It honestly felt like there were razors under my skin trying to get out. It was absolutely horrible.' Hughes rapidly weakened. Fifteen minutes after the bite, he couldn't raise his shoulders or speak coherently. His condition deteriorated further as he was transported by helicopter to a hospital where, one hour after the bite, he arrived unconscious. Massive infusions of antivenom and mechanical ventilation [respirator] saved his life.
- Brian Fry, the Melbourne-based herpetologist, said that one of the classic reactions to elapid venom is hypoxia: 'There's a sense of disconnection, of sensory disruption – a floaty feeling.' He said that when he was bitten by the common death adder [Acanthophis antarcticus], a close relative of the krait, 'It was one of the most pleasant highs I've ever experienced.' [cited in James 2008]
- Shortly after being bitten by a black mamba in the ankle, Jack Seale was driven to the hospital. He had to be carried in. 'Though the assistant was frantic, Jack himself no longer cared whether he lived or died. "It's a pure neurotoxin, and it gives you a buzz. It's the nicest feeling. First you get a sense of lightness. Then you start getting tingling sensations, like pins and needles. Then you get a very warm feeling over your body, like when you haven't eaten all day, and you have a beer. Your tongue gets kind of funny, and it's a lovely feeling." Jack's sense of well-being notwithstanding, only immediate application of a heart-and-lung machine kept him alive.' [Lee, 1996]

For the rest of Jack's 7-day ordeal, see below under Dendroaspis polylepis, Losing control over everything – Locked in, Buried alive.

| Homeopathic name | Common name | Abbreviation | Symptoms |
|---|---|---|---|
| *Family Boidae – Constrictors* | | | |
| Antaresia perthensis | Pygmy python | Anta-ps. | – |
| Boa constrictor | Boa constrictor | Boa-co. | ++ |
| Corallus hortulanus | Amazon tree boa | Cora-h-s. | – |
| Eunectes murinus | Green anaconda | Eun-mur. | – |
| Eunectes notaeus | Yellow anaconda | Eun-not. | – |
| Morelia spilota variegata | Carpet python | More-sp. | – |
| Morelia viridis | Green tree python | More-vir. | – |
| Python molurus | Indian python | Pyth-mo. | – |
| Python regius | Ball python | Pyth-re. | ++ |
| Python reticulatus | Reticulated python | Pyth-rt. | ++ |
| | | | |
| *Family Colubridae – Colubrids* | | | |
| Chironius carinatus | Amazonian whipsnake | Vip-a-c. | + |
| Cyclagras gigas | False water cobra | Cyc-gig. | + |
| Dispholidus typus | Boomslang | Dis-ty. | + |
| Drymarchon corais | Yellowtail cribo | Drymar-cr. | – |
| Drymarchon couperi | Indigo snake | Drymar-cp. | – |
| Elaphe guttata | Corn snake | Ela-gt. | + |
| Elaphe longissima | Aesculapian snake | Ela-lo. | – |
| Lampropeltis calligaster calligaster | Prairie king snake | Lamp-c-c. | – |
| Lampropeltis calligaster rhombomaculata | Mole kingsnake | Lamp-c-r. | – |
| Lampropeltis getula cal. | California king snake | Lamp-g-c. | – |
| Lampropeltis triangulum | Milk snake | Lamp-tr. | – |
| Natrix natrix | Grass snake | Natr-n. | + |
| Pantherophis obsoletus | Red rat snake | Panth-obs. | – |
| Thamnophis sirtalis sirtalis | Eastern garter snake | Tham-ss. | + |
| Vipera acustica carinata | Amazonian whipsnake | Vip-a-c. | + |
| | | | |
| *Family Elapidae – Elapids* | | | |
| Bungarus caeruleus | Common krait | Bung-cl. | + |
| Bungarus candidus | Blue krait | Bung-cd. | + |
| Bungarus fasciatus | Banded krait | Bung-fa. | ++ |
| Bungarus multicinctus | Many-banded krait | Bung-mc. | + |
| Dendroaspis angusticeps | Eastern green mamba | Dendr-ang. | ++ |
| Dendroaspis polylepis | Black mamba | Dendr-pol. | ++ |
| Dendroaspis viridis | Western green mamba | Dendr-vir. | – |
| Elaps corallinus | Brazilian coral snake | Elaps | +++ |
| Hemachatus haemachatus | Rinkhals | Hem-ha. | ++ |
| Maticora bivirgata | Blue Malayan coral snake | Mat-bv. | – |

| | | | |
|---|---|---|---|
| Micrurus lemniscatus | South American coral snake | Micru-ln. | + |
| Naja anchietae | Anchieta's cobra | Naja-an. | + |
| Naja annulifera | Snouted cobra | Naja-annu. | + |
| Naja haje | Egyptian cobra | Naja-hj. | ++ |
| Naja kaouthia | Monocled cobra | Naja-k. | + |
| Naja melanoleuca | Forest cobra | Naja-me. | + |
| Naja mossambica | Mozambique spitting cobra | Naja-mo. | ++ |
| Naja nigricollis | Black-necked spitting cobra | Naja-n. | + |
| Naja nivea | Cape cobra | Naja-niv. | + |
| Naja pallida | Red spitting cobra | Naja-pa. | ++ |
| Naja tripudians | Indian cobra | Naja | +++ |
| Notechis scutatus occident. | Western tiger snake | Note-st-o. | + |
| Notechis scutatus scutatus | Eastern tiger snake | Note-st-st. | + |
| Ophiophagus hannah | King cobra | Ophiop-ha. | ++ |
| Oxyuranus microlepidotus | Inland taipan | Oxyurn-mi. | + |
| Oxyuranus scutellatus | Coastal taipan | Oxyurn-sc. | ++ |
| Pseudonaja textilis | Eastern brown snake | Pseud-ts. | + |

*Family Hydrophiidae – Sea snakes*

| | | | |
|---|---|---|---|
| Hydrophis cyanocinctus | Annulated sea snake | Hydroph. | ++ |
| Laticauda colubrina | Banded sea krait | Latic-co. | + |
| Pelamis platurus | Yellow-bellied sea snake | Pelam-pl. | + |

*Family Viperidae, subfamily Crotalinae – Pit vipers*

| | | | |
|---|---|---|---|
| Acrochordon chocoe | = Lachesis acrochorda | Acro-c-f. | + |
| Ancistrodon piscivorus | Cottonmouth | Ancis-p. | ++ |
| Bothriechis schlegelii | Eyelash pit viper | Bothri-sg. | + |
| Bothrocophias colombianus | Colombian toadh. pitviper | Vip-l-f. | + |
| Bothrops alternatus | Crossed pit viper | Both-a. | + |
| Bothrops asper | Asper | Both-as. | + |
| Bothrops atrox | Common lancehead | Both-ax. | ++ |
| Bothrops caribbaeus | St. Lucia pit viper | Both-car. | + |
| Bothrops colombiensis | = Bothrops atrox | | |
| Bothrops insularis | Golden lancehead | Both-in. | – |
| Bothrops jararaca | Jararaca | Both-jara. | + |
| Bothrops jararacussu | Jararacussu | Both-jasu. | ++ |
| Bothrops lanceolatus | Fer-de-lance | Both. | ++ |
| Bothrops neuwiedi urutu | Neuwied's lancehead | Both-n-ur. | + |
| Cenchris contortrix | Copperhead | Cench. | +++ |
| Crotalus adamanteus | Eastern diamondback | Crot-ad. | + |
| Crotalus atrox | Western diamondback | Crot-atr. | + |

| | | | |
|---|---|---|---|
| Crotalus cascavella | South American rattlesnake | Crot-c. | +++ |
| Crotalus cerastes cerastes | Mojave Desert rattlesnake | Crot-cer. | + |
| Crotalus enyo | Baja California rattlesnake | Crot-eny. | – |
| Crotalus horridus | Timber rattlesnake | Crot-h. | +++ |
| Crotalus lepidus | Rock rattlesnake | Crot-le. | + |
| Crotalus mitchellii | Speckled rattlensnake | Crot-mi. | + |
| Crotalus molossus | Black-tailed rattlesnake | Crot-mo. | + |
| Crotalus polystictus | Mexican lance-headed rattlesnake | Crot-po. | + |
| Crotalus viridis viridis | Prairie rattlesnake | Crot-vir. | + |
| Deinagkistrodon acutus | Sharp-nosed pit viper | Dein-ac. | + |
| Lachesis acrochorda | Chocoan bushmaster | Acro-c-f. | + |
| Lachesis muta | Bushmaster | Lach. | +++ |
| Sistrurus catenatus caten. | Eastern massasauga | Sist-cc. | – |
| Trimeresurus flavoviridis | Habu | Trim-fl. | + |
| Trimeresurus mucrosquamatus | Brown-spotted pit viper | Trim-mu. | + |
| Trimeresurus puniceus | Flat-nosed pit viper | Trim-pu. | – |
| Trimeresurus purpureomaculatus | Mangrove pit viper | Trim-pur. | – |
| Trimeresurus stejnegeri | Green tree viper | Trim-st. | + |
| Trimeresurus wagleri | Temple pit viper | Trim. | + |
| Vipera lachesis fel | = Bothrocophias colombianus | Vip-l-f. | + |

*Family Viperidae, subfamily Viperinae – True vipers*

| | | | |
|---|---|---|---|
| Atheris squamigera | African bush viper | Ather-sq. | + |
| Bitis arietans | Puff adder | Bit-ar. | ++ |
| Bitis atropos | Berg adder | Bit-atr. | ++ |
| Bitis caudalis | Horned adder | Bit-ca. | + |
| Bitis gabonica | Gaboon viper | Bit-ga. | ++ |
| Bitis nasicornis | Rhinoceros viper | Bit-nas. | + |
| Cerastes cerastes | Horned viper | Ceras-ce. | ++ |
| Daboia russelii | Russell's viper | Vip-d. | + |
| Daboia siamensis | Eastern Russell's viper | Vip-ds. | + |
| Echis carinatus | Saw-scaled viper | Echis-ca. | ++ |
| Proatheris superciliaris | Swamp viper | Proa-su. | + |
| Vipera ammodytes meridionalis | Eastern nose-horned viper | Vip-am-m. | + |
| Vipera aspis | Asp viper | Vip-a. | ++ |
| Vipera berus | Common European viper | Vip. | +++ |
| Vipera daboia | = Daboia russelii | Vip-d. | + |
| Vipera lebetina | Blunt-nosed viper | Vip-ll. | + |
| Vipera palaestinae | Palestine viper | Vip-pal. | + |

| Vipera redi | Central Italian asp viper | Vip-r. | + |
| Vipera torva | = Vipera berus | Vip. | |
| Vipera xanthina | Ottoman viper | Vip-x. | + |

## SNAKE THEMES

*According to Farokh Master [India]:*

1 Competitiveness & Power.
  The central theme of snake remedies is one of competitiveness and gaining power over others and their environment. Whatever they do in life they must be the first to achieve it.

2 Attack & Defence.
  The theme of attack and defence is seen in most of the snake remedies. For example, the patient may say: "I want to kill him," "These people are my enemies" or "I cannot defend myself." This also may be reflected in the dreams.

3 Passionate & Workaholic.
  In order to achieve their goals, they work very hard. The snake remedies are known to be more active at night. They can't sleep due to a rush of ideas and plans.

4 Seduction & Eroticism.
  Seeking attention or trying to be the centre of attraction is an important feature. They may wear attractive clothes, watches, etc. It helps them to develop contacts with others and influence people. They can flatter others to get their work done. They can also flatter the physician, for example, they may say: "You are the world's best doctor."

5 Egotism.
  The feeling of being superior to others and possessing power is common to snake remedies. They can appear over-confident and have a habit of boasting. They cannot take a joke and are easily offended.

6 Duality & Secretiveness.
  Most snake remedies have a secret life or a darker side, which they don't want to reveal to others. They live a dual life. The dark side could be completely repressed, and they can appear to be spiritual, peace loving, having love for animals, etc. They can also be aware of their deceptive nature and may use it at the right time for their selfish motives. They are hypocrites with a lot of contradictions within themselves. In certain situations, when strict authorities or rules restrict them, they may develop into a weak-willed and confused personality.

7 Drug & Alcohol Abuse.
  Affection of liver due to alcoholism is an important pathology in snake remedies.

8 Affection of Speech.

Speech is one of the main modes of attracting the attention of others. But a deeper study of snake remedies will reveal their power to cause and cure a lot of speech disorders and also affections of speech after cerebrovascular accidents.

9 Suspiciousness & Deception.

Mistrust is a very common feature. They cannot trust friends, people working with them, or even family members. They have a strong fear of being betrayed. Usually this fear of being deceived has its roots in some past experiences. But this theme has another variation. The snake remedies can be deceptive, and they can project their traits onto others.

10 Forsaken Feeling.

The feeling of being deprived or of not getting what they deserve is common to snake remedies. They have a great need for multiple relationships and to connect with others in order to fill their inner vacuum. Subtle differences between snake remedies create variations in clinical presentations.

11 Death.

Death-related themes are very common in snake remedies. Similar themes are also seen in cases of children requiring a snake remedy. The fear of incurable diseases and death are very prominent in snake remedies.

12 Spirituality & Religiousness.

Related to the theme of death is the spiritual path taken by snake remedies. They are concerned about their fate after death. They adopt religion to cover their dark side. Religion and spirituality can help them to overcome their guilt. The study of religious scriptures can also be due to curiosity and a need to experience spiritual bliss.

13 Clairvoyance & Magnetism.

Intuition is an important feature of snake remedies. Some of them can look into the future and foresee events. Some of them can predict the lifespan of people; others can foresee something bad that might happen. They can tap into the lives of others in a magnetic way. Some snake remedies use intuition to protect or defend themselves against danger.

14 Sensation of Constriction.

Snake remedies have the component of constriction at a physical and mental level. The feeling of being restricted or suppressed causes a lot of tension in the individual as he cannot develop his personality with his free will. He feels constricted by society, ethical rules, orthodoxy, religious dogmas, authorities, etc.

15 Swollen Sensation.

16 Discharges >.

17 Sleep <. Touch <.

[Snakes to Simillimum]

*According to Massimo Mangialavori [Italy]:*

1 Seduction.
   Seduction in snakes implies that one must be seen by others and appreciated as a 'special' person. It has to be clear what their value is and how much better they are than others.
2 Forsaken.
   The main feeling is that they deserve something that they don't get. It is not an objective forsaken situation. Very often, for a snake to be left is not a concern about losing the person they love. It is more about an injury to their narcissism. Very often, they are the first to leave someone because they cannot deserve to be left. "Nobody leaves me!" Then they report this as if they are forsaken.
3 Congestion.
   We can see in the cases plenty of symptoms of fullness. It is interesting to see where the sensation of fullness is. More or less they feel constricted by themselves and by society around them. Symbolically, it is like the snake with this inelastic skin in which they cannot grow. They would like to enlarge themselves. In any critical situation it is as if they have the sensation of enlarging in their system and they cannot hold all this stuff in their system.
4 Persecution.
   They cannot trust those around them. But it is not a real paranoia. It is a clear classical projection because this is what they do. They know how much they are untrustworthy.
5 Knowledge.
   They have to achieve a very high point. They need explanations. They cannot stand mysteries and unexplained stuff. This life is too short to understand, clarify and be able to go deep in every situation.
6 One-sided symptoms.
   It can be one side or one part of the body.
7 Duality.
8 Haemorrhages [esp. haemotoxic snakes].
9 Discolouration.
10 Betrayal.
11 Eroticisation of feelings.
12 Clothing <. After sleep <. Swallowing <.
[RefWorks]

*According to Rajan Sankaran [India]:*

1 Issues of superiority versus inferiority.
2 Manipulative.
3 Jealousy.
4 Suspicion.
5 Delusions of mind split in two.
6 Antagonism with self.
7 Vulnerability.

8 Close-mindedness.
9 Clairvoyance.
10 Fear of attack.
11 Fear of being attacked from behind.
12 Feeling of being pursued.
13 Desire to hide.
14 Increased sexual drive.

*According to Jayesh Shah [India]:*

1 Demand attention.
2 Must be attractive.
3 Love of colours, music.
4 Clairvoyance.
5 Strong fear and dreams of snakes.
6 Marked PMS.
7 Strong fear of water, of drowning.
8 Dreams about dead people.
[Hom. Links 2/94]

*According to Konstantinos Pisios [Greece]:*

1 Duality; opposite viewpoints; 2 ways to view life.
   'There is the good and the evil way. They believe that everyone is capable of doing both. No matter which side they choose to be, they know that they could easily cross over if they wanted. If they don't, it's because they learned so from a young age and they believe that it's not true.'
2 Loquacity vs Taciturnity.
   'Although there is a general belief that snakemen talk too much, some are just the opposite. They don't speak at all, due for example, to a stroke, or they speak with difficulty, with dysarthria, with a stammer.'
3 Power vs Insecurity. Quick and energetic or Slow and passive.
4 Fear or Love of snakes.
5 One-sidedness of physical symptoms – right side or left side.
6 Issues with injustice and betrayal. Feeling alone and abandoned. Feeling wronged.
7 Persistent suspicion and mistrust of the opposite sex since a negative experience.
8 Jealousy. Selfish; ask for much more than they are willing to give in relationships or at work. May leave partner out of feeling not having received what they thought or claimed they deserved.
9 Violent response to feeling threatened.
   'If the threat is intense, they immediately react in a violent way. The 'hit' can be obvious, usually sudden, or it may be premeditated and insidious but accurate and 'deadly'. Their goal is always to belittle the enemy.'

10 Need to feel unique; hungry for recognition from their environment [to make feelings of being wronged and vulnerability go away]. Will try different strategies to get others to notice them.

'They show off and try to differ. They seek attention through sexuality and art [theater, music, dance, painting, etc.]. Even when it seems that they have nothing in common with art and appear very strict and composed, they choose nice colours for their clothes, their home, and their car in order to differ from the norm.'

11 Clairvoyance. Intuition. Premonitions. Déjà vu feelings.

'They have knowledge of things and people without knowing where it comes from. When you ask them how they know, their answer is 'I just know'. Snakemen tend to use their knowledge and power gained from their clairvoyance to put others at a disadvantage and to diminish their own insecurity and vulnerability.

12 Religion. God. Devoted and committed; strong in their faith. Or shaken in their faith.

13 Dreams of death.

14 Skeptical about doctors and medication. Search the web or read books about their health problems.

15 Aversion to change. Become more conservative and rigid with age and as their level of health reduces.

16 Sensation of tightening and pressure.

17 Congestion; sensation of warmth, burning or boiling.

18 Sensitivity to environment.

19 Generally loves eating. May have weight problems.

20 PMS.

21 Frequent symptoms.

'Regardless of the basic problem they come to address, 'snake people' quite often have problems in one of the following organs or systems:

Heart – palpitations, heart attack, chest pressure.

Neck – lump in throat.

Hormonal system – ovarian cysts, thyroid problems.

Arteries and veins – bleeding, epistaxis, phlebitis.

Nervous system – paralysis, dysarthria.

Digestive System – constipation, bloating.

[Essence of homeopathic snake remedies]

# Family Boidae, subfamilies Boinae and Pythoninae – Constrictors

### Biological Profile

- Constrictors, such as boas [subfamily Boinae] and pythons [subfamily Pythoninae], capture large prey. Whether terrestrial, arboreal, aquatic, or burrowing, constrictors wrap their body around the prey, constricting and suffocating it. Recent research shows that the enormous pressure created by the coils of such snakes can also stop circulation and even stop the heart, quickly cutting off the blood supply to the victim's brain. In addition, the force of the coils can snap an animal's neck or spine. Constriction may also break other bones, making the prey easier to swallow.

- The head of constrictors is clearly differentiated from the trunk, except in the burrowing species, and the mouth is large, with jaws that are longer than the skull [the burrowing species excepted again]. The upper jaw moves easily in relation to the skull; the mandibles can part easily. Large scales cover the stomach.
- The constrictor's powerful digestive juices can break down bones, horns and teeth as well as hide and flesh. It may take a constrictor days or even weeks to completely digest a large meal, leaving the snake potentially vulnerable because of the bulky bulge in its body. The snake may not need to eat again for months. Constrictors can *temporarily increase the size of their hearts* to improve the blood supply needed in digestion.
- Pythons have 2 functioning lungs, one large and one small – more advanced snakes have only a single lung.
- Boas and pythons are very similar. The principal difference between them is that pythons are oviparous [reproduce by laying eggs], while viviparous boas give birth to live young [with no eggs involved at any stage of development]. Boas, in addition, are usually less stocky than pythons and are more often arboreal.
- Python eggs are particularly temperature sensitive and, if incubated at insufficient temperatures, many young fail to develop or develop birth defects such as spinal kyphosis.
- Pythons and some boas [3 out of 8 genera in subfamily Boinae] have thermosensitive labial dimples on each side of the mouth, which allow them to locate a warm-blooded animal found in close proximity.
- Family name derives from Latin *bos*, 'cow', based on an old myth that boas pursue cows and suckle them until they are drained to death.
- Pythons and boas are sometimes regarded as belonging to separate families, Pythonidae and Boidae, respectively.

## Inclusion Body Disease
Inclusion body disease of boid snakes has been recognized since the mid 1970s. It is named for the characteristic intracytoplasmic inclusions that are seen in epidermal cells, oral mucosal epithelial cells, visceral epithelial cells and neurons. The affection occurs worldwide in captive boid snakes. Its prevalence in the wild is not known.

'Inclusion body disease [IBD] has been increasingly diagnosed in boas and pythons ["boids"]. It is believed to be a retrovirus. The way it affects these 2 groups of snakes is slightly different, but the long-term effects are the same: the disease is terminal in those animals who exhibit symptoms of the disease.

'Pythons, although their symptoms may be somewhat less, are just as affected as boas. There are asymptomatic carriers, so the fact that a boa or python within an infected collection does not show signs of the illness should not be taken to mean that it is immune to it. Boas are most associated with being asymptomatic carriers.

'Signs of infection in boas include central nervous system disorders such as paralysis, being unable to right itself when turned over, 'star-gazing', inability to strike or constrict. Other signs include chronic regurgitation, extreme weight loss, respiratory infections, and dysecdysis due to the inability to control body movements enough to rub off the old skin. The disease is rapidly fatal in young and juvenile boas, typified by rapid onset of flaccid paralysis.

'In pythons, the disease progresses much more rapidly than in boas. Along with the above symptoms [excluding the chronic regurgitation], pythons also tend toward infectious stomatitis ["mouth rot"], heightened or exaggerated reflex responses, disorientation [which may be precipitated by the onset of central blindness] and loss of motor coordination.' [Melissa Kaplan]

## BOIDAE IN HOMEOPATHY

| Homeopathic name | Common name | Abbreviation | Symptoms |
|---|---|---|---|
| Antaresia perthensis | Pygmy python | Anta-ps. | – |
| Boa constrictor[1] | Boa constrictor | Boa-co. | ++ |
| Corallus hortulanus[2] | Amazon tree boa | Cora-h-s. | – |
| Eunectes murinus | Green anaconda | Eun-mur. | – |
| Eunectes notaeus | Yellow anaconda | Eun-not. | – |
| Morelia spilota variegata | Carpet python | More-sp. | – |
| Morelia viridis | Green tree python | More-vir. | – |
| Python molurus | Indian python | Pyth-mo. | – |
| Python regius | Ball python | Pyth-re. | ++ |
| Python reticulatus | Reticulated python | Pyth-rt. | ++ |

1 Listed as Boa constrictor [Boa-co.] and Adeps boae constrictoris [Adeps-boa.].
2 Listed as Corallus hortulanus sebium [Cora-h-s.].

# ANTARESIA PERTHENSIS

## Systematics
• Scientific name: Antaresia perthensis [Stull, 1932].
• Synonyms: Liasis perthensis [Mitchell, 1965]. Morelia perthensis [Welch, 1994].
• Common names: Pygmy python. Anthill python.
• Family: Boidae, subfamily Pythoninae.

## Biological Profile

- Non-venomous constrictor. World's smallest python; average length of 50 cm. Head short and wedge shaped; neck and body thick and muscular. Dorsal side dark brick red; may bear a conspicuous pattern of dark dorsal bars. Belly creamy white.
- Range: NW Australia.
- Habitat: Flat land with sparse vegetation; rocky areas. Often found in large termite mounds, where they spend almost all daylight hours. Shares the mound with species of venomous snakes, constrictors & lizards. Curls inside the mound into what looks like a large ball with other snakes.
- Solitary. Aggregations with other snakes in termite mounds are opportunistic, with little interaction.
- Nocturnal.
- Preys on frogs, small lizards, bats. Uses scent to track prey.
- Oviparous; 5–8 eggs per clutch; mother stays coiled around her eggs to provide protection and warmth.
- At high risk of predation. Preyed upon by a variety of birds, carnivorous mammals, large frogs, spiders, and other snakes.
- Specific epithet derived from Perth, the capital city of Western Australia, where the original type specimen was mistakenly believed to have come from. The genus is named after the reddish star Antares in the scorpion's tail of the constellation Scorpius.
- Popular exotic pet, usually docile, easy to handle and rarely biting.

## Materia Medica

- No symptoms.

# BOA CONSTRICTOR

## Systematics

- Scientific name: Boa constrictor [L., 1758].
- Common name: Boa constrictor.
- Family: Boidae, subfamily Boinae.

## Biological Profile

- Heavy-bodied non-venomous constrictor ranging in length from 50 cm as neonates to 4 m as adults. Weight 27–45 kg. Depending on the habitat they are trying to blend into, their bodies can be tan, green, red, or yellow, and display cryptic patterns of jagged lines, ovals, diamonds, and circles.
- Range: Northern Mexico to Argentina.
- Habitat: Highly diverse, ranging from deserts and wet tropical forests to open savannah and cultivated fields, and from sea level to moderate elevation. Shows little inclination towards water. Excellent swimmer, but prefers to stay on dry land, living primarily in hollow logs and abandoned mammal burrows.

- Aggressive, solitary, nocturnal ambush hunter in the rain forests of Central and South America that kills its prey by coiling its robust body around the victim and squeezing the life out of it, swallowing it whole once it is unconscious or dead. Jaws lined with small, hooked teeth for grabbing and holding prey while it wraps its body around the victim.
- Uses thermal-sensitive facial scales to locate prey.
- Preys on lizards, birds, small mammals – possums, mongooses, rats, squirrels, and bats; the latter are its preferred prey, which it catches by hanging from the branches of trees or the mouths of caves, snatching the flying mammals right out of the air.
- Small individuals may climb into trees and shrubs to forage, but they become mostly terrestrial as they become older and heavier. It is said that specimens from Central America are more irascible, hissing loudly and striking repeatedly when disturbed, while those from South America tame down more readily. [Wikipedia]
- Females emit a scent from the cloaca to attract males. Male and female join together at the cloaca in order for the male to fertilize the eggs. Fertilization is internal. Ovoviviparous; 15–50 live young.
- Five recognized subspecies [constrictor, nebulosa, occidentalis, orophias, ortonii].

### Anecdotal Superlatives

'The boa constrictor is a cross between an animal and a parade. It is found in the hot, moist countries, which are favourable to luxuriant growths of all kinds, and attains a length varying from 789 feet, as viewed by the startled eye, to 30 feet, when stretched out and measured with a tape line.

'The boa constrictor is a snake but acts more like a railway collision. When it has gotten its growth it is as big around as a beer keg and its constant outdoor life gives it large muscles and great endurance. It has neither arms nor legs, but its educated and versatile tail makes up for this lack. When the boa constrictor wraps itself around a personal enemy, gets a half hitch with its tail around a tree and then begins to contract, its victim's ribs fold up like an accordion.

'The boa constrictor travels by chasing itself along the ground and climbs trees without bothering to hunt for a toe hold. Its favourite occupation is to festoon itself gracefully from the branch of a tree and wait for something to pass underneath. When this happens, the extensive and hungry snake drops itself swiftly about its dinner and squeezes once with a loud-cracking noise.

'After this nothing remains for the boa but to eat its meal. This is a very serious matter with it, however. Nature, for the protection of the rest of us, makes it hard for the boa to eat. He has to unjoint his jaws and swallow his meal whole. To see a hungry constrictor tucking away a pig twice his size is an interesting but painful sight. When the boa constrictor has finished his meal, he has a knot as large as a barrel half way between his head and tail, and is all in.

'For the next month or more the boa is as sleepy and indifferent as a political party after it has won an election and has gotten all the offices. He will not move and can be sawed into cord lengths with impunity.' [Fitch, 1916]

# MATERIA MEDICA BOA CONSTRICTOR

## Sources
1 Proving Uta Santos [Austria], 10 provers [7 females, 3 males], 12c; 1996.
2 Degroote, Dream Repertory.

## Mind
∞ Delusion being followed when driving car & trembling all over.[1]
∞ Delusion being pursued in dark.[1]
∞ Delusion being pursued by a man with a knife.[1]
∞ Delusion being watched.[1]
∞ Explosive temper, no desire for sex.[1]
∞ Quick tempered, wants to decide everything, bossy and dictatorial.[1]
∞ Irritability and despair, feeling of failure. Hopelessness, > weeping, suicidal thoughts, throwing self in front of train.[1]
∞ Cheerful in [late] evening.[1]
∞ Rebellious and indignant with spouse.[1]
∞ Finding fault. Impatient and offensive to everyone.[1]
∞ Fear of suffocating the person one is cuddling.[2]

## Dreams
∞ Attacked by cats.[2]
∞ Beauty.[1]
∞ Betrayal and jealousy.[1]
∞ Big flying bats.[2]
∞ Clothes too large.[2]
∞ Constrictor snake.[2]
∞ Detected by enemy while being hidden.[2]
∞ Father.[1]
∞ Grasped, being.[2]
∞ Grip, having no.[2]
∞ Hide, desire to.[2]
∞ Jealous, being.[2]
∞ Religious faith.[1]
∞ Spoiled daughter.[1]
∞ Transformation.[1]
∞ Treated with contempt.[1]

## Generals
∞ Great chilliness.[1]
∞ Exhaustion between 6 and 8 p.m. [1 pr.]. Complete exhaustion in evening, falls asleep at 8 p.m. while reading [1 pr.].[1]
∞ Attacks of binge eating: bread and mustard. Bingeing on snacks; doesn't want regular meals [1 pr.]. Strange warm feeling of nausea before mealtimes with a desperate need to eat [1 pr.].[1]
∞ Craving for beer, due to dryness mouth; black tea.[1]

∞ Aversion to bathing.[2]
∞ Right side more affected [4 pr.].[1]

## Sensations
∞ Right side face numb, as if it doesn't belong there.[1]
∞ Lips as if bloody.[1]
∞ Lump in throat-pit > drinking or eating.[2]

## Locals
∞ Frontal headache, stabbing, & very sensitive to draughts, esp. cold wind on forehead.[1]
∞ Stabbing earache and irritation, left, especially when chewing.[1]
∞ Dryness mouth at night.[1]
∞ Throatache, left or right, at night.[1]
∞ Hiccough from eating hurriedly.[2]
∞ Violent and sudden urging for stool; gushing, brown, watery stool; stool and anus burn like fire, > warm footbath.[1]
∞ Dragging pain in breast during menses.[1]
∞ Cough > lying on right side.[2]
∞ Spicy smell of sweat in armpits.[1]
∞ Dragging pain in groin radiating over thigh to shin.[1]

## Guiding Symptoms
• Anger and resentment that is suppressed and finds no vent.
• Children from over-caring parents who when grown up are bound to social rules and expectations.
• Obsessive compulsive behaviours.
• Overprotective and pushy parents who curb the freedom of their child so as to make them timid, spineless, and childish.
• Quite suffocative in relationship and situations like marital, commercial, familial, etc. Unable to breathe a sigh of relief . . . no space for one's self.
• Self-destructiveness as a result of suppressed anger.
• Strict black and white boundaries with no grey areas. [Uta Santos; Farokh Master]

# CORALLUS HORTULANUS

## Systematics
• Scientific name: Corallus hortulanus [L., 1758].
• Synonyms: Boa hortulana [L., 1766]. Boa merremii [Sentzen, 1796].
• Common names: Amazon tree boa. Common tree boa. Garden tree boa.
• Family: Boidae, subfamily Boinae.

## Biological Profile

- Non-venomous, slender, ambushing constrictor with long, prehensile tail. Average length 1.5–2 m [5–6.5 ft].
- Base colour varies from pale tan to black, with yellowish and reddish tinges. Marked by a series of blotches or bands that are often broader in the middorsal area. Head large, wider than neck; has 5 dark stripes that extend from the eyes. Belly colour also variable, from cream to reddish brown, and either with or without darker markings. Tongue black. Males and females similar in size and markings.
- Eyes yellowish, greyish, or reddish; have a reflective membrane that results in eyeshine at night.
- Range: Central America [Costa Rica] and upper half of South America.
- Habitat: Arboreal regions with high humidity; common along rivers; also in dry areas, savannas or dry forests.
- Has particularly large infrared sensitive receptors in labial pit organs, which allow it to sense heat well. Also has good eyesight, necessary for hunting during the day.
- Sensitive to vibrations [common to snakes generally].
- Has good chemoreception, which is often used in communicating reproductive information.
- Hunts mostly at night using its infrared sensitivity or sometimes during the day using vision.
- Feeds on birds, bats, frogs, rodents, lizards, marsupials.
- Viviparous; 5–20 young; after birth immediately independent of their mother.
- Solitary.
- Notoriously aggressive; bites and makes an s-coil when approached. May form into a ball, constrict and rotate the body when manipulated. Its very long needle-like teeth can inflict a painful bite.
- Popular pet for snake hobbyists; fairly common export in the pet trade.

## Materia Medica

- No symptoms.

# EUNECTES MURINUS

## Systematics

- Scientific name: Eunectes murinus [L., 1758].
- Synonyms: Boa murina [L., 1758]. Boa anaconda [Daudin, 1803].
- Common name: Green anaconda.
- Family: Boidae, subfamily Boinae.

## Biological Profile

- Non-venomous ambushing constrictor, stocky and exceptionally muscular, growing to a length of 6–9 m, rivaled only by Python reticulatus as the world's longest snake. Females much larger than males, having about 5 times their size.

- World's heaviest snake. Present an incredible change in body size from birth [200 gram] to adulthood [104 kg average weight; reported maximum weight 250 kg]. With this 500- to 1250-fold increase its change in biomass is much higher than the increase found in any other species of snake.
- Background colour olive to dark green with alternating oval black spots; and similar spots with yellow-ochre centres along length of body. Belly yellow with black markings; underside of lower tail yellow. Head narrow compared to rest of body, usually with distinctive orange-yellow striping on either side behind the eyes. Eyes set high on head, allowing the anaconda to see out of the water while swimming without exposing its body.
- Range: South America east of the Andes, from Venezuela to Brazil.
- Habitat: Primarily aquatic. Prefers slow-moving, still or murky waters over clear, swift-flowing streams. Can often be found in the shallow caves beneath undercut banks. Usually spends its time lying in shallow waters or basking in the sun on a nearby tree branch.
- Has a well-defined 'home range', i.e. an area with which it is intimately familiar.
- Viviparous; 20–40 young.
- Nocturnal. *Master of disguise*, its colouration and pattern blending in with aquatic vegetation. Ambusher lying in wait in murky waters; *crafty, stealthy*, sleek stalker seizing prey from below.
- Preys on almost anything it can manage to overpower, incl. fish, birds, a variety of mammals, caiman, turtles and other reptiles. Tends to float atop the surface of the water with the snout barely poking out above the surface. When prey passes by or stops to drink will snatch it [without eating or swallowing it] and coil around it with its body. Cannibalism is also known, most recorded cases involving a larger female consuming a smaller male. Male anacondas looking for water and/or females appear to be especially vulnerable to *cannibalism by females*. After mating, pregnant females do not eat for 7 months. It is possible that breeding females eat their mating partners in order to help them survive the long fast associated with pregnancy.
- Slow-acting digestive system; often takes days or weeks to digest food; may not eat for weeks or months after a meal.
- A striking feature in many anacondas of all sizes is the number of old and recent wounds and scars they have. Many come from piranhas, which appear to bite and release anacondas, leaving nasty wounds. Other wounds are by spectacled caimans, which put up a good fight before falling prey to the anaconda.
- Releases a horribly smelling musk from its cloaca when attacked.

## Breeding Balls
'Courtship often extends over several months. The mating period typically is from April to May. The female is thought to lay down a pheromone trail, which attracts the male to her. Another possibility is that the female herself emits some sort of air-born chemical signal. This is supported by the observation that the mating female does not move around much, yet males flock to her from all

directions. The males also constantly lick the air in order to pick up chemical traces signaling the female's presence.

'Though multiple males do not appear to be necessary in order for breeding to take place, often the snakes cluster in a breeding ball that may consist of 2 to 12 males coiled around 1 female. They may stay like this for up to 2 to 4 weeks. This breeding ball appears to be a slow-motion wrestling match amongst the males for an opportunity to mate. The strongest often wins; however, the female, being larger and stronger, may herself choose or deflect certain males. Courtship and copulation frequently take place in water. The gestation period for the green anaconda is about 6 months. A gravid female may feed during this period. However, males kept together during breeding season may refuse food.

'The male uses its spurs to stimulate the female during mating. The male presses his cloacal region against the female while scratching her with his spurs. This makes a scratching sound. The end of the courtship comes when the stimulus of the male's spurs induces the female to raise her cloacal region, allowing the 2 cloacas to come together. The male wraps his tail around the female while they copulate.' [Animal Diversity Web, website University of Michigan Museum of Zoology]

### Polyandry – Many Males
The mating of one female with more than one male while each male mates with only one female is known as polyandry, literally 'many males'. In *birds* polyandry is a rare mating system, occurring in less than 1% of all bird species, and then found mostly in shorebirds. Polyandry in birds is often accompanied by a reversal of sexual roles in which males perform all or most parental duties and females compete for mates.

Polyandry in reptiles is even rarer. Herpetologist Jesus Rivas describes the mating system of green anacondas as polyandrous, based on over 45 mating aggregations in an intensively studied population with hundreds of marked individuals in Venezuela. Prior to the work by Rivas, the closest other authors have come to acknowledging polyandry is by using the word '*promiscuity*'.

'One female lies on the mud or in shallow water and males, up to 13, approach and coil around her to court and attempt to mate. Such mating aggregations may last for up to a month and males that find a female tend to stay with the same female until the end of her attractive period. There is no evidence of the males going out to look for other females after they mate. While the female mates multiple times, there is thus no evidence of males mating with more than one female in a given season. Perhaps this is because the females are dispersed in the landscape and difficult to find.' [Rivas & Burghardt, 2005]

### Materia Medica
• No symptoms.

# EUNECTES NOTAEUS

## Systematics
- Scientific name: Eunectes notaeus [Cope, 1862].
- Common name: Yellow anaconda.
- Family: Boidae, subfamily Boinae.

## Biological Profile
- Non-venomous ambushing constrictor growing to an average length of 3–4 m. Females larger than males, the latter rarely exceeding 2.3 m. Colour pattern consists of a yellow, golden-tan or greenish-yellow ground colour overlaid with a series of black or dark brown saddles, blotches, spots and streaks.
- Range: South America – Northern Argentina, Bolivia, Brazil, and Paraguay.
- Habitat: Prefers mostly aquatic habitats including swamps, marshes, and brush-covered banks of slow moving rivers and streams.
- Does not regularly bask. Only pregnant females do.
- Viviparous; up to 30 live young.
- Forages predominately in open, flooded habitats, in relatively shallow water, preying on wading birds, ducks, fish, turtles, small-sized caimans, lizards, birds' eggs, small mammals and fish carrion. Simply drowns prey by holding them underwater.
- Generic name *Eunectes* means 'good swimmer' in Greek and reflects the snake's mainly aquatic habits.

## Mating & Cannibalism
'Female anacondas give off a special scent called a pheromone that males can detect with their flicking tongues. Like some other types of snakes, anacondas sometimes form breeding balls [also called mating balls] in which many males swarm over a single female to attempt to mate. Up to a dozen or more male anacondas may wrap themselves around a much larger female, trying to insert their sex organs into the female's cloaca. The males scratch with their tiny hind leg spurs to stimulate the female to mate. A successful male leaves a waxy plug in the female's cloaca to block other males from mating. Anaconda breeding balls take place in shallow water and can last for weeks. Females may also breed with single males they encounter.

'Two forms of cannibalism are reported with female anacondas. Large females sometimes kill and eat male anacondas, more than often following mating. Like other live-bearing members of the boa family, female anacondas also eat stillborn offspring and undeveloped eggs expelled when giving birth. Since females do not feed while carrying developing young, both behaviours may be related to nutritional needs. The females may eat adult males as a ready protein source before they stop feeding. Consuming stillborn young and unhatched eggs likely allows the females to recover more quickly from a long period without food.' [Encarta.msn.com]

SNAKES

## Uses

Anacondas figure prominently in the religions of native peoples of the Amazon region, often as spirits that protect forests or rivers. The skin of anacondas is sold to shoe and purse making factories. The flesh, although edible, is not preferred by local people and anacondas are not killed for it. Other than the skin, the only product of the anaconda that people seek [and more so than the skin] is the fat. Anaconda fat, melted under the sun in a closed container or in a fire, is considered a medicine for throat problems, asthma and other respiratory problems.

## Anaconda as Pet

'A variable species that can be either kitten tame or a spastic chainsaw serpent [wild caughts and mishandled captives]. Hardy as long as humidity requirements are met and tolerant of cooler ambient temperatures than many other boids, this species is often nocturnal [active at night]. Young animals tend to be nervous but with frequent, gentle handling in captivity they often calm and make reasonable pets. Anacondas have an odd biting method, instead of the typical forward lunging they may lash out sideways in rapid succession leaving the handler with several wounds to mull over! One thing we've observed about anacondas is the fact that they hate to be put in bags or containers. Regardless of the fact that they may be tame, they seem to freak out when put through this and often come out with a less than splendid disposition. . . . Yellow anacondas can make a herp keeping experience a rewarding challenge or a complete nightmare, with little middle ground. When a yellow anaconda is bad [i.e. wild caught import or poorly started CB] it can take a miracle to turn the snake into a healthy captive.' [reptile-community.com]

## Materia Medica
• No symptoms.

# MORELIA SPILOTA VARIEGATA

## Systematics
• Scientific name: Morelia spilota [Lacépède, 1804].
• Subspecies: M. s. variegata [Gray, 1842].
• Common name: Carpet python. West Papuan carpet python.
• Family: Boidae, subfamily Pythoninae.

## Biological Profile
• Non-venomous, slender, semi-arboreal constrictor ranging in length from 1.2–1.8 m [subspecies variegata] to 2.5–3 m [subspecies mcdowelli]. Females larger than males.
• Ground colour reddish-brown with darker cream edged bands along length of body. Regional colour variations can include bright yellow, gold, rust, and clear greys. Hatchlings have red or orange colouration, which will continually change throughout most of their lives.

- Range: Australia, New Guinea.
- Habitat: Savannah woodland, monsoon forest and dry forest.
- Oviparous; 10–20 eggs per clutch. Female coils around eggs to protect them and keeps them warm through using muscular contractions to generate heat. Maternal care ceases once hatchlings have emerged.
- Nocturnal, occasionally active during the day.
- Preys on small mammals, bats, birds and lizards.
- Seven recognized subspecies [cheynei, harrisoni, imbricata, mcdowelli, metcalfei, spilota, variegata]. M. spilota spilota is known as the diamond python.

### Behaviour & Temperament
'Male carpet pythons will battle in the spring, during mating season, with their bodies coiled and heads over 1m off the ground. They often savagely attack each other by biting and can seriously injure other males. They often will aggregate and will fight every day. The temperament of these snakes is widely variable. Some will hiss and strike if approached, with a painful bite that requires medical attention. Others are quite docile, however, and will allow themselves to be handled.' [2001 Queensland Term Wildlife Field Guide]

### Materia Medica
- No symptoms.

# MORELIA VIRIDIS

### Systematics
- Scientific name: Morelia viridis [Schlegel, 1872].
- Common name: Green tree python.
- Family: Boidae, subfamily Pythoninae.

### Biological Profile
- Non-venomous, nocturnal, arboreal constrictor with an average length of 1.2 m, maximum 1.8 m. Vividly green with a broken vertebral stripe of white or dull yellow. Spots of the same colour, or blue spots, may be scattered over the body. Eyes large with a vertical pupil; heat-sensing pits in upper and lower labial shields. Juveniles mostly bright yellow throughout, but in some areas may be dorsally red, orange or green.
- Range: New Guinea, Indonesia, and Cape York Peninsula in Australia.
- Habitat: Dry forests, swamp forests, cultivated areas.
- Nocturnal hunter, often returning to same nighttime hunting location.
- Lies *motionless* during daylight hours in a tree, looping a coil or 2 over the branches in a saddle position with its head in the middle, or secures a daytime resting place in a secluded ground location.
- Preys on small mammals, such as rodents, and sometimes reptiles. Prey is captured by holding onto a branch using the prehensile tail and striking out from an s-shape position.

- Oviparous, 12–25 eggs per clutch. Eggs are incubated and protected by the female, often in the hollow of a tree.

## Colour Changes & Camouflage

'The green python [Morelia viridis] is an iconic rainforest species in Australia. It is used to promote values of pristine wilderness and helps attract many people to zoos and reptile parks in Australia. The species is also famed for having some of the brightest colours and one of the most amazing colour changes in the animal kingdom. When young are born they are either a bright yellow or a brick red colour, but both morphs change to a vivid green later in life. This has made them one of the most popular snakes in the captive pet industry, increasing demand for wild individuals for private collections.

'Surveys revealed that the population at Iron Range is large and long-lived. Over 200 individuals were caught in the study area, which equates to a density of approximately 4 per hectare. They preferred primary lowland rainforest, but a few individuals were found in mature regrowth areas. Males mature in their third year, while females wait until their fourth year and both can live for at least 12 years. Juveniles hatch in late November, but reproduction is low in any given year. Only yellow juveniles were caught, with the colour change occurring at approximately 55 cm, which equates to animals that are about one year old.

'Radio-tracking showed that males and females have different behaviours. Both sexes move slowly [an average of 7 m per day], however females have a home range while males appear to randomly roam throughout suitable habitat. Juveniles move less [an average of 3 m per day] and are restricted to the edge of the rainforest or in tree-fall gaps. Juveniles also feed mainly during the day – for ground dwelling lizards and small invertebrates near the ground. Green individuals hunt primarily at night for terrestrial rodents, but sometimes they would hunt in the canopy for birds attracted to flowering trees. Juveniles are too small to physically swallow rodents – the minimum size this is possible corresponds to the size at which they change colour.

'Measuring the colour of the pythons and that of their background allowed us to determine how camouflaged each colour is, both against its natural background, and against other backgrounds in the rainforest. This showed that yellow individuals were most camouflaged near the ground in open areas than anywhere else. Green individuals were most camouflaged in the canopy, but importantly relatively more camouflaged than yellow individuals in open areas. I was also able to measure captive red juveniles, and these were most camouflaged near the ground in the closed canopy rainforest. This it appears that the 2 juvenile morphs have evolved to best survive in different environmental conditions, while the colour change has evolved to decrease the risk of predation once individuals are able to hunt at night.

'After 3 years we now know much more about the ecology of the green python in the wild, and the reasons behind both its amazing colours, and the remarkable colour change. We also know that the species is common in suitable habitat and not threatened with extinction.' [Hermon Slade Foundation]

Materia Medica
• No symptoms.

# PYTHON MOLURUS

## Systematics
• Scientific name: Python molurus [L.,1758].
• Synonyms: Boa ordinata [Schneider, 1801]. Python tigris [Daudin, 1803].
• Common names: Indian python. Black-tailed python.
• Family: Boidae, subfamily Pythoninae.

## Biological Profile
• Non-venomous constrictor generally reaching up to 4 m and in extreme cases over 6 m in length. Girth exceeds that of all other snakes; average weight 35–60 kg. Females longer and heavier than males.
• Background colour typically pale grey or tan with yellow-edged brown rectangular markings. Distinctive lighter, forward-pointing, V-shaped marking on top of head. Head flattened and long, large nostrils directed upwards and situated high on snout.
• Range: Southern Asia to Indonesia. Has been introduced in South Florida, USA, where it is rapidly expanding since 2002.
• Habitat: Rocky hillsides, scrubland, forests. Usually found in habitats that can provide both sufficient cover and permanent water sources.
• Adept at both swimming and climbing trees.
• Nocturnal.
• Oviparous; up to 100 eggs per clutch. During incubation females use muscular contractions or 'shivers' to raise their body temperatures slightly higher than the surrounding air temperature. Females rarely leave their eggs during the 100-day incubation period. Once the eggs hatch, the young quickly become independent.
• No subspecies.
• Endangered; often killed for its fine skin.

## Behaviour & Temperament
Python molurus is a solitary species. Mating is the only time that these snakes are commonly found in pairs. Indian pythons will generally move only when food is scarce or when threatened. They may stalk prey, first locating it by scent or by sensing the body heat of the prey with their heat pits, and then following the trail. To compensate for its very poor eyesight, the Indian python has a highly developed sense of smell, and heat pits within each scale along the upper lip, which sense the warmth of nearby prey.

'Lethargic and slow moving even in its native habitat, they exhibit little timidity and rarely try to escape even when attacked. Locomotion is usually rectilinear, with the body moving in a straight line. They are very good swimmers and are quite at home in water. They can be wholly submerged in water for many minutes if necessary, but usually prefer to remain near the bank.

'These snakes feed on mammals, birds and reptiles indiscriminately, but seem to prefer mammals. Roused to activity on sighting prey, the snake will advance with quivering tail and lunge with open mouth. Live prey is constricted and killed. One or 2 coils are used to hold it in a tight grip. The prey, unable to breathe, succumbs and is subsequently swallowed head first. After a heavy meal, they are disinclined to move. If forced to, hard parts of the meal may tear through the body. Therefore, if disturbed, some specimens will disgorge their meal in order to escape from potential predators. After a heavy meal, an individual may fast for weeks; the longest recorded duration being 2 years.' [Wikipedia]

## Materia Medica
- No symptoms.

# PYTHON REGIUS

## Systematics
- Scientific name: Python regius [Shaw,1802].
- Synonym: Boa regia [Shaw, 1802].
- Common names: Ball python. Royal python.
- Family: Boidae, subfamily Pythoninae.

## Biological Profile
- Non-venomous constrictor growing to 1.2 m in length, occasionally reaching 1.9 m. Stocky body with relatively small head. Colour pattern typically black with light brown or gold sides and dorsal blotches. Belly white or cream-coloured with or without scattered black markings. Both females and males have 'anal spurs' that look like small claws on either side of the vent.
- Range: Western to Central Africa.
- Habitat: Grasslands, savannahs, sparsely wooded areas.
- Mainly crepuscular, active around dawn and dusk, and nocturnal; relatively inactive during dry season.
- Preys mostly on small mammals, such as rats, shrews, and striped mice. Juveniles may feed on birds.
- Oviparous; 3–14 eggs per clutch. Female pythons remain tightly coiled around their eggs throughout incubation, adopting a defensive posture when disturbed. In cool climates, brooding females maintain high and constant temperatures within the clutch by shivering thermogenesis. In addition, brooding females do not feed during incubation.
- Generally docile and easy to handle. Ball pythons are probably the most commonly kept snake in the United States and are quite popular in Europe as well.

- Name *ball python* refers to the animal's tendency to curl into a ball, with its head and neck tucked away in the middle, when stressed or frightened.
- No subspecies.

### Sacred Python

'Within the Afife Traditional Area it is believed that, if a python is killed, it will not rain. If anybody does kill a royal python, he/she must purchase a new cooking pot and carry the "corpse" to Afife for burial. The culprit's hair on head, armpits, anus and genital area are shaven. He/she must carry the corpse on the shaven head and walk barefooted to Afife for the burial and ceremony. The programmed ceremonies for purification and for royal python burial are tedious and would discourage any person[s] who would have wished to kill them. . . . Christianity has eroded this belief to a certain degree. The royal python is the god, which led this particular group of Ewes from Togo to Ghana about 150 years ago.

'Worshipers cover "road-kills" with clothes or leaves if they come across a royal python "corpse". . . . Not all Ewes hold the royal python to be sacred but they "know that it is friendly, so it is not killed." Villages adjacent to the Afife Traditional Area do not kill royal pythons out of respect for their neighbours. . . . The second area where the royal python is considered sacred was Somanya and the adjacent towns, which together have a population of more than 20,000. . . . As with Afife they have a python festival at the beginning of the year. The youth of the Christians also have respect for the fetish because it is strongly linked with the annual festival of the Krobos called "Dipo". "Dipo" is a virginity right and transition to womanhood celebration. The fetish shrine is called "Ayerbida". By their tradition, there are certain localities where people are not even permitted to touch or otherwise bother a royal python. It is a taboo to kill one. A royal python entering the house is regarded as a blessing and a libation ceremony has to be performed.

'Ruvell has reported similar reverence for royal pythons in Benin. This author wrote that the "main temple and python high priest are in Ouidah, Dahomey [the python Vatican so to speak], is an early example of sustainable use and conservation. Grain is stored by villagers in granaries raised on stilts. Rodents are a persistent problem. For at least the last 600 years pythons have been venerated as god, with local priests exhorting villagers to bring them into the villages as sacred animals where they are kept in a kind of religious farming. No python worshipper would ever harm a ball python or think of eating one. The village python collections and their offspring keep the rodent population down and protect the village grain stores. The python cult is so strong that the Portuguese in the 17th century built a cathedral directly across the square from the python temple. Sustainable use may be a difficult concept for some today, but the Dahomeans in their corner of Africa have been practicing species protection through value for hundreds of years to their advantage and that of the pythons."' [Gorzula, & Oduro, 1997]

## The God to Whom All Things Are Known

Danh-gbi is the python god, the heavenly serpent, the good snake; his name implies 'life-giving snake', deriving from *danh*, snake, and *agbi*, life. He is the god of wisdom, to whom all things are known, and who opened the eyes of the first man and woman, who were blind. White ants are the messengers of the python. Whenever a native sees a python near a nest of white ants, he places round the reptile a protecting circle of palm leaves.

In his 'A New and Accurate Description of the Coast of Guinea' [1703], Dutch trader Willem Bosman describes the python worship of Whydah, in Dahomey, as follows: "Their principal god is a certain sort of snake, which professes the chief rank among their gods. They esteem the serpent their extreme bliss and general good." In Bosman's day there was a superstition to the effect that the sacred snake appeared to the most beautiful girls in order to induce madness. Such girls had then to enter the service of the snake temple. Bosman states that the priests persuaded the girls to feign frenzy so that they might be sent to the snake house.

The punishment for a native who kills a python accidentally is burial alive. For the same offence a European was to be decapitated.

'Visitors to Dahomey in the 19th century noted that the large numbers of snakes kept there were better fed and cared for than the human inhabitants. A special house situated in the centre of the town was provided for their exclusive use to which they were returned if they happened to stray. When a Dahoman caught sight of one of the reptiles, he immediately prostrated himself on the ground. Every python was treated with profound respect and addressed as "master, father, mother and benefactor."

'He [Dahn-gbi] was attended by a large priesthood nominally headed by the king, who consulted the python about government problems. Women were very prominent in the cult of Dahn-gbi. . . . Numerous wives were provided for the python. When the millet began to sprout, the old priestesses rushed round the village seizing and carrying off young girls between the age of 8 and 12 to be his brides. Some pious parents deliberately left their female offspring out in the streets. After due instruction, the snake's wives took part in licentious rites with the priests and eventually became public prostitutes whose services were eagerly sought by the male worshipers when crops were germinating. Since the god directed his wives' activities, which were thought to assist him in his efforts for the community's welfare, no disgrace was attached to their profession. The snake's wives were not allowed to marry, and any children born to them belonged to the god.' [Morris, 1968]

## MATERIA MEDICA PYTHON REGIUS

### Sources

1 Proving Brigitte Klotzsch [Germany], 6 provers [5 females, 1 male], 30c; also meditative proving with 32 persons who held a vial of 200c against their

thymus gland for 20–30 minutes. Bracketed numbers indicate number of provers experiencing the symptom.

2 Degroote's Dream Repertory.

## Mind
∞ Delusion something bad will happen after something good [2].
∞ Delusion daughter/mother will destroy her [2].
∞ Delusion being controlled by partner or other person [5].
∞ Delusion being abandoned by wife [4].
∞ Delusion partnership being a prison [7].
∞ Delusions body having a life of its own [2].
∞ Delusion hovering in air [3].
∞ Delusion being rooted to the spot.
∞ Delusion being a snake [2].
∞ Fear bleeding to death during menses [3]
∞ Fear of death by heart-attack or stroke [2].
∞ Fear to go to sleep lest she would die.
∞ Fear of high places [3]
∞ Fear of hurting others [5] or being hurt [4].
∞ Fear of injections, syringes [7], sharp objects [4].
∞ Fear losing partner or parents [3].
∞ Fear of marriage [2].
∞ Fear of starving [3].
∞ Fear of suffocation, strangulation [3].
∞ Sociable [4]. Tendency to sacrifice with idea that mothers exist only for their children [1].
∞ Depression [7], feels alone, forsaken and unsupported by family [4].
∞ Shameful; ashamed of being strange [3], poor [4], fat [6].
∞ Clairvoyance, foresees negative events [4].

## Dreams
∞ Attacked by cats.[2]
∞ Betrayal by family.
∞ Catastrophes.
∞ Divorce.
∞ Flooding.
∞ Losing one's way.
∞ Monster, changing into a.[2]
∞ Sex hell with pale and naked people.
∞ Snakes.

## Generals
∞ Pain pressing – head, eyes, throat, stomach, chest, shoulders, elbows, arms, pelvis.
∞ Desire for fresh air; being outdoors > [5].
∞ Right side more affected.

∞ Morning <, evening >.
∞ Desire for apples [4], chocolate [3], cold food [2], fruit [3].

## Sensations
∞ Objects as if spinning in all directions, & vertigo.
∞ Waves of heat in head [2].
∞ Eyes as if turned downwards [2].
∞ Right socket as if empty, eye as if absent.
∞ Left eyelid as if twitching [2].
∞ Right lower eyelid as if swollen.
∞ Numbness around eyes.
∞ Roaring in ears, shifting from right to left ear.
∞ Tongue as if thick and furred.
∞ Teeth as if dissolving [2], becoming loose and being pulled downwards [2].
∞ Lump in throat.
∞ Throat as if constricted when swallowing.
∞ Stones in stomach, falling from side to side [4].
∞ Uterus as if turned inside out and as if losing all one's blood [5].
∞ Enormous stone on chest.
∞ Enclosed as if in a corset on breathing deeply.
∞ Arms and legs as if paralysed.
∞ Weight on shoulders, as of a yoke [2].
∞ Shoulders as if pulled out of sockets.
∞ Arms and hands numb, as if paralysed [5].
∞ Right arm as if longer than left arm.
∞ Heaviness right elbow [3].
∞ Right hand as if without muscles and as if blood were flowing out [2].
∞ Hands as if in too tight gloves.
∞ Pelvis as if pulled downwards [3].
∞ Right leg as if lame, anaesthetised [2].
∞ Right leg as if longer than left leg.
∞ Right ankle as if chained.
∞ Someone as if pulling at toes of right foot [3].
∞ Left side as if extended, right side as if contracted [4].
∞ Right side as if paralysed [4].

## Locals
∞ Dizziness & nausea in waves from stomach to head [2].
∞ Pressing headache [8], above nose [3], against top of skull [4], occiput [2], temples [2].
∞ Itching of eyes, alternating sides [7]. Puffy eyes in morning [2].
∞ Field of vision increased [4]. Dim vision at dusk [3].
∞ Tip of nose icy cold [2].
∞ Clenching teeth [3].
∞ Dryness mouth alternating with salivation.
∞ Pressing pain in stomach [5], radiating to heart.

∞ Menses painful [4], too early [5], very heavy [5]; reappearing after menopause.
∞ Itching fingertips.[2]
∞ Itching scars [cicatrices].[2]

## Interdependence

'The essence of Python regia is that the powerful and the powerless exist in a mutually dependent relationship where the former smothers the latter. The python is dependent on her rodent prey, but in order to use them she must smother them. There is a state of clinging to/being addicted to their partner and in the relationship one is powerful and one is powerless. The partners may lose their own feelings and take on those of the other.

'The powerful feels as bracketed together and dependent as the powerless, so it is a remedy to consider giving to both partners. The child may feel totally addicted to the parents and have to visit them frequently. There is also a male/female power struggle. There may be too much responsibility expected at a young age, or a refusal to accept responsibility.

'Other themes that emerged included; The need to bear another's burden and hence lose your own energy. Depending on others for your energy. Inability to act. Abandoned and betrayed by family. There is an interesting rubric "her arm doesn't belong to her". This implies that she can't use her arm for her own needs but only for others.' [Geoff Johnson, cited in B. Klotzsch, 2001]

# PYTHON RETICULATUS

### Systematics
- Scientific name: Broghammerus reticulatus [Schneider, 1801].
- Synonym: Python reticulatus [Schneider, 1801].
- Common names: Reticulated python. Netted python.
- Family: Boidae, subfamily Pythoninae.

### Biological Profile
- Non-venomous constrictor with a complex net-like [reticulated] colour pattern. Average length 3–6 m, maximum 7 m; world's longest snake. Weight up to 150 kg. Females larger than males.
- Underlying colour light yellowish-brown or olive; head and neck ornamented by a dark brown line passing from tip of snout backwards, on each side of which are 2 bands passing from eyes to angles of mouth. Along the back a series of black rings bordered with white, spotted scales gives the animal a netted appearance, from which it has received its specific name, *reticulatus*.
- Range: SE Asia to Philippines and Indonesia.
- Habitat: Hot, tropical jungles; heavily dependent on water, thus can often be found near small rivers or lakes.
- Usually active during both day and night in the wild and other areas with few people; tends to be more nocturnal in more densely populated areas.
- Ambush predator, on occasion also actively foraging.

- Preys on mammals [rodents, primates, pigs, deer, dogs] and birds. Prey located by heat-sensitive pits in the labial scales lining the lips.
- Excellent swimmer; has been reported far out at sea and has consequently colonised many small islands within its range. Excellent climber, can often be seen in trees, where it also rests. Commonly rests in sheltered areas such as the roots of trees, hollow logs, or burrows that are created by other animals.
- Oviparous; 25–80 eggs per clutch. Females remain tightly coiled around their eggs throughout incubation and will defend their eggs against predators. In cool climates, brooding females maintain high and constant temperatures within the clutch by shivering thermogenesis. Brooding females do not feed during incubation.

## Behaviour & Temperament
'Reticulated pythons have a reputation of being aggressive. Because of their large size alone this animal should be given great respect. They are relatively non-social animals, as are most snakes, and prefer to be solitary. However, reticulated pythons have an aggressive feeding response, not aggressive behaviour and are not generally confrontational. Wild caught snakes have a hard time adjusting to captivity and *often bite to avoid interaction*, leading to the misinterpretation that this is an aggressive animal. Also, mistreated captive animals or those that are not handled regularly are often referred to as being aggressive. However those reticulated pythons that are captive born and raised properly show no signs of aggression.' [Todd Mexico, Michigan State University]

## Having a Familiar Spirit
'Spirit of divination. Literally, a spirit, a *Python*. Python, in the Greek mythology, was the serpent that guarded Delphi. According to the legend, as related in the Homeric hymn, Apollo descended from Olympus in order to select a site for his shrine and oracle. Having fixed upon a spot on the southern side of Mount Parnassus, he found it guarded by a vast and terrific serpent, which he slew with an arrow, and suffered its body to *rot* in the sun. Hence the name of the serpent *Python* [rotting]; *Pytho*, the name of the place, and the epithet *Pythian*, applied to Apollo. The name *Python* was subsequently used to denote a prophetic *demon*, and was also used of soothsayers who practised *ventriloquist*, or speaking from the belly. The word *ventriloquist* occurs in the Septuagint and is rendered *having a familiar spirit*. The heathen inhabitants of Philippi regarded the woman as inspired by Apollo; and Luke, in recording this case, which came under his own observation, uses the term which would naturally suggest itself to a Greek physician, a *Python-spirit*, presenting phenomena identical with the convulsive movements and wild cries of the Pythian priestess at Delphi.' [Vincent, 1887]

## The Pythoness
'No, it was not a serpent; it was a woman; a priestess at the Temple of Apollo, at Delphi, where the great Delphic Oracle was located. The *Pythoness*, sometimes called the Pythian, took her name from the python, a huge snake that, according to mythology, haunted the caves on Mt. Parnassus. The python was slain by

Apollo, who, for this reason, was afterwards called the Pythian Apollo. It was natural, therefore, to call the priestess, who ministered in his temple, the Pythoness or the Pythian.

'The ancients, especially the Greeks, were great believers in oracles. The most celebrated of these were the oracles of Apollo, of which there were about 22. The alleged revelations were made to a person called a medium, who was not unlike the so-called medium of the spiritualists of today. This medium generally spoke in unintelligible words, which were afterwards interpreted through the agency of the priests.

'The most celebrated of the oracles of Apollo was the one at Delphi, which possessed a reputation greater, even, than that of Jupiter at Olympia. At this oracle, and, indeed, at oracles in general, the revelations, or the answers, were always so obscure that it was often impossible to know what the prediction was until the event occurred. This was so especially the case in the oracle at Delphi, that in our time the adjective Delphic is frequently employed to mean ambiguous, uncertain, or double; as, a Delphic answer, meaning an answer that can be construed in different ways according to convenience.

'The Delphic Oracle was questioned through the Pythoness. The room where the oracles were delivered was in a grotto, or cave. The Pythoness took her seat on a tripod, placed over an opening in the ground. The applicant was not permitted to put the question until the Pythoness fell under the influence of the gods, or became partially unconscious, or semi-conscious. The words she then spoke were written down. They were generally arranged in verse and great skill was required to interpret them.

'There is a close resemblance between the methods employed by the Delphic Oracle and those used today in clairvoyancy, in which it is claimed that the medium, generally a female, is able, while in a semi-conscious condition known as a trance, to see objects that would otherwise be invisible, and thus be able to answer difficult questions or predict coming events.

'At the Delphic Oracle the Pythoness, before she was able to predict the future, had first to be thrown into this mesmeric state. While, of course, it would have been far easier to pretend to be in the condition of a trance, it appears that the priests preferred to bring about this semiconscious condition by means of gases, which, escaping from the ground, near the priestess, would, when inhaled, throw her into a condition closely resembling a fit, which was assumed to be the mesmeric state. During this time she was supposed to be in consultation with the gods.

'Now, while the exact means employed for this purpose are unknown, it is quite possible that the stupefying gas was carbonic acid gas, which as you perhaps know is often given off in large quantities from fissures in the ground in certain parts of the world. . . . If people today should similarly submit themselves to the action of carbonic acid gas, they would be affected in a manner very like that said to have been exhibited by the Pythoness. They would experience dizziness, faintness, and possibly nausea, and, if they continued breathing this poisonous atmosphere too long, these symptoms would be followed by convulsions and even by death.' [Houston, 1907]

# MATERIA MEDICA PYTHON RETICULATUS

## Sources
1 Proving Chetna Shukla [India], 4 provers [2 females, 2 males], c. 1995.

## Mind
∞ Aversion to take any advice. Aversion to being disturbed. Aversion to react.
∞ Aversion to communication. Doesn't talk, communicates only by gestures, if at all.
∞ Remains quiet when angry.
∞ Desire to crush opponents.
∞ Desire to stay in dark places.
∞ Delusion he is dangerous, majestic, mighty, strong; insulted by surrounding.
∞ Desire for strenuous work, working out, body-building, muscle-building, pumping iron.

## Dreams
∞ Accidents.
∞ Animals – dead cow; elephants; rats; snakes.
∞ Being cautious.
∞ Fearless.
∞ Ghosts.
∞ Meditation.
∞ Snakes wound around body.

## Generals
∞ Desire for buttermilk; chilies; chili sauce; curds; spicy; tangy.
∞ Rice and curds > digestion and dulness.
∞ Aversion to chocolate.
∞ Thirst for cold water.
∞ Sleep position on back with hands balled into tight fists overhead.
∞ Sleeping in sun >.

## Sensations
∞ Eyes as if cold.
∞ Eyes as if enlarged.

## Locals
∞ Headache, & stiffness neck, < slightest movement, > hard pressure.
∞ Itching eyes < open air, winking.
∞ Dryness upper lip, desire to moisture lip.
∞ Pain right side of sternum on breathing deeply.

## Symptoms from a cured case
Man with asthma.
Likes name and fame, appreciation, to be always first.

Desire to move fast.

Desires work.

Desires an idyllic life.

Disturbed, aversion to being.

Dogmatic, rigid, inflexible, obstinate: wants things to be his way.

Desires exercise, walking long distances.

Fearless.

In-depth know-how into everything, desire for.

Fights with authority, with superiors, with people in powerful position. Does not bow down to anyone.

Ready to bear consequences of any of his actions.

Conscientious.

Sun, desires for and amelioration from.

Seaside, desire for and amelioration from.

Cold, winter aggravates.

Suicidal with anger.

Humiliation, cannot bear.

Countryside desires to go, to go away from modern life.

[Chetna Shukla]


# Family Colubridae – Colubrids

### Biological Profile

The Colubridae have a venom-producing gland and enlarged, grooved rear fangs that allow venom to flow into the wound. The inefficient venom apparatus and the specialised venom is effective on cold-blooded animals [such as frogs and lizards] but not considered a threat to human life.

The composition of the venoms from colubrid snakes is largely unknown, even though this exceptionally diverse family contains with 2000 species well over half of the described extant species of snakes, and perhaps half of these produce toxic secretions from the Duvernoy's gland. [Protein-producing oral gland located in the temporal region of colubrids. The gland is widely understood to be the homologue of venom glands in elapids and vipers.]

A vast body of literature exists on venoms from elapids, pit vipers and true vipers, collectively termed front-fanged snakes. In contrast, the venoms of rear-fanged colubrids are rarely investigated, the major reasons of which are the typically low venom yields of most colubrids, and the time-intensive collection techniques required to obtain venom.

Colubrid venoms that have been studied to date appear to lack a number of enzymatic properties that are characteristic of most front-fanged snake venoms.

Two properties common to colubrid and front-fanged snake venoms are haemorrhagic and caseinolytic protease [casein splitting] activities, and these activities are widely distributed among colubrids.

| Homeopathic name | Common name | Abbreviation | Symptoms |
|---|---|---|---|
| Chironius carinatus | Amazonian whipsnake | Vip-a-c. | + |
| Cyclagras gigas[1] | False water cobra | Cyc-gig. | + |
| Dispholidus typus | Boomslang | Dis-ty. | + |
| Drymarchon corais | Yellowtail cribo | Drymar-cr. | – |
| Drymarchon couperi | Indigo snake | Drymar-cp. | – |
| Elaphe guttata[2] | Corn snake | Ela-gt. | + |
| Elaphe longissima | Aesculapian snake | Ela-lo. | – |
| Lampropeltis calligaster calligaster | Prairie king snake | Lamp-c-c. | – |
| Lampropeltis calligaster rhombomaculata | Mole kingsnake | Lamp-c-r. | – |
| Lampropeltis getula cal. | California king snake | Lamp-g-c. | – |
| Lampropeltis triangulum | Milk snake | Lamp-tr. | – |
| Natrix natrix | Grass snake | Natr-n. | + |
| Pantherophis obsoletus | Red rat snake | Panth-obs. | – |
| Thamnophis sirtalis sirtalis | Eastern garter snake | Tham-ss. | + |
| Vipera acustica carinata[3] | Amazonian whipsnake | Vip-a-c. | + |

1 = Hydrodynastes gigas. 2 = Pantherophis guttatus [Panth-gt.]. 3 = Misspelled as Vipera acustica carinata by Swan, who did a proving with it.

# CYCLAGRAS GIGAS

## Systematics
- Scientific name: Hydrodynastes gigas [Duméril, Bibron & Duméril, 1854].
- Synonym: Cyclagras gigas [Cope, 1885].
- Common names: False water cobra. Water queen. Brazilian smooth snake.
- Family: Colubridae.

## Biological Profile
- Rear-fanged, heavy-bodied, semi-aquatic, venomous colubrid with an average length of 2 m, maximum 3 m. Females heavier than males.
- Dorsal colour yellowish or reddish brown, with broad black cross-bands or rings. Black stripe from eye to side of neck. Anterior part of belly with 3 longitudinal series of brown dots or small round spots.
- Range: South America – Guianas, Colombia, Brazil, Bolivia, Paraguay, northern Argentina.
- Habitat: Rainforest, borders of gallery forests or patches of savannas near water.
- Primarily diurnal; very active and inquisitive, spending most of its days foraging, burrowing, and swimming.
- Preys on toads [favourite food], rodents, birds, lizards, and fish.

- Can flatten its neck in cobra-fashion in order to look larger and more intimidating when threatened. It stays in a horizontal position when flattening its neck, unlike the characteristic upright position of true cobras. Does not coil back like a rattlesnake would, but generally just strikes extremely fast. When acquiring prey, it both constricts and delivers venom. Venom delivery consists of a slashing strike followed by a side to side chewing motion.
- Tends to lash out with its tail when annoyed or startled, instead of biting as its first line of defense.
- Known as a hostile snake among reptile keepers and breeders, commonly displaying a very aggressive feeding response and frequently attempting to eat everything in sight. May even give chase to keepers.

## MATERIA MEDICA CYCLAGRAS GIGAS

### Sources
1 Effects of bite; clinical manifestations.

### Clinical Manifestations
1. 'From discussions with Paul Rowley at Liverpool School of Tropical Medicines it would appear that recent studies have likened the potency of the venom to the Timber Rattlesnake, Crotalus horridus. I personally have only seen the results from one bad reaction from a False Water Cobra bite. The late John Foden was unfortunate to receive a bite from an adult on his arm. He told me he thought little of it at the time, until the arm swelled dramatically. Within a couple of hours, he felt very poorly with a fever and severe nausea. Over the following days tissue damage occurred around the area of the bite, and a feeling of being generally unwell lasted for several days. Sometime later he still complained of discomfort and was left permanently with a disfigured arm. . . . Temperament can vary from gentle and placid to violent and intimidating.' [Kevin Stevens, False Water Cobras; www.zoo-logic.co.uk]

2. 'Manning et al. [1999] described a case in which an 18-year-old male pet store employee was bitten on the wrist by a specimen that hung on for 1.5 minutes. There was some mild swelling as a result, but after 9 hours the victim claims to have experienced 3 bouts of muscle paralysis, during which he fell and was unable to move or speak. However, a medical examination did not produce any unusual results. It's possible the symptoms described were the result of anxiety.' [Wikipedia]

3. 'Reported here is a case of envenoming in a 25-year-old male that occurred after the bite of a juvenile H. gigas. The victim was bitten on the fourth digit of the left hand while processing the snake for sex determination, and the snake remained attached to the digit for approximately 30 seconds; there was no jaw advancement [chewing]. Within 5 minutes, intense local pain developed, and at 4-hour post bite the entire dorsal aspect of the hand was significantly oedematous, the local effects progressed and involved the entire forearm, and the local pain referred to the axillary region. Mild paraesthesia and local blanching

['pallor'] were noted in the affected digit but resolved within 7 days. The clinical course in the patient showed that moderate localized symptoms may result from the bite of a juvenile H. gigas.' [Keyler, 2016]

4. 'An adult male Caucasian provided the following description of a bite by H. gigas in Paraguay. The victim was bitten on the left inner thigh by a 1.8 m specimen that maintained its bite for an undefined period. Three deep puncture wounds resulted, and the wounds bled profusely. After 6 h the wound was painful and slightly swollen, but there was no discolouration. The thigh became very painful after 24 h, and there was oedema and red discolouration at the site of envenomation. The immediate area was hard and swollen after 48 h with a slight yellow discolouration, and a burning sensation occurred when the envenomated area was touched. The yellow discolouration and soreness remained for 4 days after the envenomation, and after 7 days there was no pain, swelling or discolouration. The fang puncture marks remained red, and there was never any sign of infection.' [Hill, 2000]

# DISPHOLIDUS TYPUS

## Systematics
- Scientific name: Dispholidus typus [Smith, 1829].
- Synonym: Bucephalus typus [Smith, 1828].
- Common name: Boomslang.
- Family: Colubridae.

## Biological Profile
- Large, slender, rear-fanged, arboreal colubrid, venomous, with a distinctive egg-shaped head and enormous emerald-green eyes. Scales strongly keeled and overlapping. Average length 1.2–1.5 m, maximum 2 m.
- Sexes often coloured differently. Adult females typically olive-brown; adult males brownish-black, bright green, or bluish green. Juveniles change colour, becoming darker and duller as they become adults.
- Range: Throughout most of sub-Saharan Africa, except continuous rain forests of the Congo basin or true deserts [treeless].
- Habitat: Most common in wooded habitats; dry woodlands, thorn scrub, savannahs, and swamps bordering or close to streams, rivers, and lakes.
- Mainly diurnal, strongly arboreal, spends most of time in trees and shrubs. However, will descend to the ground or even cross water and roads in its quest for prey, but will always return to the trees to consume it.
- Preys mainly on tree lizards [esp. chameleons], birds and eggs, arboreal snakes [also its own kind], sometimes on arboreal rodents and bats. Has very long fangs and can open its mouth a full 180 degrees to bite.
- Large eyes, superior vision, believed to be binocular; can spot prey before it moves.
- Very mobile, always on the move, very agile.
- Males engage in ritual combat for breeding rights and establishing dominance.

- Oviparous; up to 25 eggs per clutch. Unlike most other snakes, which couple on the ground, boomslangs mate in trees.
- Name from Dutch and Afrikaans *boom*, tree, and *slang*, snake.
- Three recognized subspecies [typus, kivuensis, punctatus].

## Behaviour & Temperament
Notably non-aggressive and shy; quickly retreats if surprised. If cornered, inflates neck to more than twice usual size showing bright yellow or orange skin beneath.

## Challenging to Capture
'I also rescue snakes from people's homes before they are battered to death with a shovel, and I've been called out to remove the odd boomslang from someone's yard. I have never found it to be an aggressive snake, and when approached it will move away to avoid confrontation. One minute you are looking at it square in the face, but if you blink, you've lost it. However, as soon as you show any inclination to capture it, it will put up an impressive warning display to get you to back off. It is a challenging snake to capture.

'When provoked, a boomslang can exhibit a very convincing threat response. It inflates its neck and the forepart of the body, displaying the contrasting interstitial skin. This is a different type of display than that seen in cobras, as the neck is not inflated by compression of the ribs, but an expansion of the throat. At the same time, the tongue moves up and down in a slow, deliberate motion. If this warning is disregarded, the boomslang may administer a swift sideways-motion bite, after which the snake may move off, or it may retain its threat posture until the perceived threat has passed.' [Donovan, 2019]


## MATERIA MEDICA DISPHOLIDUS TYPUS

### Sources
1 Effects of bite; clinical manifestations.
2 Effects of bite; close resemblance to Phosphorus symptoms.
3 Effects of bite; faintness, giddiness & mental torpor in hot weather.
4 Effects of bite; bleeding to death.

### Clinical Manifestations
Venom potently *haemotoxic*; can cause severe bleeding internally, within critical organs, and from mucous membranes. Even a glancing scratch will bleed profusely. A bite victim's body may also develop bruising and take on a bluish tinge due to extensive internal bleeding that takes place. Other signs and symptoms include headache, nausea, sleepiness, and mental disorders. Because the venom is slow to act, symptoms may not be manifest until many hours after the bite.

This may lead victims to underestimate the seriousness of the bite. The effects of the bite rapidly distinguish a mamba from a boomslang. A mamba's venom acts with extreme rapidity in a curare-like manner, while the boomslang's bite seldom causes immediate serious effects.

A famous boomslang victim was herpetologist Karl P. Schmidt of the Field Museum of Natural History in Chicago in 1957, who died 24 hours after a bite. The wound bled profusely, but Schmidt was not concerned because the snake was a young specimen. On the train home he experienced nausea and by the evening his gums were bleeding. [*see* below]

'Patients often present very late: only when haemorrhagic symptoms occur, probably being misled by the *apparent triviality* of the bite, with *little local pain or reaction and the relative mildness of the initial symptoms* as compared with those caused by front-fanged elapid or viperine bites.

'Nausea, vomiting, malaise and *severe occipital headache* often occur after 1 hour, with occasional drowsiness and confusion. Haemorrhagic signs due to DIC [disseminated intravascular coagulation] may be seen occasionally within 1 hour of envenomation, but usually much later. Bruising is often widespread, sometimes with bulla or haematoma formation. Gastrointestinal bleeding with blood in vomitus and stools or bleeding from the mouth, nose and even conjunctivae occurs. Haematuria and haemoglobinuria may be gross while a haemolytic-uraemic syndrome, due to renal tubular necrosis with oliguria, uraemia, and deepening coma, may ensue. This syndrome occurs in most recorded cases to a greater or lesser degree.' [D.M. du Tout, 1980]

## Close Resemblance to Phosphorus Symptoms

During November 1907 we had occasion to transfer our collection of live snakes to their new apartments and Mr. Williams was carrying a large variegated Boomslang when it suddenly buried its teeth in the muscles of his bared forearm, just below the elbow-joint. It gripped with great power and held on firmly. We disengaged its jaws and I suggested treating the wound, but he would not hear of such a thing, and believing, as I did at the time, that it was practically a non-poisonous snake, I did not insist. The wound smarted a little and he went on working. Within an hour a throbbing headache had manifested itself, accompanied by oozing of blood from the mucous membranes of the mouth, followed by vomiting.

Meanwhile the wound was slowly oozing blood, and the muscles in the vicinity were somewhat swollen. He was then taken to Dr. Bruce, who declared him to be suffering unmistakably from the effects of virulent poison, which was seriously affecting the blood and mucous membranes. During the night Williams' condition gradually became more alarming and he was taken to the Provincial Hospital the following day in a state of utter collapse. He steadily grew worse and blood oozed continuously from all the mucous surfaces, viz. the mouth, nose, stomach, bladder and bowels. Then the blood began to accumulate in the tissues and caused *large blackish-purplish swollen patches* under the skin. One eye and its surrounding tissues, both forearms for two-thirds their length, a portion of the abdomen, hip, and thigh, were all charged with *extravasated* blood, presenting a dreadful sight. Other parts, incl. portions of the back, left eye, and cheek, were slightly discoloured.

Williams rapidly grew worse after the second day in hospital, *severe abdominal pains* setting in and *inability to retain even water in the stomach*. From this time he rapidly grew worse, and on the evening of the third day after being bitten I went to the hospital, accompanied by Mr. William Armstrong, J.P., who took what he believed to be his dying deposition, the doctor declaring him to be in an extremely critical condition, which might result in death before the morning. He lingered on in this state, *bordering between life and death*, till about the 6th day, when a slow improvement began to manifest itself.

From this time onward his condition rapidly improved, and in 3 weeks he was discharged from the hospital still in a weak, debilitated state, and although he gradually regained strength, he had relapses of slight bleeding from the mucous membranes of the mouth, and one eye was occasionally affected. Even 3 months after the accident, slight discolouration in the tissues surrounding one of his eyes showed itself for a few days.

I closely cross-questioned Williams and he admitted, that within half an hour of being bitten he *felt a curious, restless, dizzy, and languid feeling*, but refused at the time to own it, thinking it to be due to some other cause and believing so fully that a Boomslang was perfectly harmless. [Fitzsimons, 1912]

### Faintness, Giddiness & Mental Torpor in Hot Weather

Mr. G.W. Pretorius was one day walking among some prickly pear bushes at Uitenhage, when he disturbed a Brown Boomslang in the grass. It struck out at him and gripped the calf of his leg. He endeavoured to kick it off but failed. Stooping down he seized it by the body, plucked its head away and threw it from him. Although he had ordinary trousers on, the fangs penetrated them and made 2 punctures in his skin. He improvised a ligature and applied it. Dr. McPherson, the District Railway doctor, was soon in attendance. He scarified the wound freely and otherwise treated him. Some hours after the infliction of the bite, Pretorius *fainted away and remained insensible for some time*.

The ligature was kept on for some days, being slightly loosened at short intervals. The bitten limb swelled considerably and *extensive haemorrhage* occurred in it. Blood slowly oozed from all the mucous surfaces, particularly the nose and mouth. For a month Pretorius lay in bed in a critical condition. For the first week *his stomach rejected all food. For some days water was vomited when swallowed.*

For 10 days and more, he suffered severely from pains in the bowels. In fact, his symptoms were similar to those described in the case of James Williams, except that the haemorrhage was chiefly confined to the leg that was bitten; also the mucous membranes. This was doubtless due to the ligature, which prevented the venom passing into the general circulation in sufficient strength to cause subcutaneous haemorrhage in other parts, as was the case with Williams.

For 2 years after recovery, Pretorius *suffered from giddiness and mental torpor whenever the weather was unusually warm*. To prevent himself falling he was obliged to lie down for hours at a time. These symptoms grew less and less severe as time wore on and have now almost disappeared, although at times when he is out for long in the hot summer sun, he feels faint and dizzy. [Fitzsimons, 1912]

## Bleeding to Death

'September 25, 4:30–5:30 p.m.: Strong nausea, but without vomiting, during trip home on train.

5:30–6:30: Strong chill and shaking, followed by fever of 101.7°F [38.7°C], which did not persist [blankets and heating pad]. Bleeding of mucous membranes in the mouth began about 5:30, apparently mostly from gums.

8:30 p.m.: Ate 2 pieces of milk toast.

9:00–12:20 a.m.: Slept well. No blood in urine before going to sleep, but very small amount of urine. Urination at 12:20 a.m. mostly blood, but small in amount. Mouth had bled steadily as shown by dried blood at both angles of mouth.

A good deal of abdominal pain, mostly from gas, only inadequately relieved by belching.

A little fitful sleep until 4 a.m., when I took an enema [bowels having failed to move the previous day].

Took a glass of water at 4:30 a.m., followed by violent nausea and vomiting, the contents of the stomach being the undigested supper. Felt much better and slept until 6:30 a.m.

Sept. 26. 6:30 a.m. Temperature 98.2°F [36.8°C].

Ate cereal and poached egg on toast, and applesauce and coffee for breakfast at 7.

Slight bleeding is now going on in the bowels, with frequent irritation at the anus. No urine, with an ounce or so of blood about every 3 hours [instead of the several ounces of urine to be expected]. Mouth and nose continuing to bleed, not excessively.'

The report is completed by Clifford H. Pope:

'After breakfast Dr. Schmidt was up and active. In fact, he felt so well at about 10 o'clock that he telephoned to the Museum to expect him at work the next day. He got up to eat at noon but vomited after lunch and soon began to have difficulty in breathing. This grew worse until his laboured efforts could be heard all over the house. At the onset of these alarming symptoms, Mrs. Schmidt called the inhalator squad and the family physician. Attempts at resuscitation at first brought warmth back to Dr. Schmidt's hands and normal colour to his face, but his restoral was of short duration. He was transported to the hospital where he arrived shortly before 3:00 p.m. and was promptly pronounced dead from *respiratory paralysis*.

'The autopsy performed on September 27 at 9:30 a.m. . . . . revealed extensive internal bleeding. Massive haemorrhages were found in the lumen of the lower two-thirds of the small intestine, and the ascending and transverse colon. Subserous haemorrhages of the small intestines were from 1–5 cm in diameter. The contents of the descending colon were blood-stained, and the oral mucosa was bloody. The 4 cc of haemorrhagic urine resembled pure blood.

'Bleeding had occurred in the subarachnoid space over the lateral aspect of the left-brain hemisphere and anteriorly over the right one. There was free blood in the cerebral ventricles, and an additional haemorrhage over the right side of the cerebellum. Smaller haemorrhages were evident in the eyes and along the thoracic aorta. The renal pelvis of both sides contained fluid blood and clots. The spleen appeared to be enlarged. . . . Small bleedings had occurred also in the heart wall and in the lungs, but there was no blood in the bronchial lumina. The autopsy report emphasised that capillary damage with peri-capillary haemorrhages appeared to be the main pathological lesions [endothelial injury]. Post-mortem blood clots were not prominent features. Death was ascribed to cerebral haemorrhages caused by "venom from the snake bite."' [Pope, 1958]

# DRYMARCHON CORAIS

## Systematics
- Scientific name: Drymarchon corais [Boie, 1827].
- Synonym: Coluber corais [Boie, 1827].
- Common names: Yellowtail cribo.
- Family: Colubridae.

## Biological Profile
- Large, non-venomous, heavy-bodied but still swiftly moving terrestrial colubrid distinguished by the gradual transition in colour of its scales from black to yellow or orange on the tail end of its body. Up to 3 m in length.
- Range: Central America, Caribbean [Trinidad and Tobago], South America [Colombia, Venezuela, Brazil, Ecuador, Peru, Bolivia, N Argentina, Paraguay].
- Habitat: Typically found in forested areas.
- Solitary; shelters in underground burrows of other animals as well as naturally formed spaces.
- Diurnal, semi-arboreal, fast moving and aggressive.
- Relies on sheer strength and will feed on just about any animal that it can subdue with its powerful jaws.
- Feeds on a range of species and appears to have a generalist diet, with commonly known prey species such as frogs, lizards, birds, mammals and other snakes. Known to prey on venomous snakes such as pit vipers like the bushmaster [Lachesis muta], the venom of which they appear to be immune to, as well as poisonous frogs and toads such as the cane toad [Rhinella marina].
- Forages for nocturnal prey during the day when they are resting, both on the ground and in elevated vegetation, ingesting prey head-first.
- Males engage in ritual combat for breeding rights, defending territory and establishing dominance.
- Oviparous; 4–12 eggs per clutch.
- Has a reputation of being tame when handled properly, but a defensive or feeding response bite could be significant, due to its strong jaws and large sharp teeth. Has the tendency in both defensive bites and feeding response bites to hold on and not immediately release the victim. A bite release must

be initiated by the snake and not the handler or victim to prevent additional bite wound trauma.

## Materia Medica
- No symptoms.

# DRYMARCHON COUPERI

### Systematics
- Scientific name: Drymarchon couperi [Holbrook, 1842].
- Synonyms: Coluber couperi [Holbrook, 1842]. Drymarchon corais [Stejneger, 1899].
- Common names: Eastern indigo snake. Blue gopher snake.
- Family: Colubridae.

### Biological Profile
- Large, non-venomous, glossy black colubrid with iridescent blue highlights in sunlight. Chin, throat, and sides of head may be reddish or [rarely] white. Largest non-venomous snake in the U.S., reaching up to 8 ft [2.4 m] in length.
- Sexually dimorphic, with males growing to larger lengths than females.
- Range: Restricted to Florida and southern areas of Georgia, Alabama, and Mississippi.
- Habitat: Xeric pine-oak sandhills, hardwood forests, moist hammocks, pine flatwoods, prairies, and around cypress ponds.
- Uses gopher tortoise burrows as shelter during the winter and during the warmer months for nesting and refuge from intense summer heat.
- May move long distances during the active season and often forages along wetland margins. Summer home ranges can be as large as 273 acres [229 ha].
- Diurnal.
- Relies on sheer strength. Most snakes have a relatively weak bite force, but eastern indigo snakes have unusually muscular jaws that are used to physically overpower their prey.
- Forages during the summer in wetland areas; preys on mammals, birds, frogs and other snakes, including rattlesnakes, copperheads and cottonmouths.
- Shifts to drier habitats in winter to breed.
- Oviparous; 4–12 eggs per clutch.
- More active in cold weather than most other snakes. Does not hibernate.
- When cornered, flattens its neck vertically, hisses and vibrates its tail, which produces a rattling sound. Intimidates but rarely bites.
- Has a reputation of being tame when handled properly, but a defensive or feeding response bite could be significant, due to their strong jaws and large sharp teeth. Has the tendency in both defensive bites and feeding response bites to hold on and not immediately release the victim. A bite release must be initiated by the snake and not the handler or victim to prevent additional bite wound trauma.

## Materia Medica
- No symptoms.

# ELAPHE GUTTATA

## Systematics
- Scientific name: Pantherophis guttatus [L., 1766].
- Synonym: Coluber guttatus [L., 1766]. Elaphe guttata [Stejneger & Barbour, 1917].
- Common names: Corn snake. Eastern corn snake. Red rat snake.
- Family: Colubridae.

## Biological Profile
- Medium-sized, slender, constricting colubrid to 1.8 m long, often mistaken for a copperhead [Agkistrodon contortrix].
- Body colour pale red, reddish-brown, orange or brownish-yellow, with large, black-edged red saddle-like blotches down middle of back. Belly has alternating rows of black and white marks, resembling a checkerboard pattern. Dark arrowhead mark on top of head. Considerable variation occurs in colouration and patterns of individual snakes.
- Range: Eastern and central USA, most abundant in Florida.
- Habitat: Overgrown fields, wooded groves, rocky hillsides, meadowlands, woodlots, barns.
- Mostly nocturnal during hot and dry weather. Generally very secretive and spending most of its time underground prowling through rodent burrows, or remaining under cover of rocks, logs, surface debris during daytime. May be diurnal if more favourable temperature and moisture conditions are available.
- Adept climber.
- Preys on rodents, birds, young snakes; particularly fond of lizards. A proficient climber, it may scale trees in search of birds and bats. May enter abandoned or seldom-used buildings and farms in search for prey.
- Hibernates during winter in colder regions.
- Oviparous; 10–30 eggs per clutch. Once laid the female abandons the eggs and does not return to them.
- Males engage in combat bouts for the attention of receptive females.
- No subspecies.
- Name in allusion to similarity of the markings on the snake's belly with the checkered pattern of kernels of maize, and because it is found in corn fields and/or inhabits barns where mice and rats feed on corn and other grains.
- Popular pet snake due to its docile nature, reluctance to bite, and splendid colours and patterns.

## Behaviour & Temperament
Generally speaking, the corn snake is a bold and strong reptile, in the experience of Ditmars [1907], 'showing considerable bravery when cornered and a little

of the rush and flutter of most snakes when taken unawares. Either lazy or figuring quiet is a better safeguard than flight, they lie alert, with quivering tongue, watching developments.'

'Armed only with relatively small teeth, the corn snake, like most serpents its size, is no match against a large adversary. In the face of danger, it ordinarily does not seek to escape by dashing for the nearest shelter [a strategy used effectively by such species as the coachwhip, racer, and ribbon snake, amongst others].

'Instead, when suddenly confronted by man, especially in the open, it is likely to pull its entire body together slightly into a series of short, lateral, wavelike kinks and remain that way without taking any further action. An aroused corn snake is not so passive. When closely approached, it gathers its forebody into several tight, elevated S-loops, pulls its head back to somewhere near the top of the coils, then often leans backward so that a portion of its boldly checkered belly is visible to its foe. In this position, its body tense and waiting, the snake holds its ground, sometimes vibrating its tail as a further signal of its intentions.

'At the first threatening move, the snake delivers a quick strike that is often punctuated with a brief, sharp hiss, but seldom do the reptile's jaws engage the intended victim, for the attack is intended primarily to discourage the snake's adversary, not to injure it. When first picked up, some corn snakes bite with determination and expel faeces on their captor; others are more docile, never showing hostility, even when initially captured.

'Virtually all corn snakes become tractable soon after their first few days in captivity, which [in addition to their usual stunning roseate colouration and ease of maintenance in captivity] is why they are typically the snake of choice among reptile hobbyists around the world.' [Werler & Dixon, 2000]

## Star Gazing

Corn snakes may suffer from a genetic defect called 'star gazing'.

'At rest, a Star Gazer may appear just as normal as any other hatchling. When stimulated to move about, they seem to have difficulty with balance, swinging their heads to and fro as they slither. If agitated, they get more animated and swing their heads faster, more wildly, and may even flip their heads over in a loop. As the name implies, Star Gazers may throw their heads back and appear to gaze towards the stars at times. They may lie in odd positions with their heads upside down. Sometimes they will get themselves flipped over and slither along on their backs for a time before righting themselves. The more intensely focused on something they are, the more difficulty they have [such as when they're excited about eating, they may miss a strike or swing their heads wildly.]

'Mentally, these snakes are normal. They respond just as any hatchling would with excitement at feeding, gripping of your hand as they crawl on you, and curiosity and exploring while "tongue sniffing." They can eat normally [albeit sometimes upside down or in a weird position], they can shed normally. They don't appear to suffer any pain or discomfort and are perfectly content to go about their daily duties, even if a bit wobbly.

'Clinically, the condition is very similar to an animal that is bilaterally vestibular [meaning an animal that doesn't have balance sensation from either side of its inner ear].' [Star Gazing Information Sheet; cccorns.com]

## MATERIA MEDICA ELAPHE GUTTATA

### Sources
1 Self-experimentation; C4-trituration.

### Mind
∞ Clear-headed; emotional side as if closed down, intellectual side as if enhanced.
∞ Pent-up frustration, esp. with amount of work to do. Feeling spikey and irritated; waves or ripples of irritation coming up throat, causing cough. Must exert self-control to stay polite.
∞ Del. time is passing slowly.

### Generals
∞ Great desire for fresh air due to feeling of constriction and restriction.
∞ Feeling as if a cold is coming on or just having had the flu.
∞ Thirsty for cold water.
∞ Overpowering sleepiness.
∞ Right side more affected.

### Sensations
∞ Congestion in centre of head, as from a block of wood.
∞ Intense tingling all over scalp or below, as if skull bones are shifting.
∞ Tightness head, band sensation from ear to ear going round at back of head.
∞ Tip of tongue feels numb/tingly. Tongue feels as if quivering, vibrating.
∞ Fullness in ears, with slight bulging sensation in left ear drum.
∞ Expanding lump in throat, swelling outwards.
∞ Feet feel compressed, as if shoes are too small.

### Locals
∞ Shooting pain from right jaw to right ear.
∞ Jaw muscles cramped.
∞ Itching around nose.
∞ Ears sensitive to sound and pressure.
∞ Itching fingers and palms of hands. Aching fingers.
∞ Restless legs.
∞ Weak tiredness of limbs.

# ELAPHE LONGISSIMA

## Systematics
- Scientific name: Zamenis longissimus [Laurenti, 1768].
- Synonym: Elaphe longissima [Laurenti, 1768]. Coluber esculapii [Sclater, 1891].
- Common names: Aesculapian snake. Aesculapian rat snake.
- Family: Colubridae.

## Biological Profile
- Dark, long, slender, non-venomous, constricting colubrid with small, pointed head. Up to 2 m long. Among the largest European snakes. Males significantly longer than females.
- Olive-yellow, brownish-green, greyish-brown, sometimes almost black or bronzy in colour, with smooth scales that give it a metallic sheen. First 20–40 cm can be a lighter colour. White dots on scale edges, esp. on mid-body. Belly plain yellow to off-white.
- Range: France, Italy, Balkans, Greece; central and eastern Europe, Asia Minor.
- Habitat: Dry habitats, dense vegetation, thickets, brambles, meadows with bushes and high grass, but also stone walls, rocky terrain and hay.
- Inhabits a relatively small area and uses the same shelter for years. Hibernates. Mobility considerably increases during the reproduction period.
- Diurnal; sometimes active into the night during hot days.
- Adept climber; capable of ascending even vertical, branchless tree trunks.
- Can be very fast.
- Feeds on mice, rats, voles, squirrels, lizards and nesting birds. May forage in roof of buildings.
- Oviparous; 2–18 eggs per clutch.
- Males engage in courtship combats.

## Materia Medica
- No symptoms.


# LAMPROPELTIS CALLIGASTER CALLIGASTER

## Systematics
- Scientific name: Lampropeltis calligaster [Harlan, 1827].
- Subspecies: L. c. calligaster [Harlen, 1827].
- Synonym: Coluber calligaster [Harlan, 1827].
- Common names: Prairie kingsnake. Yellow-bellied kingsnake.
- Family: Colubridae.

## Biological Profile

- Medium-sized, slender, non-venomous, constricting colubrid with rounded head, smooth scales and relatively short tail. Light brown or grey in colour, dark grey, brown or reddish-brown blotches that run down its body length. Belly pale cream or yellowish with brown, square-shaped blotches. Average length 75–102 cm [2.5–3.3 ft].
- Range: Found primarily throughout the Midwestern and Southeastern United States, from Nebraska to Virginia, Texas and Florida.
- Habitat: Favours prairies and pasturelands; also likes to reside along edges of crop fields, hay fields, rocky woodlands and near farm buildings.
- Generally takes shelter inside mammal burrows, located near riverside plantations and open grasslands.
- Shy and reclusive; spends most of its time underground in burrows or under rocks. Can easily adapt to habitat alterations as many have found the species residing in abandoned buildings, barnyards, barrier beaches and sawdust piles.
- Generally seen while it is out foraging, around dusk during spring and fall months, but switching to night during hottest summer months. Basks on rocky surfaces on warm days.
- Feeds on rats, mice, lizards, frogs, bird eggs, and other snakes. Immune to the venom of several species of snakes like copperheads and cottonmouths. Can catch the scent of its potential prey and follows it relying on its tongue to enhance its sensing capabilities.
- Vibrates its tail if harassed, emitting a rattling sound against dry litter that sounds quite similar to a rattlesnake's rattle. Emits a foul-smelling musk and/or flattens its body when threatened.
- Generally gentle and placid, rarely biting even when first caught.
- Hibernates.
- Mates for life instead of mating with multiple partners [like most other snakes do].
- Oviparous; 5–17 eggs per clutch.
- Three recognized subspecies [calligaster, occipitolineata, rhombomaculata].

## Materia Medica

- No symptoms.


# LAMPROPELTIS CALLIGASTER RHOMBOMACULATA

## Systematics

- Scientific name: Lampropeltis calligaster [Harlan, 1827].
- Subspecies: L. c. rhombomaculata [Holbrook, 1840].
- Synonym: Coluber rhombo-maculatus [Holbrook, 1840].
- Common names: Mole kingsnake. Brown kingsnake.
- Family: Colubridae.

## Biological Profile

- Medium-sized, slender, non-venomous, constricting colubrid with rounded head, smooth scales and relatively short tail. Light/dark brown to reddish in colour with dark brown or reddish-brown blotching. Belly whitish or yellowish with red, grey or brown mottling. Average length 75–102 cm [2.5–3.3 ft].
- Range: Throughout the southeastern United States and the Mid-Atlantic States.
- Habitat: Pinelands, hardwood hammocks, sandhills, prairies, agricultural fields. Prefers loose dry soil near permanent water.
- Shy and reclusive; spends most of its time underground in burrows as the name 'mole' kingsnake indicates. Rarely seen above ground during the day unless forced out by heavy rains.
- Active mainly at night.
- Feeds on rodents, lizards, frogs, birds and other snakes.
- Vibrates its tail rapidly when harassed.
- Oviparous; up to 17 eggs per clutch.
- Three recognized subspecies [calligaster, occipitolineata, rhombomaculata].

## Materia Medica
- No symptoms.

# LAMPROPELTIS GETULA CALIFORNIAE

## Systematics
- Scientific name: Lampropeltis californiae [Blainville, 1766].
- Synonyms: Coluber californiae [Blainville, 1835]. Lampropeltis getula californiae [Blainville, 1835]. Lampropeltis getulus californiae [Seufer & Jauch, 1980]
- Common name: California king snake.
- Family: Colubridae.

## Biological Profile
- Non-venomous, constricting colubrid to 1.2 m long with smooth, shiny, unkeeled scales.
- Highly variable. Most commonly seen with alternating bands of black or brown and white or light yellow, including the underside, where the light bands become wider. Can also be striped or a combination of striped and ringed. All shades of black, brown and chocolate patterns are known with a ground colour ranging for brilliant white to nearly coal black.
- Range: Western USA – Oregon to southern Utah. Arizona, Nevada, California and Baja Peninsula of Mexico.
- Habitat: Deserts, forests, farmland, river bottoms and brushy areas.
- Active during daylight in cooler weather and at night, dawn, and dusk when temperatures are high.
- Will usually go deep underground in wintertime and enter a hibernation-like state called brumation, which is characterised by a slowed metabolism and reduced activity.

- Eats a wide variety of prey, including rodents and other small mammals, lizards, snakes [including rattlesnakes], turtle eggs and hatchlings, frogs, salamanders, birds' eggs and chicks, and large invertebrates.
- When disturbed, generally not aggressive, but sometimes vibrates the tail quickly, hisses, and rolls into a ball, hiding the head and showing the vent with its lining exposed.
- A powerful constrictor, coiling tightly around its prey, and immune to snake venom, the king snake has the reputation of being fierce, quarrelsome and aggressive to a degree seldom found even in venomous snakes.
- Oviparous; 4–20 eggs per clutch.
- Males engage in courtship combats.
- Popular pet snake. Many unusual colour phases have been bred, including albinos.
- No subspecies.
- Name from Gr. *lampros*, shiny, and *pelta*, shield, referring to the smooth, shiny dorsal scales characteristic of this genus.

## Fearless & Self-reliant

'They [Lampropeltis spp.] may all be classed as truly land snakes; so far as known none seek their food in the water. They have not the stout body of the snakes that depend for safety upon inconspicuousness or poison, nor the attenuated body and tail of the tree snakes and racers, but rather a well-proportioned body and short tail, adapted to life on the ground and more or less in the open. They seem in general to be fearless and self-reliant. Their immunity to snake venom and their powerful constricting ability render them truly kings among the reptiles of North America. Much remains to be learned about the food preferences of the various forms, but in general it may be said that they are the enemies of all small rodents and of all snakes and lizards; fledgling birds are undoubtedly eaten on opportunity.' [Blanchard, 1921]

## Bold & Courageous

'Of the grand army of harmless snakes inhabiting North America, the King Snake is unquestionably the king. It is also called the Chain-Snake and Thunder-Snake. It is the most courageous of all snakes, and in proportion to its size it is also the strongest. Toward man it is by no means especially vicious; but on the contrary, its manner is quite tolerant.

'Toward all other serpents, however, it manifests as great aversion as any snake-hating woman, and it is pugnacious and aggressive to an astonishing degree. The King Snake is, for its size, the most powerful of all the constrictors, and does not hesitate to attack a snake of another species several times larger than itself. It is cannibalistic in its tastes, and not only attacks and kills other snakes, but devours them.

'In our Reptile House, a snake of this species once attacked a Cuban boa, fully 3 times its own size, and tried to swallow it! Had not the boa been rescued, it would undoubtedly have been quickly suffocated by the coils, which its antagonist had wrapped tightly around its body. On another occasion a King Snake that was placed for a very short time in the cage of the water moccasins, attacked one of the latter, wrapped around it, and killed it. Several times the moccasin bit its assailant, but the King Snake is immune to the venom of serpents and paid no attention to the counter-attack.' [Hornaday, 1904]

## Refusing to Budge

'The king snake is equally hostile to rats and mice. He is not of great length, but thick and muscular; and is perfectly harmless to man. He is regarded in a friendly light, and no one troubles him. He is a bold fellow too. In passing through an extensive wood, I met with one coiled up so near the carriage track that one of my wheels actually grazed his skin; and yet he disdained to move. Backing my sulkey, I touched him pretty smartly with the 'snapper' of my whip, probably 20 times in the course of 10 minutes. He would, each time, raise his head, look at me, and writhe his body; but absolutely refused to budge an inch. I left him there. I should judge him to have been about 5 feet long, as he crossed the road just before I came up with him.' [Providence Journal, 1843]

## Duels to the Death

Lampropeltis getulus getulus, the typical form of the king snakes, is a large, powerful, and fearless snake. It does not appear to be secretive or to avoid an encounter. In fact, as Ditmars remarks, 'besides the promptings of its appetite this snake exhibits a pugnacious interest in other serpents that may be considerably larger than itself, engaging these creatures in a duel to the death, during which, however, they are able to make but little resistance, when encircled by the wonderfully strong constricting coils of the enemy. . . . If in its wanderings it meets a rattlesnake, there is certain to be trouble for the latter unless it continues on its way without hesitation, for the king snake likes to pick quarrels and, once aroused, will coil tightly about its astonished adversary and begin to squeeze. Slowly the grip grows tighter and the victim, if it is venomous, uses its fangs upon the body of the tormentor, but to no effect, *as the king snake is immune to snake poison*. But the wounds enrage it. Winding the lithe body round and round the doomed creature, until every part of the shining length is engaged, it tightens with such strength that the victim is benumbed, unable to bite, and is strangled. So strong is this snake in proportion to its size, and aided as it is by agility of motion, even the strong constricting snakes of other species fall victims when attacked.

'Despite its hostility toward other snakes, the king snake shows a very mild nature with man. Specimens captured by the author . . . when first caught, they strike vigorously, emitting a short hiss which sounds more like a sneeze; at such times the majority of specimens eject a powerful musky odour from glands near the base of the tail. These symptoms pass away within a few minutes, when most specimens may be handled without the least signs of bad temper. As captives, few reptiles are more gentle or devoid of nervousness. . . . When handled, these snakes will usually coil firmly about one's fingers to keep them from falling. During these actions the muscular development may be noted and will be found to exist to surprising degree in a creature of moderate size. If frightened, some

SNAKES

specimens coil into compact knots until they form a spherical mass; in this position they may be rolled about without relaxing.' [Ditmars, 1907]

### Venting its Spleen

'King snakes take their name from their ability to dominate other serpents; in fact, they eat them. . . . Common king snakes are non-venomous and often fail to bite when first encountered, so we didn't hesitate to grab our visitor on the deck to study and photograph it. As we reached for the king snake, it vibrated its tail rapidly – a common response that reaches perfection among the rattlesnakes. This scare tactic didn't deter us, and we grasped the king snake tightly behind its head. With just as firm a grip, it wrapped its strong, sinewy body around our hand – probably not an attempt to constrict and kill us but rather to provide stability in an unfamiliar situation.

'The snake's next ploy was not unexpected, but it was unpleasant: out spewed a semi-liquid substance that undoubtedly is one of the vilest odours in nature. The smell – a mixture of musk and urine and faeces – is indescribable, but once it has graced your olfactory nerves, you will never forget it. You also will wash your hands several times with perfumed soap after handling any snake that so anoints you. Most potential snake-eaters – including unnatural ones such as dogs and cats – are inclined to release any snake that "vents its spleen," especially if the predator gets a sudden mouthful.

'This odoriferous material emanates from the snake's cloaca. . . . After taking our close-up photos, we placed the king snake on the ground, where it formed into a tight ball. This behaviour may be another defensive mechanism or may simply be the safest thing to do until the snake gets its bearings; it even stayed in a ball temporarily when we rolled it over on its back to photograph the ventral side.' [Hilton, 2002]

### Materia Medica
- No symptoms.

# LAMPROPELTIS TRIANGULUM

### Systematics
- Scientific name: Lampropeltis triangulum [Lacépède, 1789].
- Synonyms: Coluber triangulum [Lacépède, 1789]. Ophibolus doliatus triangulus [Cope, 1875]. Lampropeltis doliatus doliatus [Hay, 1902].
- Common names: Milk snake. Spotted adder. House moccasin. House snake.
- Family: Colubridae.

### Biological Profile
- Moderately-sized, slender-bodied, constricting colubrid, its head but slightly distinct from the neck, tapering from the temples forward and truncate at the end. Average length 80 cm, maximum 1 m.
- Ground colour dorsally whitish, yellowish or greyish with blotches or saddles of brown, grey, or red [juvenile and some adults] from head to tip of tail,

extending down to sides, where they alternate with 1 or 2 series of roundish spots. Blotches narrowly edged with black; upper row of roundish spots brown edged with black, lower row mostly black. Belly checked with black and white, sometimes suffused with red. Y-shaped or oval spot of white on back of head.
- Range: Eastern North America.
- Habitat: Upland situations, woods and fields, not uncommon near dwellings and stables.
- Nocturnal.
- Preys on small rodents, preferably mice, as well as on snakes [also its own kind], lizards and birds. Better than a cat, it can follow a mouse to its nest and eat the whole brood of young. The fact alone that it eats so many destructive rodents 'should be sufficient to assure its protection at the hands of farmers and others; and, when one considers that it is a perfectly harmless, non-aggressive, unfearing creature, he may well wonder why it is so persistently persecuted. Its lack of fear is one cause of its great decrease in numbers. As a farmer will say, "You have to kick it out of the way."' [Blanchard, 1921]
- From the habit of prowling about stables and dairies in search of mice and rats, this prettily coloured snake has acquired the reputation of stealing milk from the cows; hence its common name.
- Oviparous; 8–13 eggs per clutch.

### Behaviour & Temperament
'The milk snake is a secretive species, hiding under flat stones or debris and preferring to prowl late in the day or at twilight. . . . In captivity this snake is indifferent in feeding and seldom lives long. It prefers mice, which are quickly constricted to death in the reptile's strong coils. Young specimens can seldom be induced to take food of any character. Although rather a quiet reptile, the milk snake will sometimes resent handling in a curious and rather treacherous manner. Without a pretense of striking it will swing the head about suddenly and grasp the hand, when it deliberately chews in such a manner that the fine, recurved teeth lacerate the flesh sufficiently to bring the blood, although the minute punctures are but very superficial wounds and heal at once, like a scratch from a fine point.' [Ditmars, 1907]

### Materia Medica
- No symptoms.

# NATRIX NATRIX

### Systematics
- Scientific name: Natrix natrix [Laurenti, 1768].
- Synonyms: Coluber natrix [L., 1758]. Natrix vulgaris [Laurenti, 1768].
- Common names: Grass snake. Ringed snake. Water snake.
- Family: Colubridae.

## Biological Profile

- Non-venomous colubrid, typically dark green or brown in colour with a characteristic yellow collar behind the head, which explains the name ringed snake. Average length 1.5 m, maximum 1.9 m. Females considerably larger than males, which are about 20 cm shorter and much smaller in girth.
- Colour may range from grey to black, with darker colours being more prevalent in colder regions, presumably owing to the thermal benefits of being dark in colour. Underside lighter colour.
- Range: Europe, NW Africa, W Asia.
- Habitat: Open woodland, field margins, woodland borders affording both adequate refuge and opportunity for basking.
- Diurnal; hunt/ambush predator, consuming prey live without using physical constriction.
- Preys almost exclusively on amphibians, especially the common toad and the common frog, but may occasionally eat rodents and fish.
- Although the Grass Snake rarely bites, it can put on a seemingly aggressive defence if cornered, inflating the body, hissing loudly and striking with the mouth closed. On occasion an individual will adopt a completely different form of defence by feigning death. This very convincing display involves the snake writhing onto its back, the body becoming flaccid and the mouth open with the tongue hanging out. If further provoked or caught, they will struggle violently and discharge an evil-smelling fluid from their vent. [www.bto.org]
- Oviparous; 8–40 eggs per clutch. Young immediately independent on hatching.
- Hibernates. Covers significant distances in search of suitable hibernation sites or feeding areas and may sometimes be found in gardens or parks.
- Nine subspecies.


## MATERIA MEDICA NATRIX NATRIX

### Sources
1 Self-experimentation Gaby Rottler [Germany], 30c; 2003.
2 C3-trituration proving conducted in Bristol [UK], 3 female, 3 male provers; 2011.

### Mind
∞ Feeling calm when active; restless and anxious when not doing something.[2]
∞ Annoyed at people not doing things properly.[2]
∞ Anxiety, being ready. Waiting, edge of seat feeling. Ready to pounce or be pounced on.[2]
∞ Sense of straightforward competitiveness.[2]
∞ Road rage; chasing another car right on its tail.[2]
∞ Feeling unsafe in car. Not concentrating.[2]
∞ Mistakes. Coming in on wrong day; missing appointments. Missed messages. Forgetting to do things.[2]

∞ Wants to go camping in the wild.[2]
∞ Del. not needing people, nature is enough. Ideals vs practicality. Nature vs society. Letting go of things, of possessions.[2]

## Dreams
∞ Eating a bird.[2]
∞ Enjoying causing pain.[2]
∞ Envisaging people being cut and stabbed, lots of blood and real pain to come.[2]
∞ Monster coming down from attic.[2]
∞ Preparing for battle in medieval times.[2]
∞ Seized upwards into attic by monster.[2]
∞ Sticking sharp needles into ankles and heels.[2]

## Generals
∞ Desire for fresh air; to be outside.[2]
∞ Desire for large amounts of white wine and to sing.[1]
∞ Desire for chocolate in evening.[1]
∞ Left side more affected.[2]
∞ Sensitivity to smells.[2]
∞ Aches and pains, esp. in morning.[2]

## Sensations
∞ Eyelids as if thinned, as if only a fragile papery left that could easily be torn.[2]
∞ Pain across top of left shoulder. Contracted or tightened.[2]
∞ Pain in joints of right hand, as if sprained.[1]
∞ Left leg feels numb, floppy and out of control when compared to the right.[2]

## Locals
∞ Headache. Heads feels full. Very hot.[2]
∞ Head quite groggy, wants the windows open.[2]
∞ Boring pain in forehead above left eyebrow.[1]
∞ Eyes sticking together, in morning.[1]
∞ Vision impaired, > violent rubbing for some time.[1]
∞ Nausea in throat when climbing on something high.[1]
∞ Flatulence when walking.[1]
∞ Raspy, squeaky bowel sounds in afternoon, while sitting.[1]
∞ Sudden and painful urge to stool.[2]
∞ Frequent urination.[2]
∞ Breasts swollen and tense, 3 days before menses.[1]
∞ Menses unusually scanty.[1]
∞ Sudden cutting, shooting pain in spinal column, lumbar region, < bending forward; not affected by walking.[1]
∞ Pressing pain side of left patella when walking, extending down tibia, > continued motion.[1]
∞ Pressing pain in left patella when walking.[1]

# PANTHEROPHIS OBSOLETUS

## Systematics
- Scientific name: Pantherophis obsoletus [Say, 1823].
- Synonyms: Elaphe obsoleta [Say, 1823]. Coluber obsoletus [Say, 1823].
- Common names: Western rat snake. Black rat snake.
- Family: Colubridae.

## Biological Profile
- Large, powerful, slender, non-venomous, constricting colubrid with wedge-shaped head and keeled scales. Black, except for its white or cream chin. Belly patterned with grey or brown over a background of yellow or white. Up to 1.8 m [6 ft] in length; record length 2.57 m [8.5 ft].
- Range: Central USA.
- Habitat: Forested wetland, riparian, heavily wooded areas, rocky canyons. Can be considered arboreal, as it seeks food and refuge inside hollow limbs as well as on exposed branches. Also can be found associated with human habitations, as it may take up residence in barns and associated farm structures.
- Diurnal in spring and fall, nocturnal in summer.
- Excellent climber; uses its angular ventral scales to climb straight up the trunk of a tree.
- Being able to access many different habitats, feeds on a variety of mammalian, avian, reptilian [mainly lizards] and amphibian [mainly frogs and toads] prey.
- Shy, avoids being confronted; tends to freeze and remain motionless when confronted by danger. Its colour variation, the Texas rat snake, however, is described as "Easily one of the most ill-tempered snakes found in Texas, it is non-venomous but will bite any aggressor voraciously." [Herps of Texas]
- Oviparous; 5–30 eggs per clutch.
- Hibernates.
- No subspecies. A revision of Pantherophis obsoletus has recommended the elimination of the various subspecies entirely, considering them all to be merely locality variations.

## Materia Medica
- No symptoms.

# THAMNOPHIS SIRTALIS SIRTALIS

## Systematics
- Scientific name: Thamnophis sirtalis [L., 1758].
- Subspecies: T. s. sirtalis [L., 1758].
- Common name: Eastern garter snake.
- Family: Colubridae.

## Biological Profile

- Highly variable colubrid in both colour and pattern, but normally with 3 yellowish stripes, 1 medial and 2 lateral ones; stripes may be brownish, greenish, or bluish. There is usually a double row of alternating back spots between stripes. Ground colour mostly black, but can be brown, green, or olive. Belly greenish or yellowish, with 2 rows of indistinct black spots. Scales keeled.
- Average length 50–70 cm, maximum 1.2 m.
- Range: Eastern USA and Canada.
- Habitat: Hardwood and pine forests, lowland and upland grasslands, abandoned fields, along margins of creeks, rivers, ponds, and lakes, agricultural and urban areas, freshwater marshes.
- Diurnal; active during the cooler parts of the day – early morning, late afternoon, early evening.
- Viviparous; 10–60 young per litter.
- Preys on earthworms, millipedes, spiders, various insects, salamanders, frogs, and toads.
- Congregates in large numbers at good places to hibernate over the winter.
- First to appear in spring from hibernation and the last to hibernate in the autumn.
- Will discharge a foul-smelling musky secretion and strike when cornered.


## MATERIA MEDICA

### Sources
1 Effects of bite; clinical manifestations.

### Clinical Manifestations
'The salivary secretions of the common garter snake [Thamnophis sirtalis] are elaborated from mandible glands and serve as evidence of a venom delivery system. Several cases of envenomation have resulted from bites by the garter snake species *Thamnophis sirtalis* and *Thamnophis elegans vagrans*. The victims of these bites suffered local swelling, oedema, haemorrhagic vesicles, and ecchymosis, to the extent that they required hospital admission. Systemic symptoms did not occur, but the clinical presentation was likened to that observed with pit viper envenoming. Thus, even colubrid species considered to be totally harmless are capable of causing some degree of toxinological insult.' [Hayes, 2007]

# VIPERA AQUATICUS CARINATA

### Identity Uncertain
This snake is not Echis carinatus, although the name would suggest so. Swan gave it the name *Fel vipera acustica carcinata* [sic], referring to 'the serpent galls brought by Dr. Higgins from South America.' Higgins, however, was all but clear

about its origins. He categorised a snake, which he named *Vipera echis carinata*, as occurring in both India and South America. Since snakes of the genera Vipera and Echis only occur in the Old World, the location South America obviously cannot be correct. Aside from the first mentioned V. echis carinata, Higgins also speaks of one with the enigmatic name *Vipera acuaticus [colubriformis] carinata*, which would explain Swan's misspelling of the name as *acustica* instead of acuaticus. This snake seems to be native to South America, the Colombian 'curers' [snake handlers] claiming that its gall acts as an antidote to poisoning, if we are to believe Higgins. The drawn-out name of the snake is difficult to trace back to something scientifically acceptable and accepted.

Thus, if Higgins brought the preparation with him from South America, and according to Swan he did, it cannot have been obtained from the Indian species Echis carinata. On the other hand, if the snake's local name *Lomo de Machete* [misspelled by Swan as 'Loina de machete'] would be anything to go for, the mystery will be solved. It would explain the addition of *colubriformis*, meaning 'colubrid-like', since Lomo de Machete is the non-venomous snake Chironius carinatus in the family Colubridae. It is large and known for its aggressive behaviour and goes by the names Amazonian whipsnake, keeled whipsnake, machete savane and yellow machete. It opens its mouth in vigorous threat display, meanwhile inflating its neck region to expose the white skin between the scales and biting readily when given the chance. When caught it will whip at the capturer's face or hand like an uncoiling spring, which often helps its release and subsequent escape. The specific epithet *acuaticus* refers to *aquaticus*, in allusion to this snake readily taking to water and feeding on frogs.

Higgins deemed it venomous. While highly truculent and pugnacious, it is not venomous, as Mike Boston's encounter with a large specimen in a Costa Rican rainforest demonstrates.

' "You never see snakes, huh!" remarked one of the women as the taxi driver pointed out a large, electric blue keel-backed racer, Chironius carinatus, on the road a short distance ahead. I just can't resist catching snakes and, despite the protests from the women, I burst out of the taxi and ran towards the snake. Keel-backed racers are fast diurnal hunters, with large eyes and keen vision. They are wary snakes, and one cannot afford finesse when attempting to catch them. So I lunged at the snake, just as it was about to disappear into the undergrowth and seized it by the tail. The snake turned and struck at my face, but with reflexes of a prize boxer I dodged, and the snake missed.

'I now had 6 feet of angry snake suspended from my grasp. Meanwhile, protests from the taxi were reaching fever pitch: "No, Mike!" "Please don't, Mike!" The snake then bit my knee, released and struck again at my chest. In the process of getting the snake into a more manageable position it bit me several times more on my left arm. With the snakes head now under control and my knee, chest and arm oozing rivulets of blood, I approached the taxi. I had a huge grin on my face – my prayers were answered, I thought! By the time I reached the taxi the snake had settled down in my gentle grasp. The expressions on the women's faces were ones of total disbelief. They were aghast and speechless. My enthusiastic dissertation on snakes, extolling their abundant virtues, went largely unheard!

'I released the snake, wiped the blood from my arm, chest and knee, and jumped into the taxi. The women were amazed that I was still alive, and examined my bite wounds minutely, and repeatedly. They said I was a complete lunatic and begged me to desist from such activities lest I die and leave them abandoned in the jungle. But, of course, I didn't!' [Mike Boston, Tales from the Jungle: Snakes; www.osaaventura.com]

## Systematics
- Scientific name: Chironius carinatus [L., 1758].
- Synonyms: Coluber carinatus [L., 1758]. Natrix carinatus [Merrem, 1820].
- Common name: Amazonian whipsnake. Keeled whipsnake. Machete savane.
- Family: Colubridae.

## Biological Profile
- Very large but slender colubrid varying in colour from dark olive green to brown or black. Back sharply ridged with a lighter stripe along the middorsal region that contrasts with the darker colouring on the upper side of its body. Chin and underside of forebody bright yellow; yellow spots on body and tail along first row of dorsal scales. Head large and distinct from the slim neck. Tail very long and thin. Up to 3 m [10 ft] in length.
- Range: Costa Rica, Venezuela, Trinidad and Tobago, French Guiana, Suriname, Guyana, Colombia, Peru, Ecuador, Brazil.
- Habitat: Terrestrial and arboreal, but also readily takes to water.
- Active hunter; preys on frogs, lizards, mice and birds.

# MATERIA MEDICA VIPERA AQUATICUS CARINATA

## Sources
1 Proving Swan [USA], 1 female prover, 1M; 1885.

## Mind
∞ Feels like crying, esp. when spoken to, not from pain, but from being generally miserable all over. Feels miserable in morning.
∞ Very little patience; small matters annoy.

## Generals
∞ Restless sleep wakes with a start; cramps in limbs during sleep, < in right, in popliteal space.
∞ Thirst all the time; takes one goblet of cold water after another.
∞ Sick and miserable all over; awfully tired. Feels fatigued all the time.
∞ At times feels hot, yet chills crawl over her. Chilly only if uncovered. Alternate heat and crawling chills.
∞ Appetite poor; after eating a little, has suddenly a sense of fullness, and more food nauseates.

## Sensations

∞ When walking, momentary dizziness, as if she would fall backward [occiput as if very heavy].

∞ Head seems so heavy as to cause neck to ache.

∞ Sensation of a hair across nose; felt it yesterday across the hand, about third and fourth fingers.

∞ When lying down, noises in head like summer insects and frogs, etc., such as is heard in the country when all is quiet.

## Locals

∞ Headache in spells, first over left side, then stops entirely; then returns on right side; alternates.

∞ Face swollen on right side, and looks red.

∞ Saliva stringy, frothy, thick, sticky.

∞ Cramps in bowels, immediately after drinking cold water.

∞ Pains of menses, but no flow.

∞ Menses 12 days too late; profuse and very liquid, colour bright.

∞ Both breasts sore; cannot bear pressure or when lying on them.

∞ Can't draw a deep breath, it hurts so in left side and round to back, and for 2 hours cannot speak without catching a stitch in this side.

∞ Dry cough while sitting; cannot reach mucus, which seems low down under sternum; on lying down it becomes loose.

∞ Lungs very sore when coughing or inhaling air.

∞ Pains in 2 middle fingers of left hand, but most in back of hand; the pain is shooting, needle-like, going up the fingers; also aching in back of hand.

∞ At night, hands itch as if bitten by insects; commences about 8 p.m. and continues till toward morning; itching is on joints of fingers and wrists, and also on ankles.

∞ Pain in sacrum in region of the dimples and down back of left leg to popliteal space; it then appears midway down outside of calf through ankle to underside of foot.

∞ Soreness all through both feet; a tired pain, < standing. Feet so lame and sore, has trouble to walk. On walking, sharp pain from outer left malleolus back into heel.

## Clinical Notes

W.H. Leonard, calling the remedy 'Viperia acontica carinata', claimed its successful use in:

'Climacteric haemorrhages, flow red with dark clots, excessive flowing to prostration and faintness. There exists a small fibroid in uterus. A few doses of the remedy changed matters for the better, and the excessive haemorrhages did not return.

'Same remedy in case of a lady nursing child one year old; much prostrated from flowing for several weeks, not profusely but continuously; nearly every day nosebleed; weaning brought no relief. A prescription of China 200 did no good. Gave Vipera CM; 3 doses cured.'

[Proceedings of 11th annual session of the International Hahnemannian Association, 1891]

# Family Elapidae – Elapids

## Biological Profile

- Elapidae have short, permanently erect fangs so that the venom must be injected by repeated bites, in contrast to the viperids, which can envenomate with only a quick, stabbing motion. The maxilla is intermediate in length and mobility between typical colubrids [long, less mobile] and viperids [very short, highly mobile]. When the mouth is closed, the fangs fit into grooved slots in the buccal floor.
- All elapids are venomous [predominantly neurotoxic] and many are potentially deadly.
- Distribution: Worldwide in tropical and subtropical regions except for Europe.
- Habitat: Fossorial [burrowing] to terrestrial [coral snakes], arboreal [mambas], savannah-scrubs-grassy woodland [taipans, tiger snakes], semi-fossorial [shield-nosed cobras, Asian coral snakes, New World coral snakes] or surface foragers [kraits, cobras].
- Behaviour: Primarily diurnal [coral snakes, tiger snakes, mambas, taipans, king cobra] or nocturnal [African and Asian cobras, death adders, kraits]. Defensive display of hood in cobras.
- Elapids and sea snakes are closely related. They have been considered both as separate families and combined within the family Elapidae.
- The left lung is greatly reduced or absent; a tracheal lung is commonly present in sea snakes and absent in terrestrial ones.
- "Outwardly, terrestrial elapids look similar to the colubridae: almost all have long and slender bodies with smooth scales, a head that is covered with large shields and not always distinct from the neck, and eyes with round pupils. In addition, their behaviour is usually quite active, and most are oviparous. There are exceptions to all these generalisations: e.g. the death adders [Acanthophis] include short and fat, rough-scaled, very broad-headed, cat-eyed, live-bearing, sluggish ambush predators with partly fragmented head shields." [Wikipedia]
- "One of the most common myths about elapids is that they can be 'charmed' or controlled through playing music. Film clips show snake charmers playing the flute and cobras rising from their baskets because they have been 'hypnotised' or put into a trance, by the music. Actually, cobras cannot even hear music. Like all elapids, they can hear low sounds, like the vibrations made by a person stomping on the ground, but they cannot hear musical notes, which are much higher sounds. The cobra sways back and forth not because it is listening to the musical beat but because it is following the movements of the snake charmer, who is swaying to the music." [animals.jrank.org]
- "Most elapids reproduce in the spring. In general, males fight with one another and the winners mate with the females. Many elapids lay eggs, but others give

birth to live young. The egg-laying females usually place their eggs under a rock or a log or in some other hiding place. The eggs hatch in about 3 months. The females that give birth to live young do so in a hiding place. Scientists believe that the king cobras are the only elapids that provide any care for eggs or young. These snakes remain with their eggs and will strike out at anything or anyone who approaches too closely." [animals.jrank.org]

## Neurotoxins – Paresis & Paralysis
Neurotoxins are produced by snakes in the families Elapidae and Hydrophiidae [sea snakes] and by some pit vipers [Crotalinae].

Pharmacologically divided in pre-synaptic [or beta-] neurotoxins and post-synaptic [or alpha] neurotoxins, these toxins interfere with the pre-synaptic release or the post-synaptic binding of acetylcholine. The net result is the same: no activity of acetylcholine mediated nerve function.

Pre-synaptic neurotoxins are found in Bungarus [krait], Oxyuranus [taipan], Notechis [tiger snake], and some pit vipers [e.g. Crotalus cascavella].

Post-synaptic neurotoxins are particularly found in Naja [cobra], Ophiophagus [king cobra], and Dendroaspis [mamba].

The elapid genus Micrurus [Elaps in homeopathy] produces both pre- and post-synaptic neurotoxins.

Neurotoxins have a high preponderance for the peripheral nervous system because most do not or only minimally cross the blood brain barrier due to the molecular size of snake venom neurotoxins. Following envenomation, the *cranial nerves are usually affected first*, which results in ptosis, ophthalmoplegia [paralysis or weakness of one or more of the muscles that control eye movement], dysarthria, dysphagia, and drooling. This progresses to weakness of limb muscles, paralysis of the respiratory muscles, and ultimately death if prompt treatment is not initiated. Descending paralysis is typical of snakebite neurotoxicity.

## Hypertension & Autonomic Dysfunction
Autonomic dysfunction in victims of elapid snakebites has been under reported. AD can present as unexplained abnormalities in heart rate [tachycardia or bradycardia] or rhythm, hypertension or hypotension, pupillary abnormalities, episodes of unexplained sweating, lachrymation, salivation, vomiting, abdominal pain, paralytic ileus and constipation. AD, most often, is not a dominant clinical manifestation and is overshadowed by other serious neuro-paralytic manifestations. In a study of common krait bites, 139 of 210 victims [66%] exhibited AD, which was more marked in those with severe enveno-mation. [Vinod, 2013]

'Elapid envenomation predominantly gives rise to neurotoxicity, a conse-quence of neuromuscular blockade, which manifests as paralysis of the bulbar, ocular, limb, and respiratory muscles, leading to respiratory failure. Predomi-nantly, presynaptic neurotoxins present in the venom of the Bungarus species are highly potent and suppress the capacity of neuron endings to release biochemical transmitters. Transmitter release is primarily blocked subsequent to envenomation with such bungarotoxins [giving rise to a brief paralysis], a process followed by a period of substantial overexcitation [incl. cramps, spasms, and tremors], which, in turn, leads to further paralysis.

'Hypertension in our cases was probably ascribable to snake venom [Bungarus caeruleus], as the secondary causes of hypertension were ruled out. Moreover, blood pressure levels normalized following ASV [antisnake venom] therapy, and the recoveries from neuromuscular paralysis observed indicate that krait venom might have contributed toward hypertensive episodes in such cases.

'Autonomic dysfunction following snakebite may induce various symptoms such as abdominal pain, vomiting, sweating, and mild-to-moderate hypertension or hypotension, and cardiac arrhythmia. In a previous study, it was observed that more than 50% of the patients with krait bite had elevated blood pressure. However, severe hypertension subsequent to snake envenomation and requiring intravenous NTG is under-reported. The pathogenesis for autonomic dysfunction in snakebite is unclear.

'However, it may be attributable to the presynaptic alpha-2 adrenoreceptor inhibition by elapid neurotoxin, thereby blocking inhibition of the neutrally mediated release of norepinephrine. Hence, this process gives rise to sympathetic overactivity and decreased parasympathetic stimulation. A patient who was bitten by a Malayan krait experienced sweating, tachycardia, dilated pupils, and hypertension arising from parasympathetic abnormalities.' [Meenakshisundaram, 2013]

## Locked-In Syndrome – Inability to Communicate

'Neurological manifestations are caused by the Elapidae group [cobras, kraits]. The common krait is nocturnally active snake with *painless bite*; so many patients with neurological manifestations present to emergency without history of snakebite. In 60%–70% of cases, snakebite occurs when the patients were asleep, and site of bite is undetectable in 17% cases.

'Locked in syndrome [LIS] is a neurological syndrome in which despite being conscious patient is *unable to communicate*. It is rarely reported in snakebite. We report 4 children with LIS following snake bite.'

# CASES

1 A 2-year-old child presented with bleeding from ear, followed by altered sensorium and respiratory failure within 2 hours of initial complaints. At admission, child had respiratory arrest with severe bradycardia, absent peripheral and central pulses, and Glasgow coma scale [GCS] score of 3; pupils were fixed and dilated and doll's eye movements [oculocephalic reflex] were absent. After initial resuscitation, he was noted to have some movement of right toe. Seven hours later, snakebite was suspected and polyvalent antisnake venom [ASV] was administered. Thirty hours later, after receiving 25 vials, child had spontaneous respiration, movements of lower

limbs and eye opening but pupils were still fixed and dilated. Pupillary reactions became normal on day 3, doll's eye movement appeared a day later, and the child was discharged in premorbid condition on day 10.

2 A 10-year-old boy presented with history of anxiety, pain abdomen and vomiting *appearing acutely early morning* while sleeping on the floor of his cottage. His sister had died an hour back with similar complaints. Parents did not report any venomous bite. At admission, he had bradycardia, gasping respiration and GCS of 3. Pupils were fixed and dilated, and doll's eye movement were absent. He was put on respiratory support. There was no improvement over next 48 hours. Detailed examination revealed fang marks on one foot so ASV was given. On day 6, parents noted fluttering of eyelids and next day he had spontaneous respiration and limb movements. After 1 week, doll's eye movements appeared but internal ophthalmoplegia persisted. CT head was normal and fundus examination did not show features of optic neuritis. At discharge, 5 weeks later, internal ophthalmoplegia was persisting.

3 A 1½-year old child with history of snake bite presented to the emergency department with breathing difficulty. At admission, she had gasping respiration, bradycardia, GCS of 3, fixed dilated pupils and absent doll's eye movement. There was no response to ASV. After 36 hours, she started having spontaneous respiration and occasional movement of limbs. She used to cry on looking at parents. On day 4, pupillary size and reaction became normal. She was discharged on day 10 in premorbid condition.

4 A 7-year-old boy presented with history of *sudden onset of pain abdomen* and vomiting while in the playground. At admission, he had gasping respiration. Two hours later, he was atonic, areflexic; pupils were fixed and dilated with absent doll's eye movements. After ruling out other causes [normal cerebrospinal fluid examination, CT head, and liver function tests]; possibility of snake bite was entertained and ASV was given. After 10 vials of ASV, ptosis resolved and child started responding using eye movements; 25 vials later, spontaneous limb movements appeared but internal ophthalmoplegia persisted. Three weeks later, at discharge, internal ophthalmoplegia was persisting.

'In LIS, patient is conscious yet unable to communicate. It can be of 3 types: classic, in which patient has quadriplegia and anarthria with preservation of consciousness and vertical eye movements. Incomplete LIS is similar to classic except remnants of voluntary movement other than vertical eye movement are present. In total LIS, there is total immobility and inability to communicate, with *preserved consciousness*. Usual causes of LIS are stroke, trauma or encephalitis of ventral pontine area but it can also be caused by extensive bilateral destruction of corticobulbar and corticospinal tracts in the cerebral peduncles. LIS can also be caused by peripheral causes such as severe *Guillain-Barré syndrome*, neuromuscular junction blockade [*myasthenia gravis*, toxins, snakebite], etc.

'LIS in snakebite occurs due to neuromuscular paralysis of voluntary muscles, which in turn is caused by neuromuscular transmission blockade [krait venom acts pre-synaptically while cobra venom acts post-synaptically]. Irreversible binding of toxin to presynaptic portion makes clinical recovery slow in krait envenomation as recovery occurs only with the formation of new neuromuscular junctions, as seemingly in our cases, especially case 2.

'Fixed dilated pupils and absent doll's eye movement can easily be interpreted as *brain death*, if possibility of LIS is not considered.' [Azad C. et al, 2012]

## Suspected Brain Death

Anadure [2018] reported the case of a 38-year-old driver who had an alcohol binge with his friends in the evening and fell asleep in the courtyard at home around 11 p.m. He woke up at morning 3 a.m. complaining of abdominal pain and vomiting, which was attributed to alcohol by his wife and managed with lemon juice and antacids at home. However, he could not go back to sleep and remained restless throughout the night. By 6 a.m. he complained of difficulty in swallowing and double vision and was taken to a local doctor.

There he was noted to have *neck muscle weakness* and respiratory distress and was referred to nearby medical college in Aligarh, state of Uttar Pradesh, in northern India. He became stuporous during the road journey and was intubated on arrival at the medical college as he was found drowsy with a low GCS [Glasgow coma scale] of 8/15 along with pupillary abnormalities and was desaturating despite oxygen therapy.

His initial hematological and biochemical parameters were normal, and a CT head did not reveal any abnormality. He was managed with broad spectrum antibiotics, anti-malarials and ventilatory support. However over the next 2 days he became deeply comatose with a GCS of 3/15, dilated fixed pupils and absent respiratory efforts.

An initial diagnosis of brain death was reversed since the patient did not have a clear cause of brainstem dysfunction, had normal neuroimaging, and therefore did not meet the first basic criteria for potential brain death testing. as brain dead and almost went under the transplant surgeon's knife before timely diagnosis. It was decided to give the patient 1.5 mg IV neostigmine to test for reversible neuromuscular blockade, immediately after which he for the first time showed eyelid movements along with few weak inspiratory efforts on the ventilator tracing. This raised the suspicion of a possible *elapid bite* with severe neuroparalysis. The patient recovered steadily after starting ASV [antisnake venom] with complete reversal of neuroparalysis in 6 weeks.

## Signs & Symptoms of Neurotoxic Snakebites

- Drowsiness.
- Headache.

- Ptosis; heavy eyelids, external ophthalmoplegia [paralysis or weakness of extra-ocular muscles that control eye movement].
- Blurred vision or difficulty seeing.
- Pupils dilated and fixed.
- Paralysis of facial muscles and other muscles innervated by cranial nerves.
- Inability to open mouth and protrude tongue.
- Drooling.
- Abnormalities of taste and smell, transient or permanent, sometimes leaving the victim with permanent complete anosmia.
- Difficulty speaking or swallowing.
- 'Broken neck sign' – weakness/paralysis of cervical flexor muscles.
- Aphonia.
- Respiratory arrest or dyspnoea.
- Convulsions or epileptiform seizures.
- Sudden loss of consciousness.
- Flaccid paralysis.
- Limb weakness – usually ataxic gait first, then inability to walk, then stand or even sit up.
- Paraesthesias.
- See also Venomous Phenomena, page 185.

## ΕLAPIDAΕ IN HOMΕOPATHY

| Homeopathic name | Common name | Abbreviations | Symptoms |
|---|---|---|---|
| Bungarus caeruleus | Common krait | Bung-cl. | + |
| Bungarus candidus | Blue krait | Bung-cd. | + |
| Bungarus fasciatus | Banded krait | Bung-fa. | ++ |
| Bungarus multicinctus | Many-banded krait | Bung-mc. | + |
| Dendroaspis angusticeps | Eastern green mamba | Dendr-ang. | ++ |
| Dendroaspis polylepis | Black mamba | Dendr-pol. | ++ |
| Dendroaspis viridis | Western green mamba | Dendr-vir. | – |
| Elaps corallinus | Brazilian coral snake | Elaps | +++ |
| Hemachatus haemachatus | Rinkhals | Hem-ha. | ++ |
| Maticora bivirgata | Blue Malayan coral snake | Mat-bv. | – |
| Micrurus lemniscatus | South American coral snake | Micru-ln. | + |
| Naja anchietae | Anchieta's cobra | Naja-an. | + |
| Naja annulifera | Snouted cobra | Naja-annu. | + |
| Naja haje | Egyptian cobra | Naja-hj. | ++ |
| Naja kaouthia | Monocled cobra | Naja-k. | + |
| Naja melanoleuca[1] | Forest cobra | Naja-me. | + |
| Naja mossambica | Mozambique spitting cobra | Naja-mo. | ++ |

| Naja nigricollis | Black-necked spitting cobra | Naja-n. | + |
|---|---|---|---|
| Naja nivea | Cape cobra | Naja-niv. | + |
| Naja pallida | Red spitting cobra | Naja-pa. | ++ |
| Naja tripudians | Indian cobra | Naja | +++ |
| Notechis scutatus occidentalis | Western tiger snake | Note-st-o. | + |
| Notechis scutatus scutatus | Eastern tiger snake | Note-st-st. | + |
| Ophiophagus hannah | King cobra | Ophiop-ha. | ++ |
| Oxyuranus microlepidotus | Inland taipan | Oxyurn-mi. | + |
| Oxyuranus scutellatus | Coastal taipan | Oxyurn-sc. | ++ |
| Pseudonaja textilis | Eastern brown snake | Pseud-ts. | + |

1 Symptoms mistakenly assigned to Naja tripudians in Allen's Encyclopedia.

# BUNGARUS CAERULEUS

## Systematics
- Scientific name: Bungarus caeruleus [Schneider, 1801].
- Synonyms: Boa lineata [Shaw, 1802]. Pseudoboa caerulea [Schneider, 1801].
- Common names: Common krait. Indian krait.
- Family: Elapidae.

## Biological Profile
- Black or bluish-black, highly venomous elapid with white narrow cross-bands and narrow head. Average length 90 cm, maximum 1.5 m.
- Range: South and southeast Asia, particularly India, Sri Lanka, and Pakistan,.
- Habitat: Open fields, human settlements, dense jungle. Known to reside in termite mounds, brick piles, rat holes, or inside houses.
- Ophiophagous, preying primarily upon other snakes [incl. venomous varieties] and cannibalistic, feeding on other kraits. Will also eat small lizards.
- Nocturnal; active at night.
- Males engage in ritual combat during mating season.
- Oviparous; 8–12 eggs per clutch.
- Typically kraits are more docile and mellow during daylight hours, becoming aggressive demons at night. However, they are rather timid and will often hide their heads within their coiled bodies for protection. When in this posture, they will sometimes whip their tail around as a type of distraction.

## Behaviour & Temperament
This krait is of special concern to man. It is deadly, about 16 times more deadly than the common cobra. It is active at night and relatively passive during the day. The native people often step on kraits while walking through their habitats.

The krait has a tendency to seek shelter in sleeping bags, boots, and tents. Its venom is a powerful neurotoxin that causes respiratory failure.

## MATERIA MEDICA BUNGARUS CAERULEUS

### Sources
1 Effects of bite; clinical manifestations.
2 Effects of bite; abdominal colic, amnesia & autonomic disturbances.
3 Effects of bite; abdominal pain.
4 Effects of bite; bitten in the night.
5 Hypokalemia & metabolic acidosis.

### Clinical Manifestations
Bungarus species contain neurotoxic venom that is 16 times more potent than cobra venom. Krait venom is extremely powerful and quickly induces *muscle paralysis*. Clinically, their venom contains mostly pre-synaptic neurotoxins. These affect the ability of nerve endings to properly release the chemical that sends the message to the next nerve. Following envenomation with bungarotoxins, transmitter release is initially blocked [leading to a brief paralysis], followed by a period of massive overexcitation [cramps, tremors, spasms], which finally tails off to paralysis. Not all these phases may be seen in all parts of the body at the same time.

'Fortunately, since kraits are nocturnal they seldom encounter humans during daylight hours, so bites are rare. Nonetheless, any bite from a krait is potentially life threatening and must therefore be regarded as a medical emergency. Note that there is frequently little or no pain at the site of a krait bite and this can provide false reassurance to the victim. Typically, victims start to complain later of severe abdominal cramps accompanied by progressive muscular paralysis, frequently starting with ptosis. As there are no local symptoms, a patient should be carefully observed for telltale signs of paralysis [e.g. the onset of ptosis, diplopia and dysphagia] and treated urgently with antivenom. Before antivenom was developed, there was an 85% mortality rate among bite victims. . . .

Cause of death is often respiratory failure i.e. suffocation via complete paralysis of the diaphragm. Even if patients make it to a hospital subsequent permanent coma and even brain death from hypoxia may occur given potentially long transport times to get medical care.' [Wikipedia]

### Abdominal Colic, Amnesia & Autonomic Disturbances
'Common krait [Bungarus caeruleus] is the deadliest snake found commonly in the dry zone of Sri Lanka. In Anuradhapura, 210 farmers bitten by the common krait over a 3-year period were investigated prospectively from 1 January 1996. One hundred and one [48%] patients were severely envenomed and needed mechanical ventilation from 12 hours to 29 days [mode 2 days]. The bite occurred at night while the victims were asleep on the floor. The cardinal symptom was *abdominal pain* developing within hours of the bite. Alteration in

the level of consciousness was observed in 150 [71%] patients: drowsy in 91 [43%], semiconscious in 24 [11%], and deep coma in 35 [17%]. Autonomic disturbances included transient hypertension, tachycardia, lacrimation, sweating, and salivation. These manifested in 139 [66%] patients with moderate to severe envenomation. One hundred and forty-nine [71%] had hypokalemia and 105 [50%] metabolic acidosis, *anterograde memory loss** in 84 [40%], and delayed neuropathy in 38 [22%] patients. Polyvalent antivenom had no significant benefit in reversing respiratory paralysis and preventing delayed neurological complications. Sixteen [7.6%] patients died and a submucosal haemorrhage in the stomach was seen at necropsy in 3 cases. Mortality could be minimized with early and free access to mechanical ventilation.

'A significant number of patients 65 [31%] had not been aware of the bite but had *woken up with colicky abdominal pain [mainly in the epigastrium]*. In 35 [17%] patients the site of the bite was undetectable, and they presented with abdominal pain, dyspnoea, dysphagia, and signs of neuromuscular paralysis.

'Abdominal pain was the first symptom to manifest with a range of minutes to a few hours. Other common clinical features were *weakness of limbs, inability to stand up, drooping of eye lids, double vision, difficulty in breathing, and changing sensorium*; all progressed rapidly to severe neuromuscular paralysis. Less commonly, myalgia, paraesthesia at the site of bite, *decreased hearing and vision*, and faintness were observed. Very often the site of the bite and fang marks were indistinct, and the local reaction was faint. Bites on fingers and hands invariably produced a significant local reaction with swelling and pain.

'Patients in deep coma had absent brainstem and spinal reflexes; pupils remained fully dilated and light reflexes were absent. The onset of deep coma ranged from 2 hours after the bite up to 48 hours and the persisted from 6 hours to 5 days. Patients in deep coma developed more complications than others during assisted ventilation. These included collapse of lung segments in 10 patients, hypostatic pneumonia in 8, ileus in 23, ventricular arrhythmia in 2, atrial tachycardia in 18, and adult respiratory distress syndrome [ARDS] in 6 patients [5 died]. Twenty-two patients in deep coma made a complete recovery. The level of consciousness had a direct and significant correlation to the duration of respiratory paralysis as patients in deep coma needed longer duration of ventilation.

'There was no change in heart rate or blood pressure with changes in position or to pharyngeal stimulation during physiotherapy. Paralytic ileus leading to abdominal distension and absent bowel sounds was manifested in 42 patients. Sixty-six patients with severe envenoming had semi-dilated pupils with positive light reflex and the remaining 35 had completely dilated fixed pupils during the stage of deep coma.

'Eighty-four [40%] patients who recovered had a variable duration of memory loss. The range was 12 hours to 8 days.

---

* Anterograde amnesia is the loss of the ability to create new memories, leading to a partial or complete inability to recall the recent past, even though long-term memories from before the event that caused the amnesia remain intact.

'Thirty-eight patients had delayed neurological deficits. Fourteen of them had nerve conduction defects in the ulnar, median, and common peroneal nerves that lasted for 2 weeks to 6 months before complete recovery. Sensory loss at the site of bite was observed in 34 patients; this lasted for 2 weeks to 6 months. One patient had bilateral ulnar nerve palsy with wasting of small muscles of the hands, 4 patients had glove type sensory motor neuropathy, and 1 patient developed cerebellar ataxia that persisted for 2 years.'

*Incidence of symptoms & signs on admission*
Dyspnoea 68% of all 210 patients – 90% of severe patients.

| | |
|---|---|
| Abdominal pain | 68%–82%. |
| Dysphagia | 64%–73%. |
| Chest pain | 52%–60%. |
| Faintness | 46%–46%. |
| Giddiness | 32%–32%. |
| Myalgia | 30%–36%. |
| Vomiting | 16%–18%. |
| Ptosis | 70%–82%. |
| Weakness of limbs | 64%–78%. |
| Decreased consciousness | 64%–78%. |
| Weakness of neck flexors | 60%–68%. |
| Blurred vision | 53%–65%. |
| Decreased respiration | 45%–77%. |
| Local reaction | 30%–18%. |

*Recovery of functions in severely envenomed patients*
Function. Number of patients. Average number of days for full recovery of function.
Cough reflex. 53 patients. 2.6 days.
Gag reflex. 54 patients. 2.8 days.
Normal consciousness. 90 patients. 2.8 days.
Ophthalmoplegia. 101 patients. 3.6 days.
Memory. 78 patients. 4.0 days.
Neck to power grade 2–3. 96 patients. 4.0 days.
Normal respiration. 101 patients. 3.0 days.
Facial muscles. 101 patients. 5.0 days.
Ptosis. 101 patients. 5.1 days.
Distal muscles [hand grip/foot]. 101 patients. 6.0 days.
Proximal muscles [hip/shoulder]. 101 patients. 7.5 days.
Sitting up, unsupported. 96 patients. 7.0 days.
Neck to full strength. 101 patients. 8.7 days.
[Kularatne, 2002].

## Abdominal Pain

Common kraits [B. caeruleus] were identified as the snakes responsible for 88 [11.5%] of the 762 bites by venomous species. All the bites occurred during the hours of darkness; the highest incidence [76 patients, 86%] was between 11 p.m. and 3 a.m. Local symptoms at the site of the bite were rare: paraesthesia [numbness] in 4 cases and pain in 2 cases. Slight local swelling was detectable in only 8 patients [9%]. The remaining 80 patients [91%] had no signs or symptoms of local envenoming. Neurotoxic signs, such as partial or complete ptosis, external ophthalmoplegia, difficulty in breathing, and dysphagia were observed in 84 patients [95%].

Fifty-six patients [64%] developed respiratory failure. Ptosis, the earliest sign of neurotoxicity, was first detected 30 minutes to 4 hours after the bite. Respiratory failure developed between 30 minutes and 13 hours after the bite. Abdominal pain, which was non-colicky, often severe, and increased in intensity over several hours and vomiting, was reported by 91% of patients. None showed any evidence of spontaneous bleeding or incoagulable blood.

Although none of the bites in this series was provoked intentionally by the victim, involuntary movement during sleep may have been sufficient to incite the krait to strike. Hati and others noted that most of the 22 cases of identified krait bite in Raidighi, West Bengal, were bitten in the third quadrant of the night when episodes of rapid eye movement [REM] sleep, associated with dream anxiety attacks and involuntary movements, become more prolonged. However, among our patients, the incidence of bites remained constant from 23:00 to 03:00 hours and then declined.

The clinical syndrome of krait bite envenoming was characterized by negligible local envenoming, vomiting, abdominal pain that could be very severe and was frequently the presenting symptom, and descending paralysis that started as soon as 30 minutes after the bite but was sometimes delayed for up to 4 hours. Progression to respiratory paralysis requiring mechanical ventilation was observed in 64% of cases.

*Abdominal pain has long been recognized as a characteristic symptom of Bungarus caeruleus envenoming* but has never been explained adequately. It is not invariably associated with vomiting, is not colicky in pattern, but gradually increases in intensity. It is not attributable to rhabdomyolysis of abdominal muscles or to acute gastrointestinal haemorrhage but seems more likely to be caused by stimulation of the autonomic nervous system, perhaps the biliary tract. [Ariaratnam, 2008]

## Neurological Symptoms Preceded by Abdominal Pain

The classic symptoms observed in krait bite [which is often described as painless] are early morning symptoms such as abdominal pain or cramps, together with progressive muscular paralysis which often commences with ptosis.

'One early morning in August 2011, a previously healthy girl of 17 years was brought to the emergency medicine department of our hospital with a history of sudden onset drooping of upper eyelids, diplopia, difficulty in speaking, swallowing and breathing and weakness of limbs for 2 h. These symptoms were preceded by abdominal pain and vomiting. She was apparently alright the previous night and had slept outside her kutcha house [house built of mud brick] on the ground. There was no history of similar illness in family or deliberate self-poisoning.

'On admission, she was found to be unconscious, cyanosed with poor respiratory efforts. Pupils were normal and reactive to light. She was intubated immediately and mechanically ventilated. After an hour, she regained consciousness and was noticed to have ptosis, complete external ophthalmoplegia and quadriparesis [muscle power: grade 2/5], with preserved tendon jerks and *neck muscle weakness*. With suspicion of neurotoxic snake bite, 10 vials of freeze dried polyvalent antisnake venom [ASV] antitoxin were administered, although no fang marks could be made out. Later, mechanical ventilation was continued in medical intensive care unit [MICU] under sedation and analgesia. Ten more vials of ASV were repeated 2 h after first dose. Serum potassium, calcium, phosphates, magnesium, arterial blood gas, renal, liver function, coagulation tests and serum cholinesterase levels were normal.

'During the first 3 days in MICU, she had multiple unexplained episodes of dysautonomia, each lasting about 5–15 min, characterized by unexplained tachycardia [heart rate 110–150 per minute], hypertension [BP: 150/100–190/110 mm Hg], profuse sweating and pupillary mydriasis. Hypoglycaemia and hypoxia were ruled out during these episodes. These episodes were managed conservatively, without drugs.

'Electrocardiogram, chest radiograph, abdominal sonography and cardiac echocardiography were normal. She had complete recovery of muscle power and was extubated on day 6. Urinary porphobilinogen measurement [done on day 2], thyroid function tests [day 6], nerve conduction and repetitive nerve stimulation studies [day 7] were normal. Upon recovery, patient could recollect some bite on her right leg but was not aware of what had bitten her. Autonomic function tests done on day 12 and repeated at 6 weeks, 3 and 6 months follow-up were normal.'

'Other differential diagnoses such as myasthenic crisis, Grave's disease with ophthalmopathy, botulism, Guillain-Barré syndrome [Miller Fisher variant] and acute porphyria were considered. These were excluded based on clinical features, course of illness and relevant investigations. [Vinod, 2013]

# CASES

### Bitten in the Night

1 Case reported by Major S. J. Rennie, Meerut, India.

'A 12-year old Hindu boy, named Moraddy, was brought to me at 6 p.m., on July 10, in a semi-comatose condition, with commencing paralysis of the respiratory muscles. I was told that the child was sleeping on the ground, when he was bitten in the left hand. He immediately felt very great pain and giddiness, and his arm began to swell. Two small wounds were clearly visible, corresponding to the marks of the fangs of a krait, or Bungarus caeruleus.

'The child had salivation, and ptosis of both eyelids. Respiration was difficult, and deglutition impossible; the pulse was 110 and dicrotic. The patient's breathing was of an abdominal character; the surface of the body was covered with cold sweat. The child soon became lethargic and collapsed; his condition appeared absolutely desperate. I gave a subcutaneous injection of 12 cc of antivenomous serum, and commenced artificial respiration, which I continued for half an hour in order to give the serum time to take effect. In 48 hours the symptoms gradually disappeared, and the child became quite well. Diplopia of the left eye persisted for a few days, but this also entirely passed away.' [cited in *Venoms* by A. Calmette, 1908]

2 Fatal case reported in the Madras Quarterly Medical Journal, vol. 1, 1839: 'A stout muscular man about 30 years of age, was awoke when sleeping in his tent by a snake crawling over his face, and in the act of suddenly springing up, was bitten somewhere in the forehead. He instantly killed the snake and soon after, finding no ill effects from the wound, lay down and went to sleep again; between 11 and 12 p.m., or in 2 or 3 hours after, a person passing through the tent accidentally observed that the man appeared convulsed and *when spoken to he was unable to answer*; he was therefore at once conveyed to the Hospital tent and immediately seen by me. The symptoms were as follows: the entire body was in a state of violent spasm, the limbs being stretched at full-length and quite rigid, the muscles of the throat and fauces seeming to be most violently effected. Pulse very quick and weak, extremities cold, *appears to understand questions but cannot speak*, makes an exertion to point to his forehead as the seat of pain when asked where he was bitten; the wound however could not be discovered, owing to the very dark colour of the skin, and probably the small size of the puncture. An attempt was made to exhibit a draught containing spt. ammoniae, but the effort of swallowing induced such violent and general convulsions of the entire body that several men were required to hold him, and a *distressing sense of suffocation*, lasting for several minutes, threatened the immediate extinction of life. The head, particularly the front part was constantly rubbed with the liquor ammoniae and some stimulating frictions to the limbs were kept up by the several attendants, whilst life remained. All attempts at introducing medicine into the stomach completely failed, the vital powers gradually sunk, and he died in about 30 or 40 minutes after admission into Hospital.'

3 Fatal case reported in the Edinburgh Medical and Surgical Journal, Vol. 47, 1837.
'John Lynn, of stout make and sanguineous temperament, was suddenly awakened by a pricking sensation over the sacrum and on looking around, he perceived a snake gliding along the floor. He instantly got out of bed, and, with the assistance of his comrades, killed it. This was about 2 o'clock

in the morning. About 15 minutes after receiving the bite, he was seized with a disposition to syncope, accompanied with a *cold clammy perspiration* and followed by nausea and vertigo. A draught composed of a dram of spiritus ammoniae, the same quantity of sulphuric ether, and of 2 drams of camphor mixture, was administered, to be repeated every half hour; and potassa fusa [caustic potash or potassium hydroxide] was freely applied to the bitten part.

At 3 a.m. the pulse became very quick [160 in the minute] and small; the skin cold and clammy; the *vertigo increased with dimness of sight.* At 4 a.m. he was suddenly seized with spasms in the muscles of the throat, with *inability to speak*, difficult deglutition, hurried respiration, and tendency to coma. The medicine was continued, with the addition of a dram of laudanum to each dose. At 5 a.m. all the symptoms became worse; the spasms of the throat more severe, *extending to the abdomen and loins*; the clammy perspiration general and profuse; the countenance expressive of great anxiety; and the pulse weaker. The cold affusion was now applied to the head, neck, shoulders, and spine; the draught continued with hot brandy and water, and a stimulating enema was administered. At 6 a.m. after the cold affusion, the spasms were less severe; the coma had increased; the pupils were dilated; he was unable to swallow; made frequent attempts to vomit; there was frothing at the mouth; and the skin continued to be covered with a cold clammy sweat. At 7 a.m. the coma was complete; the pulse at the wrists scarcely perceptible; the respiration laborious. At 9 a.m. he died.'

## Hypokalemia & Metabolic Acidosis

Significant hypokalemia [serum potassium <3.5 mmol/l and U waves on the electrocardiogram] was observed in 149 [71%] patients during early stages, esp. in the first 48 hours post-bite. Hypokalemia was not related to respiratory alkalosis and needed replacement therapy, depending on the severity. Furthermore, metabolic acidosis within first 24 hours was seen in 105 [50%] patients [hypokalemic acidosis].

The effects of hypokalemia regarding the renal function can be metabolic acidosis, rhabdomyolysis [in severe hypokalemia] and, rarely, impairment of tubular transport, chronic tubulointerstitial disease and cyst formation. Nervous system is affected, the patient can suffer from leg cramps, weakness, fatigue, paresis or ascending paralysis. Constipation or intestinal paralysis and respiratory failure often present as signs of severe hypokalemia. Hypokalemia can have detrimental effects on the cardiovascular system, leading to electrocardiographic [ECG] changes [U waves, T wave flattening and ST-segment changes], cardiac arrhythmias and heart failure.

Symptoms of metabolic acidosis include varying degrees of dyspnoea. chest pain, palpitations, headache, confusion, generalized weakness, bone pain, nausea, vomiting, and anorexia.

# BUNGARUS CANDIDUS

## Systematics
- Scientific name: Bungarus candidus [L., 1758].
- Synonyms: Coluber candidus [L., 1758]. Bungarus semifasciatus [Boie, 1827]. Bungarus javanicus [Kopstein, 1932].
- Common names: Blue krait. Malayan krait.
- Family: Elapidae.

## Biological Profile
- Slender, highly venomous elapid with black and white banded colouration. Black bands wider than white bands, esp. towards head. Black bands do not completely encircle body. Belly white. Maximum length 1.6 m.
- Range: SE Asia, ranging from Thailand to China, and south to Indonesia.
- Habitat: Predominantly found in flat land, frequently in close proximity to water. Also found close to rice fields and rice dams, where it uses the many holes of rats and the nests of mice to hide in.
- Active hunter.
- Ophiophagous, preying primarily upon other snakes [incl. venomous varieties] and cannibalistic, feeding on other kraits. Will also eat small lizards.
- Nocturnal; active at night.
- Males engage in ritual combat during mating season.
- Oviparous; 4–10 eggs per clutch.
- Typically kraits are more docile and mellow during daylight hours, becoming aggressive demons at night. However, they are rather timid and will often hide their heads within their coiled bodies for protection. When in this posture, they will sometimes whip their tail around as a type of distraction.

## MATERIA MEDICA BUNGARUS CANDIDUS

### Sources
1 Effects of bite; clinical manifestations.
2 Effects of bite; neurological & cardiovascular effects.
3 Effects of bite; ptosis, myalgia, dysphagia & muscle weakness.
4 Hyponatremia.
5 Hyponatremia & the brain.
6 Chronic effects.
7 Symptom in MM from Boericke [unspecified as to the exact species of krait]: Generals, Poliomyelitis.

### Clinical Manifestations
Of 5 patients bitten by Bungarus candidus in eastern Thailand or NW Malaya, 2 were not envenomed ['dry bite'], while the other 3 developed generalised paralysis which progressed to respiratory paralysis in 2 cases, 1 of which ended

fatally. The first patient was breathless and unable to open his mouth or swallow; 4 hours after the bite he had to be intubated and ventilated manually.

On admission to the hospital, 7½ hours after the bite, the patient was fully conscious but almost completely paralysed and had bilateral ptosis. *He replied to questions by flexing fingers and toes.* When manual ventilation was stopped briefly he became distressed, sweaty, and cyanosed. The pulse was 120/min and regular, and blood pressure 140/70 mm Hg. The abdomen was moderately tender. There was flaccid tetraparesis with total bilateral external ophthalmoplegia, pronounced ptosis, *inability to open the mouth, protrude the tongue, or swallow, and no gag reflex*. On the third day after the bite the eyes were divergent but capable of slight movement in the horizontal plane and downward but not upward. Ptosis hooded two-thirds of the pupil. On admission the pupils had been fixed and dilated but the patient could see. The patient recovered after antivenom and other treatment.

The second patient complained 2 hours after the bite of blurred vision and *generalised numbness in addition to increasing breathlessness.* Two hours later she suffered a respiratory and cardiac arrest from which she was resuscitated but required artificial ventilation. Anoxic brain death was suspected, and she died 17 hours later.

The third patient was bitten on the ankle while farming. He walked home, and 2 hours later headache and giddiness were soon followed by difficulty in keeping his eyes open and swallowing. Pains in the trunk and limbs started 4½ hours after the bite. *Movement aggravated the pains*, which progressively increased precluding sleep. On admission to the hospital, 19 hours after the bite, he was conscious and responded to questions by grunts or slight hand movements.

Pulse was 90/min, respiration 25/min, and blood pressure 130/70 mm Hg. There was bilateral ptosis, total external ophthalmoplegia, and paralysis of facial muscles. Maximal jaw opening was 1 cm between teeth margins. He could not protrude his tongue or swallow. Pupillary responses were normal. There was generalised paresis. *All muscles were tender, and passive movements were very painful.* Muscle twitches were evident in the legs. Antivenom treatment resulted in full recovery. [Warrell, 1983]

### Neurological & Cardiovascular Effects

Previous studies have shown that phospholipase A2 [PLA2] and three-finger toxins [3FTxs] are the major components of Malayan krait venom and responsible for the neurotoxicity following envenoming. In addition, non-neurotoxic symptoms such as rhabdomyolysis and cardiovascular disturbances [e.g. hypertension and shock] were observed following Malayan krait envenoming in Vietnam.

'Between 1998 and 2007, 42 patients admitted to Choray hospital, Ho Chi Minh City, and to 2 hospitals in adjacent regions in southern Viet Nam brought the Malayan kraits [Bungarus candidus] that had been responsible for biting them. Half of the patients had been bitten while they were asleep. Fang marks and numbness were the only local features of the bites. Common signs of neurotoxic envenoming included bilateral ptosis, persistently dilated pupils, limb weakness, breathlessness, hypersalivation, dysphonia and dysphagia.

Thirty patients [71.4%] required endotracheal intubation of whom all but one were mechanically ventilated. Fourteen patients [33.3%] developed hypertension, 13 [31.0%] shock, 31 [73.8%] hyponatremia [plasma sodium concentration < 130 mEq/L] and 30 [71.4%] showed evidence of mild rhabdomyolysis [peak plasma creatine kinase concentration 1375 ± 140 u/l]. None developed acute kidney injury. All the patients were treated with a new monospecific B. candidus antivenom. There were no fatalities.' [Kiem Xuan Trinh et al., 2010]

## Ptosis, Myalgia, Dysphagia & Muscle Weakness

A 47-year-old Thai snakekeeper was bitten twice on his right thumb while he was demonstrating the snake to students. The snake was an adult Bungarus candidus, 3 feet long, and had been fed. The last venom extraction had been 2 months previously. The bite was virtually painless. Approximately 30 minutes later, the patient noted headache, nausea, vomiting, and myalgia that was most marked in his neck. On admission to Chulalongkorn University Hospital, there were barely visible fang marks on his thumb with adjacent minimal erythema and swelling.

His pulse, respiratory rate, blood pressure, and temperature were normal, but he complained of double vision and had difficulty in keeping his eyes open. The following laboratory studies yielded normal results: hematocrit, complete blood count, prothrombin time, urinalysis, BUN, creatinine, SGOT [serum glutamic-oxaloacetic transaminase], SGPT [serum glutamic-pyruvic transaminase], alkaline phosphatase, serum bilirubin, and serum sodium, chloride, and potassium. His clinical course is summarized as follows as time elapsed after the bite.

30 minutes: Headache, nausea, vomiting, myalgia.

1 hour: Ptosis of eyelids, diplopia, difficulty swallowing, increased myalgia, but respiration and vital signs still normal.

3½ hours: Tightness of chest, increasing ptosis of both eyelids, still able to move eyes, normal vital signs and respiration.

6½ hours: Myalgia now extending to abdominal muscles; patient experiencing blurred vision, oculomotor palsies and dysarthria; respiration and tidal volume remain normal.

8½ hours: Dysphagia, aspiration of fluids, diffuse muscle weakness, peak air flow now only 180 L/min; patient intubated and mechanically ventilated.

24 hours: Myalgia of back, chest, and abdomen; patient conscious and can open eyes to 1.0–1.5 mm; motor power, grade 4/5; and no response to intravenous injection of 8 mg of edrophonium chloride.

48 hours: Less myalgia, able to open eyes to 2 mm but cannot move eyes; motor power diminished at 4/5.

72 hours: Mild swelling around fang marks gone; mild myalgia present, motor power 4/5; patient still on respirator.

96 hours: Myalgia gone, good consciousness, able to open eyes fully and move them; motor power restored; patient extubated.

On extubation, the patient's temperature was 39°C [102.2°F] and he had crepitations over the left lower lung fields. A chest radiograph revealed atelectasis or pneumonitis of the left middle lobe and a patchy infiltration at the apical posterior segment of the left upper lobe. Sputum examination after acid-fast staining revealed evidence of active pulmonary tuberculosis. The pneumonitis of the left middle lobe responded to suction and amoxicillin. His incidentally discovered pulmonary tuberculosis was treated using the British Medical Research Council protocol of isoniazid, rifampin, pyrazinamide, and ethambutal. The patient ultimately made a full recovery and is working again at the Queen Saovabha Memorial Institute snake farm.

Symptoms of intoxication in our patient began with ptosis, myalgia, dysphagia, and muscle weakness. They started 30 minutes after the bite and progressed over the next 8 hours to respiratory failure. At 72 hours, muscle power began to improve, and the patient could be extubated at 96 hours after the bite. His clinical course was complicated by aspiration pneumonia and the incidental discovery of active pulmonary tuberculosis. The patient exhibited no cardiac arrhythmias and no hypotension. He experienced myalgias that started within 1 hour after the bite and lasted 96 hours. [Pochanugool, 1997]

## Hyponatremia
Your blood sodium level is normal if it's 135 to 145 milliequivalents per liter [mEq/L]. If it's below 135 mEq/L, it's hyponatremia. Bungarus candidus envenomation caused in the blood sodium level of 31 people to drop below 130 mEq/L.

*Signs and symptoms of hyponatremia may include:*
Nausea and vomiting.
Headache.
Blurred vision.
Confusion.
Loss of energy, drowsiness and fatigue.
Generalized malaise.
Restlessness and irritability.
Muscle weakness, spasms or cramps.
Seizures.
Coma.

- Aside from blue krait bite, a low sodium level has many other [and more common] causes, incl. consumption of too many fluids, diarrhoea, vomiting, pancreatitis, diabetes, severe burns, hypothyroidism, kidney failure, congestive heart failure, cirrhosis, cerebrovascular accident [CVA], adrenal insufficiency and chronic obstructive pulmonary disease [COPD].
- Disorders, such as kidney disease, cirrhosis, and congestive heart failure, can cause the body to retain sodium and fluid. Often the body retains more fluid than sodium, which means the sodium is diluted.
- Drugs known to be associated with hyponatraemia include diuretics, NSAIDs, carbamazepine, cancer chemotherapy, calcium antagonists, angiotensin converting enzyme [ACE] inhibitors.

- The brain is particularly sensitive to changes in the sodium level in blood. Therefore, symptoms of brain dysfunction, such as sluggishness [lethargy] and confusion, occur first.

## Hyponatremia & the Brain

'The link between hyponatremia and brain is strong and mutual; in fact several neurologic diseases frequently are associated with hyponatremia and hyponatremia itself causes serious clinical consequences that involve the central nervous system. Therefore, it is not surprising that hyponatremia is very frequently encountered in neurosurgical and neurocritical care settings, where it is present in up to 50% and 38% of patients, respectively. Common neurological pathologies, incl. subarachnoid haemorrhage, cerebrovascular accidents, brain tumour and head trauma, result in hyponatremia secondary to the syndrome of inappropriate secretion of antidiuretic hormone [SIADH] or to the cerebral salt wasting syndrome [CSW], which are a consequence of the release of ADH or natriuretic peptides, respectively, from the brain as a response to an injury. Furthermore, several drugs acting on the nervous system and frequently used in neurosurgical or neurologic/psychiatric patients, i.e. antidepressants and anti-epileptic drugs, may cause hyponatremia secondary to SIADH.

'Hyponatremia is a very common electrolyte disorder, esp. in the elderly, and is associated with significant morbidity, mortality and disability. In particular, the consequences of acute hyponatremia on the brain may be severe, incl. permanent disability and death. Also chronic hyponatremia can affect the health status, causing attention deficit, gait instability, increased risk of falls and fractures, and osteoporosis.' [Giuliani & Peri, 2014]

## Chronic Effects

Prolonged decreases in parasympathetic functions [i.e. mydriasis, tachycardia, hypertension, constipation, or difficulty in urinating] lasting for months to years, have been reported in patients with Bungarus candidus envenomation who were not given antivenom.

# BUNGARUS FASCIATUS

## Systematics

- Scientific name: Bungarus fasciatus [Schneider, 1801].
- Common name: Banded krait.
- Family: Elapidae.

## Biological Profile

- Stout, highly venomous elapid with alternate black and yellow bands, triangular body cross-section and marked vertebral ridge consisting of enlarged vertebral shields along its body. Head broad and depressed; arrow-head-like yellow markings on otherwise black head; black eyes; yellow lips, lore, chin and throat. Average length 1.5 m, maximum 2.1 m.

- Range: Indian Subcontinent and SE Asia, south to Indonesia.
- Habitat: Ranging from forests to agricultural lands. Inhabits termite mounds and rodent holes close to water; often lives near human settlements, esp. villages because of supply of rodents and water.
- Ophiophagous, preying primarily upon other snakes [incl. venomous varieties] and cannibalistic, feeding on other kraits. Will also eat small lizards and rodents.
- Nocturnal; active at night.
- Males engage in ritual combat during mating season.
- Oviparous; 4–14 eggs per clutch; female remains with the eggs until the young have hatched.

### Behaviour & Temperament

'Though venomous the banded krait is a shy snake, not typically seen, and is mainly nocturnal. When harassed they will usually hide their head under their coils, and do not generally attempt to bite, though at night they are much more active and widely considered to be more dangerous then. During the day they lie up in grass, pits or drains. The snakes are lethargic and sluggish even under provocation. They are most commonly seen in the rains.' [thainationalparks. com]

## MATERIA MEDICA BUNGARUS FASCIATUS

### Sources

1 Proving Farokh Master [India], 5 provers [2 females, 3 males], 6c and 30c; 2002–03. Unmarked symptoms.
2 Degroote, Dream Repertory.
3 Effects of bite; clinical manifestations.

### Mind

∞ Desires activity, in morning, or when sleepless.
∞ Touchy. Extremely sensitive, either gets angry or weeps.
∞ Outbursts of violent anger; at trifles; abusive; with quick repentance [cooling down].
∞ Wants to fight.
∞ Striking from anger, when quarrelling.
∞ Angry with "those who ask questions or with those who tend to lie."
∞ Morbid impulse to argue and to use abusive language.
∞ Talks a lot and argues about trivial matters.
∞ Snappish and impatient.
∞ Irritability when questioned, from contradiction.
∞ Very irritable when hungry; has to eat something.
∞ Irritability > eating.
∞ Irritability < consolation.
∞ Depressed and low; dwelling on past disagreeable things.

∞ Easily affected and weeping from small things.
∞ Feeling exposed, unable to control or hide emotions.
∞ Lack of self-control. Strong impulse to say things that will spoil relationships.
∞ Lack of self-control. Can't stop hand from hitting someone when angry.
∞ Lack of self-control. Can't control feeling of hunger and tendency to eat.
∞ Uncontrollable, violent anger.
∞ No control over one's tears.
∞ Desire for black or for black and white colours.
∞ Desire for sad music/sad songs.
∞ Awareness of breast; preoccupied with breast.
∞ Shameless; exposes breasts.
∞ Aversion to talking and to noise. Wants to sit quietly.
∞ Extreme forgetfulness; for names; recent events; when writing; for what one has said minutes before.
∞ Talks loudly. Speaks out boldly ["abrupt or open-hearted"].
∞ Afraid to go to sleep and not wake up.
∞ Nervous and anxious during menses.
∞ Anxiety > music.
∞ Inquisitive and talkative; constantly wants to know what's happening.
∞ Avarice, greed.[2]
∞ Want of self-confidence; self-depreciation.[2]

## Dreams
∞ Abused sexually.
∞ Animals, hedgehog.[2]
∞ Ants, red.[2]
∞ Bad news, getting; death of a child.[2]
∞ Caressing male genitals.
∞ Critized or blamed, being.[2]
∞ Death of relatives; husband.
∞ Death penalty by hanging.[2]
∞ Embarrassment and feeling ashamed.
∞ Executed, will be.[2]
∞ Exposing [left] breast to attract men.
∞ Exposing genitals.
∞ Exposing thighs to attract men.
∞ Food, cannot swallow.[2]
∞ Forsaken, being or feeling; not being helped/served.[2]
∞ Hit from behind by a car.
∞ House open from all directions.
∞ Being laughed at.
∞ Loss of control over hands, tripping mother up.
∞ Menses.
∞ Naked people.
∞ Being neglected.
∞ Sharing possessions [instead of being possessive].

∞ Throwing things out of anger.
∞ Wedding.

## Generals
∞ Left side more affected.
∞ Desire for butter; cheese; cold drinks; ice cream; tea.
∞ Desire for passion fruit; raisins.[2]
∞ Aversion to warm food.
∞ Decreased appetite during menses.
∞ Great hunger, uncontrollable, at around 3 p.m., even after having lunch at 1 p.m.
∞ Wants to eat all the time. Gaining weight.
∞ Constant hunger; has to nibble on something.
∞ Hungry feeling unchanged by eating; wants something more to eat.
∞ Cannot remain hungry, "otherwise I get angry and also get a headache and cannot concentrate."
∞ Sensation of strength.
∞ Active and fresh in morning and throughout day. Needs less sleep.
∞ Constant feeling of sleepiness and drowsiness throughout day, since morning.
∞ Hard pressure > headache; pain nape of neck; pain limbs.
∞ Lying on back >.[2]
∞ Pain muscles at transition to tendon, from exertion.[2]
∞ Problems with tendons – inflammation [tennis elbow], injury [Achilles tendon] or pain [quadriceps tendon].

## Sensations
∞ Tongue as if thick and swollen.
∞ Throat as if swollen; swallowing difficult.
∞ Stomach as if empty.
∞ Heaviness stomach > lying on back.[2]
∞ Heat in upper part of left thigh.
∞ Lower legs, from calves to ankles, very heavy.
∞ Hands as if paralysed.

## Locals
∞ Headache, forehead or left temple, < noise, writing; > eating, lying quietly, pressure, sitting still; extending to cervical region; & pain in neck and nausea.
∞ Frontal headache in morning, extending to occiput.
∞ Frontal headache > lying on back [occiput].[2]
∞ Lachrymation in hot room.
∞ Diminished sense of smell, for perfumes/fragrances, for food overcooked or burnt.
∞ Dryness mouth awakening one from sleep.
∞ Dryness mouth, unchanged by drinking water.
∞ Lips bluish from straining at stool.[2]
∞ Pain left side tongue < eating.

∞ Has to keep clearing throat before being able to speak.
∞ Pain stomach > lying on back.[2]
∞ Pulsation [visible] abdomen, during gastric and abdominal complaints.[2]
∞ Constipation; no urge. Hard stools, taking much time to pass.
∞ Ovarian pains during ovulation and during menses.
∞ Pain in left breast before menses.
∞ Backache cervical region, < during menses; extending to head, occiput, down back.
∞ Pain coccyx on ascending stairs.[2]
∞ Pain coccyx when sitting long.[2]
∞ Left hand hot, right hand cold.[2]
∞ Pain knee, left, < bending, beginning motion, walking, > pressure.
∞ Pain knees < walking, beginning motion, > pressure, sitting, flexing leg.
∞ Pain ankles when walking.

## Lack of Control

'In the afternoon, I was in my clinic and was feeling very sleepy, so took a nap sitting on a chair. I do not know how but this happened in front of a patient who entered in, but even after seeing that patient entering the clinic, I could not wake up or move myself. My hands and legs were as if paralyzed; even though I wanted to move for a few seconds I thought, "What is happening?" Though my eyes were open and I was watching the patient, still I could not control my body parts. My hands were not moving. I couldn't get up from my seat. This happened for the first time in my life; as I have never slept this way in the afternoon at any time. After a few moments I came back to my normal position. I felt very embarrassed in front of the patient. I don't know what exactly happened, but one thing I do know is that this was a very unique experience in my life. After this incident I think I am really afraid to go to sleep.' [Proving Farokh Master]

## Themes of Proving
- Loss of impulse control.
  Suddenly overcome by a force that does not allow rational thinking and prompts irrational acts.
  Feels vulnerable and exposed, not in control of emotions.
  Delusion being observed by people around.
  Too much boldness and audacity; behaviour that can land one in trouble.
- Embarrassment. Doing things and feeling very self-conscious.
- Anger that is either masked due to fear or expressed very aggressively.
- Feeling of injustice and Loss of control over the situation.
- Feeling exposed and unprotected.
- Free regarding sexuality. Self-exposure.

## Guiding Symptoms
- Ailments from being a victim of social violence, esp. gang rape, marital abuse, torture by in-laws.

- Guilt feelings after anger.
- Heightened awareness about the body, esp. the breasts.
- Poor control over animal qualities such as anger, aggression and irritability. Morbid impulse to fight, argue and say nasty things.
- Violent anger after suffering molestation or indecent acts.

### Clinical Manifestations
- The composition of Bungarus faciatus venom is essentially neurotoxic. Symptoms develop very rapidly and most often the bites are painless and marks are invisible in the body. The major clinical effects include vomiting, abdominal pain, diarrhoea, and dizziness. Severe envenomation leads to rapid respiratory failure and death.
- Wall, in experimenting upon animals with the poison of Bungarus fasciatus, found that in some cases symptoms were caused by it exactly resembling those seen in cobra-bite, while in others the first effects of the poison on the nervous system were slight, and soon passed off, but, after an interval of 2 to 5 days, were followed by a fresh set of constitutional symptoms. The animal became weak, purulent discharges took place from the eyes, nose, and rectum, the urine became albuminous, and death occurred from exhaustion several days after the bite. In these cases, however, there was no tendency to haemorrhage.

### Bitten in a Tree
'A 13-year-old boy from Thephyu Chaung village, Meikhtila township, Mandalay Division, was bitten on the middle phalanx of the right middle finger by a 1-metre long banded krait [Bungarus fasciatus] while climbing a tree at 19:00 on 20 October 1991. He was admitted to the station hospital of Mahlaing township. On arrival, 2 h after the bite, his swollen eyelids were drooping, and he was unable to open both eyes. He was drowsy and could not speak, open his mouth, or swallow saliva, but he responded-to questions by moving his limbs. His pulse rate was 110/min and his blood pressure was 11070 mmHg.

'Forty mL of monospecific Russell's viper antivenom was given because of the prolonged clotting time [15 min]. Locally, 2 fang marks were visible, and a slight swelling of the finger was noted. Later the dead snake was identified. The boy had complete ptosis and remained drowsy; his pupils reacted to light, but he could not open his eyes and mouth. A slow intravenous infusion of 5 dextrose-saline was given. No improvement in neurological signs was observed following the antivenom. Since no specific antivenom was available, the patient was kept under observation only. Ventilatory support was not available at the station hospital. The boy died of respiratory failure 14 h after the bite.' [Pe, 1997]

# BUNGARUS MULTICINCTUS

### Systematics
- Scientific name: Bungarus multicinctus [Blyth, 1861].
- Synonym: Bungarus semifasciatus [Günther, 1858].

- Common names: Many-banded krait. Chinese krait. Taiwanese krait.
- Family: Elapidae.

## Biological Profile
- Slender, highly venomous elapid with alternate black and white bands, and 15–17 rows of smooth and glossy scales. Head broadly ovate. Belly dirty white or cloudy grey; progressively darker toward short tail.
- Range: Taiwan, S China [incl. Hong Kong, Hainan], Myanmar [Burma], Laos, N Vietnam, Thailand.
- Habitat: Humid environments on mountain slopes and in agricultural areas.
- Nocturnal; active at night.
- Preys on frogs, lizards, fish, mice, snakes [even those of its own species] or snake eggs.
- Although primarily terrestrial, also preys on arboreal snakes.
- Males engage in ritual combat during mating season.
- Oviparous; 3–20 eggs per clutch; female remains with the eggs until the young have hatched.
- Produces the most powerful venom of any terrestrial snake outside Australia.

## Deceptively Slow & Surprisingly Quick
Active at night and mainly hunts other snakes. Generally docile when approached but capable of striking from multiple directions and will normally do so without taking much of a defensive stance, which can be surprising. Normally slow and deliberate in their movement, they are capable of moving quickly if fleeing. This species is also known to have a jaw capable of twisting sharply, even when held behind the head, increasing the risk of a bite. As the most venomous snake in Hong Kong the many-banded krait should never be approached. Its venom is notorious for its delayed effect, often taking over an hour before symptoms present, leading many bite victims to assume they were not envenomated. [www.hongkongsnakeid.com]


## MATERIA MEDICA BUNGARUS MULTICINCTUS

### Sources
1 Effects of bite; ptosis, paralysis & retention.
2 Effects of bite; resembling Guillain-Barré syndrome.
3 Effects of bite; waking at 4 a.m. with tingling legs.
4 Effects of bite; general overview.

### Ptosis, Paralysis & Retention
In northern Vietnam, Bungarus multicinctus is the only krait of medical importance. We report 60 consecutive patients admitted to an ICU in Hanoi during 2000–2003 because of envenoming by B. multicinctus. 69% of the snakebites occurred during the night. The mean length of time until the first symptom

developed was 3 hours [range 0.5–24 hours]. The only sign at the site of the bite was fang marks, which were noted in 90%.

The most common neuromuscular symptoms were ptosis and mydriasis [93%], ophthalmoplegia [82%], jaw weakness [90%], pharyngeal pain [83%], palatal palsy with inability to swallow [90%], neck muscle paralysis [85%], limb paralysis [85%], dyspnoea [87%], absent or diminished deep tendon reflexes [78%], diaphragmatic palsy [82%], intercostal muscle paralysis [87%], general myalgia [68%], urinary retention [67%] and absent or decreased bowel movements [45%].

Respiratory failure was either a result of respiratory muscle paralysis and/or palatal paralysis leading to accumulation of secretions. No antivenom was available. Fifty-two patients [87%] needed mechanical ventilation for a mean of 8 days. The most surprising laboratory finding was a high rate of significant hyponatremia [42%]. The mean duration of the ICU stay was 12 days and the hospital mortality was 7%.

*The first symptom developed after envenomation*
Pharyngeal pain – 22%.
Ptosis – 20%.
General myalgia – 15%.
Dyspnoea – 13%.
Dysphagia – 10%.
Difficulty in opening the mouth – 5%.
General weakness – 5%.
Blurred vision – 3%.
Limb paralysis – 2%.
Abdominal pain – 2%.

The cardiovascular signs most often documented were tachycardia [defined as a heart rate faster than 100 beats per minute during > 6 hours during the first 2 days] and hypertension [above 140/90mmHg during > 6 hours during the first 2 days]. Conjunctivitis as a result of dry eyes was also commonly noted. The dilatation of the pupils was often maximal and was extremely persistent in some cases.

The most severely affected patients developed generalized muscle paralysis and became completely unresponsive. This situation, combined with apnoea and dilated pupils, may easily be misdiagnosed as *brain death*.

The envenomed patients in the study often experienced general myalgia. Some patients still had pain and numbness several months after discharge, requiring analgesic therapy. [Ha Tran Hung et al., 2009]

## Resembling Guillain-Barré Syndrome

A 36-year-old man was in good health after having had a traumatic left above-knee amputation secondary to a motorcycle accident in 1989. He was bitten by a poisonous snake on his left index finger on July 14, 1995. He warned his brother, who killed the snake and identified it as Bungarus multicinctus. About

1 hour after the bite, he had difficulty speaking and swallowing; moreover, bilateral ptosis, vomiting, and blurred vision also developed progressively.

He was unconscious with cardiorespiratory arrest upon arrival at the emergency department of a general hospital. He was resuscitated and given bungarotoxin-specific antivenom serum. Three days later, he was discharged and experienced only slight numbness at the site of fang puncture.

It was not until August 10, 1995 that he developed weakness in the upper and lower limbs, blurred vision, difficulty swallowing, and weak facial expression, and then he lost consciousness. He was sent to our hospital's emergency department in a cyanotic and comatose state. On examination, he was unresponsive, flaccid, and areflexic. His pupils were fixed and dilated without light reflex.

Computed tomography [CT] of his brain was unremarkable. General supportive treatment, mechanical ventilation, and antibiotics were administered. A complete blood count, comprehensive serum biochemical analysis, immunoelectrophoresis of cerebrospinal fluid [CSF], antinuclear antibody levels, human immunosuppressive virus survey, and serum antibody screening results were all within normal limits with the exception of a mildly elevated CSF protein level. No bacteria, fungus, or tuberculosis grew in the CSF acute and convalescent cultures. Blood and urine cultures were also unremarkable.

The patient regained consciousness *after 8 days*, and motor testing of upper and lower limbs showed 0/5 proximally but 1/5 distally. Sensory examination demonstrated mild deficits in pain, temperature, and light touch with fading glove-and-stocking hypaesthesia. All deep tendon reflexes were lost, and bilateral facial palsy was noted. Electrophysiology performed on day 12 in the acute care unit indicated severe axonal degeneration of motor and sensory fibers; needle electromyography [EMG] showed numerous fibrillation potentials and positive waves in both proximal and distal limb muscles with voluntary motor unit action potential [MUAP] absent in proximal but discrete in distal.

At 3 weeks after admission, he was treated with a total of 5 sessions of plasmapheresis over a period of 10 days and methylprednisolone, 500mg/d for 5 days. After the third plasmapheresis, the patient noticed increased strength and decreased numbness in both hands and feet. After the fifth plasma exchange, he was successfully weaned from the ventilator.

At 5 weeks after admission, repeated electrodiagnostic tests showed progressive improvement. abnormal, somewhat diminished, spontaneous activity, and motor unit potentials returning, indicating considerable reinnervation signs. The facial muscles showed mild membrane instability and short-duration lowamplitude MUAPs, which imply early states of reinnervation of muscle. Repetitive stimulation assessment, recorded from hypothenar muscles, failed to reveal defects in neuromuscular transmission.

Single-fiber EMG demonstrated a mild increase in fiber density, which represents initial motor unit remolding in patients with axonal loss, and the mean jitter for distal/proximal muscles was slightly elevated. The sympathetic skin response was persistently absent in the beginning and follow-up investigations.

At the start of his rehabilitation program he was dependent in all activities of daily living [ADL], and was non-ambulatory. After 4 weeks of intensive inpatient rehabilitation, his functional status improved from being wheelchair-bound to being to ambulate independently with a pair of crutches and a left above-knee prothesis. Also, his transfers, dressing, and ADL were independent. [Tien-Yow Chuang, 1996]

## Waking at 4 a.m. with Tingling & Numbness of Lower Limbs

'A 32-year-old woman living 5.4 km from Yangon, Myanmar, felt a scratch on the right upper arm while sleeping in bed at about midnight on 15 June 1993. Not knowing it was a snakebite, she went to sleep again but woke at 04:00 with tingling and numbness of the lower limbs. She could not open her eyes or swallow saliva. Her speech became slurred and she was admitted to North Okkalapa General Hospital. A snake found nearby was killed and identified as B. multicinctus; it measured 970 × 60 mm. She received 40 mL of Naja kaouthia antivenom, since specific antivenom was not available. Locally, she had only a small scratch. Nine hours after the bite, she became drowsy, confused and cyanosed. She was intubated, manually ventilated and transferred to the intensive care unit of Yangon General Hospital. On arrival [14 h after the bite] she had ptosis, her pupils were reactive to light, and muscle power was reduced in all 4 limbs. Her blood pressure was 110/80 mmHg, pulse rate 88/min, and respiratory rate 22/min. Intravenous administration of prostigmine [0.5 mg] and atropine [0.2 mg] failed to improve the neurological symptoms. Her dilated stomach was deflated through a nasogastric tube. Spontaneous respiration was maintained with oxygen therapy at low flow rate. Repeated injections of neostigmine and atropine failed to improve the neurological symptoms. The patient began to recover from ptosis 152 h after the bite and resumed normal feeding. She was discharged from the hospital 14 d after the bite with no neurological deficit.' [Pe, 1997]

## General Overview

Because wound site reactions are minimal in Bungarus multicinctus envenomation, the signs and symptoms were arbitrarily organized by motor or sensory effects. Motor effects were identified in 33 [75%] patients, sensory effects in 38 [86.4%], and miscellaneous effects in 35 [79.5%]. Twelve patients [27.3%] developed respiratory failure 1.5–6.5 hours post-bite. Moreover, 12 patients experienced severe general pain 1–12 hours post-bite, causing disability, such as *inability to get out of bed, cough without distress, or turn the head*. The estimated duration of general pain was 3.5–24 hours.

'Local' [pain or numbness] describes effects that did not extend beyond the affected limb. 'General' pain or numbness] describes effects spreading to the head/neck, trunk, and/or contralateral limbs. 'Numbness' was defined as a feeling of decreased sensation, tingling, but might have included subtle weakness. 'Pain' was defined as muscle soreness, ache, pain, or their combination. 'Motor effects' included general weakness, respiratory failure, ptosis, diplopia, difficulty in opening the mouth, chewing, or swallowing, and dysarthria. 'Sensory effects' included numbness or pain [incl. eye, throat, head, facial, neck, abdomen, back, or general pain]. Miscellaneous effects included dilated pupils, abnormal taste, nausea or vomiting, urinary retention, sweating, hypertension [> 140/90 mm of Hg], tachycardia [> 100 beats/minute], and bradycardia [< 60 beats/minute]. Laboratory findings were recorded on arrival in the emergency department and included *hyponatremia* in 3 patients [≤ 135 mEq/L], hyperglycaemia in 7 patients [≥ 200 mg/dL], and rhabdomyolysis in 1 patient.

After discharge from the hospital, 9 patients had persistent limb or body numbness, pain, soreness, or weakness. Two patients had persistent GI effects, including GI upset or constipation.

The hallmark of B. multicinctus envenomation is neuromuscular blockade caused by bungarotoxins.

The second most frequent distinct symptom of Bungarus snakebite is *pain* remote from the bite site of undetermined mechanism, which has been described in cases of Bungarus spp. envenomations incl. abdominal pain, generalized burning sensation or muscle pain. A significant proportion of our [44] patients developed severe general pain. Patients described the pain as *similar to myalgia after heavy exercise* but much more intense, esp. in the head and neck and trunk in addition to the limbs. Patients usually did not experience pain relief after nonsteroidal anti-inflammatory drugs [NSAIDs] administration. Instead, the pain was ameliorated by tramadol treatment. [Mao, 2017]

# DENDROASPIS ANGUSTICEPS

## Systematics
- Scientific name: Dendroaspis angusticeps [A. Smith, 1849].
- Synonyms: Naja angusticeps [Smith, 1849]. Dendraphis angusticeps [Günther, 1858].
- Common name: Eastern green mamba.
- Family: Elapidae.

## Biological Profile
- Very slender, highly venomous elapid with narrow, elongated head distinct from the neck and long, thin tail. Emerald green to lime green dorsally with sometimes a few scattered blue or yellow scales. Belly mostly pale green or yellowish green. Edges of mouth are often yellowish. Inside of mouth white to bluish white [bluish-grey to blackish in black mamba]. Average length 1.8–2.4 m [6–8 ft]; maximum 2.7 m [9 ft]. Males larger than females.
- Range: East coast of Africa, from Kenya southward to southern Natal and northeastern Cape Province.
- Habitat: Coastal bush, evergreen coastal forests, bamboo thickets. Also found in closer proximity to humans, when residing in farm trees, such as citrus, mango, coconut, and cashew.
- Mostly arboreal, seldom venturing to the ground, unless following prey or to bask.
- Relies on vision and olfaction to locate prey.

- Preys on adult and juvenile birds, bird eggs, frogs, lizards, snakes, rodents, and other small mammals.
- Males engage in ritual combat.
- Courtship and mating takes place in trees.
- Oviparous; 8–15 eggs per clutch.
- Smallest of the 4 species in genus Dendroaspis [angusticeps, polylepis, viridis, jamesoni].

## Behaviour & Temperament
'In my opinion, this species is one of the most dangerous elapids to work with. Besides possessing and extremely potent neurotoxin, it *doesn't readily show aggression*. Its calm demeanour is often very *misleading* and amateur herpetologists could become victims of envenomation simply because they will drop their guard. Unlike its cousin the black mamba, this species uses *no threat display* and will strike out without warning. I would advise anyone keeping this species to constantly be on guard when working with these animals. When handling this species, use slow deliberate movements. Never become jumpy or overexcited when tailing this species on a hook as they seem to react to fast movements. Be careful of using holding bins that open from the top, if the specimens gets startled when the bin is opened, they may strike. They have very potent venom." [Michael Burmeister; www.venomousreptiles.org]

## Polycystic Kidney Disease
'Polycystic kidney diseases [PKDs] are genetic disorders in which multiple cysts grow in kidneys, leading to end-stage renal failure. Vasopressin antagonists [vaptans] currently used to treat PKDs have side effects due to liver toxicity. We report the characterization of Mambaquaretin-1, a Kunitz-fold polypeptide isolated from green mamba venom that selectively and fully inhibits 3 major signaling pathways of the vasopressin type-2 receptor. Mambaquaretin-1 induces a purely aquaretic effect on mice and reduces cyst development in a mouse model. We produced mambaquaretin-1 by peptide synthesis and determined its X-ray structure, its binding mode, and functional properties. With high selectivity and without toxic metabolic byproducts associated with its peptidic nature, mambaquaretin-1 could become the preferential treatment for these disorders." [Ciolek, 2016]


# MATERIA MEDICA DENDROASPIS ANGUSTICEPS

## Sources
1 Proving by Sharad Hansjee, Dept. of Homoeopathy, Durban University of Technology [South Africa], 13 female and 11 male provers, 30c, 2010.
2 Effects of bite; clinical manifestations.

## Mind

∞ Haughty and vain. 'I am the best and I am always right.' 'Not my job description to sweep and dust.' 'I want to show myself off to the world.'

∞ Attractive.

∞ Self-indulgent. Feels best when focusing attention on self and one's beauty. 'I love myself.'

∞ Sensual. Overweening. Flirtatious.

∞ Oozing confidence; exuding sensuality; feels like a force to be reckoned with. Self-admiration; claims to 'own the world'.

∞ Provocative. Teasing. Playful. Seductive.

∞ Lascivious; passion and lust. High sex drive; desire for other men.

∞ Sex relieves stress.

∞ Not a slave to anyone, disliking taking orders from others.

∞ Suspicious.

∞ Territorial; doesn't want anyone in one's space.

∞ Crafty. Manipulative. Deceitful. Misleading.

∞ Wants to be alone in a cool dark room.

∞ Ailments from suppressed emotion; domination; restraint.

∞ Aversion to authority.

∞ Feeling confined; trapped in a cage. Energy feels pent up or caged up.

∞ Looking for space and freedom.

∞ Wants to escape, leave, run away.

∞ Aggressive, confrontational; wants to argue, wants to start a fight. Ready to pounce. Impulse to kill. 'This is war.'

∞ Consumed by rage; angry at everything and everyone. Enraged like a dragon. Wants to hit or break something to release anger and frustration.

∞ Anger when misunderstood.

∞ Prepares to retaliate.

∞ Wants to win at all costs. Competitive.

∞ Aggression worse during headache.

∞ Delusions: Impression of danger; evil; forsaken by friends; everyone is looking at her; seeing green lights; seeing red lights; seeing snakes in corner of eye.

∞ Desire to be held, cuddled, caressed.

∞ Praying; feeling close to God. Spiritual. Meditating.

∞ Depressed, feeling as if being dead inside.

∞ Wants to die or feeling as if going to die.

## Dreams

∞ Abandoned by friends.

∞ Accusations.

∞ Being an actor.

∞ Affairs.

∞ Amorous, young boys; old boyfriends; fallen in love.

∞ Beautiful scenery.

∞ Blackmail.

∞ Pools of blood.

- ∞ Bribery.
- ∞ Car, driving fast.
- ∞ Changing places.
- ∞ Chased.
- ∞ Unsuccessful coition.
- ∞ Changing colours.
- ∞ Death of relatives.
- ∞ People on fire.
- ∞ Flirting.
- ∞ Forsaken by friends.
- ∞ Old friends.
- ∞ Own funeral.
- ∞ Driving a green car.
- ∞ Green eyes.
- ∞ Green light.
- ∞ Green snake.
- ∞ Horror movies.
- ∞ Injections.
- ∞ Being invisible.
- ∞ Killing.
- ∞ Lizards fighting.
- ∞ Giant praying mantis.
- ∞ Mother Mary.
- ∞ Movie star.
- ∞ Promiscuity.
- ∞ Prostitutes.
- ∞ Red riding hood.
- ∞ Chased by snakes.
- ∞ Killing snakes.
- ∞ Strippers.
- ∞ Vampires.

## Generals

- ∞ Ravenous appetite [8 pr.]. Eating every 2 hours. Devouring food. Eats like not having seen food for months. Can't stop eating; just seem to eat and eat.
- ∞ Increased appetite on waking.
- ∞ Very thirsty for large amounts of water [9 pr.].
- ∞ Throbbing, bursting, pounding pains.
- ∞ Weak and easily fatigued during menses; generally < heat > cold, cool winds, esp. to feet and head.
- ∞ Sleep position on left side.
- ∞ *Tightness* – head, jaws, epigastrium, testicles, chest, back. Eyes tightly shut.

## Sensations

- ∞ Night in bed, as if floating on closing eyes, as if drifting from side to side, as if on the ocean. Floating and bobbing up and down.

∞ Dizziness, as if head were turning round.

∞ Head as if a balloon full of pressure, ready to burst.

∞ Head as if separated from body; as if too much air and water were moving from back to front in head.

∞ Cap on top of head.

∞ Heat on top of head.

∞ Lightning strike in head from ears to centre of head and from ear to ear; < light.

∞ Itchiness of scalp as from ants crawling on scalp.

∞ Eyes as if forced out, during headache.

∞ Eyes as if too big for sockets, < looking up; during headache.

∞ Iron taste in mouth on drinking water.

∞ Tongue as if swollen, rough, and burnt by hot tea; < talking, sugar.

∞ Jaws as if locked on going to sleep.

∞ Tightness of jaws. [3 pr.]

∞ Jaws as if tightening on opening mouth.

∞ Throat as if closing up, & difficulty swallowing.

∞ Left side of pharynx as if dead.

∞ Sinking feeling all the way from chest to navel.

∞ Tight knot in epigastric area, making deep breathing impossible.

∞ Ovarian pain as from 2 big sponge balls in pelvis.

∞ Heavy menstrual flow; as if draining the life out of her.

∞ Uterus as if going to burst.

∞ Great heavy weight on chest.

∞ Punched on sternum, bruised ache; > breathing.

∞ Heart as if sinking.

∞ Back as if crushed.

∞ Pins and needles in soles of feet.

∞ Soles of feet and toes as if swollen; feet as if bound by heavy shackles; < standing, touch, wearing shoes; > massage, feet in cold water.

## Locals

∞ Pounding, bursting headache in temples on waking in morning; > closing eyes, lying down, sleeping; < opening eyes, applying cold water; & sore pain around eyes.

∞ Pounding, bursting headache in temples & heavy, drooping eyelids and pain in nape of neck as if overstretched.

∞ Throbbing headache < sun, < noise, < movement; > hard pressure, > placing hand over right eye; & nausea, felt in pit of stomach.

∞ Throbbing headache < thinking of food.

∞ Throbbing headache & nausea < sweets.

∞ Headache < coffee.

∞ Severe occipital headache > hard pressure; > keeping very still and quiet, motionless.

∞ Upper eyelids painful and heavy, hurts to open eyes, in morning on waking; < light.

∞ Subconjunctival haemorrhage during throbbing headache; eyes sensitive to light.

∞ Pain ovaries > after stool.

∞ Constant throbbing pain in pelvis and hip bones during menses, & pulling throb in lower back, > hot applications, stretching.

∞ Pain nape of neck/cervical region, extending to head, clavicles and/or shoulder.

∞ Pressing pain lumbar region.

## Remedy Overview

'Provers experienced a wide range of symptoms particularly on the mental and emotional spheres including feelings of powerful assertion and confidence; cheerful and excited energy; spiritual and prayerful feelings; seductive, sensual and extravagant mannerisms; desire to dance and heightened energy; clairvoyance and desire to be in nature as well as pronounced irritability, anger and sadness. Other symptoms included desire to be alone and withdrawn feelings; quarrelsome nature; desire to kill; deceitful ways; intolerance to injustice; poor concentration; thoughts of the past; confusion and antagonism of the will and anxious thoughts. Delusions, fears and thoughts of death also manifested in provers.

'On the physical sphere there were marked symptoms produced in the head area with a wide range of headaches. Eye symptoms were also vast in the inflammation, heaviness and ptosis of the eyes. Throat symptoms manifested as pharyngitis and sore throat. Toxicological symptoms included vertigo, ptosis, pain in different areas, inflammation, vomiting, blurred vision, slurred speech, difficulty breathing and difficult swallowing. Back pain and lower back pain were also key symptoms. Sleep difficulties and sleepiness were experienced by provers.

'Dream symptoms were the most prevalent in this proving. Dreams were repetitive in provers in the dreams of changing places and being in many places and unfamiliar places. There were marked dreams of sexuality, death, spirituality, friendships, colours, snakes, weddings, fighting and killings and past recollections.' [Sharad Hansjee, Introduction to proving]

## Clinical Manifestations

Venom primarily neurotoxic, with some cardiotoxic factors. Unique mamba toxins are the so-called fasciculins, potent inhibitors of acetylcholinesterase that produce severe, generalised and long-lasting fasciculations [muscle twitching]. The green mamba moreover produces calcicludine, a protein toxin that inhibits high-voltage-activated calcium channels, esp. L-type calcium channels, resulting in decreased cardiac contractile force, decreased heart rate, vasodilation and hypotension.

The first systemic sign of elapid venom poisoning is usually drowsiness, followed by ptosis, blurring of vision, and difficulties in speech and swallowing. In bites by mambas a similar clinical picture may be seen, except that there is often *intense abdominal pain*, with weakness, nausea and vomiting. Other characteristics are blurred vision, slurred speech, excessive salivation, and headache;

these manifestations are frequently followed by hypotension, respiratory distress, and shock.

# DENDROASPIS POLYLEPIS

## Systematics
- Scientific name: Dendroaspis polylepis [Günther, 1864].
- Synonym: Dendraspis antinorii [Peters, 1873].
- Common name: Black mamba.
- Family: Elapidae.

## Biological Profile
- Slender, highly venomous elapid with narrow, elongated head and long thin tail. Body colouration dark olive, olive green, grey brown, or metal colour. Inky black lining of mouth. Average length 2.5 m, maximum 4.5 m. Often found in pairs or small groups.
- Range: Africa.
- Habitat: Prefers arid environments such as semi-arid dry bush country, light woodland, and rocky outcrops. Prefers open bush country.
- The world's fastest land snake, able to reach speeds in excess of 20 km per hour. It uses this speed to escape danger, rather than catch prey.
- Diurnal; active during daytime. Often sleeps in hollow trees, burrows, rock crevices, or empty termite mounds, and will come back to the same place every night.
- Relies on vision and olfaction to locate prey.
- Preys on small mammals and birds, such as voles, rats, squirrels, mice, rats, or bush babies [galagos]. Will strike a large animal, release it and then stalk it until it becomes paralysed. With smaller animals it will strike and hold on until the animal becomes paralysed.
- Adept at climbing trees.
- Its proclivity for travel contributes to its frequent contact with humans.
- Oviparous; 6–17 eggs per brood.
- Black mambas have fast metabolisms by snake standards and generally consume quite a bit more food than similarly-sized individuals of other species. Hatchlings have been known to reach 6 feet in length within 1 year. *Hunger* can therefore sometimes be used to manipulate them.
- Name from Gr. *dendron*, tree, and *aspis*, shield, also used to describe the shape of a snake coiling itself thus resembling a shield; *poly,* many, and *lepis*, from Gr. *lepidos*, scale.
- The name *black mamba* may be somewhat misleading as it does not refer to the colour of this species, but rather to the pitch black lining of the mouth.

## Behaviour & Temperament
When feeling threatened, it will raise its front and head about 1 m off the ground, open its mouth, spread a flat hood, and shake its head. When attacking

it will make several quick strikes and escape as fast as it can. Black mambas can strike from 1–2 m away. Before antivenoms were developed, a black mamba bite was almost 100% fatal.

'Wild Dendroaspis polylepis are easily the most feared animals in the bush, by man and animals alike. I have seen even lions and elephants back away from a large Dendroaspis polylepis with its characteristic black mouth lining, and the reflecting silver tips. Adult Dendroaspis polylepis over 8 feet have no natural predators in Southern Africa.

'Dendroaspis polylepis are creatures of habit. They frequent the same basking spot, hiding spot and hunting spot for as long as they aren't forcibly removed. They travel by the same pathways, generally avoiding game trails. If you get within 40 feet you are very lucky, or it is still early morning. This combination of habits and nervousness make this species a rare find in houses, barns etc., although it does happen from time to time, in particular the younger specimens. Catching this species is precarious at best, utilizing enormous skill and patience. In the wild, Dendroaspis polylepis is not used to interacting with people, and will voice their displeasure rather vehemently. Its first option is always escape. If this option is not given, it will stand its ground. The chain of events usually takes 2 paths from here:

'First: – If the snake is still cold or cool it usually stays in 1 spot, lifts its head and front third of the body. It then flattens the neck, opens its mouth to show the black lining and emits a hollow hiss. Any further antagonizing will result in a few rapid and unerringly accurate strikes.

'Second: – If the snake is warmer the game changes a whole lot! Here is where the typical "Mamba" comes from. The snake moves forward at pace, starts raising the front part of its body [sometimes up to two-thirds] and strikes out without slacking off in the forward pace. The rule of thumb here is to make sure you are 1 foot back for every 1 foot the Mamba is in length. After the initial lunge, the snake usually stops, and hisses with the mouth open. Any movement at this stage will encourage the snake to strike out.

'This species rarely, if ever, delivers a dry bite. A bite from a large specimen will more than likely be on the head or chest area. Standing still is not an option, it's a necessity!

'I have caught many Dendroaspis polylepis in the bush and there are various methods of doing this, one of them is very, very risky indeed. First off, out of personal experience, Dendroaspis polylepis are true solar machines. Catching one or trying to do so in the late afternoon is dangerous, very dangerous. . . . Bagging this species without a bagging frame etc. is very difficult. The snake tends to wrap as much of its body as it can around yours, making it very difficult to let go.' [Joe Switalski & Martin Smit, 2007]

## Beauty & Menace Greatly Dreaded

Many and varied are the stories told of the terrible Mambas. Sitting within the cheerful glow of camp fires, after a day's tough riding and climbing, I have passed many a happy hour listening to thrilling, if legendary tales, of the evil powers and fierce aggressiveness of the Mamba. I think there is no happier life than to live for months at a time away from all the cares, bickerings, conventionalities and empty vanity with which town life is so permeated, and with a companion or 2, a favourite horse, a few affectionate and devoted dogs, and a couple of trusty Zulu servants, to go right into the wilds, away from all civilization, and live surrounded by Nature, and study the ways of her creations.

So great is the dread of the Mamba in the native mind that if one be known to inhabit any particular locality, few, if any, natives will venture there. In fact, a wide detour is always made. As a general rule, the more we learn about snakes and their ways, the less fear we have of them. This is usually not so with the Mamba. The more one learns of his ways, the greater grows the dread of him. He, without doubt, is the king of snakes in South Africa. For quickness, aggressiveness and the deadly nature of his venom, he has no equal.

After 2 or 3 encounters with large Black Mambas, I learned to be wary. I found that even a gun was not always a protection, so quick and sinuous were his movements. A Black Mamba should never be attacked in the bush or long grass. I have frequently startled Mambas out of a nap on the Kafir paths in the bushy parts of Natal. Sometimes they would glide off and away into the undergrowth, but as likely as not the Mamba would slide up a shrub at the side of the path and remain on the defensive. If a stone be thrown at him, or if he be wounded, he will, as likely as not, make straight at his aggressor and with body raised, bite him.

The quickness of movement, grace and ease with which the Mamba glides about in his native habitat is very lucidly summed up by Mr. W.F. Jones, of Zululand. "The Mamba is essentially partial to trees, and thorns make no difference to the ease of its movements. Our large dongas are matted in places with a dense network of bramble-like growths, which extend searchingly in long, sinuous branches, which are studded with formidable thorns, curved like the claws of a cat. Whatever road he elects to take, whether on the top or along and through this cruel maze of brake, it is the same to this graceful creature. To see a startled Mamba making for his home along the crown of one of these thickets is a marvel of perfected movement. The small head, with its full prominent eyes, the long body, partially raised and sweeping from side to side with a forward throw, so swift and sudden as to bewilder one into believing that the creature is bounding along with 10-feet gaps between the curves.

"And as the tail disappears into the dark cavity edging the donga, there follows immediate stillness and peace. But, on the first sunny day, some person steals along with a gun charged with No. 6 shot, and midway in the passage home this time there is a sharp decisive pause. We are using smokeless powder, and, without taking the eye off the line of the barrels, the lightning turn of the head can be followed as it darts viciously back at the gaping wound halfway down the body. Realizing its impotence, it strikes hither and thither at leaf or branch. In a few moments we see the jaws opening widely, the writhe of the contorted body showing the clean white belly, and we know that the end of so much beauty and menace has come."

The Black Mamba, as a general rule, has some secure retreat to which it decamps when alarmed. If a Mamba be surprised when out in the open and if you happen to be between it and its retreat, it will not rush off in an opposite direction, as most animals would do, but will instantly dart off at terrific speed, apparently charging right at you. If a Mamba should act in this manner and if you are not prepared to defend yourself, your safest plan is to sprint off without an instant's delay. Whilst travelling at great speed, a Mamba can strike right and left with consummate ease, without apparently abating its speed in the slightest. To stand in the path of a Mamba rushing off to its lair, is fraught with the gravest danger, even if well-armed. At such times the nerves are none too steady and it is as likely as not that even an expert with the gun will miss his aim. There is no time for reloading and often not even time to take a second aim should the gun be a double-barreled one, before the snake has swept past and in passing deposited its death-dealing venom.

When making off through the bushveld, the Black Mamba, with a rapid and continuous succession of forward propulsions, glides over the stubble, the head and anterior part of its body being sometimes several feet off the ground. When a bush fire is raging Mambas may be seen escaping in this way at a swift pace. Viewed at a distance they seem to be gliding over the tops of the long grass and low shrubs. Cases are on record of men being bitten as high up as the thigh, when mounted on horseback. [Fitzsimons, 1912]


## MATERIA MEDICA DENDROASPIS POLYLEPIS

### Sources
1 Proving Rajan Sankaran [India], 21 provers [13 females, 8 males], 30c [?]; 1994. Unmarked symptoms.
2 Degroote, Dream Repertory.
3 Effects of bite; clinical manifestations.
4 Effects of bite; sudden death.
5 Effects of bite; tightness, numbness & twitching.
6 Effects of bite; losing control over everything.
7 Effects of bite; taken for dead.
8 Effects of bite; fading in & out of consciousness.

### Mind
∞ Forsaken feeling; cannot depend/rely upon others, must do everything oneself.
∞ Black depression, as if surrounded by a black cloud, as if going into a narrow, black tunnel; overwhelmed by thoughts of death and accidents, esp. of relatives. Nothing can be done; nothing is left; no one understands; no point to try.
∞ Unfeeling, insensitive; blunt, rude, malicious, abusive; deliberately mean; untouched, uncaring. Easily provoked, leading to violent impulses and desire to kill. Eager and ready to retaliate.
∞ Aggressive. Quarrelsome. Ready and prepared to take on anyone for a fight.
∞ Wants to fight for defenseless, helpless people.
∞ Forceful. 'Proves' to be right when wrong; makes others apologize.

∞ Anger, increasing and decreasing suddenly.

∞ Anger with paleness face.[2]

∞ Irritability when someone is standing in front of one; wants to strike that person.

∞ Speaks loudly.

∞ Contemptuous.

∞ Impulsive, rash; morbid impulse to climb out of running train; to hurt others; to sexually harass women; to do violence.

∞ Impulsive, alternating with fear of losing control.

∞ Hurried, runs instead of walks; sense of being short of time.

∞ Demanding that others listen and agree but refusing to listen to anyone himself.

∞ Delusion of someone behind one that would touch or harm one.

∞ Delusion of trying to escape from a crowd of people crushing each other.

∞ Delusion being caged up, closed up, trapped, locked up, restrained.

∞ Delusion of everything being monotonous/boring.

∞ Delusion being isolated, cut off from others.

∞ Delusion of conspiracies; being spied upon.[2]

∞ Suspicion others would deliberately do things to harass or harm.

∞ Deceitful, lying; avoids blame, or feels wrongly accused.

∞ Risky behaviour. Careless, reckless in driving.

∞ Goes to extremes.

∞ Indolence, aversion to work.

∞ Tells beautifully fabricated lies deliberately, just for the fun of it.

∞ Feeling of mind not working; mental block; < mental exertion, > sleep.

∞ Inability to remember or understand what was said. Blank mind.

∞ Boasting, loud-mouthed but small-hearted.[2]

∞ Desire to climb in top of trees; in children.[2]

∞ Fear of flies and ants.[2]

∞ Thinks being always right.[2]

∞ Strikes oneself when becoming hysterical.[2]

## Dreams

∞ Accidents, unaffected by.

∞ Accused of having bad intentions.

∞ Accused wrongly of murder.

∞ Accused wrongly of rape.

∞ Bad news, getting; of loved ones having died.[2]

∞ Battles; being beaten.

∞ Bitten by shark; snake.[2]

∞ Cannibals, threat of being eaten.[2]

∞ Cheated, feeling or being.

∞ Crocodiles.

∞ Dancing.

∞ Death of relatives.[2]

∞ Deceitful, being.

∞ Exploited, being.[2]
∞ Falling off a mountain.
∞ Forsaken, being or feeling; castaway; excluded.[2]
∞ Funeral, own, assisting in preparation of.[2]
∞ Gun fights.
∞ Homosexuality amongst boys.
∞ Ignored, being.[2]
∞ Murder.
∞ Murdered by skeletons and devils.[2]
∞ Nakedness.[2]
∞ Pursued by murderers.
∞ Pursued by snakes.
∞ Pursued to be stabbed.[2]
∞ Saving someone from drowning in sea.
∞ Sexual assault.
∞ Stabbed from behind.
∞ Threats of rape.
∞ Unwanted, feeling.

## Generals
∞ Desire for cheese; cold food; ice cream; oranges; spices.
∞ Desires very cold food, icecream; even ice-cream is not cold enough.
∞ External numbness.
∞ Right side then left – pains.
∞ Sensation of strength.
∞ Increased ability to walk long distances without fatigue.
∞ Short sleep >.
∞ Sleeplessness before menses; exhaustion on first day of menses.
∞ Sleeplessness in dark room.[2]
∞ Weakness from 12:30 to 15:30; > sleep.
∞ Extreme weakness during menses.
∞ Cold sweat all over.
∞ Pains coming on suddenly.
∞ Bodyache < morning.
∞ Great agility of limbs.[2]
∞ Warm bathing >.[2]
∞ Lack of vital heart in evening and in bed.[2]
∞ Body piercings – chin; tongue.[2]

## Sensations
∞ Sinking into ground from weakness and weight of own body.
∞ Head as if numb, as if about to fall down, must support forehead with hand.
∞ Heaviness heart region, causing dyspnoea.[2]
∞ Heart as if having stopped beating, followed by tumultuous rebound.[2]
∞ Bones as if hanging vertically from joints, while lying.

## Locals

∞ Dizziness and fear at high places.

∞ Headache, bursting, pulsating or sharp, from loss of sleep; dull pain < talking.

∞ Desire to close eyes. Falling of lids.

∞ Protrudes tongue when coughing.[2]

∞ Teeth sensitive to cold.

∞ Cracking of jaw when talking.[2]

∞ Throat pain < empty swallowing, drinking, eating, > warm drinks, finger in ear.

∞ Pain stomach when lying on back.[2]

∞ Tendency to masturbation in males.

∞ Backache cervical region > circular head movements.

∞ Perspiration nape of neck/cervical region morning on waking.[2]

∞ Walks on toes.[2]

## Clinical Manifestations

Injecting fast as lightning a highly potent neurotoxic venom, the black mamba can strike so quickly that the victim may be unaware he has been bitten.

'The symptoms and signs of envenomation may include early dyspnoea and a feeling of tightness in the throat, dysphagia, slurred speech, and muscle spasms and fasciculations, followed by marked weakness or paralysis, respiratory difficulty, and increased salivation. The pulse may be normal or increased, while blood pressure may be normal at first but then falls to shock levels in severe poisoning. There may be some nausea and vomiting, and ptosis, but pain and swelling are usually minimal.' [Russell, 1980]

After a black mamba bite, symptoms can occur as quickly as within 10 minutes. A tingling sensation at the site of the bite may be the only initial sign of envenomation. Other neurological symptoms include miosis, ptosis, blurred vision, bulbar symptoms, paraesthesia, fasciculations, ataxia, and loss of consciousness. General signs of envenomation may include local pain, nausea, cough, and *profuse sweating* from sympathetic overstimulation. In severe cases, intubation, mechanical ventilation and circulatory support may be necessary.

After having been bitten in the right thumb, his "condition on admission was grave and he showed signs of general collapse and restlessness. He appeared as though *he had just been immersed in water*. His pulse was rapid, but respiration was depressed and in a short time only diaphragmatic respiration was visible. There was paralysis of the vocal cords and of the muscles of the pharynx with profuse salivation, the products of which had to be removed by continuous suction. He was difficult to control as, although deglutition was completely paralyzed and respiration partly so, his limbs were not affected and he was very violent, thrashing about with arms and legs and generally very distressed. Treatment was immediately instigated, and the patient gradually experienced more and more difficulty in breathing, in spite of oxygen administration; the pulse rate dropped from 120 to 48 per minute and cardiac arrest finally ensued about 1½ hour after admission. [Strover, 1967]

'Black mamba venom has rapid onset of action and symptoms have been reported to occur anywhere between 10 and 15 min post-envenomation. The clinical presentation may vary markedly owing to the array of toxic proteins that make up the venom. Initially, envenomation may be characterized by little or no swelling or bleeding, nausea, and conjunctival congestion. A few minutes later, the victim may begin to sweat profusely, hypersalivate, vomit, complain of a strange taste in the mouth, and tingling sensations throughout the body leading to paraesthesia and weakness. Thereafter, the victim may begin to appear as if he/she has just been immersed in water ['gooseflesh'] and may exhibit laboured breathing. Then, ptosis, paralysis of vocal cords, muscles of the pharynx and deglutition as well as general flaccid paralysis may be observed. Thus, victims may be conscious but unable to speak. Several hours after envenomation, victims may become restless and may violently thrash about with arms and legs. Eventually, generalized fasciculations may set in and cardio-respiratory collapse may lead to death. Clinically, tachycardia, hypotension, polyuria, and a high leucocyte count may be observed. There may also be sinus bradycardia, glycosuria, fall in Hb and creatinine levels.' [Erulu, 2018]

## Sudden Death

Mr. Hector McKenzie-Shaw, Government Land Surveyor, related to me the details of the sad death of the young farmer Claud ['Punch'] Moller. He was present when the deceased was bitten by a Mamba and remained with him till his death. His account is as follows: "We had been out hunting and on returning to the wagon, which was about a 100 yards distant, my friend trod upon a large Black Mamba, which instantly bit him on the front part of the left foot, just above the top of the boot.

Without an instant's delay we tied ligatures above and below the punctures, scarified the part and rubbed the wounds full of permanganate of potash crystals. I then put on another ligature above the knee and yet another at the top of the thigh, tightening them with a stick and screwing it round. Arriving at the wagon, I sucked the wound thoroughly and gave him half an ordinary tumbler of brandy, and placing him on a mattress, covered him up with blankets and kindled a large fire at his side to keep him warm. At intervals we gave him doses of brandy. In all, he drank about half a bottle of it. The snake inflicted the bite about 3 o'clock in the afternoon. For the first hour my friend was somewhat excited and talked and laughed with us. Then he calmed down and was perfectly normal apparently and complained of nothing except diarrhoea and an unpleasant twitching of the muscles of the mouth and tongue.

Hour after hour went by, and we chatted away beside the cheerful fire, planning out many things for the future, never dreaming for one moment that this was the last day for my friend, who seemed none the worse for the bite. A little before 9 p.m. I noticed he was less talkative and that his eyelids were getting puffy. From this time onward he seemed to be rather tired. Then, at 10 p.m. without any warning he clutched his throat desperately and sprang with a bound to his feet, threw his arms out, gripped his throat again and with a desperate effort tried to speak to me, but as he was uttering my name his breath failed and he collapsed upon the ground, struggled, and was dead in 5 minutes.

All this came upon us with such startling suddenness that we were appalled. In laying him out I noticed that the entire left side of his body was stiff and rigid, while the right side was quite relaxed. He evidently had had a paralytic stroke just before death. On removing the clothes from the body I noticed an irregular line of dark purple of varying diameter up to 2 inches, running from the site of the bite up the left side, over the left shoulder, up behind the ear to the base of the skull. There was no swelling or discolouration other than this livid band anywhere about the body, nor was there any haemorrhage from the mucous surfaces. Diarrhoea was more or less pronounced from the time he was bitten till his death.

My friend was exceptionally strong and muscular. In fact, he was remarkable for his physical strength. He was within 2 or 3 days of being 21 years of age. He was one of the most fearless and daring of men, but strange to say he had an absolute horror and dread of snakes. About a week before his death he stumbled over a Puff Adder and declared that if he should have another such experience it would be his last, he would clear out of the country, for he could not stand the sight of snakes. Poor fellow, his next experience was indeed his last. [Fitzsimons, 1912]

### Tightness, Numbness & Twitching

While feeding a 5-year-old male black mamba, a 34-year-old snake breeder suddenly noticed a tiny bloody mark on his forearm and, at the same time, a slight tingling of his lips. He immediately realized that he had been bitten and called a befriended snake expert to seek advice. . . . Within the next 5 minutes, chest tightness, generalized paraesthesia, and fasciculation occurred. Upon arrival of the ambulance, the patient was unable to walk, was tachypneic, and had prominent dysarthria. . . . Forty minutes after the bite, the patient arrived in the emergency department, complaining of worsening fasciculations and paraesthesia affecting the extremities and the face. On physical examination, he was fully conscious with a heart rate of 105/min and a blood pressure of 165/80 mmHg. He was tachypnoeic at 30/min. Pulse oximetry revealed an oxygen saturation of 95% on room air. There were 2 tiny puncture wounds with local swelling and redness on the left forearm. Motor function was normal, except for mild ptosis. Seventy minutes after the bite, the patient was given 2 vials (20 ml) of "Samir Polyvalent Snake Antivenin" together with 2.5 mg of IV midazolam for ongoing hyperventilation. . . . Upon arrival in our ICU, the patient was haemodynamically stable but still tachycardic and tachypnoeic. Fasciculations, dysarthria, and ptosis had slightly improved. ECG showed a grade 1 atrioventricular block without any other abnormalities. Initial laboratory tests were unremarkable, apart from moderate respiratory alkalosis. Over the next few hours, sweating, chills, and difficulty with swallowing as well as nausea occurred. However, the airway was never compromised, coughing reflex was intact, and respiratory failure did not occur. . . . On the next day, symptoms of envenomation had improved, but the patient developed cellulitis of the bitten forearm and rhabdomyolysis, with a peak serum creatine kinase level of 16,049 U/L. Upon treatment with intravenous fluids and amoxicillin/sulbactam, his condition gradually improved. After 4 days in the hospital, he was discharged home with muscular pain as the only residual symptom. A few weeks later, the patient had fully recovered. [Quarch, 2017]

## Losing Control over Everything – Black Mamba Bite
This is the story of a black mamba and Danie Pienaar, Head of Scientific Services in the Kruger National Park, South Africa.

'It was about midday on a Thursday in January 1998 when Danie Pienaar came face to face with a Black Mamba and its bite. He was alone and was wearing shorts. . . . He recalls feeling a burning sensation on the side of his leg, under the knee. "Subconsciously, perhaps I knew I was bitten because 2 strides on I stopped to check." He found 4 blue-purple holes and a drop of blood and had his worst suspicion confirmed. The first symptoms appeared quickly. He had a bad taste in his mouth, almost like metal, and 'pins and needles' in his fingertips and lips. It soon became worse and later it "felt like all the hair on my body stood up."

"I realised the venom was doing its damage." Being alone, far from the bakkie [pick-up truck] and with no medical equipment on hand Danie faced daunting decisions. "I was relatively sure I was not going to get to help in time." For a brief time he considered settling under a tree and writing farewell notes to friends and family. Fortunately, the desire to survive burned stronger and he decided to try and reach the bakkie. . . . He tried, knowing it was not the right thing to do, to open the bite marks with his knife – with little success. He tied his belt around his upper leg and with the tourniquet in place made a quick note of what had happened to him. Leaving all else behind, he took his gun and compass and ventured back to the bakkie. "It was extremely difficult as I deliberately forced myself to walk and breath slowly to try and slow my heartbeat down."

'He was sweating badly and by that time had tunnel vision as the poison attacked the smaller muscles. He finally arrived at the bakkie and attempted the closest route to a tourist road, using the firebreaks and, at times, almost getting stuck in streams. "They must have thought a weirdo was on the attack as I was doing 130 km an hour, forced them off the road, jumped out without a shirt and gun in hand." . . .

'He arrived at the hospital, about 2 hours after the time he had been bitten. By this time, the symptoms had intensified, but he could still communicate sufficiently to tell the doctors what had happened. Because of the time frame, they were skeptical, and told him he would be 'monitored carefully'. "Even my father, when speaking to me on the phone, tried to convince me it was not a Black Mamba." As the doctors removed the tourniquet, his condition deteriorated rapidly. Suddenly he could not swallow, and his speech slurred. He tried to tell Tom not to switch the machines off, as he remembered how a snake expert had an experience where he could hear the people contemplating switching the life-support off as they thought he was in a coma.

'The doctors put him on the ventilator, and he was briefly knocked-out. When he came to, he was completely paralysed, yet he could touch, hear and see everything. "I could only see if they lifted my eyelids to check my pupils, but there was nothing wrong with my sight," he said. It was the same situation as the snake expert. He was restrained to the bed and recalls how his sweat dammed on the plastic sheeting in the hollow of his bed. The fan was on and he was freezing but could not do anything. By 6 o'clock that night, his friend Dewald Keet visited. He urged Danie to try giving him an indication if he could hear anything.

"With great difficulty I managed to slightly move a foot," which Dewald luckily noticed. They then realised he was not in a coma. Slowly he regained more muscle function. The following morning . . . he was still on the ventilator and not fully recovered from the paralysis. . . . He never received any antivenom. Other than the sweating that continued for some time and the bite marks that remained purple for a while, Danie suffered no consequences. Danie believes he survived for a number of reasons. "Firstly, it was not my time to go." The fact that he stayed calmed and moved slowly definitely helped. The tourniquet was also essential. "It was not easy to stay calm," he says. "It was almost as if I dislodged myself from my body and was talking to someone else the entire time."' [Summarized from Lynette Strauss, Bitten by a Mamba! Kruger Times]

### Taken for Dead

After a black mamba bite, Jack Seale was rushed to the hospital. 'For a week Jack lay without moving, unable even to blink. His wife spent hours playing music and talking to his inert form. No medical precedent existed for his case. "I heard everything," Jack says. "One doctor kept saying, Pull the plug, give the poor bugger a break. I heard them say I was going to be a vegetable. I thought, Not me, my boy. I hung on the words of everyone, kept myself sane by picking up on patterns, the time of day, who was coming in and out. A week after admittance, Jack managed to twitch a finger. A few hours later he was out of bed and walking around, and he left the hospital the next day under his own steam. . . . Historically, he points out, victims in a coma-like state were often taken for dead while actually experiencing something like suspended animation – effects similar to curare's or those of the blowfish poison given to voodoo's zombies. "It's part of the folklore and fear of mambas. Sometimes the bodies didn't rot for 5 or 6 days – because they weren't dead! And sometimes they got up and walked away!" Such a reaction may occur when a striking snake delivers only a minimal dose of venom.' [Douglas Lee, 1996]

### Fading In & Out of Consciousness – Black Mamba Bite

The following is a step-by-step account of the symptoms of my black mamba bite, and time frames within which they occurred.

- Within 2 minutes the "tingling" sensation had spread throughout my arm.
- There was mild swelling at the bite site, which was slightly painful when touched.

- 6 minutes after the bite the "tingling" sensation had spread throughout my body. It feels like millions of insects crawling under your skin.
- 8 minutes into the bite I experienced increased salivation.
- I began sweating excessively.
- After about 10 minutes I could "taste" the fillings in my teeth. I experienced a "coppery" taste.
- 12 minutes after the bite I began feeling drowsy. It became difficult to keep my eyes open. It felt like someone had tied bricks to my eyelids, which prevented me from opening them fully.
- After about 15 minutes my coordination began to falter. At this point I could still walk, but it felt as if I had punished a couple of bottles of tequila.
- At this point help arrived to take me to hospital. I realised that my condition would deteriorate rapidly. I knew at some point I would lose consciousness. I informed the lady assisting me that should I pass out that the medical staff inject 8 vials of antivenom and have a respirator on hand should my breathing stop.
- 20 minutes into the bite I begin to lose the ability to control my bodily functions and I experienced incontinence of faeces and urine. Not my finest hour!
- At this point I started developing chest pains, almost as if a sumo wrestler was sitting on my chest.
- After about 25 minutes confusion and slight hallucinations begin taking over my system.
- 30 minutes into the bite. Flaccid paralysis sets in. I am unable to walk. My arms, legs and head hang limply. Although conscious I am unable to respond. My speech is slurred and responses slow.
- After about 40 minutes the real pain sets in. I began trembling and muscular seizure begins to set in. It's like having a cramp in your calf muscle except in this case every muscle in my body cramps up.
- 45 minutes, I begin to have difficulty breathing. Fortunately this coincides with me fading in and out of consciousness.
- This lasted for approximately 2½ hours with all of the above symptoms taking their turn at beating the living *** out of my system.
- These are all classic symptoms of a black mamba bite and the effects of a neurotoxic venom.

The beauty of a neurotoxic venom is that unlike a cytotoxic venom, there is no residual effect. I was bitten on Wednesday; Thursday I was out of hospital and catching snakes again. [summarized from 'Black mamba Bite' on snakesuncovered.com, website of Perry's Bridge Reptile Park, Mpumalanga, South Africa]

# DENDROASPIS VIRIDIS

### Systematics
- Scientific name: Dendroaspis viridis [Hallowell, 1844].

- Synonym: Leptophis viridis [Hallowell, 1844].
- Common names: Western green mamba. West African green mamba.
- Family: Elapidae.

## Biological Profile

- Long, thin, venomous arboreal elapid. Biggest arboreal mamba species, with an average length of 1.5–2 m; maximum 3 m.
- Large green scales outlined in black. Scales on its long tail yellow and edged in black. Skin between scales black and visible. Ventral scales pale green, yellow or bluish-grey.
- Range: Native to coastal and riverine rainforests of West Africa, incl. Liberia and Côte d'Ivoire.
- Waves its head, as is generally characteristic of tree snakes.
- Mostly diurnal and mainly arboreal, but quite often descends to the ground if disturbed.
- Preys on birds, lizards, and mammals.
- Males engage in combat dances, which can last for hours.
- Mating takes places on the ground or in trees with the tails hanging down. Mating can take 10–16 hours.
- Oviparous; 6–14 eggs per clutch.

## Behaviour & Temperament

Captive Western green mambas are alert snakes that need to be kept in a large enclosure. Most of the day they are resting on a branch or climbing around in their enclosure; they can be kept in groups without any problem.

They don't like to be touched and when tailed they can get very jumpy and wild. When cornered they flatten down their necks and opening their mouths a little while rapidly tongue flicking and loud hissing, striking is rare.

## Stricken by the Light

Black mambas are 'easily the most feared animal in the bush', and have become, according to Jeremy Seal, a 'byword for serpentine hostility, aggression, speed, and virulence'. F.W. FitzSimons, Director of the Port Elizabeth Museum and Snake Park in Durban, South Africa, related many stories about both green and black mambas, labeling the latter as the textbook exhibit of 'the diabolical ingenuity of Nature', the 'Attila of Snakes' that 'is more to be feared than the very devil himself.' Notwithstanding such univocal words of warning from a fellow member of the profession, Raymond L. Ditmars [1876–1942], the famed herpetologist and reptile expert of the Bronx Zoo in the first quarter of the 1900s, opted for the green mamba as the 'whip-like and most dreaded of the serpents of Africa'.

Ditmars bears witness to the fact how also in snakes looks can deceive, portraying the mamba's slender outlines and large eyes as *imparting a particularly innocent picture* – for a snake – yet it is one of the world's most deadly serpents. 'The chief point about mambas is their alleged disposition to attack human beings with a *bewildering rush* from which there is little chance to escape,' Ditmars explains.

'Shuddery stories tell of the downward rush of a lithe form, as quick as a released cable sliding through branches of trees and bushes, a deliberate bite, then a gliding rush away.'

In the chapter titled *Mamba* of his book *Confessions of a Scientist*, 1934, Ditmars recalls an encounter with a green mamba as 'the most thrilling experience' in his laboratory film work, making scientific movies. While working one night to create the snake's natural surroundings in the studio, accidentally touching its tail with a stick, he is attacked by the mamba, its anger rising and its 'blue-green form shot at me so that I ducked to the floor'. Although seemingly the object of the mamba's wrath, Ditmars regarded 'such transition of temperament among serpents . . . [as] . . . not unusual,' ascribing it to the lighting. 'I have noticed it with specimens long captive, when taken out of doors into a genial, spring sun. I have seen reptiles we called tame take a few breaths, and a moment later flatten out and strike. The mercury lights, rich in ultra-violet, had affected the mamba like spring sunshine. So here I was, learning something about bringing a belligerent disposition to the boiling point, coupled with chain-lightning speed.

'There was now not the remotest chance of "coaxing" this particular serpent back into the fiber case. He had it in for me, and I was earnestly wishing he was back and locked up. I kept thinking of those little fangs up near his nose, like slivers of glass, and even of some of the stories of how a mamba could descend from a tree as if it were spilled out of it.

'I sat quietly on the floor and thought it over. How could I get him into the case? Had the rays of the lamp stimulated that brain to the extent that psychological wires were crossed, and the radiance indicated Africa, during the mamba breeding season? If so, I was in for an unpleasant time and would have to step lively. . . .

'My decision was to argue with him – but with a longer pole. . . . I slid backward along the floor until I reached that pole, then picked it up and walked slowly toward the mamba. He was studying my moves, as I could see by his head being lifted higher but inclining directly at me.'

[After a chase through the studio, Ditmars manages to press the snake to the floor with the help of a long pole with a hook. Grasping the mamba by the neck, and 'for a moment . . . somewhat tangled with the protesting body,' he is 'surprised to find how easy the creature was to hold. . . . Despite this creature's remarkable aptitude to reach upward as straight as a rod a distance of more than half its length, and to strike fully that distance, its neck felt thin, soft and delicate. A blow with a Malacca walking-stick would have broken it. No wonder Nature had arranged that such a fragile type should distil a venom of highly lethal potency.'

## Materia Medica
- No symptoms.
- Venom primarily neurotoxic. Potentially dangerous, but bites of humans are rare. A few reported envenomations and human deaths due to bites by this species had symptoms very similar to those caused by black mamba venom.

# ELAPS CORALLINUS

## Systematics
- Scientific name: Micrurus corallinus [Merrem, 1820].
- Synonym: Elaps corallinus [Merrem, 1820].
- Common names: Brazilian coral snake. Painted coral snake.
- Family: Elapidae.

## Biological Profile
- Medium-sized, brightly tri-coloured coral snake. Average length 65–85 cm, maximum 1 m. Head black with a posterior yellow or white band that narrows strongly dorsally [may be incomplete]. Body pattern of broad red rings separated by a series of 15–27 [usually 17–21] fairly wide black rings narrowly bordered with greenish-white. Tail with 3–8 black and alternating yellow rings. Body rather big in proportion to head and terminating in a sharp tail.
- Range: Brazil, Uruguay, NE Argentina, Paraguay.
- Habitat: Predominantly tropical deciduous and evergreen forest at low to intermediate elevations [near sea level to about 500 m], mainly in the Amazon basin.
- Nocturnal, terrestrial or burrowing in loose soil and litter, non-aggressive.
- Preys on invertebrates, lizards, worm lizards [Amphisbaena sp.], and other snakes.
- Its defensive behaviour differs from other coral snakes. It contracts its body dorso-ventrally in order to look larger than it really is.
- Oviparous; 2–15 eggs per clutch.

## Coral Snakes
The coral snakes are a large group of elapid snakes that can be divided into 2 distinct groups: New World coral snakes and Old World Calliophis snakes. There are 16 species of Old World coral snake in 3 genera [Calliophis, Hemibungarus and Sinomicrurus], and over 65 recognized species of New World coral snakes in 3 genera [Leptomicrurus, Micruroides, and Micrurus].

In some regions, the order of the bands distinguishes between the non-venomous mimics and the venomous coral snakes, inspiring some folk rhymes – 'Red and yellow, kill a fellow; red and black, friendly jack,' and 'Red and yellow, kill a fellow; red and black, venom lack' or 'If red touches yellow, you're a dead fellow [for Coral Snakes]; if red touches black, you're ok jack [for similar looking Milk Snakes].'

However, this only reliably applies to coral snakes native to North America: Micrurus fulvius [Eastern or common], Micrurus tener [Texas], and Micruroides euryxanthus [Arizona], found in the southern and eastern United States.

## Relationship with Rain
Micrurus corallinus occurs mainly in the Serra do Mar region, SE Brazil, which is characterized by *abundant rainfall* throughout the year.

In Brazil, one most often comes across juvenile M. corallinus in the late rainy season and early dry season, esp. in March and April. Adult males and females can be spotted during all months of the year, although they are less common in the dry [April–September] than in the rainy seasons [October–March]. The frequency of capture of adult males peaks in October, whereas adult females show a peak in frequency in November.

Reproduction in Micrurus corallinus seems to be highly seasonal, with mating and vitellogenesis occurring at the onset of the *rainy season*, oviposition in mid rainy season, and hatching at the end of the rainy season and early dry season.

Amphisbaena microcephala [syn. Lepostemon microcephalum; smallhead worm lizard] is the predominant prey of both juvenile and mature M. corallinus. From years of research there is a unique relationship between coral snakes, fossorial amphisbaenians and caecilians emerging. [Caecilians are tropical, burrowing, slender-bodied, limbless amphibians resembling worms, eels or snakes.] Many amphisbaenians and caecilians are highly fossorial and live for the most part underground, rising to the surface after heavy rains where they feed on a diverse range of prey. When amphisbaenians and caecilians mobilise *after heavy rainfall*, individual Micrurus spp. have been found to forage for and capture these preys either in their underground shelters or on the ground. Coral snakes appear adept at finding the subterranean galleries built by amphisbaenians and do so by following signals left on the terrestrial surface. These signals [possibly chemical tracks] are likely to be more evident in the soil during *rainy periods* [when amphisbaenians move more frequently to the surface], and possibly incite the foraging activity of Micrurus spp. Recent studies on activity patterns are suggesting that environmental triggers such as higher temperatures and conditions of humidity may correlate directly with increased activity patterns in Micrurus spp. [www.fieldherpforum.com]

## MATERIA MEDICA ELAPS CORALLINUS

### Sources
1 Proving Mure [France–Brazil]. 'several provers and clinical confirmations', 3c trit.; *c.* 1845.
2 Proving Lippe [USA], 1 female prover, 4th dil.; *c.* 1859.
3 Clinical observations, in Hering.
4 Self-experimentation Reinhard Flick [Austria], 30x; 1991.
5 Clinical observations Boger [USA].
6 Clinical observations Mangialavori [Italy].
7 Clinical observations Farokh Master [India].
8 Clinical observations Sadhana Thakkar [USA].
9 Degroote, Dream Repertory.
10 Synthesis Repertory Treasure Edition 2009.
11 Van Zandvoort's Complete 2013 Repertory.
12 Kent's Repertory.
13 Effects of bite; clinical manifestations.

## Mind

∞ Reveries in daytime, delusion receiving blows.[1]

∞ Delusion hearing someone speak; hears talking without comprehending.[1]

∞ Absence of mind.[1]

∞ Strange illusion of hearing; hears whistling and ringing and rises to see where it is.[1]

∞ Desire to strike and pick a quarrel.[1]

∞ Desire to go to the country and play about in the grass. Plans about traveling.[1]

∞ Desire to be alone; remains for days in corner of anti-chamber. Retires to a distant room to work.[1]

∞ Wants to withdraw and to be left alone.[4]

∞ Depression of spirits; desire to be in a deep cavern, where nobody can be seen.[1]

∞ Wants to leave house at moment when she is going to bed.[1]

∞ Strong aversion to light; prefers to be in the dark.[1]

∞ Excessive horror of rain.[1]

∞ Fretful about herself, does not want to be spoken to.[2]

∞ Fear of being alone due to feeling that something would happen or that rowdies [roughnecks, ruffians, thugs] would break into the house.[2]

∞ Delusion being neglected.[6]

∞ Delusion / anxiety being friendless.[9]

∞ Forsaken feeling.[6]

∞ Jealousy.[6]

∞ Bashful timidity.[6]

∞ Intense rage as if blood boils, as if she must shriek loud. Desire to break things, destroy property, yell, quarrel.[8]

∞ Peacemaker between parents.[9]

∞ Affectionate. Craves attention.[9]

∞ Children imitating adults – parents, teachers.[9]

∞ Benevolence.[9]

∞ Making fun >.[9]

∞ Witty.[9]

∞ Loves cats.[9]

∞ Ambition, hard worker.[9]

∞ Answers, says 'I know everything'. Smart answers. Delusions: Knowing everything. Others seeing his confusion. Overestimation of self; exaggerated opinion of oneself; boasting. Loud-mouthed boasting; big mouth, small heart. Squandering. Superiority.[9]

∞ Pedantic, hair-splitting, schoolish. Defiance, with an air of triumph.[9]

∞ Aphasia, ability to speak but comprehension of speech lost.[10]

∞ Fears: Being alone, during menses. Cats. Rain. Robbers. Snakes. Solitude.[10]

∞ Fears: Apoplexy. Crowds. Disease, being incurable. High places.[11]

∞ Difficulty expressing herself when speaking; cannot think of the words; cannot think of the names of the things she looks at. [Effects of Elaps CM, observed by Berridge]

∞ Enormous irritability, feeling as if everything is too much; can't stand it, violent outbursts of anger, every trifle that does not fit irritates extremely.[4]

∞ 'Strong attitude of having to defend myself against threat and attacks from the outside. This aggressive attitude is directed mainly against my wife, a mixture of impulses to fight or to flee, anxiety, aggression and hatred mingled together. The best way to describe it is as a feeling of wanting to jump out of my own skin. I feel myself standing with my back to the wall and cannot bear to look into people's eyes.'[4]
∞ Highly creative persons interested in art, nature, aesthetics, etc. often using creativity as a tool to attract attention.[7]
∞ Globetrotters, like Marco Polo or Captain Cook, persons who love to walk, travel and explore the world and nature. Others are occupied with family responsibilities and others are preoccupied with a love for traveling to any countryside if given the opportunity.[7]
∞ Unwanted by mother; orphaned feeling, independent at an early age. Different from siblings and family members in opinions, taste, hobbies and world view. Instead of feeling wronged like Lachesis and Naja, feel separate, ignored, unrecognized, unappreciated, disrespected, stepped on, pushed out of the way. Aversion to be domesticated, wanting to be free and independent.[8]
∞ Slowness while eating.[9]

## Dreams
∞ Abyss, near an.[9]
∞ Accused falsely, wrongly.[9]
∞ Beating someone in face; from indignation; in self-defence.[9]
∞ Betrayal.[6]
∞ Burying a dead person and digging about in his wounds with a knife; following by great remorse and a flood of tears.[1]
∞ Cats. Red-haired cats.[9]
∞ Cheated, being.[9]
∞ Countryside, enjoying, walking.[9]
∞ Danger of flooding through dike break.[9]
∞ Danger from water.[9]
∞ Dead persons.[1] Kissing dead people.[1]
∞ Dominated, being.[9]
∞ Drowned person with wide open eyes.[9]
∞ Events of the day.[1]
∞ Excelling in swimming.[9]
∞ Falling in pits where feet get entangled.[1] Falling into an abyss.[12]
∞ Fighting with a man condemned to the galleys.[1]
∞ Foggy weather.[9]
∞ Forsaken, being or feeling; in a group; overlooked, not being offered something.[9]
∞ Grief, weeping.[9]
∞ Ill-used like Cinderella; has to work whole others can amuse themselves.[9]
∞ Kidnapped, being.[9]
∞ Privacy, infringed.[9]
∞ Proud, being.[9]

∞ Pursued by robbers.[9]
∞ Rain, hard.[9]
∞ Remorse.[9]
∞ Resurrection during funeral.[9]
∞ Saving somebody out of water.[9]
∞ Selected as fashion model.[9]
∞ Sexual obtrusiveness.[9]
∞ Swimming against the current.[9]
∞ Threatened, being; with knives; by malicious men; by terrorists.[9]
∞ Times of war, being surrounded by 2 enemy armies in a neutral country.[4]
∞ Underground corridor, garage, room.[9]
∞ Walking sideways.[1]
∞ Walking underwater.[9]

## Generals

∞ Right side more affected.[1] Right side feels paralysed, weak or insensible.[5]
∞ Desire for cold water and ice. Unquenchable thirst. Very thirsty; desire for milk.[1]
∞ Fruit and cold drinks lie in stomach like ice.[1]
∞ Aversion to meat, bananas, and particularly bread[1]; tomatoes and vegetables[6].
∞ Desire for oranges, acids, salads, and esp. for sour beef. Eats nothing but oranges.[1]
∞ Desire for sweetened buttermilk.[3] Marked desire for pork.[4]
∞ Loathing of food, acidity after every mouthful of food. Or is hungry but unable to eat [due to continual vomiting].[1]
∞ Drowsy the whole day, but sleepless nights.[1]
∞ Discharges bloody, dark blood, blackish.[1]
∞ Profuse cold sweat all over body.[1]
∞ Clothing as if too tight, loosening it >.[6]
∞ Before menses <.[6]
∞ Perspiration from excitement.[9]
∞ Lying on abdomen >.[9]
∞ Great agility of movement.[9]
∞ In mountains >.[9]
∞ Likes swimming with head above water surface.[9]
∞ Static electricity shock on touching anything.[9]

## Sensations

∞ Brain as if loose & pain in vertex and nausea, cannot hold head still.[2]
∞ Weight in right parietal region and pain which penetrates to nape of the neck.[1]
∞ Foreign body in right temple.[1]
∞ Long and white filaments floating before eyes. On closing eyes, everything looks red, dotted with black points.[1]
∞ Greyish veil before eyes, like a cloud, which becomes thicker; at first it is of the size of a penny, and spreads until finally it covers the whole field of vision.[1]

∞ Can scarcely tell light from dark; everything seems white, even at night.[3]
∞ Objects seem to be moving to and fro before the eyes.[12]
∞ Eyeballs as if sticky under lids and as if rough.[3]
∞ Continual buzzing as from a fly in ear.[1]
∞ Pressive constriction in throat.[1]
∞ Increased awareness of throat, it feels narrow, & increased disposition to swallow, at same time oppression in chest, with a bit of dyspnoea, especially when walking upstairs.[4]
∞ Food descends in oesophagus as if turned round like a screw. At other times soup falls heavily and precipitately, as if through a metallic tube into stomach, which trembles violently.[1]
∞ Stoppage in oesophagus after eating, as if a sponge had lodged there.[1]
∞ Weight at stomach after eating.[1]
∞ Liquid as if poured into abdomen through a valved tube.[1]
∞ Intestines as if twisted and strung together with a cord.[1]
∞ Great weight at uterus when rising, < during a walk.[1]
∞ Sensation in chest and at sternum as if pleurae would be torn off, and as if lungs would be separated from each other by force.[1]
∞ Tearing pain, as if lungs were forced apart. Lungs as if forcibly separated.[10]
∞ Chest as if cold inside after drinking.[1]
∞ Thorax as if constricted by a corset.[1]
∞ Heart as if swollen, chest as if too narrow.[9]
∞ Heart as if being torn out.[5]
∞ Throbbing at regular intervals in nape of neck, like ticking of a clock.[1]
∞ Cerebellum as if settling downwards, causing pressing pain in nape of neck.[1]
∞ Iron bar as if pressing on lumbar region.[1]
∞ Right hand as if paralysed.[1]
∞ Knee joints as if stiff and sprained.[1]
∞ Something as if rising and descending in left tibia.[1]

## Locals
∞ Dizziness < during menses.[12]
∞ Congestion head during menses; < stooping.[12]
∞ Violent headache if desire for food is not satisfied at once.[1]
∞ Pain occiput < mental exertion.[10]
∞ Pain occiput when lying on back.[9]
∞ Holds head with hands when coughing.[9]
∞ Violent throbbing of external carotid. Horrid pains when inclining head backwards; less when inclining it forwards. Tension in nape of the neck.[1]
∞ Desire to close eyes as in fever.[1]
∞ Dryness/burning eyes morning on waking.[12]
∞ Eyes sensitive to cold water.[12]
∞ Constant deafness.[1]
∞ Nasal discharge smelling like fish brine, as of herring pickle, esp. on blowing nose.[12]
∞ Coryza when exposed to least current of air; sneezing.[1]

∞ Obstruction nose, nose stopped up, in wet weather.[12]
∞ Epistaxis: sudden, profuse, while walking; after a blow. Nose bleeds when violently blown [in nasal catarrh].[3]
∞ Salivation while talking.[9]
∞ Choking throat < clothing external throat.[10]
∞ Must drink in order to swallow.[10]
∞ Indigestion after drinking ice water; after fruit.[10]
∞ Pain anus in the act of sitting down and when rising from sitting.[9]
∞ Urging to urinate after urination. Chill during start of urination.[9]
∞ Something as if bursting in womb, followed by a continuous stream of dark-coloured blood, on attempting to urinate; flow very profuse, venous, and containing some clots.[3]
∞ Itching of breasts during pregnancy.[9]
∞ Spitting of black blood clot, & painful tearing as if proceeding from heart. Almost constant cough.[1]
∞ Tearing pain in heart region during cough.[12]
∞ Palpitations from wine.[10]
∞ Heart complaints accompanied by dizziness.[9]
∞ Cannot bear draft of air on nape of neck, cervical region.[9]
∞ Impelled to crack nape of neck/cervical region by moving head sideways.[9]
∞ Violent pains in lumbar region, like a band extending to uterus.[1]
∞ Pain lumbar region ext. to abdomen; pain > walking.[9]
∞ Sciatica pain during menses.[9]
∞ Itching urticaria on legs and feet after showering.[9]

## Clinical Manifestations

Venom shows a high neurotoxicity associated with pre- and post-synaptic toxins, inducing neuromuscular dysfunction and diaphragm paralysis, which may result in death. Coral snake venom has little enzymatic activity or necrotic potential compared with true vipers and pit vipers.

Pain and swelling may be minimal or absent and are often transitory. The absence of local symptoms and signs may erroneously suggest a dry bite, producing a false sense of security for both victim and clinician. Weakness of the bitten extremity may become evident within several hours. Systemic neuro-muscular manifestations may be delayed for 12 h and include weakness and lethargy; altered sensorium, including euphoria and drowsiness; cranial nerve palsies causing ptosis, diplopia, blurred vision, dysarthria, and dysphagia; increased salivation; muscle flaccidity; and respiratory distress or failure.

Once the neurotoxic venom effects manifest, they are difficult to reverse and may last 3 to 6 days. Untreated patients may die of respiratory failure. Mechanical ventilation may be necessary. [Merck Manual Online]

Micrurus venoms are known to possess neurotoxic properties. In most symptomatic cases neuromuscular paralysis is the most prominent and is caused by postsynaptic motor end-plate blockage of acetylcholine receptors, which produces *similar effects to those seen in myasthenia gravis and curare poisoning*. This prevents nerves from stimulating muscle contraction and leads to paralysis.

Similar actions are described for other Elapidae venoms, such as Naja and Bungarus spp.

# CASES

**Case 1**
'Case SD 2832

'Recurring problems for 2 years after her daughter was born; has irritation on the inside of the thigh and had treatment from her GP for fungal problem; if uses the cream the irritation goes. Patient was wearing black and red and wears black, white and red a lot. Problem with right ear for 2 years painful worse from touch. Two years ago had surgery on the jaw since then does not breath properly through the nose GP gave Beconase, which did help – the right nostril is blocked. Had her bottom jaw moved forward because of problems with roof of the mouth she did have pain in the ear before jaw surgery and it may have improved it this was because her bottom jaw stopped growing at the age of ten.

'The last 2 summers keeps coming out in boils gets them all year round every 4/6 weeks under the arms in the groin vagina face etc. Now they are draining her emotionally. They come up with a huge white head and start as a hot lump they seem to appear at mid cycle and last until her period comes which is 10 days. They leave a purple scar on her face. Acne as a teenager on her chin and in the first 3 months of each pregnancy. No migraines until pregnant but did have them during both pregnancy and they continued after her daughter was born. Headache no visual disturbances. Nausea has to go to bed in a dark room and they can last up to 2 days used to take Migraleve. Head worse smoking. Wakes up with headache.

'Family history Mother migraines varicose veins died heart attack, palpitations and terrible menopausal problems. Father diabetic shock of sons death gangrene 76. Past history: Age 4 severely burnt was hospitalised for 3 months and still has scarring on the abdomen and thighs used to be very shy but is not now. As a child people used to stare.

'Food: Loves aubergines [3] sweets [2] seafood [2].

'Psyche: Is terribly moody [3], becoming more intolerant as gets older. Takes on family problems from extended family, they affect her badly; her brothers tend to phone her. Has a lot of anger towards her husband and niece. Was married before; most of the time became violent. 21 – first married; 26 – separated; 31 – second marriage. Very strict with children; was bought up strictly herself. Shout and screams about things at times. Husband is the opposite to her.

Feels angry if does not get enough time with husband. Hates housework but has to have it tidy. Suppressed by her father; her parents were upset by the stigma of her divorce. Used to worry a lot about what people thought about her. At 26 realised she had to change and take control of her life. Her second husband had an affair for 1.5 years was when her son was young went to counselling because of it. Was unable to forget about it. Things were so bad that they did not talk at all.

'Fears: Heights [3], cannot stand the sea, did not learn to swim until age 36, Snakes [3]. Determined; husband says thinks she is always right. Cynical never sees the best in people at first; about herself; stems from her father; he did not think that women should be educated.

March 96 Rx Elaps 30/1xD [once daily].

April 96 No spots or boils; emotionally terrible this month. Rx Elaps 30/1xD.

May 96 Feeling wonderful no spots or boils the longest she has been for 2 years without. Less moody, not blowing her top, been less irritable, feels happier. More assertive with her husband and her niece. She knew all about coral snakes and their imitations, cannot stand to watch sidewinders. Rx Elaps 30/1xD.

June 96 OK until last week had lump under right arm again. More in control emotionally; she and her husband think wonderful. Rx Elaps 50/1xD.

8/96 Husband thinks he is living with another woman. Menses are still a problem; every other one comes too soon, and they are also heavier. Both mother and grandmother had early menopauses. Rx Elaps 200/1xW.

[Case Michael Thompson, from Thompson's Snakes; RefWorks]

## Case 2
Initial Visit: March 10, 1991
Female. Age 23.

She is a single mother who had brought her son in earlier for eczema and behavioural problems. The son responded nicely to Sulphur.

She is an attractive, mild-mannered blonde woman of medium build and fair complexion who has an air of naiveté or vulnerability.

Chief Complaint: Allergies [2], mostly affecting her nose.

Cold air [2] or a change of temperature [2] hurts the inside of her nose.

There's pain behind her eyes, a sharp pain [2].

Has a stuffy nose with nasal obstruction, which is worse when she's lying down [2].

Suffers from sneezing, watery eyes, and an itchy throat [2], which are worse when she's around cats [2] and damp places [2].

Has always had allergies. She had sneezing, stuffiness, and weepy eyes even as a baby.

Had asthma once.

Her symptoms were worse with pregnancy and she has taken a lot of anti-histamines.

Can get irritable and grouchy. Things can drive her 'nuts' and she loses patience. At other times she can be depressed and serious.

Poor self-confidence.

Very indecisive and can't decide where to go to school.

Wants a serious relationship in order to have more children. She used to live with her child's father in Hawaii [he is a native there]. He started bossing her around. He was violent, very physically violent, and took drugs. He beat her a lot. She did not fight back. She knew the abuse was wrong but did not leave. She felt lonely. To end the relationship she had her friend call the police. She got away and came back to California. She would like her son to see his father, but she is afraid if she goes to Hawaii this man will talk her into staying and she won't be able to get away.

She is not assertive. Internalizes instead. Gets angry with herself because she doesn't fight back.

She couldn't disagree with her father. Never got anywhere with him. Can't say no to men. As a teenager it was horrible for her, with ongoing fights with her father. When she was angry she wouldn't speak to him. He thought she was a devil worshipper.

She was molested by her uncle.

She was raped by a baby sitter. She wants to kill this person and is absorbed with a murder plan. She wants it to be the most painful way possible.

Keeps all her feelings inside.

Wants to be alone when she's depressed.

Has low-to-average sexual interest, which increases with good conversation.

Deep sleeper. Sleeps on her abdomen [2] and clenches her jaw at night [2]. Gets a stiff neck and headache from the clenching [1].

Fears snakes [3]. She tapes together the pages in her biology book that show pictures of snakes, so she won't see them by accident. Seeing a picture of a snake makes her clench her teeth. Used to have nightmares of snakes and still has recurring dreams of snakes.

Fears spiders [2] and insects [2].

Claustrophobic [2].

Fears being attacked [3]. Starts to perspire walking to her car at night. Needs to look in the back seat for attackers. [She lives in a small town where such attacks are extremely rare.]

She gets chilly [2] when it's cold.

Her feet perspire [2].

Always thirsty [3], for juice and tea, and has dry, chapped lips [2].

Her teeth are sensitive; worse in the cold [2].

Her ears hurt in the cold [2].

Regular menses.

[Case Eric Sommermann, IFH 1993; RefWorks]

# HEMACHATUS HAEMACHATUS

## Systematics
- Scientific name: Hemachatus haemachatus [Bonnaterre, 1790].
- Synonyms: Aspidelaps haemachates [Jan, 1859]. Naia capensis [Smith, 1826]. Naja haemachates [Schlegel, 1837]. Sepedon haemachatus [Merrem, 1820].
- Common names: Rinkhals. Ringhals.
- Family: Elapidae.

## Biological Profile
- Medium-sized, stocky, hooded elapid with short, pointy head and highly modified fangs to defensively eject or spit venom at the eyes of adversaries. Has keeled scales [smooth in Naja spp. and other elapids]. Average length 1 m, maximum 1.5 m.
- Body colour may vary but is usually a spotted black to brown with yellow to white crossbars with 2–3 large bands on throat. Head rather broad, flattened, not distinct from neck; snout obtusely pointed.
- Fangs fitted out with spiral grooves, which function as riflings [spiral grooves] in a gun barrel, forcing a spin on the emerging liquid and enhancing accuracy.
- Has to rear up in order to spray its venom, unlike spitting cobras, which can spray venom from the ground without rearing up.
- Range: Southern Africa.
- Habitat: Grassland areas, open country with ample rainfall. Also found in swamps or marshy fields, moist lowlands and wetlands.
- Primarily diurnal.
- Inactive during cold temperatures.
- Preys on frogs, toads, rodents, birds and their eggs, lizards and other snakes. Will raid chicken runs; often found near homesteads in search of prey or water.
- Indiscriminate feeder; will eat food rejected by other species, leading to obesity in captivity.
- Males engage in dominance combats.
- Territorial during the mating season.
- Ovoviviparous; 20–35 live young per brood.
- When threatened it is very quick to disappear down a hole but if cornered it will stand its ground, form a hood and is quick to spit, throwing the head forward when doing so.
- Name derived from Dutch 'ring hals', ringed neck.

## Intimidating & Pretending
Similar to the European grass snake [Natrix natrix], the American hognose snakes [Heterodon], the Egyptian cobra [Naja haje] and a few other cobras, the rinkhals has the ability to sham death. If presented with no possibility to flee, and faced with a predator unfazed by its spitting, it will roll over on its back melodramatically, open its mouth and let the tongue hang out, all this to discourage whoever may be hovering over it. Soon after the assumed predator has walked away, the animal will roll over on its belly and slide carelessly away. Like in the other

species, death feigning in the rinkhals comes at the end of a repertoire of other defensive activities, including intimidation, spitting, and odour production. [See above, Feigning death]

## Body Temperature Regulation

'All snakes are ectothermic, and their body temperature is dependent on their surroundings. They have no internal temperature-regulating method and succumb if exposed to extremes of below 7°C [44.6°F] or above 38°C [100.4°F] for any length of time. Most snakes prefer a range of 20°–32°C [68°–89.6°F]. Hemachatus haemachatus displays a relatively wide thermal tolerance. They are highly effective thermoregulators and are able to raise their body temperature rapidly, even when the ambient temperature is low.

'Under some circumstances, they select low body temperatures – so low that Alexander refers to them as 'hypothermic'. Hypothermic snakes use only a fraction of the energy of 'normothermic' snakes to stay alive, so there is a clear benefit for snakes to cool themselves down. Under other circumstances, such as when radiant heat is available, rinkhals selects body temperatures that are more typical of snakes but are at the upper limit of 'normality' for snakes [32°C; 89.6°F].

'Alexander has observed specimens basking in the sun with spread hood to increase surface area. Alexander explains that it has to do with the costs and benefits of low and high body temperatures: snakes save energy when cool but are better at defending themselves or making a hasty retreat when their body temperature is high. Snakes, including rinkhals, hibernate, or more accurately ruminate, during cold winter months. In the temperate areas such as South Africa, they hibernate intermittently by retiring during the cold spells. In the sunny days between cold fronts, they come out of their holes to bask in the sun between 10 a.m. and 3 p.m. They stay right at the entrance of the hole, and retreat at any sign of danger, as they cannot lift their body temperature sufficiently to be able to move actively.

'They do not eat while ruminating, as they cannot digest prey if their body temperature is below 20°C [68°F]. A substantial reserve of body fat is stored before the onset of cold to see them through these long periods without food. Nevertheless, they emerge thin and emaciated when the hibernation is over.' [Lize de la Rouvière]

# MATERIA MEDICA HEMACHATUS HAEMACHATUS

## Sources
1 Proving Lize de la Rouvière and Jodi Cahill [South Africa], 24 provers [14 females, 10 males], 30c; c. 2007.
2 Effects of bite; clinical manifestations.
3 Effects of bite; pains on any change of weather.

## Mind

∞ Depression in morning, elation in evening.
∞ Happy, positive and enthusiastic. Sense of inner joy.
∞ Great activity mentally and physically until late in night.
∞ Alert, focused, productive, purposeful **or**:
∞ Forgetful, foggy, absent-minded.
∞ Mistakes in speaking; mixes up words, uses wrong words.
∞ Delusion as if looking through someone else's vision while driving car in morning.
∞ Delusion of being watched, as if others could look into one's mind or soul.
∞ Delusions: not being appreciated; laughed and mocked at; neglected; persecuted; trapped.
∞ Absorbing, picking up mood from others [3 pr.].
∞ Anxiety as if something bad were going to happen [5 pr.].
∞ Empty and sad, as if having lost or missing someone or something.
∞ Sadness from disappointed love; about past events.
∞ Heightened sense of danger on the roads during rainy weather.
∞ Frustration and anxiety from interruption of routines.
∞ Avoids reality and responsibilities; unconcerned and disinterested.
∞ Awkwardness; stumbling, tripping, bumping, knocking, dropping things.
∞ Feels home to be the safest place.
∞ Great sensitivity to noise, < crowds, > solitude.
∞ Takes things really personally and takes offence easily.
∞ Scolding others, aware of short fuse but can't help shouting; feels bad about it but doesn't apologise.
∞ *Extreme irritation* regarding what is felt to be incompetence, inefficiency, stupidity etc. [see below].

## Dreams

∞ Accusations.
∞ Attacked, being.
∞ Battles.
∞ Body deformed.
∞ Cats.
∞ Chased and pursued.
∞ Chased by bears; dinosaurs; people; police.
∞ Danger; friends in danger; escaping from danger; protecting others from danger.
∞ Deceit.
∞ Embarrassment.
∞ Erotic, sex with 2 women.
∞ Fights.
∞ Hiding.
∞ Homosexuality.
∞ Journeys by water.
∞ Obese, being.

∞ Prostitutes.
∞ Rape.
∞ Sexual.
∞ Ships.
∞ Snakes.
∞ Spiders, huge.
∞ Stuck.

## Generals
∞ Morning on waking < – no energy, difficulty waking up, bad mood, headache, runny nose, pallor, sore throat, stomach pain, abdominal bloating, backache, stiffness [> stretching].
∞ Tired, listless, drained, lethargic; can't get out of bed.
∞ Tired feeling > exercise.
∞ Evening between 5 and 7 p.m. <.
∞ Heat of sun < – vertigo, occipital headache, general.
∞ Cold, rainy weather <.
∞ Great thirst [9 pr.], for cold water [3 pr.]; & dryness mouth [2 pr.]; at night.
∞ Craving for black coffee; oily food; red meat; red wine; salty, savoury things; seafood pasta; sweets [chocolate]; yoghurt.
∞ Aversion to vegetables. Fruit = stomach pain, indigestion.
∞ Pain burning.

## Sensations
∞ Body and limbs as if light.
∞ Feeling of lightness, as if wading through water or through really thick air or clouds.
∞ Head as if made of feathers [dizzy feeling], < sun heat, > cold water.
∞ Head as if in cloud on waking, & thirst for ice cold water.
∞ Head as if wrapped in cotton wool or as if submerged.
∞ Head as if gradually and slowly inflating like a balloon, > closing eyes.
∞ Headache as if having a brick on head.
∞ Nail driven in left temple.
∞ Base of occiput as if heavy.
∞ Needles poking in eyes from light.
∞ Eyes puffy on waking, as if bags filled with water under eyes, & face feeling as if bloated.
∞ Eyes heavy, as if held down by weights.
∞ Nose as if heavy, during slight dizziness.
∞ Tip of nose as if numb, extending to forehead.
∞ Face as if bloated, & swelling under eyes, in morning on waking.
∞ Sand in mouth.
∞ Tongue as if numb, > sips of cold water.
∞ Something stuck on root of tongue that can't be swallowed.
∞ String in back of throat that can't be swallowed.
∞ Ball stuck in left side of throat.

∞ Food as if sitting in throat in chunks.
∞ Nausea as if food were sitting in throat in chunks.
∞ Stomach as if hollow, intestines as if squeezed.
∞ Huge hole in pit of stomach.
∞ Something hard and heavy pressing into stomach [epigastric area].
∞ Hot burning coals in abdomen 10 minutes after eating.
∞ Something stuck in left iliac fossa.
∞ Anus as if open and cold after passing stool.
∞ Pressing down / bearing down in uterus & heavy flow of darkish red blood.
∞ Steel pole as if stuck up into uterus.
∞ Left breast as if squashed in a vice.
∞ Rope around chest that is being tightened, constricting breathing.
∞ Fullness behind sternum.
∞ Hard ball pressing against left calf muscles, < touch, > standing upright.
∞ Muscles as if frozen in morning on waking, > coffee and stretching.
∞ Body heavy on rising as if upper and lower limbs are weighted down by lead, > stretching, < lying down.

## Locals
∞ Dizziness when getting up or moving quickly [4 pr.], > closing eyes.
∞ Dizziness while driving car, < heat of sun, > cold water.
∞ Dizziness by quick movement of head.
∞ Slight light-headedness from drinking fizzy drinks.
∞ Headache on waking in morning as if head were hit by a blunt object; > application of ice to neck and black coffee.
∞ Headache < bending head forward, > coffee, cold drinks, darkness.
∞ Occipital headache radiating to both temples & slight tinnitus, < noise, > lying down and cold water.
∞ Occipital headache & aversion to tobacco smoke.
∞ Occipital throbbing headache < heat of sun.
∞ Sharp pain radiating up back of head from protuberances of the occipital bone.
∞ Eyes extremely sensitive to slightest amount of light, > covering eyes and cold water.
∞ Eyes very sensitive to fluorescent lights.
∞ Photophobia during headache.
∞ Blowing nose = blocking of ears, coughing, loss of urine.
∞ Heartburn, burning rising up in throat, after eating, > pressure.
∞ Nausea from smell of tobacco.
∞ Abdomen very tender to touch, bruised feeling.
∞ Urging to pass stool ineffectual or absent.
∞ Involuntary urination < cough, motion, sneezing.
∞ Menstrual blood dark red, dark brown, almost black.
∞ Pain in left breast, < jar, < exhaling, > hot water, > being still.
∞ Lumbar backache < leaning forward, lifting, rising from sitting, > sitting.

## Spitting it Out

'Irritability was one of the most characteristic symptoms in this proving. Fourteen provers experienced marked irritability. This irritability was mainly directed towards people, accompanied by feelings that others were inefficient. Provers became aware of the increased use of foul language and insults. Provers experienced feelings of impatience and short tempers. In most cases this anger was not externalised, but rather internalised with the prover retreating away from society into their safe place.' Symptoms were expressed thus:

∞ Felt irritable with whoever, but held back; mustn't spew it on others.
∞ Irritability causes me to be sarcastic.
∞ Shouting at everyone. Irritable at night.
∞ Very argumentative.
∞ Got into huge debate with someone about something stupid and insignificant.
∞ Taking things really personally and taking offence readily.
∞ Hitting wall out of irritation.
∞ Rushed irritated feeling toward co-workers, taking frustration out on them.
∞ Irritable when asked stupid questions.
∞ Irritated by the same stupid comments made by the same people.
∞ Irritated when people are useless.
∞ Irritated with inefficiencies and bad service.
∞ Irritability after 13:00, esp. with people and children not part of my immediate family, who are in my space.
∞ Frustrated with laxness of others.
∞ Low tolerance and snappy; feeling that people 'just don't get it'.
∞ Borderline road rage, especially to incompetent slow drivers.
∞ Annoyance with things 'so poorly planned'.
∞ Deep irritation welling up at inconsiderate drivers and family's noisy, distracting antics.
∞ Irritated by 'boorish comments' of others, causing one to withdraw to room.
∞ Feeling angry at selfishness of people and need to let them know.
∞ Exploding and incensed when not being believed, followed by trading insults.
∞ Almost immediate fight with father, as he is extremely critical and tries to correct me, again and again.
∞ Want to rip someone's head off.
∞ Enraged by cutting remarks; must concentrate to swallow anger; urge to punch her in the face.
∞ Mean things to say are just coming out of mouth.
∞ Frustrated when people interrupt routine, hate it.
∞ Sick of customers, draining and irritating me; cannot deal with people questioning me about everything.
∞ 'After what seems like an eternity of disrupting queries from my parents, there is peace.'
∞ 'Parents give me annoying little chores to do.'

## Extremities

'There was marked muscle tension throughout the proving, especially in the neck, shoulders and calves affecting mainly the left side. There was a general feeling of weakness, tiredness and heaviness in the limbs. A vast majority of provers experienced painful joints especially those of the wrist and fingers. The joint pain was described as sharp, electrical and stabbing; another described it as a bruised feeling. The joint pain was also aggravated by motion. The limbs were itchy and dry in many of the provers and were ameliorated by the cold and by scratching. They were hot to touch and aggravated by heat and covering. One prover in particular had exceedingly hot feet, especially in the morning and seemed to be ameliorated by having wind on them or being exposed to cold air. It is also noted that there were blisters and eruptions experienced. One prover had a peculiar sensation of their limbs feeling light and floating. An observation was also made of increased nail growth.' [Jodi Cahill]

## Clinical Manifestations

Venom both cytotoxic and neurotoxic. Effects not as potent as those of true cobras [genus Naja]. Actual bites from Hemachatus are fairly rare, and deaths in modern times are so far unheard of. Local symptoms of swelling/bruising is reported in about 25% of cases. General symptoms of drowsiness, nausea, vomiting, violent abdominal pain or cramps and vertigo often occur, as does a mild pyrexia reaction.

Neurotoxic symptoms may include solely diplopia and dyspnoea. Ophthalmia has been reported but has not caused as severe complications as in some of the spitters in the genus Naja [especially N. nigricollis and N. mossambica].

'FitzSimons described immediate local tingling and burning, followed within half a minute by tightness of throat, paralysis of tongue and vocal cords, nausea, blurring of vision, weakness of the arms and legs and, 2 minutes later, unconsciousness that lasted for 4 hours. When he recovered consciousness, he noticed chest tightness, dyspnoea, blurred vision, and vomiting.' [Meier & White, 1995]

Venom in the eyes causes conjunctivitis, extensive chemosis, prolonged corneal oedema, corneal cloudiness, marked miosis, and blindness [usually temporary].

## Effects of Bite – Pains on Any Change of Weather

'We were told here that a colonist had been bitten in the foot some time before by a serpent, of the species called Ringhals [or Ringneck] as he was walking along in the grass barefoot, as is the custom here, in default of shoes and stockings, which the peasants seldom wear, except when they go up to Cape Town or to church.

'I informed myself accurately of the symptoms produced by the bite. It seems the man was several miles distant from home when he met with this accident. He then immediately dispatched his slave to his house to bring him a horse with all speed, on which he went home, after having bound up his leg tight, in order to prevent the poison from spreading upwards.

'On his return home he grew so sleepy that his wife could not, without great difficulty, keep him awake. He also became quite blind in an instant and remained so for the space of a fortnight. His leg was swelled to such a degree that the flesh covered the bandage over, like a sheath, insomuch that it could not easily be removed. An incision was made round the wound with a knife, and the foot washed with salt water.

'He drank new milk copiously and that to the quantity of several pails-full in a night, but cast it all up again. After this the serpent-stone was applied to the wound. By means of this he gradually recovered; but still, though it is now several years since the accident happened, he has pains in the part on any change of weather, and at times the wound breaks completely out again.' [Thunberg, An account of the Cape of Good Hope; 1795]

# MATICORA BIVIRGATA

## Systematics
- Scientific name: Calliophis bivirgatus [Boie, 1827].
- Synonyms: Elaps bivirgatus [Boie, 1827]. Maticora bivirgata [Stejneger, 1922].
- Common name: Blue Malaysian coral snake. Long-glanded blue coral snake.
- Family: Elapidae.

## Biological Profile
- Medium-sized, slender, semi-fossorial coral snake, dark iridescent blue or black, with large bluish-white stripe on each flank. Head, belly and tail bright coral red. Average length 1.4 m; maximum 1.8 m.
- Range: Indonesia, Malaysia, Singapore, Thailand.
- Habitat: Found in leaf litter of primary and secondary forests.
- Nocturnal, but may be diurnal on rainy and cloudy days. Emerges early to mid-morning when night-time rain has made the leaf litter wet.
- Terrestrial.
- Preys on lizards, birds and esp. on fast-moving, venomous snakes [incl. kraits and young king cobras] that have both a high likelihood of prey escape but also the potential for lethal retaliatory actions, representing significant danger to the predator itself.
- Oviparous.
- Maxillary venom glands extend one quarter of the snake's body length and nestle within the rib cavity.
- Three recognized subspecies [flaviceps, bivirgatus, tetrataenius].

## Stuck in Contraction
Venom produces spastic paralysis, in contrast to the flaccid paralysis typically produced by neurotoxic snake venoms. According to Bryan Frey, the venom "turns on all the nerves of their fast-moving prey at one time, almost instantly resulting in a frozen state." The venom's mechanism of action resembles that of cone snail and scorpion venoms. It works by preventing nerves from turning off their sodium channels, keeping the nerves firing continuously, thereby preventing muscles to go back to the resting state. The net effect is that muscles are stuck

in the contracted activated state, fully tensing the muscles in a tetanus-like spasm, instead of the typical elapid effect of being stuck in the non-contracted resting state. [Yang, 2016]

## Materia Medica
- No symptoms.

# MICRURUS LEMNISCATUS

## Systematics
- Scientific name: Micrurus lemniscatus [L., 1758].
- Synonym: Elaps lemniscatus [Duméril & Bibron, 1854].
- Common name: South American coral snake.
- Family: Elapidae.

## Biological Profile
- Medium-sized, slender-bodied, brightly marked 3-coloured coral snake with small, rounded head barely distinct from neck and very short tail. Average length 60–90 cm; maximum 1.45 m. Dorsal scales smooth and glossy without apical pits.
- Front of head black, with narrow white ring in front of eyes; remainder of head red. Body pattern consists of moderately broad red rings separated by 7–17 triads of 3 black & 2 white rings, tail with no more than 2 black triads alternating with white rings.
- Range: Northern South America, east of the Andes, from Bolivia to Trinidad. Dominant in the Amazon.
- Habitat: Lower montane wet forest, lowland rainforest, savannah, gallery forest, secondary forest, lowland flood plains, cleared regions and rocky regions. Frequently found near human settlement in humid environments or watercourse regions.
- Terrestrial and nocturnal. Will enter the water to hunt for prey.
- May burrow in loose soil or leaf litter
- Preys mainly on swamp eels, small snakes and legless lizards.
- Oviparous; 5–6 eggs per clutch.
- Four recognized subspecies [lemniscatus, carvalhoi, frontifasciatus, helleri].

## Food Frenzy
Large coral snakes [M. lemniscatus diutius; now L. diutius] are noted to be active and aggressive and are decidedly so when uncovered at night beneath a termite's nest. Its large size allows its cannibalistic nature or the preying on other coral snakes, esp. on much smaller species of coral snake. The large coral snake uses something called 'jaw walking' for the swallowing of prey. It identifies reptile prey head first, by the overlapping scales, and moves toward the head. Very rarely tails are swallowed first. The head is swallowed by alternating of the jaws and pauses are made in swallowing until the entire organism is ingested. To hasten

the process of swallowing it may rub its heads on hard surfaces, e.g. the ground, to assist in pushing down the prey. When the prey is swallowed, the head is raised off the ground. After consumption of food a "feeding excitement" occurs in captivity. Increased alertness is achieved due to increased hormonal levels, response and reaction time to stimuli is heightened, tongue flicking is increased as well as the lateral head movements. It is this food frenzy that may be a factor that promotes cannibalism in this species. [The Online Guide to the Animals of Trinidad and Tobago]

## MATERIA MEDICA MICRURUS LEMNISCATUS

### Sources
1 Effects of bite; clinical manifestations.
2 Pain control.

### Clinical Manifestations of Coral Snake Bite
'Local effects of a coral snake bite may include scratch marks or fang puncture wounds; minimal to moderate oedema or tissue reaction; erythema; and pain. If present, pain is usually minor and confined to the bite site but may radiate throughout a bitten extremity. In contrast to crotalid bites, in which moderate to severe envenomation usually can be predicted by rapid onset of local effects, severe and even fatal envenomation from a coral snake bite can be present without signs and/or symptoms of a substantial local tissue reaction. This fact, combined with the relative lack of local findings, may lead to a false sense of security on the part of the inexperienced treating physicians. The earliest signs may be *euphoria* or *drowsiness,* followed by nausea and vomiting, excess salivation, bulbar paralysis, fasciculations, and later peripheral weakness progressing to paralysis.

'Systemic signs and symptoms usually begin 1–7 hours after envenomation, although they may not occur for as long as 18 or more hours. . . . Once evident, systemic signs and symptoms may progress rapidly and precipitously. Paralysis has occurred within 2–3 hours after a bite and appears to be a bulbar-type paralysis, involving cranial motor nerves. Death from respiratory paralysis has occurred within 4 hours after a bite.

'Systemic signs and symptoms of envenomation may include euphoria; anxiety or apprehension; lethargy' drowsiness; headache; weakness; nausea; vomiting; bulbar signs such as fasciculations of the tongue, dysphagia, and paresis of the extraocular muscles; diplopia or blurring of vision; dysphonia; dyspnoea; abnormal reflexes; seizures; motor weakness or paralysis, incl. complete respiratory paralysis, weak and irregular pulse, and occasional hypotension. Children appear to be prone to seizures following coral snake envenomations.' [Bryson, 1997]

Bucaretchi et al. [2016] analyzed literature reports of *coral snake bites* in Brazil from 1867 to 2014. Thirty published reports describing bites caused by Micrurus spp. in Brazil were identified and involved 194 distinct cases. Since no information on the clinical manifestations was available in 44 cases, the analysis was restricted to 25 reports [150 cases]. The offending snakes were described in 59 cases [Micrurus corallinus 36, M. frontalis 12, M. lemniscatus 5, M. hemprichi 2, M. filiformis 1, M. ibiboboca 1, M. spixii 1 and M. surinamensis 1]; in 22 cases only the genus [Micrurus spp.] was reported.

The main clinical features were local numbness/paraesthesia [52.7%], local pain [48%], palpebral ptosis [33.3%], dizziness [26.7%], blurred vision [20.7%], weakness [20%], slight local oedema [16%], erythema [16%], dysphagia [14.7%], dyspnoea [11.3%], inability to walk [10.7%], myalgia [9.3%], salivation [8%] and respiratory failure (4.3%). Fang marks were described in 47.3% of cases and 14% of bites were classified as asymptomatic.

## Pain Control

The therapeutic potential of snake venoms for pain control has been previously demonstrated. In the present study, the antinociceptive effects of Micrurus lemniscatus venom [MlV] were investigated in experimental models of pain. The antinociceptive activity of MlV was evaluated using the writhing, formalin, and tail flick tests. . . . In a screening test for new antinociceptive substances – the writhing test – oral administration of MlV [19.7–1600 μg/kg] produced significant antinociceptive effect. The venom [1600 μg/kg] also inhibited both phases of the formalin test, confirming the antinociceptive activity. The administration of MlV [1600 μg/kg] did not cause motor impairment in the rota rod and open field tests, which excluded possible non-specific muscle relaxant or sedative effects of the venom. . . . In this test, the MlV-induced antinociceptive effect was long-lasting and *higher than that of morphine*, an analgesic considered the gold standard. In another set of experiments, the mechanisms involved in the venom-induced antinociception were investigated through the use of pharmacological antagonists. The MlV [1600 μg/kg] antinociceptive effect was prevented by naloxone [5 mg/kg], a non-selective opioid receptor antagonist, suggesting that this effect is mediated by activation of opioid receptors. . . . The present study demonstrates, for the first time, that oral administration of M. lemniscatus venom, at doses that did not induce any motor performance alteration, produced potent and long-lasting antinociceptive effect mediated by *activation of opioid receptors*. [Leite dos Santos, 2012]

# GENUS NAJA – TRUE COBRAS

Of the 28 true cobra species in the genus Naja, 14 are of the non-spitting kind and 14 are spitters. The majority of species is found in Africa, with the remainder in Asia. The word comes from the Portuguese *cobra de capello*, which means 'hooded snake'.

## *Neurotoxic non-spitting cobras*

Bites by these species may cause some local swelling but necrosis does not develop. Classical neurotoxic symptoms appear as early as 30 minutes after the bite and can evolve to the point of fatal respiratory paralysis within 2–16 hours of the bite.

There are signs of progressive descending paralysis, starting with ptosis drooping eyelids], external ophthalmoplegia [causing diplopia] and weakness of the muscles innervated by the cranial nerves so that the victim cannot open the mouth, clench the jaws, protrude the tongue, swallow, protect the airway from secretions, speak, flex the neck and eventually cannot breathe. When the respiratory muscles become affected, the pattern of breathing is initially abdominal or 'paradoxical': the abdomen expands during inspiration due to contraction of the diaphragm. Respiratory distress increases, the patient becomes anxious, sweaty and cyanosed and will die unless ventilated artificially.

Electrophysiological features are similar to those of **myasthenia gravis**.

- The following neurotoxic non-spitting cobras have a listing in homeopathic materia medicas/databases and/or are available from homeopathic pharmacies:
  Naja anchietae. Angolan cobra. Primarily neurotoxic with cytotoxic factors.
  Naja annulifera. Snouted cobra. Primarily neurotoxic with haemotoxic factors.
  Naja atra. Chinese or Taiwan cobra. Primarily neurotoxic with cardiotoxic factors.
  Naja haje. Egyptian cobra. Primarily neurotoxic with cytotoxic factors.
  Naja kaouthia. Monocled cobra. Primarily neurotoxic with cytotoxic factors.
  Naja melanoleuca. Forest cobra. Primarily neurotoxic with cardiotoxic factors.
  Naja nivea. Cape cobra. Primarily neurotoxic with cardiotoxic factors.
  Naja tripudians. Indian or Spectacled cobra. Primarily neurotoxic with cardiotoxic factors.

*Spitting cobras*
Spitting cobras tend to aim for the eyes while spitting out the venom, which is often a combination of neurotoxins and cytotoxins.

When venoms of the spitting elapids enter the eye, there is intense local pain, blepharospasm, palpebral oedema, epiphora and lachrymation. In Nigeria, slit-lamp or fluorescein examination revealed corneal erosions in more than half the patients spat at by N. nigricollis.

Secondary infection of the corneal lesions may result in permanent opacities causing blindness or panophthalmitis with destruction of the eye. Rarely, venom is absorbed into the anterior chamber causing hypopyon and anterior uveitis. Seventh [facial] cranial nerve paralysis is a rare complication which results from tracking of venom from the conjunctival sac through lymphatics posteriorly to the superficially situated VIIth cranial nerve.

- The following spitting cobras have a listing in homeopathic materia medicas/ databases and/or are available from homeopathic pharmacies:
  Naja mossambica. Mozambique spitting cobra. Cytotoxic and neurotoxic.
  Naja nigricincta. Western barred spitting cobra. Cytotoxic and haemotoxic.
  Naja nigricollis. Black-necked spitting cobra. Cytotoxic and neurotoxic.
  Naja nubiae. Nubian spitting cobra. Cytotoxic and neurotoxic.
  Naja pallida. Red spitting cobra. Cytotoxic and neurotoxic.

Naja philippinensis. Northern Philippine cobra. Neurotoxic.

Naja samarensis. Samar or Southern Philippine cobra. Neurotoxic and cytotoxic.

Naja siamensis. Indo-Chinese spitting cobra. Neurotoxic.

Naja sputatrix. Javan spitting or Indonesian cobra. Neurotoxic and cardiotoxic.

Naja sumatrana. Equatorial or Golden spitting cobra. Neurotoxic and cardiotoxic.

# NAJA ANCHIETAE

## Systematics
- Scientific name: Naja anchietae [Bocage, 1879].
- Synonyms: Naja haje anchietae [Mertens, 1937]. Naja annulifera anchietae [Broadley, 1995].
- Common names: Anchieta's cobra. Angolan cobra.
- Family: Elapidae.

## Biological Profile
- Large hooded elapid with broad, flattened head slightly distinct from the neck, rounded snout and medium length tail. Average length 1–1.2 m; maximum 2–2.3 m.
- Two colour variations occur: a plain variation, which can be brown, orange-brown, purple-brown or very dark brown, nearly black; and a banded variation with dark brown and yellow bands; the yellow bands are the same width as or wider than the darker bands. Broad, dark brown band on the throat. Spreads a wide hood.
- Range: Angola, Zambia, Zimbabwe, Namibia, Botswana.
- Habitat: Arid savannah, esp. in wooded areas along river and wetlands.
- Terrestrial. Occasionally found in small shrubs.
- Permanent home base. Often takes up residence in the same retreat for years.
- Nocturnal; active at night, foraging for food from dusk onwards; feeds on a variety of vertebrate prey, mostly rodents, birds, reptiles and toads; often ventures into poultry runs.
- Oviparous; 8–30 eggs per clutch.
- More aggressive than closely related species such as the snouted cobra [Naja annulifera], but otherwise similar in habits. Will posture in a hostile way when provoked but will flee when given the chance. May also play dead. Bites readily when confronted.

## MATERIA MEDICA NAJA ANCHIETAE

### Sources
1 Effects of bite; clinical manifestations.

## Clinical Manifestations

Venom neurotoxic and cytotoxic, affecting breathing and in severe cases leading to respiratory paralysis and death. Initial symptoms include burning pain and swelling that may result in blistering.

# NAJA ANNULIFERA

## Systematics

- Scientific name: Naja annulifera [Peters, 1854].
- Synonyms: Naja haje var. annulifera [Peters, 1854]. Uraeus annuliferus [Wallach, 2014].
- Common names: Snouted cobra. Banded cobra.
- Family: Elapidae.

## Biological Profile

- Large hooded elapid with short, broad head, large eyes and rounded snout Average length 1.5 m; maximum 2.5 m. Males larger than females.
- Colouration dorsally yellowish to greyish-brown, dark brown or bluish-black. Belly yellowish with darker mottling. Banded phase blue-black with 7–11 yellow to yellow-brown crossbars. Spreads a wide hood.
- Range: Zambia, Malawi, Zimbabwe, Mozambique, Botswana, South Africa, Swaziland.
- Habitat: Arid and moist savannah; common in bushveld and lowland areas.
- Permanent home base. Often takes up residence in the same retreat for years.
- Active at night, foraging from dusk onwards; preys on small mammals, birds and their eggs, lizards and other snakes [esp. puff adders]. Often raids poultry runs and can become a nuisance.
- Oviparous; 8–33 eggs per clutch.

## MATERIA MEDICA NAJA ANNULIFERA

## Sources

1 Effects of bite; clinical manifestations.

## Clinical Manifestations

Accidents involving N. annulifera are considered severe. The envenomed individuals experience swelling, pain and local burning at the site of the bite, followed by pain throughout their entire body. Beside these clinical findings, affected individuals can present with dizziness and palpebral ptosis. Some can progress to respiratory arrest and, without a specific treatment, death. The treatment for envenomated individuals is serum therapy and in respiratory arrest cases, mechanical ventilation.

Some studies have also reported that envenomed individuals in South Africa may develop necrosis at the site of the bite as well as haematologic disturbances.

Veterinary epidemiologic data demonstrated that approximately 60% of dogs poisoned by snakebites in South Africa were bitten by N. annulifera. These dogs presented with various clinical findings, incl. haematologic alterations, such as leukocytosis and thrombocytopenia, and disturbances in the coagulation system.

The venom promoted lung haemorrhage, an event that may also occur in cases of human envenomation, since death by respiratory arrest can be the result of the sum of neurotoxin activity and lung haemorrhage. [Silva-de-França, 2019]

# NAJA HAJE

## Systematics
- Scientific name: Naja haje [L., 1758].
- Synonyms: Coluber haje [L., 1758]. Cerastes candidus [Laurenti, 1768]. Coluber candidissimus [Lacépède, 1789]. Vipera haje [Daudin, 1803]. Uraeus haje [Wallach, 2014].
- Common name: Egyptian cobra.
- Family: Elapidae.

## Biological Profile
- Large hooded elapid with a large, depressed head, large round eyes, broad snout and broad neck. One of the largest snakes of African continent. Average length 1.5 m, maximum 2.5 m.
- Colouration highly variable, but mostly some shade of brown, often with lighter or darker mottling, and often a 'tear-drop' mark below the eye. Specimens from NW Africa almost entirely black.
- Range: Most of Africa [except for central part above equator and lower third], Arabian Peninsula.
- Habitat: Wide variety ranging from steppes, dry savannahs, semi-deserts with some vegetation and water to oases, agricultural areas, hills with sparse vegetation, grassland and human habitations. Often enters houses.
- Permanent home base. Establishes its territory and adopts a shelter where it normally lives for many years.
- Terrestrial, but has also been found climbing up trees.
- Nocturnal.
- Preys on a wide variety of vertebrates, incl. other snakes.
- Oviparous; 17–22 eggs per clutch.
- Three recognized subspecies [haje, legionis, viridis].
- Of great fame as the alleged instrument of Cleopatra's suicide in 30 BC, the Egyptian cobra's venom causes generalised paralysis progressing to respiratory paralysis. Envenomation may cause symptoms like those of *myasthenia gravis*.

## Behaviour
'The Egyptian cobra is terrestrial and nocturnal in the wild, though in captivity they seem to tend towards diurnality. It can, however, be seen basking in the sun at times in the early morning. It shows a preference for a permanent home

in abandoned animal burrows, termite mounds or rock outcrops and the like, sometimes entering human habitations to hunt domestic fowl. It will generally attempt to escape when approached, at least for a few meters, but if threatened it assumes the typical upright posture with the hood expanded.' [Wikipedia]

## MATERIA MEDICA NAJA HAJE

### Sources
1 Proving Farokh Master [India], 8 provers [6 females, 2 males], 30c and 200c; 2009–10.
2 Effects of bite; clinical manifestations.

### Mind
∞ Feeling of being a dead body or a robot just following instructions.
∞ Absorbed in own thoughts when being spoken to; aversion to talk; irritation when forced to answer.
∞ Likes to be alone.
∞ Sadness when listening to sad stories.
∞ Delusions: Being watched; house having become very small.
∞ Confused in taking decisions. Indecisive. Regrets decisions taken.

### Dreams
∞ Being a criminal fearful of being caught by police.
∞ Bomb attacks.
∞ Clairvoyant.
∞ Criminals out to kill.
∞ Drowning people.
∞ Escaping from water and drowning.
∞ Ghosts.
∞ Having an incurable skin disease.
∞ Hiding and attempts to escape from criminals.
∞ Incurable skin disease with thickening of skin.
∞ Scolded, being.
∞ Searching for own safe place.
∞ Someone dear turning into an angry, arrogant person.
∞ Trying to hide and escape from criminals intent on killing.
∞ Water rising, spreading all over beach.
∞ Weddings.

### Generals
∞ During menses < [2 pr.].
∞ Morning, after sleep <.
∞ Short sleep suffices to feel refreshed in morning.
∞ Drowsiness. Sleeping doesn't decrease sleepiness.
∞ Numbness, tingling and heaviness.

## Sensations

∞ Heaviness head and heaviness eyes < after sleep.
∞ Heaviness forehead with prostration.
∞ Eyes as if bruised, beaten up.
∞ Menses as if about to appear [2 pr.].
∞ Waist region as if tight.
∞ Tingling numbness left palm extending to forearm; heaviness left hand.
∞ Left hand as if weak, no strength.
∞ Left hand as if heavy.
∞ Numbness left hand and left leg.
∞ Tingling numbness both legs.
∞ Left thigh as if hot.
∞ Numbness left foot.
∞ Numbness soles of feet.
∞ Numbness entire left side and right leg.
∞ Numbness entire left side of body & heaviness left breast during menses.

## Locals

∞ Dizziness after getting up from sleep.
∞ Eyes itching and tired > application of ice.
∞ Photophobia – sunlight.
∞ Stomatitis, aphthae, burning, smarting pain, lower lip, < drinking, eating, night, talking, touch; > keeping mouth open; disturbed sleep from pain.
∞ Sneezing [4 pr.] with profuse watery coryza dripping from the nose.
∞ Sneezing < exposure to cold air.
∞ Nausea < while eating, brushing teeth.
∞ Pain lower abdomen after hard, unsatisfactory stool radiating to genitals and rectum.
∞ Pain uterus radiating to rectum.
∞ Pain right side of chest extending to left shoulder, < pressure.
∞ Tenderness breasts < after menses.
∞ Palpitation < first day of menses.
∞ Pain right wrist joint, < morning on waking, movement of wrist or hand.
∞ Itching legs when undressing.
∞ Pain left leg < standing for long.
∞ Pain legs < standing.
∞ Pain left foot < slightest touch, slightest movement, hanging leg; cannot put foot on floor; & crying from pain, sleeplessness from pain; & fear that left leg will be paralysed.

## Clinical Manifestations

Venom mainly neurotoxic with some cytotoxic factors.

Death due to complete respiratory failure. Envenomation causes local pain, severe swelling, bruising, blistering, necrosis and variable non-specific effects which may include headache, nausea, vomiting, abdominal pain, diarrhoea, dizziness, collapse or convulsions along with possible moderate to severe flaccid paralysis.

# NAJA KAOUTHIA

## Systematics
- Scientific name: Naja kaouthia [Lesson, 1831].
- Synonyms: Naja tripudians var. fasciata [Gray, 1830]. Naja naja kaouthia [Smith, 1940].
- Common name: Monocled cobra. Thai cobra. Monocellate cobra.
- Family: Elapidae.

## Biological Profile
- Medium-sized to large hooded elapid. Average length 1.3 m, maximum 2.3 m.
- Hood mark O- or mask-shaped ['eye' or monocle]; dorsal colour yellow, brown, grey or blackish; plain or with ragged or clearly defined cross-bands; throat pattern usually clear; one pair of lateral throat spots. Colour belly usually similar to dorsal colour, may be light.
- Hood patterns vary greatly and can have the design of spectacles, hollow discs, single or double monocles, or just white bands or wavy lines.
- Range: Bangladesh, Myanmar, Cambodia, NE India, Laos, N. Malaysia, S. China, Thailand, S Vietnam.
- Habitat: Wide variety of habitats, incl. forest and shrub areas, plantations, rice fields, pastures, villages and cities.
- Terrestrial, but climbs and swims very well.
- Nocturnal, most active at dusk and at night; sometimes also diurnal.
- Preys on rodents, birds and amphibians.
- Oviparous; 25–45 eggs per clutch.
- Major cause of snake bite mortality and morbidity throughout Thailand.
- Exploited in Thailand for skin [luxury products], meat [food], and gall bladder [medicine].

## A Man Respected & Feared
'Using as his medium ink that has been infused with snake venom and Chinese herbs, and a 16 inch split metal syringe with sharp needle tips, the Abbot elevated tattooing to a mystical art. . . . The first man to submit to the needles had been harassed by his neighbours. He feared their designs upon his wife, his young daughters, and his little farm. He begs the Abbot to inject into his body the spirit of the great Naga, Muchalinda, the immense cobra who coiled his body 7 times around the meditating Buddha and flared his great hood to protect The Blessed One from a violent rainstorm. As the monks chant, the Abbot begins to entwine the man's body with a long blood-puddle that, as an attendant monk blots the serpentine form into recognition, culminates in the center of the man's chest in a hooded, fang-bared cobra's head.

'The ink does its work and the man begins to hiss and writhe on the ground, raising his chest and turning his head, open mouthed with his lips drawn back to reveal teeth that are ready to bite . . . incisors, lateral incisors, and canines surround a flicking tongue imitating that of the bifurcated snake tongue, in what are truly terrifying gestures. He flails and slithers uncontrollably as several attendant monks attempt to subdue him. Their efforts are in vain. The man has received the power of the great naga and only exhaustion will bring him to rest.

' "What will happen to him now?" I ask a spectator monk. "He'll sleep it off and go home and his neighbourhood will buzz with the news that he's someone not to be trifled with. It's all in the belief, isn't it? He believes that the protective strength of the cobra has been put into him and they believe that the protective strength of the cobra has been put into him. As they fear and respect the cobra, they will fear and respect him. And he'll be a better person, too. His body, in a very real sense, is the great Naga's temple." . . .

'The central image has traditionally been the Naga, the Snake, which plays such an important role in Thai culture. . . . In Thailand the Naja naja kaouthia or the Monocled Cobra, is this venerated serpent. . . .

'Asian cobras are also seen as fertility symbols, phallic symbols, and emissaries of various gods. In China, the snake's organs are believed to have medicinal value – the gall bladder, for example, is used for ophthalmic disorders. . . .

'As I watched the devotees of the Tattoo Festival I thought about the entrancements experienced by members of other religions, the "speaking in tongues," the "holy rolling" and the fainting when receiving the "laying on of hands" of faith healers. There may be differences in degree in all of these experiences, but there are not differences in kind. These spiritual responses come from deep within our psyches. . . . The physical changes witnessed in these tattooing rituals are likewise mysterious, but they also deserve our respect. Our talismans and good luck charms are as much a part of sympathetic magic as these totem animal tattoos. They all serve a purpose that transcends logic. . . .

'By late afternoon there was an uncountable number of spiritually possessed devotees writhing, jumping, hissing, slithering, clawing, pawing and swaying rhythmically as they advanced towards the source of the chanting music they danced to. . . . The cobra tattoos seemed to inspire the most violent behaviour.'
[Yin Shan Shakya, The Cobra Spirit; Zen and the Martial Arts; zatma.org]


## MATERIA MEDICA NAJA KAOUTHIA

### Sources
1 Effects of bite; case report of 3 bites.
2 Effects of bite; case report of 69 bites.
3 Effects of bite; overview.

### Case Report of 3 Bites
'In 1964, an investigation of 47 patients bitten by Malayan cobra Naja naja subspecies observed the occurrence of neurotoxic symptoms in only 4 of the 47

cases; whereas a study in 1986 showed 14 of 24 cases exhibited neurological deficiencies after a bite by the Thai cobra Naja kaouthia. In both publications mentioned all patients who exhibited a local necrosis at the area of the bite wound developed signs of neurotoxicity.

'Our 3 patients were all hospitalised as emergencies and monitored in the intensive care unit. The time interval between the snakebite and the first detectable neurological symptoms varied from a few minutes to 4 hours. All patients had a local inflammation and a swelling around the bite wound; laboratory findings documented an elevation of inflammatory parameters.

Patients 1 and 3 exhibited ptosis, dysphagia, dysarthria, and somnolence after 4 and 2 hours respectively. One of them had to be intubated and ventilated mechanically because of a respiratory insufficiency resulting from an increasingly shallow breathing. Patient 2 developed signs of anaphylactic shock a few minutes after the snakebite. During the transport to the hospital a cardiac arrest occurred. The patient was successfully resuscitated, intubated and ventilated mechanically.

'In the patient who had the anaphylactic shock at the initial phase, extubation was delayed despite regained consciousness and spontaneous breathing activity because of an extensive swelling of the tongue and the pharyngeal area. The third patient developed a deep vein thrombosis. All our patients recovered completely without further sequelae.' [Bernheim, 2001]

## Case Report of 69 Bites

Of the 70 cases of monocled cobra [Naja kaouthia] bite admitted to Chittagong Medical College Hospital, Bangladesh, 69 patients were envenomed.

Nonspecific signs/symptoms included vomiting, seen on admission in 43 patients and fainting experienced by 10 patients. Neurotoxic signs present on admission included bilateral ptosis [58 patients], difficulty in speaking [52], generalized weakness [49], weak neck muscles [44], difficulty swallowing [41], blurred vision [29], breathlessness [23], and cyanosis in 3.

Swelling of the bitten limb was seen in 53 patients. Localized blistering and necrosis of the skin at or close to the bite site appeared during day 1 in 4 patients, thereafter increasing to 6 by day 2, 9 by day 3 to peak at 19 by day 5. In 3 patients, there was local blistering with no signs of systemic neurotoxicity, and in 1 patient the blister first appeared 5 days after admission. Surgical debridement of necrotic skin was required in 12 patients.

A 7-year-old girl was bitten on her left ankle 10:00 pm by a "blackish/yellowish snake" formally identified as "zhawra," the local name for a monocled cobra, N. kaouthia. The patient reported immediate pain and there was localized bleeding at the bite site. The pulse rate was 104 beats/minute and blood pressure 105/80 mmHg. The patient felt faint and generally weak and had difficulty in swallowing and speaking. Five hours after the bite, neurological signs predominated with complete bilateral posies, external ophthalmoplegia, an inability to open or close the mouth or protrude the tongue, a "broken neck" sign, a weak grip, and depressed reflexes. . . . Neurotoxic signs began to diminish after 35 minutes. . . . By 2 days after the bite, all neurotoxic signs had resolved but a small area [~3 cm diameter] of blistered, necrotic tissue appeared. The blister was aspirated, and necrotic tissue debrided. The patient was discharged 8 days after admission.

An 18-year-old agriculture worker was bitten on the dorsal aspect of the right foot by a blackish snake that he identified as "zhawra." He did not vomit or feel faint but developed weakness and drooping eyelids 1 hour after the bite and had difficulty in speaking and swallowing after 90 minutes. Within 2 hours, he developed neck weakness and passed scanty, highly coloured urine. At 2.5 hours, he complained of breathlessness. Pulse rate was 120 beats/minute and blood pressure 110/70 mmHg. Bilateral ptosis was complete and was accompanied by external ophthalmoplegia, the "broken neck" sign, weak grip and depressed tendon reflexes, an inability to open or close the mouth or protrude the tongue, pooled saliva, and an absent gag reflex. . . . The patient remained on continuous assisted ventilation but was unresponsive until his death 7 days after admission. Immediately before death, oxygen saturation fell to 21% and he had an episode of status epilepticus. The cause of death was recorded as hypoxic encephalopathy. [Faiz, 2017]

## Overview Effects of Bite
Venom powerfully neurotoxic and cytotoxic.

'Cobras causing both extensive local effects, ± flaccid paralysis, such as Naja kaouthia, generally cause a painful bite, with progressive swelling and if necrosis develops, then there is often discolouration of the skin and/or blistering first. This may progress to full thickness skin necrosis over 3–7 days. Such wounds may be extensive, sometimes involve underlying tissues and be difficult to heal. There is a potential for both secondary infection and long-term morbidity. Squamous cell carcinoma can develop in such long-term sores.

'In addition to these unpleasant local effects, there may be systemic symptoms, such as headache, nausea, vomiting, abdominal pain and less commonly, evidence of mild, sometimes moderate to severe flaccid paralysis. This may develop within a few hours or be delayed > 12 hrs. Ptosis is usually the first sign, followed by ophthalmoplegia, then if it progresses, dysarthria, dysphagia, poor tongue extrusion, drooling, limb weakness, lastly respiratory paralysis. Relative rates of necrosis versus paralysis for Naja kaouthia vary between studies, but it appears necrosis will develop in about 10–40% of cases, while paralysis occurs in > 50% of cases. Infection of the bite area is also common, as high as 58% of cases.' [Snakebite Management Naja kaouthia]

# NAJA MELANOLEUCA

## Systematics
- Scientific name: Naja melanoleuca [Hallowell, 1857].
- Synonyms: Naja haje var. melanoleuca [Hallowell, 1857]. Naja annulata [Buchholz & Peters, 1876]. Boulengerina melanoleuca [Wallach et al., 2014].
- Common names: Forest cobra. Black cobra.
- Family: Elapidae.

## Biological Profile

- Large, slender-bodied, hooded elapid with blunt head and highly polished, shiny scales. Head, neck and forepart of body yellowish-brown to dark brown, heavily flecked with black, becoming dark brown to shiny black towards the rear and tail. Belly creamy white to yellow belly, often with dark blotches. Average length 1.5–2 m; maximum 2.7 m.
- Range: West Africa [and into Central, Eastern and Southern Africa].
- Habitat: Closed-canopy, coastal, lowland forest and moist savannah, where it favours coastal thickets and riverine bush.
- Very active; climbs and swims well. Equally at home in trees, on ground, or swimming in lakes or rivers.
- Primarily active at night, but often encountered during day, esp. in overcast weather.
- Rears to a great height when disturbed, raising its body usually to more than two-thirds off the ground. Spreads a narrow hood.
- Preys on small mammals, birds, frogs, and snakes.
- Males engage in ritual combat during the mating season.
- Oviparous; 15–25 eggs per clutch.
- Quick to disappear in dense thickets when disturbed; will spread a narrow hood and bite readily if cornered.


## MATERIA MEDICA NAJA MELANOLEUCA

### Sources
1 Effects of bite, in Allen's Encyclopedia.
2 Effects of bite; clinical manifestations.

Allen's Encyclopedia gives the following symptoms under authority nr. 36 as related to the Indian cobra:

Mind – His mind wandered, but at last he got better, and was able to go out again; a short time after, having an axe, going, as he said, to cut wood, *he suddenly split his own head in two;* he had become insane.
Heart and Pulse – *Complained of a great pain near the heart.*
Generals – His body became swollen.
Generals – He suffered intensely, and his life was despaired of.

Authority no. 36 is Paul du Chaillu [1835–1903], a French-American traveller and anthropologist, who explored in the late 1850s, early 1860s the regions of West Africa, particularly Gabon. He became famous as the first modern outsider to confirm the existence of gorillas and the Pygmy people of central Africa. He wrote several books 'narrated for young people' based upon his African adventures, amongst others *Wild Life Under the Equator*, published in 1861. It is from chapter IV in this book that the information in Allen is taken.

However much reliability this story has, one thing is certain: there are no Indian cobras in tropical West Africa. It is the forest cobra, *Naja melanoleuca,* also known as the black cobra.

Here is the section where a snake charmer and a large black shining naja appear on the scene:

### An Axe to Split

'This species of naja is the only one I have ever seen that could erect itself. One day I witnessed a fearful scene. A man, a native of Goree, an island on the coast of Senegambia [now Senegal and Gambia], who had the reputation of being a snake charmer and was then at the Gabon, had succeeded in capturing one of these large naja. He was a bold man and prided himself on never being afraid of any snake, however venomous the reptile might be; nay, not only was he not afraid of any of them, but he would fight with any of them and get hold of them. . . .

'That day he brought into a large open place, perfectly bare of grass, one of these wild naja that he had just captured and was amusing himself by teasing the horrid and loathsome creature when I arrived. It was a huge one! . . . Two or 3 times, as the snake crawled on the ground, we made off in the opposite direction with the utmost speed, myself, I am afraid, leading off in the general stampede; though I had provided myself with a gun. It was perfectly fearful, perfectly horrid and appalling to see that man making a plaything of this monster; laughing, as we may say, at death, for it could be nothing else, I thought. . . .

'On a sudden he threw the snake on the ground. Then the creature began to crawl away, when suddenly the Goree man came in front of it with a light stick and instantly the monster erected itself almost to half its full length, gave a tremendous whistle, which we all heard, looked glaringly and fiercely in the man's face with its sharp, pointed tongue out, and then stood still as if it could not move. The Goree man, with his little stick in his left hand, touched it lightly as though to tease it. It was a fearful sight – and if he had been near enough the snake would no doubt have sprung upon its antagonist. The man, as he teased and infuriated the snake with the rod he held in his left hand, drew the attention of the reptile toward the stick; then suddenly and in the wink of an eye, almost as quick as lightning, with his right hand he got hold of the creature just under his head.

'The same thing that I have just described again took place. The snake folded itself round his body; then he unfolded the snake, which was once more let loose, and now this horrid serpent got so infuriated that as soon as he was thrown on the ground he erected himself and the glare of his eyes was something terrific. It was indeed an appalling scene; the air around seemed to be filled with the whistling sound of the creature.

'Alas! a more terrible scene soon took place! The man became bolder and bolder, more and more careless, and the snake probably more and more accustomed to the mode of warfare of his antagonist, and just as the monster stood erect, the man attempted to seize its neck as he had done many and many a time before, but grasped the body too low, and before he had time to let it go the head turned on itself and the man was bitten!

'I was perfectly speechless; the scene had frozen my blood and the wild shrieks of all those round rent the air. The serpent was loose and crawling on the ground, but before it had time to go far a long pole came down upon its back and broke its spine, and in less time than I take to write it down the monster was killed. To the French doctor who had charge of the little colony the man went [happily he was just at hand]; all the remedies were prompt and powerful; the man suffered intensely, his body became swollen, his mind wandered, and his life was despaired of; but at last he got better, and though complaining of great pain near the heart, he was soon able to go out again. A short time after this accident, having an axe in his hand, going as he said to cut wood, he suddenly split his own head in 2. He had become insane!'

## Venom & Clinical Manifestations
Considered by many to be one of the most dangerous snakes [to humans] in West Africa, partly due to its aggressive behaviour, rapid movement, rather large size and potent neurotoxic venom. Its bite can be rapidly fatal without prompt intervention. Envenomation usually presents predominately with systemic neurological manifestations. Drowsiness, neurological and neuromuscular symptoms may develop early; paralysis, respiratory failure or death could ensue rapidly.

Neurological and neuromuscular manifestation typically appear within 15 minutes to 4 hours following envenomation. They include excessive salivation; drowsiness; restlessness; sudden hearing loss [unilateral and bilateral hearing loss have been reported]; sudden loss of consciousness; eyelid drooping; ophthalmo-plegia; palatal paralysis; glosso-pharyngeal paralysis or dysphagia; vertigo; fasciculations; limb paralysis; stumbling gait [ataxia]; head drooping [cervical muscle paresis or paralysis]; headache; local pain or numbness around bite site [tends to be only mild].

Other symptoms include hypotension; abdominal pain; nausea and vomiting; regional lymphadenopathy and lymphadenalgia; hyperpyrexia; epistaxis; flush-ing of the face; warm skin; increased sweating; pallor.

Direct toxic effects on the myocardium or conducting system have not yet been reported in Forest Cobra envenomation; in contrast to the Indian cobra, Naja naja. [toxicology.ucsd.edu/Snakebite]

# NAJA MOSSAMBICA

## Systematics
- Scientific name: Naja mossambica [Peters, 1854].
- Synonym: Naja nigricollis mossambica [Peters, 1854].
- Common name: Mozambique spitting cobra.
- Family: Elapidae.

## Biological Profile

- Medium-sized, slender-bodied, hooded, spitting elapid with blunt head, round pupils, and long tail. Average length 1.1 m, maximum 1.5 m.
- Colouring dorsally olive brown or slate grey, with each scale darkly outlined. Belly salmon pink or sometimes yellowish with black crossbars and blotches on throat.
- Range: Southern Africa.
- Habitat: Moist savannah and lowland forest, where it favours rock crevices, hollow logs, termite mounds, and animal burrows, often close to permanent water, to which it will readily take when disturbed.
- Often present in towns but remains largely unnoticed due to its small size and secretive habits.
- More active at night; juveniles can be quite active at daytime.
- Preys chiefly on toads and small mammals, or hen's eggs.
- Oviparous; 10–22 eggs per clutch.
- Shy and retiring, seldom stands its ground; will spread hood if cornered but will not hold the pose for long. Main defense, in addition to going into hiding, is to spit its venom.
- Can be very docile but also very fierce in captivity. Some specimens are very docile for a long time and then change without any apparent reason in furious snakes that will spit and strike.

## MATERIA MEDICA NAJA MOSSAMBICA

### Sources

1 Proving Lorna Smal and Liesel Taylor [South Africa], 13 provers [9 females, 4 males], 30c; 2004.
2 Effects of bite; clinical manifestations.

### Mind

∞ Feeling disjointed, distant, anti-social; desire to be alone.
∞ Short-tempered, impatient, hostile.
∞ Venting irritability and hostility on family and friends.
∞ Intense aversion to authoritive people.
∞ Irritated by being pushed around by others.
∞ Abrupt, snappish and rude.
∞ Carefree attitude, cannot take much seriously, light-hearted about everything, high spirits but semi-dazed.
∞ Indifferent, unmotivated and lazy.
∞ Enjoys lying in the sun; relaxed and lazy, as if being on holiday.
∞ Feels frustrated, restless and at the same time likes doing nothing.
∞ Feels not being able to handle life; wants to curl up into a little ball and give up; wants to sleep for a week or forever.
∞ Difficulty coping; overwhelmed, everything seems too much.

∞ Mood swings, alternation of being upset, being angry, swearing, and feeling happy.
∞ Excitement alternating with sadness.
∞ Delusions: body lighter than air; divided into 2 parts; mind and body separated; separated from the world.
∞ Delusion going mad, as if unable to keep all bits of one's mind together.
∞ Worse for crowds and social settings.
∞ Sociable and talkative.
∞ Feels on top of world and able to overcome all obstacles with a smile on face.
∞ Desires activity, which >.
∞ Anxiety about family; money matters; felt in stomach.
∞ Actions contrary to intentions.
∞ Dullness, slow in thinking, unable to think long.
∞ Hurry, haste while eating.
∞ Sadness, would like to sleep and never wake up.
∞ Sadness with heaviness body.

## Dreams
∞ Adventurous.
∞ Animals changing shape.
∞ Blood.
∞ Cats.
∞ Chased, being.
∞ Danger, escaping from.
∞ Danger of falling.
∞ Difficulties on journeys.
∞ Dogs attacking.
∞ Dogs, black.
∞ Driving recklessly.
∞ Held hostage.
∞ Hippos and crocodiles turning into humans.
∞ Parents separating.
∞ People fighting.
∞ Persecution and escape.
∞ Pools and swimming.
∞ Snakes.
∞ Stabbing someone who was bothering me to death, splitting open his skull.
∞ True on waking, dreams seem.
∞ True, dreams are coming.

## Generals
∞ Morning on waking <.
∞ Dryness mouth, lips, tongue, throat [5 pr.].
∞ Pain cramping – stomach, abdomen, left ovary, heart region, feet.

∞ Craving for chocolate [2 pr.]; chocolate cake; coffee; fizzy drinks; fruit [2 pr.]; sweets [2 pr.].

∞ Left side more affected.

## Sensations
∞ Floating feeling on waking up from a nap.

∞ Forehead as if cold.

∞ Head as if swinging around when standing still.

∞ Head as if separated from body.

∞ Squeezing all around the head.

∞ Eyes as if popping out during intense frontal headache.

∞ Mouth and tongue as if stiff and dry.

∞ Throat as if constricted, tight and narrow, > drinking anything, honey and lemon.

∞ Lump in throat.

∞ Stomach as if full after eating ever so little.

∞ Lumbar region as if weak.

∞ Legs and hands as if extremely weak and not being able to move them.

∞ Needles and pins in fingertips left hand, < pressure, moving fingers.

## Locals
∞ Loss of balance in morning; tendency to fall to left side, even when sitting; bumping into things.

∞ Headache < light, moving, watching TV; & sore eyes.

∞ Headache, sharp pain all through head, > pressure and massage.

∞ Headache between eyes < blinking, pressing teeth together; pain radiates over skull.

∞ Headache moving from frontal region to back of neck.

∞ Headache in a small spot, moving to all directions.

∞ Itching head when head becomes warm.

∞ Eyes burning < heat and sun.

∞ Sneezing attacks from dust.

∞ Coryza, < motion, > lying down or sitting up.

∞ Speech difficult from swelling of tongue.

∞ Belching on motion.

∞ Nausea after anxiety or excitement.

∞ Nausea on looking at food.

∞ Stomach pain after beer.

∞ Ovarian pain on urination or passing stool.

∞ Tightness chest and throat, battling to breathe. Feels suffocated and faintish, as if needing to breathe very deeply, although it makes no difference. Can't get enough oxygen.

∞ Difficulty breathing in a crowded room.

∞ Sharp pain under right breast in ribs, < stretching; moves to left side under breast in ribs. Comes and goes.

∞ Low backache < bending forward, sitting.

## Eyes

'Prover 42 had a severe reaction in her eyes and required antidoting. Symptoms started as a simple conjunctivitis in the left eye, which progressed to the right eye. The symptoms were similar to the clinical symptoms found in a person spat in the eyes by a Mozambican spitting cobra. The left eyeball and eyelid were extremely red, and the eyelid was swollen. The eyelids were swollen, and the upper lid was overlapping the lower lid making it difficult to open them for examination. The appearance of the eyeball could be likened to raw meat when the lids were pried open. The prover described a pressure in the left eye as if it would "pop out". The eye was sensitive to light and wind, worse for bending forward and lying down and better for rinsing with cold water. There was a yellowish secretion from the left eye indicating infection. The conjunctivitis was spreading rapidly to the right eye. Prover 42 was antidoted with Apis mellifica based on the clinical picture. The prover's symptoms improved markedly in the next 24 hours but took another few days to clear completely.'

## Clinical Manifestations

Venom predominantly cytotoxic, causing serious local tissue damage that often requires skin grafts. Slight neurotoxic symptoms such as drowsiness may occur.

'Bites result in local and extensive cytotoxic effects. Severe local pain and swelling develop immediately after the bite and may spread quickly up the affected limb. Painful, tender, enlargement of the regional lymph glands is typical. Blisters may develop as soon as a few hours to 24 hours after the bite. They are most marked at the site of the fang marks and may form a ring around a defined area of darkened or pale numb skin. The earliest signs of tissue death or necrosis are the changes in colour and sensation, the appearance of blisters and a smell of rotting flesh.

'Areas of necrotic tissue and deeper tissues may slough off spontaneously. Tissue loss may be massive, extending up the bitten limb, along the path of the lymphatics in the form of discrete "skip" lesions separated by areas of apparently normal skin. Complications can include secondary infection of dead tissue, sometimes with bacteria [Clostridia] causing tetanus or gas gangrene; this may require extensive surgical removal or even amputation. Other complications include keloid formation; chronic ulceration with or without infection of the underlying bone and in worst cases can lead to cancerous changes later [Norris, 2003].

'Vomiting is the earliest symptom of generalised envenoming in victims of bites by cobras whose venoms cause gangrene. Paralysis has not been convincingly demonstrated in patients bitten by African spitting cobras. There is absence of neurological symptoms and few fatalities. . . . Venoms may also affect the heart directly. An additional, unique form of toxicity that is found with Naja mossambica is acute ophthalmia, which occurs when venom is spit into the eyes. . . . Immediate and intense pain results, with blepharospasm, tearing, and blurring of vision. It is difficult to open the eye, tears flow copiously, membranes around the eye become swollen and inflamed and the eyeball appears very red. Without treatment the lids swell, the membranes of the eye develop haemorrhages and keratitis and ulcerations of the cornea within 24 hours, which is followed by blindness. Systemic toxicity does not occur with eye exposure, but corneal ulcerations, uveitis, and permanent visual impairment or blindness has been reported in untreated cases.' [Lorna Smal]

# NAJA NIGRICOLLIS

## Systematics
- Scientific name: Naja nigricollis [Reinhardt, 1843].
- Synonyms: Naja nigricollis atriceps [Laurent, 1955]. Naja crawshayi [Broadley & Cotterill, 2004]. Afronaja nigricollis [Wallach et al, 2014].
- Common name: Black-necked spitting cobra.
- Family: Elapidae.

## Biological Profile
- Medium to large hooded, spitting elapid. Usually 1.0–1.5 m long, maximum 2.5 m. Body colour highly variable, ranging from pinkish-tan in some geographical areas to uniformly black in others, most forms have 1 reddish and 1 black band across underside of throat. Dorsal scales smooth.
- Range: Central and southern Africa.
- Habitat: Found mainly in moist or dry savannah, where they shelter in abandoned termite mounds, rodent burrows, or hollow trees.
- Very active, needs space to move.
- Generally nocturnal [or crepuscular – coming out at dusk and dawn]; juveniles often active during day.
- Mainly terrestrial, but fairly good swimmer and climber. At home in trees.
- Preys on a wide variety of animals, incl. toads, chickens [often raiding chicken runs], other birds and/or eggs, small mammals, lizards, and snakes.
- Oviparous, usually 8–20 eggs per clutch.

## Spitting Straight in the Eye
'The performance is accomplished with the jaws slightly parted . . . The performance is very quick. . . . The snake rears and it may instantly spring to the pose. Facing the object . . . it looks intently into one's face. . . . If it seeks to direct the poison upwards it curves its rearing pose backward, thus directing the head upwards. The ejection of the poison is an instantaneous operation. The jaws are slightly opened and closed so quickly as to appear like a snapping motion and during this action the poison leaves the fangs. There is no dribbling or spilling of the fluid. It issues in twin jets and the jaws of the snake are clear of it when the feat is accomplished.

'There is every indication that, at the instant the snake prepares to eject the poison, it contracts the temporal muscle over each gland, thus producing pressure to force the toxic fluid a considerable distance. This flies with such force that its impact can be distinctly heard against ordinary glass 5 feet away. At the instant of the ejection the snake emits a sharp hiss. This ejection of air might be

an accompanying token of anger, or it may assist the travel of the poison.'
[Ditmars, 1937b]

## MATERIA MEDICA NAJA NIGRICOLLIS

### Sources
1 Effects of bite; clinical manifestations.

### Clinical Manifestations
Venom mainly cytotoxic in nature, a bite causing severe tissue necrosis. Venom entering the eyes will, as with other spitting cobras, cause severe pain and could possibly result in permanent damage to the eyes if untreated.

If the 'spat' venom enters the eyes, there is immediate and persistent intense burning, stinging pain, followed by profuse watering of the eyes with production of whitish discharge, congested conjunctivae, spasm and swelling of the eyelids, photophobia and clouding of vision. Corneal ulceration, permanent corneal scarring and secondary endophthalmitis are recognized complications of African spitting cobra venom but have not been described in Asia.

'Bites by *Naja nigricollis* give rise to pain, which is often immediate, bleeding from the wound site, localised swelling, which may spread to involve the entire limb within several hours, and some ecchymosis. Blebs and blood-filled blisters may form. Leukocytosis, a fall in haematocrit, and thrombocytopenia may occur. Clot retraction time is often prolonged. Drowsiness was present in both our patients. There was a definite muscle weakness in the affected extremity, with a slight decrease in deep reflexes in 1 patient.

'The same patient complained of a sensation of "pins and needles" over the injured part. He also had some decrease in muscle strength in that part. It is certain that both of our patients were lethargic and considerably drowsier than patients I have observed following rattlesnake bites. Deep reflexes were decreased over the involved extremity in 1 patient, and he developed paraesthesia and muscle weakness over the affected arm and forearm. . . . Warrell and Ormerod have had far more experience with treatment of bites by this species than I, but other than drowsiness, their examinations have failed to uncover any significant neurological deficits.' [Russell, 1980]

'The local effects of *bites by spitting cobras* are essentially similar to those of large adder bites. Swelling usually begins early, often within 10–30 minutes. It may become extensive, involving the entire limb and even adjacent areas of the trunk, esp. in children. Regional lymph nodes may become enlarged and painful within 30–60 minutes. The aggressive and progressive cytotoxic nature of envenoming is usually evident within hours of the bite. Blisters and bullous skin lesions, fluid or blood filled, and ecchymoses often develop, at first near the fang marks, but may later extend beyond the bite site within 6–24 hours.

'Skip lesions' [areas of necrosis separated by strips of apparently normal skin caused by proximal spread of venom in lymphatic vessels] are characteristic of spitting cobra bites. Extravasations of plasma may cause hypovolaemia, which may lead to hypovolaemic shock, esp. in children. The local cytotoxic effects may progress to necrosis, with spontaneous sloughing of dead tissue. Compartmental syndromes may develop, esp. involving the anterior tibial compartment after bites of the feet and ankles, or forearm, in bites of the hand or wrist. This complication may lead to ischaemic necrosis of the compartmental muscles and nerve damage.' [Müller, 2012]

# NAJA NIVEA

## Systematics
- Scientific name: Naja nivea [L., 1758].
- Synonyms: Vipera flava [Merrem, 1820]. Naja haje var. capensis [Jan, 1863].
- Common names: Cape cobra. Yellow cobra.
- Family: Elapidae.

## Biological Profile
- Relatively slender elapid with broad and rather rounded hood. Average length 1.5 m, maximum 1.85 m.
- Colours vary from plain yellow to yellow-brown flecked with dark patches, to dark reddish brown. Juveniles have dark band on throat, which fades with maturity.
- Range: SW Africa.
- Habitat: Dune thicket, coastal and mountain fynbos, and karroid sandveld [sparse vegetation dominated by dwarf, perennial shrubs in semi-desert Karoo region of South Africa].
- Diurnal, actively foraging during day. Rarely, if ever observed during hours of darkness.
- Preys on small mammals, lizards, toads, and snakes [including its own kind].
- Oviparous; 8–20 eggs per clutch.
- Timid, always seeking to escape when encountered, although when aroused it has been described as willing to bite readily.

## A Day in the Life of the Cape Cobra
'Emergence was a slow process. Firstly, the tip of the snout and flicking tongue would be apparent at the lip of the burrow. The cobra would then slowly move up with hood spread, fully alert, and then turn the head a full 180°. The cobra usually remained at the mouth of the burrow for a full 5 minutes or so before moving off to bask a metre or so away. The duration of basking varied little on clear sunny days with a minimum of 20 minutes, and a maximum of 28 minutes. On overcast days the basking period extended to a maximum of 42 minutes. Regardless of weather conditions the basking posture never varied; the cobra extended the body for its entire length exposing maximum surface to both ground and available sun. Following the morning basking sessions the cobra would move off slowly into the surrounding vegetation but return a short while later after a period of between 30 and 60 minutes. On returning to the site the

cobra would either engage in a brief lying out session, or retreat into the burrow using either of the 2 entrances. This behaviour was consistent for the 12-day period. . . . During the hottest part of the day both cobras remained together in retreat within the burrow for a period ranging from 2 to 3 hours. At mid-afternoon, always between 15:00 and 15:45 h, the female cobra would emerge from the right side burrow and move off immediately into the surrounding vegetation. Between 10 and 15 minutes later the male would emerge, and after a very short period of lying out would move off. On its return, never later than 17:00 h, the male went into retreat immediately. For the entire 12-day period this represented the last sightings of the day for both male and female.' [Tony Phelps, 2007]

## MATERIA MEDICA NAJA NIVEA

### Sources
1 Effects of bite, 2 cases.
2 Effects of bite; clinical manifestations.

# CASES

### Symptoms
Blaylock et al. reported 2 cases.

### Case 1
A 53-year-old man, was bitten on the right index finger. Within 5 minutes a tight tourniquet was applied to the arm. Five minutes later his mouth was dry, he began sweating and shaking, followed by ptosis and weakness of the arm. When seen by a physician 1 hour later, he was acting as if drunk. At 2½ hours he was fasciculating and sweating and had difficulty breathing. En route to the hospital he had a generalised convulsion but was not inconti-nent and did not hurt himself. In the hospital it was noted that he had complete flaccid paralysis. He later claimed that at this stage he had been able to hear and understand but could not move. On day 2 he had complete flaccid paralysis with no response to stimuli and no corneal, pharyngeal, plantar or tendon reflexes. He could move his tongue on day 3 and later that day opened his eyes and moved his left leg. After being extubated, about 5 days post-bite, he continued to improve and could be discharged on day 13, almost completely recovered.

### Case 2
A 26-year-old snake-catcher, also developed complete flaccid paralysis. On day 2 there was some movement of his hands and head. On day 3 there was

further improvement, and. he was able to communicate, open his eyes, and move his head and shoulders. The bitten hand was swollen. He showed gradual improvement in muscular power and was extubated on day 8, a full 7 days after ventilation commenced. He walked with help on day 9 and was discharged on day 15. [Blaylock, 1985]

## Clinical Manifestations
Venom strongly neurotoxic, causing areflexic flaccid paralysis, incl. respiratory paralysis requiring supportive, prolonged ventilation.

Local symptoms in the about 10 cases of envenomation reported were pain, numbness, swelling and enlargement of regional lymph nodes. Systemic symptoms included headache, dizziness, dry mouth or excessive salivation, nausea, vomiting, sweating, and fever. Early neurotoxic symptoms were visual disturbance [as early as 30 minutes post-bite], a feeling of heaviness of the eyelids, ptosis, external ophthalmoplegia and slurring of speech. Respiratory weakness or paralysis can develop as early as 2 hours or up to 12 hours after the bite. [Meier & White, 1995]

# NAJA PALLIDA

## Systematics
- Scientific name: Naja pallida [Boulenger, 1896].
- Synonyms: Naja nigricollis var. pallida [Boulenger, 1896]. Naja mossambica pallida [Broadley, 1968]. Afronaja pallida [Wallach et al., 2014].
- Common names: Red spitting cobra. African cobra.
- Family: Elapidae.

## Biological Profile
- Medium-sized, hooded spitting cobra with broad, flattened broad slightly distinct from neck, rounded snout and medium-length tail. Colouration bright salmon-red or orange-red contrasted with a broad black or dark blue throat band and subocular teardrop markings. Belly reddish; throat area may be creamy white. Other colour variations include yellow, pinkish, pink-grey, pale red or steel grey. Dorsal scales smooth and strongly oblique. Average length 0.7–1.2 m; maximum 1.5 m.
- Range: Egypt, Sudan, Eritrea, Ethiopia, Somalia, Kenya, Tanzania, Chad.
- Habitat: Dry savannah and semidesert areas; usually found near water holes.
- Terrestrial.
- Nocturnal.
- Cannibalistic.
- Prefers amphibians such as toads and frogs; also preys on rodents, birds and other snakes. Will raid chicken runs.
- Oviparous; 6–21 eggs per clutch.

- Not aggressive, but if provoked will rear up, hiss loudly, flare its hood, and if this warning is not heeded, will spray a high velocity jet of toxins into the antagonist's face and eyes.

## MATERIA MEDICA NAJA PALLIDA

### Sources
1 Proving Farokh Master [India], 7 provers [4 females, 3 males], 30c and 200c; 2009–10.
2 Effects of bite; clinical manifestations.

### Mind
∞ Violent anger at trifles, followed by repentance or sadness.
∞ Irritability at trifles.
∞ Dullness, confusion, difficulty concentrating.
∞ Mistakes in spelling.

### Dreams
∞ Big cats.
∞ Exposure of body parts.
∞ Fighting, 2 people.
∞ Head lice.
∞ Killing family members.
∞ Late, being.
∞ Missing bus or train.
∞ Mother nursing her child.
∞ Old school friends.
∞ Prostitution
∞ Religious.
∞ Repentance killing brother.
∞ Romantic scenes.
∞ Smothering.
∞ War.

### Generals
∞ During menses <.
∞ Sudden weakness & all-gone sensation in stomach.
∞ Daytime drowsiness.
∞ Low blood sugar episodes; dizziness & cold sweat.
∞ Eating >.
∞ Profuse perspiration < slightest exertion, standing.

### Sensations
∞ Worm crawling on vertex.
∞ Right tonsil as if raw and inflamed < chocolate.

∞ Heaviness sternum.

∞ Electric current flowing through left thumb when holding objects.

∞ Legs giving out as if lacking strength.

∞ Numbness of extremities, first left then right, < exertion.

## Locals

∞ Dizziness & sensation of falling to left side.

∞ Dizziness on turning head quickly.

∞ Right-sided headache, < bending head down, > vomiting.

∞ Headache < sun exposure.

∞ Headache & neck stiffness.

∞ Irritation throat, itching, tickling, urge to swallow or to clear throat constantly, > swallowing liquids.

∞ Acidity stomach < spicy food, > cold drinks.

∞ Nausea < smell of food.

∞ Diarrhoea < during menses.

∞ Diarrhoea in morning, with weakness.

∞ Itching rash on buttocks during menses.

∞ Suffocation in crowded places.

∞ Loose cough after eating.

∞ Itching chest < touch of water.

∞ Palpitations < exertion.

∞ Palpitations from slight anxiety.

∞ Stiffness lumbar region morning on waking.

∞ Cramps in calf muscles, first right then left, > pressure.

## Clinical Manifestations

Venom is composed of cytotoxins resulting in tissue destruction, localised bleeding and extensive painful swelling, and of neurotoxins causing paralysis of muscles of swallowing and respiration.

# NAJA TRIPUDIANS

## Systematics

• Scientific name: Naja naja [L.,1758].

• Synonyms: Naja fasciata [Laurenti, 1768]. Naja maculata [Laurenti, 1768]. Naja tripudians [Merrem, 1820]. Naja naja naja [Smith, 1943]. Naja nigra [Gray, 1830].

• Common names: Indian cobra. Indian spectacled cobra. Spectacled cobra.

• Family: Elapidae.

## Biological Profile

• Large, heavy-bodied, hooded elapid. Adults usually 1.5–2.0 m long, maximum 2.4 m. Body usually dark brown or black to yellowish-white above and white or yellowish below. Distinctive markings include spectacle mark on top [dorsal

surface] of expanded hood, with dark spot in middle of lighter ring, or within each 'lens' of the 'spectacles'.
- Range: Indian Subcontinent.
- Habitat: Found in a variety of habitats: flat grasslands and jungles, among scattered trees, near rice fields and other cultivated areas, and near settlements. Occurs at sea level and higher elevations to at least 300 m.
- Often lives in holes in embankments, hollows of trees.
- Mainly crepuscular; most active in evening and early morning.
- Quick-moving and agile.
- Preys on small mammals, birds, other snakes, lizards, frogs and toads.
- Oviparous; 8–32 [up to 45] eggs per clutch. Eggs laid in rat holes or termite mounds.
- Like other cobras famous for its threat display involving raising the front part of its body and spreading its hood. The distance a cobra can strike in a forward direction is equal to the distance its head is raised above the ground. Like other cobras, Indian cobras like to telegraph their strikes and throw a lot of bluff strikes at the threat, even if it is well out of range, angrily biting out at the air in its direction. When biting, holds on and chews savagely.
- Revered in Indian mythology and culture and often seen with snake charmers.

### The Cobra's Revenge

'It was a warm, sunny day in Saligao. At the seminary, it was business as usual for us seminarians. The staff were going about their daily routine and the seminarians and priests were either attending classes, or studying/praying, as was their wont were they to have an hour or so free between assignments. Suddenly, one of the kitchen helpers spotted a large snake – a cobra – slithering across one of the corridors. He shouted out loud to draw the attention of the others and soon there was quite a commotion all around.

'The helper along with another colleague scurried around trying to keep track of the movements and whereabouts of the deadly serpent in our midst. Someone went to summon Sashikant, a snake-catcher from Donvaddo. He arrived in a jiffy, carrying the simple implement of his unusual trade – a not-too-stout, specially-shaped stick. He was directed to the corner in which the cobra had coiled itself. With a deft flick of the wrist he soon had the cobra aloft on the stick, and proudly displayed his trophy to all of us. He grasped it below the head, and we marveled at his skill and fearlessness. Then he took out a white handkerchief from his pocket, apparently to remove the snake's fangs. From my vantage point at a safe distance, the cobra's large round eyes seemed to be glaring wrathfully and its nostrils widened and fuming in protest.

'Suddenly, all hell broke loose. Somehow, the cobra slipped out of Sashikant's grasp. It raised itself about half a meter from the ground, its hood – with the characteristic "U" mark – flared up, it hissed once and sprang forward and struck at Sashikant. He collapsed onto the floor and almost immediately broke out into uncontrollable convulsions. We were all terrified. Even as Sashikant was lifted into the seminary's jeep and rushed to hospital, some worked chased the snake and battered it to death [in those days 'animal lovers' and 'conservationists' were rarely heard of, and least of all in the context of a poisonous snake that had just bitten a man]. It turned out that Sashikant died on the way to the Mapuca hospital. We were of course rather distressed, and some of us, along with the seminary beadle, paid a condolence visit to Sashikant's family.

'In Indian mythology and the Hindu religion, snakes play a prominent role. The Hindu pantheon features snakes in many different ways. Lord Ganesh has a snake wrapped around his waist, almost like a belt; Lord Shiva has a snake around his neck, kind of like a scarf; and, Lord Vishnu is depicted as resting on a coiled snake.

'In the village folklore of India, there are innumerable stories of snakes seeking revenge on humans, and the cobra is especially singled out for this unnerving trait. Village elders talked of how a cobra that had lost a mate at the hands of a human would keep following the killer regardless of distance or time until it took appropriate revenge, sometimes extending that revenge to the killer's entire family! One can understand how these stories assumed credibility, in an era before antidotes to snake venom were easily available and the probability of getting bitten by a snake, and succumbing to the poison, were very much higher than today.

'The enemy of the cobra is the mongoose, romanticized in Rudyard Kipling's story *Riki Tiki Tavi*. Fiction and folklore allude to the female cobra's desire to avenge the death of a mate, but whether this is true in reality is a matter of speculation. Snakes rely mainly on their senses of smell and touch to get around, although they are not blind, as many people believe. Snakes hear by detecting vibrations of sound waves conducted through the ground [I remember elders in the house telling us that banging a stick on the ground was the best way to drive away a snake that had strayed from its natural habitat into the house]; some low frequencies of sound waves conducted through the air can also be picked up by the snake. Snakes do not have a sense of taste; in fact, the tongue serves as a secondary organ of smell. Indeed, snakes do follow the scents of their mates during the breeding season but extending that to sniffing out a human enemy for revenge is most likely far beyond the realm of reason!' [Mascarenhas, 2009]

## MATERIA MEDICA NAJA TRIPUDIANS

### Sources

1 Proving Stokes [UK] on self and his future wife, 19-year-old Rosa; inoculation with drop of venom, olfaction of 1st and 2nd dils., and ingestion of 2nd, 4th and 6th dils.; 1852–53.
2 Proving Russell [UK], 10 provers [2 female, 8 males], 1x, 2x, 3x dils. and trits.; 1853.
3 Clinical observations, in Hering.
4 Clinical observations Römer [Germany], 8 cardiac cases, 1976.
5 Clinical observations Mangialavori [Italy].
6 Clinical observations Farokh Master [India].
7 Degroote, Dream Repertory.

8 Synthesis Repertory Treasure Edition 2009.
9 Effects of bite; clinical manifestations.
10 Effects of bite; drooping, dragging, dropping dead.
11 Effects of bite; bitten in the nose.
12 Effects of bite; typical course of cobra envenomation.
13 Effects of bite; symptoms & signs.

### Wrong Snake!

In his Encyclopedia, Allen includes under Naja the following source: '28, Ireland, effects of bite of Coluber carinatus on hand, Med.-Chir. Trans., 1813, p. 396; 29, same, second case; 30, same, third case.'

Various things are wrong. A trivial error is the year, which ought to be 1811 instead of 1813. A grave error is inclusion under Naja, a neurotoxic elapid native to India, of a snake that turns out to be a haemotoxic New World pit viper. Ireland refers to Mr. J.P. Ireland, Surgeon to the 4th battalion of the 60th regiment of foot, who, when quartered on the island of St. Lucia, in the eastern Caribbean, 'was informed that an officer and several men . . . had died from the bites . . . of one of the most deadly [snakes that] . . . appears to be the Coluber carinatus of Linnaeus.'

Although wrong about its name, Mr. Ireland correctly qualified the pit viper as deadly. Coluber carinatus L., now classified as Chironius carinatus, on the other hand is non-venomous and endemic to Central and South America. Besides, it does not appear on St. Lucia. Five species of snakes have been recorded from St Lucia – one of these is extinct, 3 others are non-venomous, while the last one is the St. Lucian pit viper. The latter, highly venomous, was previously thought to be synonymous with the fer-de-lance [Bothrops lanceolatus] from the neighbouring island of Martinique but has now been assigned the status of a separate species, Bothrops caribbaeus. *See* Bothrops caribbaeus for the symptoms observed by Mr. Ireland.

### Mind

∞ Melancholic mood, images of possible wrongs and mistakes, and brooding over them.[1]
∞ Anxious to do a great many things but disinclined to come into action. Feels inclined to huddle up near the fire and brood over one's business [activities].[2]
∞ Great agony of mental suffering on another's behalf from slight causes.[1]
∞ Very excitable and playful [Rosa].[1]
∞ Frequent fits of vexed mood, & disposition to fault-finding.[2]
∞ Delusion everything is going wrong. Feeling that everything done was done in a wrong way and cannot be rectified. Feeling of having some duty to perform, but at the same a strong impulse not to do it, resulting in extreme restlessness. Increased perception of what one *ought* to do and at the same time an unaccountable inclination not to do it, to which one is irresistibly compelled to yield.[2]

∞ After walking in open air in evening, dullness making place for unusual state of excitement and energy, mental and physical lasting the night, with a lively waking state, giving feeling in morning of having been awake all night.[2]

∞ Desires company. Fear of being alone. Delusion being neglected. Want of self-confidence, feels himself a failure. Confusion as to identity, sensation of duality. Delusion divided into 2 parts.[5]

∞ Bulimia; eating > mental symptoms, eats even when not hungry and more than she should, followed by repentance [feeling of not being in control of instincts].[5]

∞ Fears: deep water; sharks; snakes; of death on going to bed and to sleep, lest he would die.[5]

∞ Duty conscious, very family oriented, full of responsibility and high morality. Self-depreciation with poor self-confidence and irresolution stemming from an experience of excessive domination or abuse and being tormented or persecuted by members of the family or at the place of work; the person feels he is a failure and has not achieved anything in life. Suicidal impulses chiefly arising from a sense or feeling of having suffered wrong or having a feeling of neglecting duty or due to disappointment in a relationship.[6]

∞ Loud-mouthed boasting; big mouth, small heart.[7]

∞ Ostentation.[7] [Unnecessary display of wealth, knowledge, etc., in order to attract attention, admiration, or envy.]

∞ Delusion being exploited.[7]

∞ Loves silver jewellery.[7]

∞ Very active memory, recalling things from babyhood.[7]

∞ Anxiety > motion.[8]

∞ Delusions: Being injured by one's surroundings. Being neglected. Being starved. Being under superhuman control. Wasting away.[8]

∞ Exaggerating her symptoms.[8]

∞ Everything seems wrong.[8]

∞ Fears: Being left behind or alone. Flying [airplane]. Poverty.[7]

∞ Fears: Deep water. Sharks. Snakes. Death, on going to bed and to sleep, lest he would die.[5]

**Dreams**

∞ Accidents, car.[7]

∞ Alone in a desert, being.[7]

∞ Animals, scorpion.[7]

∞ Attention, receiving no.[7]

∞ Bad news, getting; death, divorce, sexual abuse.[7]

∞ Bats.[7]

∞ Bitten by animal, being.[7]

∞ Black, people dressed in.[7]

∞ Blamed for being incompetent.[7]

∞ Criticized, being; of doing nothing right.[7]

∞ Disparaged by a superior.[7]

∞ Drowning of self.[7]

∞ Envy.[7]
∞ Falling from a height.[7]
∞ Fire.[6]
∞ Flood.[7]
∞ Forsaken, being or feeling; excluded by friends.[7]
∞ Funeral, sees own.[7]
∞ Grasped by throat.[7]
∞ Impending danger.[7]
∞ Inspected by police.
∞ Jealous, being.[7]
∞ Move, unable to, except for one's tongue.[7]
∞ Murder.[6]
∞ Powerless after receiving bad news.[7]
∞ Rain.[7]
∞ Rejected, being.[7]
∞ Resignation about own death.[7]
∞ Rivalry in love affairs.[7]
∞ Shot in heart by arrow.[7]
∞ Suicide.[6]
∞ Thanks, receiving no.[7]
∞ Vivid recollection of events of day with additions and new plans for next day.[2]
∞ Vivid sexual dreams.[2]
∞ Water and high waves.[5]

## Generals
∞ Easily affected by a very little wine or alcoholic drink.[1]
∞ Craving for stimulants.[1] Great desire for wine.[2]
∞ 'All-overish' feeling [uncomfortable all over], & lightness in head.[1]
∞ Lying on affected side > chest, lungs, cough, breathing.[2]
∞ Feels best when lying on left side.[4]
∞ Cold and raw fruits = indigestion [sense of fulness; empty eructations].[2]
∞ Sour fruit > nausea and faintness.[2] Pear [jargonel] = headache and abdominal ache.[2]
∞ Cannot run or walk fast, = shortness of breath, pain in chest, palpitations [3 pr.].[2]
∞ Inability to make least effort for some minutes from sheer sense of exhaustion, & frequent loss of all power of using limbs.[2]
∞ Clothing as if too tight; loosening clothing >.[5]
∞ Before menses <.[5]
∞ Change of weather <.[4]
∞ Sun exposure >.[7]
∞ Dryness – nose, compels blowing nose, but without discharge; mouth, morning on waking; throat, morning on waking.[7]
∞ Pains, ailments extending from left to right – ovarian pains, throat, joint affections.[8]
∞ Ailments after surgery – stripping of varicose veins.[7]

∞ Lack of vital heat during pregnancy.[7]
∞ Flushes of heat downward from forehead or face.[7]
∞ Static electricity shock on touching anything.[7]

## Sensations
∞ Feeling as if ether has been evaporated in room.[2]
∞ Sensation as if wasting away[2], thin and starving[2].
∞ Sensation of being smaller.[8]
∞ Tightness across vertex.[2]
∞ Skull of forehead as if too small and tight.[2]
∞ Frontal part of brain as if loose.[2]
∞ Excessive weight over upper eyelids.[2]
∞ Noise in ears, as from a mill in head.[2]
∞ External throat between larynx and top of sternum as if skinned.[2]
∞ Lump in upper part of oesophagus and stomach.[2]
∞ Ball in bladder.[8]
∞ Roused by sudden sense of choking, while dozing, as if grasped by throat.[2]
∞ Tightness in larynx as if it were stuffed, & difficulty of swallowing.[2]
∞ Broken rib as if tearing lung on left side, on attempting to walk fast.[2]
∞ Ribs as if dislocated or broken.[8]
∞ Emptiness heart region.[8]
∞ Heart as if swollen.[8]
∞ Something wanting in praecordium.[1]
∞ Uneasiness about heart while walking.[2]
∞ Someone coming up from behind and dealing a severe blow to one's neck and head.[3]
∞ Heavy dragging in spine between scapulae.[2]
∞ Pain as if lumbar region would break, during stool. Pain lumbar region > sitting erect.[7]

## Locals
∞ Shooting frontal headache from glass of wine and/or hasty eating, < moving head.[2]
∞ Headache, morning on waking; after menses; on cessation of menses; > spirituous liquors; > smoking.[8]
∞ Pain occiput when lying on back.[7]
∞ Eyelids puffy in morning.[1]
∞ Dryness eyes, frequent blinking; dim vision on reading small print, must rub eyes and look closely.[2]
∞ Great dryness of tongue and mouth on waking in night or in morning on waking.[2]
∞ Protrudes lower lip < when talking. Salivation while talking.[7]
∞ Nausea and stomach pain from eating walnuts.[2]
∞ Involuntary urination from anger.[7]
∞ Larynx sensitive to cold air; to touch.[8]
∞ Voice, hoarseness, at night; when reading aloud.[8]

- ∞ Tried to sing, but had no power to throw out the voice.[1]
- ∞ Dull heavy pain over lower half of right chest, & stabbing pain on deep inspiration; cannot lie for a minute on left side, but pain and breathing much relieved by lying on affected side.[2]
- ∞ Palpitations prevent speech, on account of choking. Nervous chronic palpitation, esp. after public speaking. Speech difficult, from choking. Choking, on going to sleep; from palpitations.[8]
- ∞ Palpitations, < lying on left side; > lying on left side; < motion of arms; < riding in carriage; unable to speak; when turning in bed; after wine.[8]
- ∞ Pain in heart ext. to nape of neck, left scapula or left shoulder.[4]
- ∞ Heart symptoms > lying on left side.[4]
- ∞ Pain heart, > lying on right side, can only lie on right side.[8]
- ∞ Short hacking cough on going from a warm to a colder room, and esp. on going out in open air.[2]
- ∞ Tingling in legs and feet while standing.[1]

# CASE

Mrs. V., aet. 33, married and the mother of one child, was under treatment last winter and spring. First began to suffer 3 years previously. Was subject to headaches and pain in cardiac region. Very easily excited; was frightened just before her illness began, and on account of the singular condition resulting therefrom was taken to St. Luke's, and afterward to Bellevue Hospital. Does not know what the physicians pronounced her disease to be. Remained in hospital only a few weeks and then returned home. Never felt well after that; suffered from pain in left temple, cardiac and left ovarian region. Patient supposed she had heart disease, but physical examination revealed nothing unusual in the sounds or action of the organ. Had sharp, stabbing pains in cardiac region. *Great mental depression*; countenance wore an expression of sadness; *aversion to talking*; indeed it was almost impossible to induce her to tell me her symptoms.

When thus gloomy her heart symptoms, viz: the stabbing pain and sudden irregular action were greatly aggravated. Had frequent attacks of violent cardiac palpitation, coming on in the night, compelling her to sit by the open window in order to get relief. Pain in left ovary, simultaneous with pain in heart. *Sensation as if heart and ovary were drawn up together; a sense of contraction or drawing together between the organs*. Numbness of head and *back of neck*; would sometimes prick herself with pins and pinch her flesh to see if sensation still remained. Momentary vanishing of sight, felt weary.

After trying many remedies, Lachesis particularly, in high and low potencies without effect, the symptoms mentioned above, esp. those italicised, corresponded so closely with those belonging to Naja I concluded to give this remedy, and did so, in the 6th potency.

Complete recovery followed in a short time. I did not see my patient after her improvement, until several months had elapsed, when her countenance was cheerful, and she was free from all unpleasant symptoms. [Danforth, 1881]

## Clinical Manifestations

The Indian cobra's venom contains a powerful post-synaptic neurotoxin. The venom acts on the synaptic gaps of the nerves, thereby paralysing muscles, and possibly leading to respiratory failure or cardiac arrest. The venom components include enzymes such as hyaluronidase that cause lysis and increase the spread of the venom.

# CASE

The following case report of a cobra bite by Dr. Hilson [Indian Med. Gazette, Oct. 1873] exemplifies the predominantly neurotoxic properties of the cobra:

'On the night of the 19th June last year, at about half-past 12 o'clock, Dabee, a Hindu punka-coolie, aged 40 years, while sleeping in the verandah of my house, was bitten on the shoulder by a snake. . . . A burning pain was complained of in the neighbourhood of the bite, which rapidly increased in intensity, and extended so as to affect a circular portion of the integument of the size of an ordinary saucer; and, judging of the description given of it by the patient, I concluded it was very similar in character to that produced by the sting of a scorpion. '. . . While waiting for the ammonia [the then current treatment of snakebites], 1 had the patient walk up and down, and small quantities of brandy and water administered to him. At 12:45, or about a quarter of an hour after being bitten, he complained of a pain in his shoulder shooting towards his throat and chest, and said he was beginning to feel intoxicated; but there was nothing in his appearance at this time to indicate that he was in anyway under the influence of the poison. On the contrary, he was quite calm and collected, and answered to all questions intelligently, while at the same time he was fully alive to the danger of his condition.

"A person bitten by a black snake never recovers," he replied to 1 of his friends, who suggested, by way of consoling him, that the snake might possibly have been a harmless one. The pupils were not dilated, and they contracted when exposed to the light of a candle; his pulse was normal, and there was no embarrassment of the respiration. About 5 minutes after he began to lose control over the muscles of his legs, and staggered when left unsupported. At about 1 o'clock, the paralysis of the legs having increased, the lower jaw began to fall, and frothy and viscid saliva to ooze from the mouth. He also spoke indistinctly, like a man under the influence of liquor. At 1:10 a.m. he began to moan and shake his head frequently from side to side. The pulse was now somewhat accelerated, but was beating regularly. The respirations were also increased in frequency.

'He was unable to answer questions, but appeared to be quite conscious. His arms did not seem to be paralysed. . . . [Five minutes later] . . . it was evident that the condition of the patient was fast becoming critical. He continued to moan and shake his head from side to side, as if trying to get rid of viscid mucus in his throat. The respirations were laboured, but not stertorous. . . . The breathing gradually became slower and slower, and finally ceased at 1:44 a.m., while the heart continued to beat for about 1 minute longer. No convulsions preceded dissolution, which took place in 1 hour and 5 minutes after the infliction of the bite.'

### Drooping, Dragging, Dropping Dead

'The Cobra, *nág*, Naja tripudians, is of 2 kinds, the black or *kála*, and the white or *pándhra*. Mr. E. Mackenzie, Assistant Surgeon, Kumta dispensary, in his report for 1873–74, gives the following details of a fatal case of cobra bite. The patient, a boy, was admitted at 11:40 a.m. and died at 2:30 p.m. Though more than an hour had passed since he was bitten, when he was brought to the hospital, the symptoms, though urgent, did not seem to point to a fatal issue. The most marked symptom was paroxysms of pain stretching up the limbs.

The boy was lively and talkative, but there was an uncontrollable drooping of the upper eyelid. The breathing and circulation were unaffected. From his admission till his death the symptoms became slowly but steadily more serious. The drooping of the eyelid became more marked, the boy dragging it up when he wanted to use his eye. In the paroxysms he shouted from pain. Next he mumbled in his speech. Then the tongue lost feeling and the speech grew dim till the tongue moved without sound. Breathing became heavy and spasmodic, the throat and tongue dried, he grew drowsy, fell in a swoon and was dead. [Bombay Gazetteer, 1883]

# CASE

### Bitten in the Nose

'The following case, by Dr. Burder, affords one of the fullest descriptions on record of the action of Cobra Poison, when altogether unchecked by treatment.

'A keeper at the Regent's Park Zoological Gardens, aged 31, of rather intemperate habits, was bitten, while partially intoxicated, on the upper part of his nose, by an Indian Cobra. For a short time after the receipt of the wound, there appear to have been no striking symptoms, apart from his agitation and alarm at the occurrence. He was able to walk and talk without difficulty. After 20 minutes, however, he began to *stagger in walking, and ceased to speak intelligibly*. At the same time, movements, apparently convulsive, of the mouth and of the limbs were observed. He made no special complaint.

'He was brought to the hospital about 35 minutes after the accident. He was then unable to speak, and consciousness was nearly or quite abolished. He moaned, grasped his throat with some eagerness of action, tossed his head from side to side and moved his arms and legs in an uneasy restless manner, not apparently convulsive. When asked, in a loud voice, if he felt pain, he made no reply, nor gave any indication of intelligence, beyond the action of placing his fingers on his throat.

'He was unable to support himself in a sitting posture. His face generally was slightly livid, his eyes fixed, the pupils rather large, acting sluggishly to light; the skin was of natural temperature and moisture; pulse 120, regular in rhythm, but unequal in force, most of the beats, however, being tolerably full and strong. On the upper part of the nose were a number of small punctured wounds, from one or more of which a small quantity of blood had flowed. The eyelids of the right eye, esp. the upper, were swollen and livid, the lividity extending to the right side of the nose. The eyelids of the left eye were not thus affected.

'There appeared to be no swelling of the tongue. Within 5 minutes, movements of the extremities had entirely ceased, the respiration was 20 per minute, very shallow, without stertor and free from any sound indicating laryngeal or tracheal obstruction. The lividity of the face had very markedly increased, a free perspiration had occurred over the body generally. The pulse continued tolerably good. In 2 minutes more [about 40 minutes after the infliction of. the bite] natural respiration had ceased [?], and, but for the continuance of the pulse, the man might have been pronounced dead. The pulse at this time was 32 per minute, remarkably regular both in rhythm and in force, some of the beats being strikingly full and bounding. Artificial respiration and the application of galvanism were now employed and continued for 50 minutes, at the end of which time all the muscular action ceased.' [Chevers, 1856]

## Typical Course of Cobra Envenomation

The special symptoms of cobra envenomation rapidly manifest themselves. 'In man it is very commonly observed that the patient cannot any longer keep his eyes open and about this time it is found that he is losing power in his legs. When he walks he staggers, and, if left unsupported, falls. The arms seem to retain their strength much longer. The order in which the symptoms occur next varies in different individuals.

'In some loss of the power of speech and of raising the lower jaw is shown and afterwards profuse salivation; but the salivation may precede. But whichever may occur first, the tongue and the larynx become speedily paralysed; the patient is unable to speak or to clear his throat or to swallow; and the saliva, which is profusely poured forth, trickles down the lips, the patient being no longer able to eject it voluntarily.

'The paralysis now becomes more general and decided. The patient lies on his back, *almost incapable of movement.* He threatens to be suffocated by the saliva running into his paralysed larynx; should however, the head be placed on one side, the abundant secretion will flow down his lips. His limbs at this time may be subject to startings and muscular twitchings. His breathing becomes slower and slower, and the respiratory excursus is lessened.

'He appears to be conscious, but is *unable to express himself,* through the paralysis of his larynx and tongue, but it is not infrequently the case for the victim to become quite unconscious. The action of the heart is somewhat quickened, but the organ acts with fair strength. At last the breathing, too slow and too slight to support life, ceases, and with or without general convulsions the heart shortly after stops.'

'That the chief action of cobra poison is on the nervous system there can be no doubt. . . . One of the most characteristic features of cobra poisoning in the human subject is paralysis of the legs. The patient is unable to walk or to stand, though his arms have not as yet experienced any loss of power. . . . It will have been observed that paralysis of the lips, tongue, larynx, and pharynx, as evidenced by inability to retain the saliva within the mouth, by incapacity to move the tongue, or to speak, or to swallow, are very prominent signs of cobra-poisoning. It is singular that the striking resemblance of these symptoms to the disease known as glosso-laryngeal paralysis has not been previously noticed. . . .

'It will be seen how rapidly and completely cobra poison, when introduced into the circulation, destroys the respiratory function, so that cobra poisoning is generally simply death from asphyxia in an acute form. . . . Cobra poison cannot be said to exercise a very great effect on the circulation. . . . In ordinary cases of cobra poisoning the heart can generally be felt beating for a short time after respiration has stopped. Absorbed in the ordinary way, cobra poison appears to slightly accelerate the heart's action, and it also seems to lessen the blood pressure – at any rate for some time. . . . Cobra poison also appears to have but little influence on the temperature of the body. Sometimes a very slight rise is to be noticed; generally there is no change, and even a slight fall has been observed. . . .

'On the secretions cobra poison appears to have considerable influence. It seems as if most secreting structures were stimulated by it. The lachrymal glands act freely during cobra poisoning. Salivation is a most marked and constant symptom; it is very rarely indeed absent in dogs and it appears to be equally common in man. In dogs the saliva often runs from the mouth literally in streams; nor in man does it seem much less copious. Should only a small quantity of poison have entered the system salivation may be the only symptom.

'The whole of the mucous tract is also apparently in an active state of secretion. After the stomach has been thoroughly emptied by vomiting, animals will often bring up repeatedly large quantities of mucus, and mucous discharges are also frequently evacuated from the rectum. The respiratory mucous membrane, too, participates. Mucous secretion sometimes flows from the nose, and the air tubes are not unusually found bathed in fluid.

'In the vast majority of cases there is no symptom of serious blood-poisoning even during the occurrence of the nerve symptoms.' [Wall, 1873]

### Symptoms & Signs

*Neurological and Neuromuscular*: These signs and symptoms will usually manifest earliest. Not all of these will necessarily develop, even with severe envenomation.

Drowsiness [over 90% of cases].
Eyelids drooping [Ptosis] [75–85%]
Respiratory paralysis or dyspnoea [70–80%]
Ophthalmoplegia [35–45%]
Palatal paralysis [30–40%]
Glosso-pharyngeal paralysis [30–40%]
Limb paralysis [20–30%]
Convulsions [10–20%]
Head drooping [cervical muscle paresis or paralysis]
Headache
Sudden loss of consciousness
Stumbling gait

*General*: These symptoms typically manifest within 1 to 4 hours following the bite if envenomation occurred. They include: Nausea and vomiting. Hypotension. Flushing of face. Warm skin. Pain around bite site. Abdominal pain.

*Cardiotoxicity*: Increased blood pressure and increased cardiac output followed by myocardial depression and asystole. Mortality approaches 100% if cardiotoxic complications occur.

*Local symptoms*: In some Cobra bites, local tissue destruction and necrosis can dominate the clinical presentation. Gangrene requiring amputation can occur. Local tissue damage appears to be less frequent and less severe in most cases of Indian cobra [Naja naja] envenomation, but may include: Localised discolouration of skin. Vesiculation [usually small and localised]. Necrosis [can be extensive, but is characteristically localised to the bite site]. Local oedema [usually minimal]. [Davidson, University of California, Snakebite Protocols]

# NOTECHIS SCUTATUS OCCIDENTALIS

### Systematics
- Scientific name: Notechis scutatus [Peters, 1861].
- Subspecies: N. s. occidentalis [Glauert, 1948].
- Synonym: Notechis ater occidentalis [Cogger, 2000].

- Common name: Western tiger snake.
- Family: Elapidae.

## Biological Profile

- Stout-bodied, short-tailed elapid; body flattened dorso-ventrally. Body variable in colour from brown, olive, grey to black. Most usual pattern is alternating light and dark bands, which gives rise to the common name. Belly cream, yellow, olive green or grey. Average length 1.2 m, maximum 2.1 m.
- Head moderately wide and deep; only slightly distinct from robust, muscular body.
- Range: Southwest corner of Western Australia.
- Forests and open grasslands.
- Unlike most other Australian elapids, tiger snakes climb well on both vegetation and human constructions and have been found as high as 10 m above the ground.
- Predominantly diurnal but becomes semi-nocturnal on excessively hot nights [over 34°C]. Likely to be out on balmy evenings, esp. after rain, because at such times frogs, its main prey, are out and about.
- Preys on small mammals, birds, and frogs.
- Ovoviviparous; 20–30 live young per brood.
- Neck and upper body can be flattened to a considerable degree when performing a threat display, exposing the black skin between the relatively large, semi-glossy scales.


## MATERIA MEDICA NOTECHIS SCUTATUS OCCIDENTALIS

### Sources
1 Effects of bite; clinical manifestations.
2 Effects of bite; general overview

### Clinical Manifestations
'20 February 1986. 4:00 p.m.; Bitten on tip of left forefinger whilst hand feeding Notechis scutatus occidentalis, i.e. bitten by 'mistake'. Consequently the Notechis scutatus occidentalis retained its hold on my finger for approximately 1 minute, believing it had hold of the lizard. Initial movements by me [moving finger] in an attempt to make it release its hold prompted 'chewing' and the injection of more venom. It eventually released its hold when I gently prised its upper jaw from my finger.
4:05 p.m.; Headache beginning.
4:12 p.m.; Finger swollen to knuckle.
5:00 p.m.; Headache. Finger swollen to knuckle. Lymph node in left armpit painful.
7:45 p.m.; Headache. Lymph node in left armpit painful. Entire left arm, except for 'middle' of forearm, sore. considerably swollen and painful.
8:30 p.m.; Went to bed.

10:50 p.m.; Awoke with severe headache, nausea and almost delirious. Hallucinating somewhat; my left hand was expanding, becoming enormous as I watched. I then realised this couldn't be so as my left hand was tucked beneath my pillow and therefore not visible. Vision blurred. Entire left arm and all lymph nodes [armpits, groin, etc.] painful.

21 February 1986.

3:50 a.m.; Awoke. Vision blurred; unable to focus on objects closer than [approx.] 1 metre, hence cannot read normal print nor what I write. Left arm still painful and finger still swollen. No sense of taste.

Daytime; Left arm painful, as are lymph nodes in neck. Took 2 Panadeine and 2 Dispirin throughout day to alleviate headache and vague feeling of malaise. Finger swollen and painful. Vision still blurred and unable to focus on nearby objects. Unable to taste food properly.

7:00 pm [approx.]; Vision clearing somewhat.

22 February 1986.

Slight, vague headache and malaise, took 2 Panadeine. Vision much improved with blurring only on very close objects, i.e. can write normally but cannot read small print closer than 30 cm. [approx.]. Finger less swollen and painful. Little else was noted at the time. My sight returned to normal after a couple of days and my sense of taste after about a week.'

[Paul Orange, Envenomation by the Western Tiger snake; cited by Michael Thompson, RefWorks]

## General Overview

The western tiger snake is seventh on the list of the world's most venomous snake using the LD50 in mice as a guide and in humans the venom causes coagulopathy, neurotoxicity and myolysis. About 50% of tiger snake bites result in significant envenoming and prior to antivenom therapy there was a mortality of 45%.

Of 23 recorded cases of western tiger snake envenomation in SW Australia, 17 [74%] suffered headache, 17 [74%] nausea/vomiting, 11 [48%] abdominal pain, 10 [43%] local pain, and 6 [26%] showed clinical signs of bleeding. Bleeding occurred at the bite site or presented as epistaxis or haematemesis. Complications included ptosis and diplopia in 2 patients [9%], respiratory arrest in 1 [4%], rhabdomyolysis in 6 [26%], and renal failure in 1 patient [4%]. [Scop, 2009]

# NOTECHIS SCUTATUS SCUTATUS ▬▬▬

## Systematics

- Scientific name: Notechis scutatus [Peters, 1861].
- Subspecies: N. s. scutatus [Peters, 1861].
- Common names: Eastern tiger snake. Mainland tiger snake.
- Family: Elapidae.

## Biological Profile
- Stout-bodied, short-tailed elapid; body flattened dorso-ventrally, olive to dark brown above with yellowish or olive belly and cross-bands. Average length 1.2 m, maximum 2.1 m.
- Head moderately wide and deep; only slightly distinct from robust, muscular body.
- Range: SE Australia, Tasmania, Bass Strait islands, New Guinea.
- Often associated with watery environments such as creeks, dams, drains, lagoons, wetlands and swamps. Can also occur in highly degraded areas e.g. grazing lands, esp. where there is water and local cover.
- Will shelter in or under fallen timber, in deep matted vegetation and in disused animal burrows.
- Unlike most other Australian elapids, tiger snakes climb well on both vegetation and human constructions, and have been found as high as 10 m above the ground.
- Predominantly diurnal but becomes semi-nocturnal on excessively hot nights [over 34°C]. Likely to be out on balmy evenings, esp. after rain, because at such times frogs, its main prey, are out and about.
- Preys mainly on frogs and mice, but will take the odd bird or lizard.
- Ovoviviparous; 14–37 live young per brood.
- Will usually act out an impressive threat display before attempting to bite. This begins with flattening of the neck and upper body and loud hissing followed by mock strikes.

## Behaviour & Temperament
Most dangerous snake in Australia. When aroused, it is aggressive and attacks any intruder. It will hold its forebody in a tense but loose curve, head raised slightly and facing directly at an intruder, inflating and deflating the body and hissing loudly. Captive tiger snakes are considered unpredictable – quiet and calm one day, evil the next.

## MATERIA MEDICA NOTECHIS SCUTATUS SCUTATUS

### Sources
1 Effects of bite, 5 cases described in Sutherland, Australian Animal Toxins [1983], and case summaries from literature reported on www.toxinology.com.
2 Effects of bite; clinical manifestations.

### Mind
∞ Speech like that of a drunken man; difficulty in articulation and swallowing.
∞ Irritable and drowsy.
∞ Confusion and disorientation.

### Generals
∞ Inability to stand or walk without assistance.

∞ Progressive weakness of lower limbs, unsteady gait.
∞ Severe hypotension.
∞ Cyanosis.
∞ Sweating.

## Locals
∞ Headache.
∞ Pupils dilated, reacting slightly to light.
∞ Diplopia and partial bilateral ptosis.
∞ Vision blurred, quickly followed by complete loss of sight.
∞ Inability to move either eye in any direction.
∞ Retinal haemorrhage.
∞ Loss of sense of smell.
∞ Swallowing difficult; impossible to drink.
∞ Vomiting of dark brownish material at intervals.
∞ Continuous desire to micturate and defaecate.
∞ Incontinence of urine and faeces.
∞ Diarrhoea and vomiting associated with apathy, tremors and blurred vision.
∞ Urine very dark, containing blood cells and haemoglobin, but no casts.
∞ Heavy heartbeat & peculiar burning sensation in mouth.
∞ Respiration short, shallow, jerky, abdominal-thoracic in type.
∞ Respiration difficult, & paralysis of palate and swelling of throat.
∞ 'Approximately 10 minutes after the bite speech was difficult and breathing was almost impossible as the lungs could be felt slowly paralyzing. I believe it was only by being sufficiently conscious to inhale deeply at regular intervals and so fully inflate the lungs that it was possible to continue breathing. I feel certain that, should go to sleep under such circumstances, it would be very difficult to avoid suffocation. Throughout the effects I would have had no difficulty in going to sleep, but this was purposely avoided.'
∞ Left forearm [bite wound midway between elbow and wrist] swollen and pitting on pressure; pain in left axilla.

## Clinical Manifestations
Venom is mainly neurotoxic with some cytotoxins and myotoxins present, as well as a coagulant with some haemolytic activity.

'There may be bleeding from the wound site, and this can persist. In most cases there is some delay in the appearance of significant clinical manifestations. In 1 case seen by the author, the first signs of envenomation were dizziness, headache and abdominal pain, approximately 30 minutes following the bite. Until that time the patient did not believe that he had been envenomated. Examination revealed slightly enlarged and tender axillary lymph nodes on the affected sides, mild weakness of the arm [at 90 minutes], and the complaint of some feeling of numbness over that extremity. Reflexes were intact at that time. The patient complained of weakness, drowsiness, and headache. Shortly thereafter, the patient developed pain in the abdomen, in the large muscle masses of the back and shoulders, and in the chest on inspiration. There was moderate weakness of the muscles of the upper extremities and shoulders. Since antivenom was given at this time, no further manifestations developed except for haematuria, which persisted for 12 hours. The patient had an increased blood-clotting time and decreased blood calcium, but these deficits disappeared within 48 hours.

'In a second case, the patient complained of headache and some muscular weakness within 15 minutes of the bite. At 30 minutes, he noted slurring of speech and onset of dull abdominal pain. At 45 minutes, he had some difficulty in breathing, some blurring of vision, difficulties in focussing, slight ptosis, and gradually developing paresis. These findings worsened over the next 8 hours. The abdominal pain became severe, and both the urine and stools contained bright red blood. Skeletal muscle paralysis developed.

'At this point, approximately 30 hours following the bite, a tracheostomy was performed, and artificial ventilation initiated. . . . The patient was given 3 pints of fresh whole blood. Electrolyte imbalance was corrected. There was no myoglobinuria. An artificial pacemaker was placed because of cardiac arrhythmia. The patient had a slow but uneventful recovery. He had a deficit of the olfactory nerve for many months following the bite.' [Russell, 1980]

Particularly in cases of tiger snake bite, the *headache may be extremely severe*. 'Patients have described it as being an overwhelming pounding pain. One victim believed that some large hospital machine had come adrift from its foundations and was causing the whole building to vibrate to its beat. The mechanism causing these severe headaches is not known.' [Sutherland, 1983]

Some snake bite victims have recovered from severe envenomation without any treatment at all. For example, at the end of a moderate drinking spree a man was bitten late in the evening by Notechis scutatus just as he reached his isolated and solitary camp in the bush., He ignored the bite and after 30 minutes felt dizzy and vomited. He had no recollection of the next 48 hours and, for the 48 hours following, could barely walk and passed very dark brown urine. It was another 4 days before he could resume work and 2 weeks later he was still "weak as a kitten." [Sutherland, 1983]

# OPHIOPHAGUS HANNAH

## Systematics
- Scientific name: Ophiophagus hannah [Cantor, 1836].
- Synonyms: Hamadryas hannah [Cantor, 1836]. Naja bungarus [Schlegel, 1837]. Dendraspis bungarus [Fitzinger, 1843]. Naja hannah [Taylor, 1922].
- Common names: King cobra. Jungle cobra. Hamadryad.
- Family: Elapidae.

## Biological Profile
- Large, powerful, majestic elapid, the world's longest venomous snake, averaging 3–4 m, maximum 5–6 m.

- Olive-green, tan, or black with faint, pale yellow cross-bands down length of body. Belly cream or pale yellow. Scales smooth. Males larger and heavier than females.
- King cobras found in darker forests are darker in colour than those found in open forests or savannahs.
- Not a true cobra, placed as monotypic in a separate genus.
- Range: South and SE Asia into Indonesia and the Philippines.
- Habitat: Near streams in both dense and open forest, as well as bamboo stands and agricultural areas, like tea plantations. Also inhabits mangrove swamps.
- Diurnal, active during daytime; has good eyesight.
- Mostly terrestrial, but is good swimmer and excellent climber and will pursue prey into trees.
- Preys on snakes [Ophiophagus = snake eater], incl. pythons, kraits, cobras and its own kind. May also feed on lizards, birds, and rodents.
- 'The female king cobra is a very dedicated parent. Before she is ready to lay her eggs, she uses the coils of her long body to gather a big mound of leaf litter. She deposits 20–40 eggs into the mound, which acts as an incubator. The female stays with her eggs and guards the mound tenaciously, rearing up into a threat display if any large animal gets too close.' [Wikipedia]
- Both male and female are reported to remain in the vicinity of the nest until hatching. They are protective of their eggs and will be very aggressive towards any human that approaches the nest.
- Males fight for a female using a 'neck-wrestling' technique. The successful male then courts the female by rubbing her with his head.
- Despite its fearsome reputation and deadly bite, the king cobra is a shy and reclusive animal, avoiding confrontation with humans as often as possible. Yet, when confronted it raises up to one-third of its body straight off the ground and still moves forward to attack. In addition it will flare out its iconic hood and emit a bone-chilling, severely intimidating hiss that sounds almost like a growling dog.
- King cobras are a favourite of the snake charmers of South Asia, in particular the female snake charmers of Burma.

## No Serpent More Clever & Curious

In *Snakes: A Natural History*, a brain-size index is presented that allows appreciation of the relative importance of the brain to the rest of the body, and to compare this development across the several groups of reptiles and amphibians. The higher the index, the more evolved the species is considered. Snakes do not score high on the listing, seemingly not being the sharpest knives in the drawer. Moreover, it is well known that long-bodied, limbless animals pay the price for their streamlined, sleek design in a regression of their brain volume. The brain-size index for snakes ranges from 32 for the Boa constrictor to 104 for the cottonmouth [Agkistrodon piscivorus]. These numbers differ relatively slightly from those found in amphibians [35 to 174], but are definitely low compared to those found in other reptiles, such as turtles [43 to 234] or lizards [72 to 337].

Worm lizards score about the same as snakes, while crocodilians are lowest in the table, their index ranging from 50 to 80. Although brain-size perhaps ought not to be equated with intelligence, Ditmars found king cobras to possess extraordinary brainpower. He notes: 'I have observed many demonstrations of the singular intelligence of the king cobra – and am using the word "singular" because other snakes do not act this way. For a day or 2 it will strike at visitors and thus bump its nose, but soon does nothing more than rear and feint at striking. Captive examples appear to recognise the persons who care for them, yet evince antagonism towards strangers. They become active at feeding intervals, usually a week apart, will come to the rear door of the cage and if there is a small crevice will peer up or down a passageway watching for the keeper.

Moreover, I have noted that specimens discovered which side of the door was the opening portion as the head keeper often rolls the door back slightly to insert a long wire to pull out fragments of shed skin. All of this demands caution in door manipulation as the inclination of these snakes would be to immediately come to an open door, "boss" the keeper out of the way by rearing and feinting a strike, then glide into a passageway. Interference would be met by bold attack. I have never seen them show much fear or nervousness. They have their favourite corners in which to coil and sleep and a king cobra I took from New York to Washington, that had invariably coiled in the left hand rear corner of its cage, prowled its new quarters and went to rest in a left rear corner.' [Ditmars, 1937b]

## MATERIA MEDICA OPHIOPHAGUS HANNAH

### Sources
1 Proving Farokh Master [India], 4 provers [3 females, 1 males], 30c and 200c; 2009–10; unmarked symptoms.
2 Clinical observations Mangialavori [Italy].
3 Effects of bite; clinical manifestations.
4 Effects of bite; king-size effects.
5 Effects of bite; locked-in syndrome.

### Mind
∞ Absent-mindedness; confusion; irresolution.
∞ Anger at trifles, & impulse to strike others.
∞ Depressed and sad; no enthusiasm; things feel sordid.
∞ Delusion being doomed.[2]
∞ Egotism, self-esteem, over-estimation of self.[2]
∞ Seeks relief in constant praying.[2]

### Dreams
∞ Missing train.
∞ Pursued by a group of people in a forest at night.
∞ Riding a horse.
∞ Satan and evil.

∞ Showing/expressing anger.
∞ Unable to finish task.

## Generals
∞ Daytime drowsiness.
∞ Waking from sleep at 2–3 a.m.
∞ Thirst for cold water.

## Sensations
∞ Heaviness root of nose, with obstruction nose.

## Locals
∞ Obstruction nose with formation of thick green crusts.
∞ Cannot tolerate hair being tied.
∞ Diarrhoea < 2 a.m. [must rush out of bed] and morning on waking.
∞ Pain behind sternum extending to left side of chest and to left arm, like an electric current passing through these areas; at night during first part of sleep.
∞ Palpitation < slight exertion, slight anxiety, any emotion.
∞ itching red rash on buttocks after menses.
∞ Low backache < bending forward; before or during menses.
∞ Weakness legs < standing.

## Clinical Manifestations
'The King Cobra's venom is primarily neurotoxic and thus attacks the victim's central nervous system and quickly induces severe pain, blurred vision, vertigo, drowsiness and paralysis. In 1 to 2 minutes, cardiovascular collapse occurs, and the victim falls into a coma. Death soon follows due to respiratory failure. There are 2 types of antivenin made specifically to treat King Cobra envenomations. The Red Cross in Thailand manufactures one, and the Central Research Institute in India manufactures the other; however, both are made in small quantities and are not widely available. Ohanin, a protein component of the venom, causes hypo-locomotion and hyperalgesia [increased sensitivity to pain] in mammals. Other components have cardiotoxic, cytotoxic and neurotoxic effects.' [Wikipedia]

## King-size Effects
'Fortunately, bites by this formidable species are rare. Its reputation for aggressiveness is unwarranted. Two out of 13 bites, which occurred in Guangxi in 1990 were inflicted while the captive snake was being handled. Three cases of bites in people involved in the famous snake dance in Rangoon Zoological Garden, Burma, were described and 32 other cases reviewed. Many of these patients were bitten by snakes, which they had greatly provoked. When the king cobra bites its natural prey, a snake or monitor lizard, it retains its grip sometimes for 10–30 minutes until the prey is immobile or dead. In 1 case, the snake held on to the human it had bitten for at least 8 minutes. Sixty-three percent of these 35 patients died but 2 of them showed no signs of envenoming.

Local envenoming has rarely been mentioned in reports of bites by *O. hannah*, but in 2 of the patients observed in Rangoon, swelling was extensive, involving the entire bitten limb and adjacent areas of the trunk and neck in one of them. Local swelling was described in 6 of the 32 cases from the literature and blistering and small areas of local necrosis in 5 out of 35 cases and in 3 of 13 patients in Guangxi. Despite its high enzyme [esp. hyaluronidase] content, the venom of *O. hannah* is clearly less necrotic than those of the Asian *Naja*, perhaps because of its low content of proteases. Neurotoxicity is the most prominent features of envenoming, reputedly leading to death "soon" or in a "few minutes."

A 30-year-old reptile housekeeper in Rangoon who was bitten by a 2 metre long specimen began to feel dizzy 15 minutes after the bite. Thirty minutes after the bite his speech was slurred and his breathing difficult; 10 minutes later he had developed bilateral ptosis and his respirations were shallow. There was a gradual deterioration in his breathing, which became slow and diaphragmatic. He could open his mouth only slightly and, 90 minutes after the bite, he had respiratory arrest and required 38½ hours of mechanical ventilation.

Two-and-a-half hours after the bite he had congested conjunctivae, ptosis, complete external ophthalmoplegia, areflexia, and generalised flaccid paralysis but was fully conscious [shown by his ability to answer "yes" or "no" to questions by flexing his fingers]. The pupils were normal and reactive to light. There was slight improvement in neurological signs before specific antivenom could finally be given 38 hours after the bite. . . . No bleeding or clotting disorders have been reliably reported in victims of *O. hannah*. . . . The interval between bite and death has ranged from a few minutes to 12 hours. In Guangxi, two-thirds of the patients developed paralytic symptoms and 7 out of 13 died.' [Meier & White, 1995]

### Locked-in Syndrome

'A patient bitten by Ophiophagus hannah may manifest local and systemic signs of envenoming. Local tissue necrosis, with or without secondary infection, is a common feature of envenoming from cobra bites. A patient may present with lethargy, nausea, vomiting and in more severe cases, victims may develop hypotension, tachycardia, altered conscious level, shock and death. Systemic neurotoxic envenoming from O. hannah could result in the early onset of ptosis, blurring of vision, paraesthesia, difficulty in speaking, weaknesses of limbs and respiratory failure. One of the infrequently documented neurological manifestations following cobra bite envenoming is locked-in syndrome [LIS]. Here, we report a case of LIS following O. hannah envenoming.

'A 30-year-old gentleman presented to an emergency department [ED] 35 mins following a bite by a 4-meter long wild-caught king cobra. According to the patient, he was bitten in the right arm while trying to capture the snake. The bite lasted approximately 10 seconds before they managed to release it. The snake was subsequently killed. The patient complained of difficulty opening the eyes, blurred vision, nausea, vomiting and dizziness during transportation to the hospital. On arrival, he had generalised muscle weakness, circumoral paraesthesia, hypersalivation and slurred speech. There was pain and swelling over the entire right forearm extending to the fingers. He was tachycardic, tachypnoeic and unable to speak or swallow. He was intubated and ventilated in the ED.

'Five vials of the O. hannah monospecific antivenom [OHAV] was administered in the ED prior to admission to the Intensive Care Unit [ICU]. An additional of 28 vials of OHAV was administered in 6 divided doses over the course of 36 hrs in the ICU. The patient only received minimal sedation and analgesia.

'The first neurological response was noted 28 hrs post incident. The patient was able to grimace and shook his head upon calls. At the 30th hr post incident the patient was able to obey simple commands and opening the eyes slightly. By the 48th hr of admission, the patient was breathing spontaneously, self-initiated eye opening and obeying command for muscle movements. . . . The oedema progressed proximally to involve the chest and supraclavicular region with clear blisters forming over the fingers, forearm and arm. Multiple enlarged and tender lymph nodes were palpable in the right axilla. The pain score was 5/10.

'The oedema, soft tissue inflammation, multiple bullae and ecchymosis at posterior right upper arm resolved over the subsequent 5 days. In a retrospective interview, the patient was able to recall the period when he was paralyzed but able to hear the conversations taking place around him. He felt severe pain in the arm and was aware of the procedures performed but *unable to response or move*. He was able to recall family members visiting him and the conversations between healthcare providers in the ICU. Following significant recovery, he was discharged home on day 12, post incidence. The patient was reviewed 1 week later with complete resolution without any adverse sequelae.' [Khaldun, 2017]

# OXYURANUS MICROLEPIDOTUS

## Systematics
- Scientific name: Oxyuranus microlepidotus [McCoy, 1879].
- Synonyms: Diemenia microlepidota [McCoy, 1879]. Pseudechis ferox [Boulenger, 1896]. Parademansia microlepidota [Kinghorn, 1955].
- Common names: Inland taipan. Fierce snake. Western taipan. Small-scaled snake.
- Family: Elapidae.

## Biological Profile
- Large elapid, closely resembling O. scutellatus, with glossy black head, black eyes, black throat and cream-coloured to yellow belly with indistinct reddish blotches. Body dark brown above, usually with dark flecking, which may merge to form V-shaped bands towards the tail. Colour tends to be lighter in summer and then changes to a brownish olive-green. All scales smooth, very glossy and without keels. Average length 2 m, maximum 2.5 m.
- Range: Australia [New South Wales, Queensland, South Australia, Victoria].
- Habitat: Vast treeless semi-arid and arid ashy downs remote from the coast. [Ashy downs or Gibber plains are vast, generally treeless plains that are waterless except after heavy rains.]

- Usually active on the surface in the morning between 8 a.m. and 10 a.m., basking and foraging in and near soil cracks. In cooler weather it is active in the afternoon and in hot weather it becomes nocturnal.
- Preys predominantly on plague rats [Rattus villosissimus; specific name in reference to its long, soft and fluffy hair], which inhabit extensive burrow systems in ashy downs areas. Searching out the dangerous rats for a meal, the inland taipan's extremely potent venom is thought to assist it in killing its dangerous prey before being injured by the prey's retaliatory bites with sharp teeth in the narrow confined spaces of the rat burrows.
- Oviparous; 9–13 eggs per clutch.
- Although highly venomous, it is very shy and secretive, preferring to escape from trouble, only biting if threatened. The most venomous land snake, its bite can contain enough venom to kill 100 human adults or 250,000 mice. Its venom is about 20 times as toxic as the king cobra and about 90 times more toxic than North America's most dangerous snake, the eastern diamondback rattlesnake.

## MATERIA MEDICA OXYURANUS MICROLEPIDOTUS

### Sources
1 Effects of bite; potentially life-threatening.
2 Effects of bite; heart stopping twice.

### Potentially Life-Threatening
Venom strongly neurotoxic. Symptoms of envenomation include headache, nausea, vomiting, abdominal pain, collapse and paralysis. The venom of the Inland taipan is extremely potent and is rated as the most toxic of all snake venoms in LD50 tests on mice. As well as being strongly neurotoxic the venom contains a 'spreading factor' [hyaluronidase enzyme] that increases the rate of absorption. The venom's toxicity coupled with its spreading action makes a bite from a Fierce Snake potentially life-threatening, and anyone suspected of receiving a bite should seek immediate medical attention. [australianmuseum.net.au]

### Little One Can Do – Heart Stopping Twice
In 1967, Australian reptile expert Athol Compton suffered a double bite on the right thumb while attempting to capture an unfamiliar, large light brown snake with a dark head in Corner Country, in far southwest Queensland. A tourniquet was applied above the elbow and the bitten area was incised and sucked.

It is interesting to compare the treating physician's case report with Compton's own experience of the bite.

- First the case report, as retrieved from www.inchem.org/documents/pims/animal/taipan.htm:

'50 minutes post-bite he collapsed, unconscious, with faecal and urine incontinence. He regained consciousness within 15 minutes. He remained stable, but with muscle pain for several hours, then developed nausea and vomiting. By 6 hours post-bite he had dysphagia and dysarthria, and the bite site was swollen and cyanosed [tourniquet still in place, with intermittent release]. During the next 3 hours he became agitated, confused, [while in transit in a Flying Doctor aircraft] and on landing, about 9 hours post-bite, suffered a cardiac arrest, from which he was successfully resuscitated. As he had [incorrectly] identified the snake as a brown snake [Pseudonaja] he was given brown snake antivenom [which is not protective for taipan bites].

'He had a past history of severe allergy to horse serum, though no anaphylaxis developed on antivenom administration. He was subsequently placed on a ventilator. Ptosis and ophthalmoplegia were present, but he could move all limbs. At 17.5 hours post-bite he had a hypotensive episode, with haematuria and bloody diarrhoea. By 24 hours post-bite the bleeding had subsided. He developed episodes of frequent ventricular extrasystoles during aspiration of his endotracheal tube, which continued intermittently, along with transient hypertension. He made a slow recovery, requiring ventilator support for several [unspecified] days.'

- Stackhouse [1972] recorded Compton's first-hand account of the bite:

'In about 15 minutes I started to feel the first effects of the bite. This was mainly lack of judgement in distance. There was no other feeling of being sick or pain. I got in a car and started driving for help and found I couldn't judge corners.

'We made it to a station about 20 miles away with the idea of using their flying doctor radio set. But this was broken down, so I had to rig my portable radio. I couldn't complete the driving, by the way. I had to hand over to one of the chaps with me.

'By the time I got on air my speech had thickened and I was feeling slightly drunk. My eyes had become bloodshot, I was quite calm. I had decided by this time from the effects and because a doctor was so far away – I was 400 miles from the base at Broken Hill – that there was only going to be a very slim chance of getting over this one.

'By this time, I was just about due to collapse. There was still no pain, but I couldn't sit up, so I handed the radio over to one of the chaps with me. My friends picked me up, then all my muscles went. I lost control of my legs, my bowels – the lot. I could still think, but I couldn't co-ordinate.

'From then on I started to lose consciousness. I felt well, which is not a good sign. This indicates that there is little your body can do to fight the venom.

'This chap who was working the radio for me kept notes. The doctor told him to take my temperature and the first reading on the case notes was that my temperature was too low to register on the thermometer. It gradually came up, however. They gave me an aspirin or something.

'Occasionally, I was conscious and felt well. I found my vision had doubled – one picture on top of the other, vertically. I was also vomiting. I can remember the doctor arriving. He got a needle out and I said: "Now, I can't take antivenene. I'm allergic to horse serum."

'I remember his saying: "Well, you're a big help." And I can remember other vague sorts of things. I can't remember the trip to Broken Hill at all. On the flight my heart stopped, and they revived me. It stopped again in the hospital in Broken Hill. I was unconscious all this time. I was flown from there to Adelaide – it was a Friday night. I became conscious again on Monday, about midday.

'There are after effects. I have no sensations of either smell or taste. I can't drink alcohol like I used to either.'

# OXYURANUS SCUTELLATUS

## Systematics
- Scientific name: Oxyuranus scutellatus [Peters, 1867].
- Synonym: Pseudechis scutellatus [Peters, 1867].
- Common names: Coastal taipan. Common taipan.
- Family: Elapidae.

## Biological Profile
- Large, fairly stout-bodied elapid sake. Body generally brown, black, coppery red, or olive; pale, creamish colour around head. Head large, oblong, almost rectangular ['coffin-shaped'], neck narrow [described as 'ridiculously thin'], body cylindrical; often with a rather wide reddish-orange vertebral stripe. Head usually lighter in colour than rest of body with a pink mouth and reddish eyes. Belly lighter, usually yellowish-brown to pale orange. Average length 2 m, maximum 2.9 m.
- Range: Along east coast of Australia from northeastern New South Wales through Queensland and across northern parts of Northern Territory to NW Australia.
- Open forests, dry closed forests, coastal heaths, grassy beach dunes, cultivated areas such as cane fields.
- Preys mainly on small mammals, sometimes on birds [and rarely on lizards].
- Fast diurnal elapid that hunts down its prey quickly and efficiently. Usually restricts its activity on the surface to the mid-morning, but may extend or change this to include late afternoon in cooler weather.
- Nocturnal in hot weather.
- Oviparous; 3–21 eggs per clutch.
- Changes colour with the seasons in captivity, becoming a bright coppery colour in summer and dull brown in winter. Presumably the change helps the snake to warm up quickly during the cooler months [when darker] and avoid overheating in the warmer months [when lighter].

## Lightning Fast

When hunting, the Taipan appears to actively scan for prey using its well-developed eyesight and is often seen travelling with its head raised above ground level. Once prey is detected the snake 'freezes' before hurling itself forward and issuing one to several lightning-fast bites. The prey is released and allowed to stagger away – this strategy minimizes the snake's chance of being harmed in retaliation, particularly by rats which can inflict lethal damage with their long incisors. After a few moments the Taipan tracks down the dying animal by following the scent trail with its flickering tongue. [australianmuseum.net.au]

## Bitten Before Realizing

The Coastal Taipan is often regarded as the most dangerous snake in Australia. They are extremely nervous and alert snakes, and any movement near them is likely to trigger an attack. Like any snake the Taipan prefers to avoid conflict and will quietly slip away if given the chance, however if surprised or cornered it will ferociously defend itself. When threatened, the Coastal Taipan adopts a loose striking stance with its head and forebody raised. It inflates and compresses its body laterally [not dorso-ventrally like many other species] and may also spread the back of its jaws to give the head a broader, lance-shaped appearance. Invariably the snake will strike, often without any warning, inflicting multiple snapping bites with extreme accuracy and efficiency. The muscular lightweight body of the Taipan allows it to hurl itself forwards or sideways and reach high off the ground, and such is the speed of the attack that a person may be bitten several times before realizing the snake is there. [australianmuseum.net.au]

## Behaviour & Temperament

Considered one of the deadliest snakes, the taipan reputedly has an aggressive disposition. When aroused, it can display a fearsome appearance by flattening its head, raising it off the ground, waving it back and forth, and suddenly striking with such speed that the victim may receive several bites before it retreats.

'Is Oxyuranus scutellatus naturally aggressive? When approached, it will almost invariably attempt to slip away quickly or 'vanish like a flash'. It is when the snake is cornered, attacked or ineffectively restrained that it quickly ceases to be shy and retiring. When angered, its behaviour warrants its evil reputation and it will attack with unequalled ferocity. Perhaps the best description is that made by Thompson [1933] as follows:

'When annoyed, the Taipan does not flatten its body dorso-ventrally, as do most Australian snakes, but depresses its sides, so that the vertebral column stands up like a keel. It has also the curious habit when about to attack of raising 1 or 2 coils of its body for several inches clear of the ground, its head slightly raised and flattened to such an extent that the angles of the jaws protrude; at the same time it erects its tail in the air and waves it to and fro, its behaviour giving it a sinister appearance. After remaining in this attitude for some seconds it strikes suddenly and with extreme rapidity. When biting, the Taipan does not seize and "chew" its victim, as does, for example, the powerful and aggressive *Pseudechis australis*, but snaps 3 or 4 times in such quick succession that there is almost no possibility for its victim escaping any of the bites. It then takes hold, snapping again at intervals.' [Sutherland, 1983]

## MATERIA MEDICA OXYURANUS SCUTELLATUS

### Sources
1 Proving Farokh Master [Homeopathic Health Centre, Mumbai, India], 6 provers [4 females, 2 males]; 2005.
2 Effects of bite; clinical manifestations.
3 Effects of bite; nearly always fatal.
4 Effects of bite; survival & recovery.
5 Effects of bite; overview typical signs & symptoms.

### Mind
∞ Playful and desire to tease family members.
∞ Irritable, unable to cope with any stress; frowning continuously; yelling and upset at trifles; desire to argue, fight, hit, smash, kill; sarcastic.
∞ Revengeful; recalls past events and slightest hurts and retaliates.
∞ Hatred and bitter feelings over slight offences.
∞ Quick tempered with immediate repentance.
∞ Desire to do the opposite of one's natural inclinations, to rebel with everyone, to do things against what is expected.
∞ Aversion to loved ones; mere sight causes hatred; wants to hurt them and take revenge.
∞ Quickly changing moods.
∞ Self-absorbed; wants to be alone all the time, aversion to company.
∞ Self-absorbed; wants to be left alone with one's thoughts.
∞ Secretive, wants to hide things and to tell lies.
∞ Death wish due to feeling of worthlessness and insignificance.
∞ Wants to die a premature natural death or through a fatal accident.
∞ Feeling of being slighted.
∞ Loves rain. Wants to walk in the rain.
∞ Hyper; wants things to be done immediately.
∞ Everybody must hurry.
∞ Wants to do the opposite of one's normal self, to rebel against everyone, to do things against what is expected.
∞ Censorious, splitting hairs, nit-picking, finding fault with others.
∞ Nothing pleases.
∞ Oversensitive to harsh words or rude tone of voice.
∞ Forsaken feeling; sensation of isolation.
∞ Loss of self-control.

### Dreams
∞ Burning right leg.
∞ Clairvoyance that something bad is going to happen to loved one.

∞ God.

∞ Old school days and old friends.

## Generals

∞ Lethargy, weakness, desire to lie down, or disinclination to get up.

∞ Chilliness; wants to be covered; feeling cold in morning on rising.

∞ Great hunger – mind only on food, anything will do.

∞ Appetite decreased, easy satiety after a few bites.

∞ Desire for chocolate; ice cream.

∞ Water retention; body swollen all over.

∞ High blood pressure.

∞ Weight gain.

## Sensations

∞ Heaviness vertex.

∞ Heaviness supraorbital region & pulling pain in eyes and lethargic feeling.

∞ Heaviness eyes.

∞ Burning mouth, and tongue.

∞ Swallowing difficult, even water, as if forcing something down a narrow pipe.

∞ Splinter in throat.

∞ Throat as if constricted.

∞ Lump in throat on swallowing.

∞ Stomach and abdomen as if empty – increased appetite.

∞ Weight on chest.

∞ Fever with pain as if bones would break.

## Locals

∞ Thick post-nasal discharge, < morning; discharge right sided, thick, watery, yellowish-green.

∞ Increased salivation; constant inclination to swallow saliva.

∞ Throat dry, parched & increased thirst.

∞ Throat pain < swallowing liquids and empty swallowing.

∞ Must clear throat before talking. Hoarse, thick voice.

∞ Urine very hot, almost piping hot.

∞ Severe dysmenorrhoea; severe cramp-like pain < sitting, > lying on abdomen.

∞ Palpitations of heart with anxiety, disturbing sleep or on waking.

## Central Idea of Remedy

*Worthless*

The feeling of a life without purpose in which one does not have a significant role is very characteristic of this remedy. They feel like a burden on their family or group.

*Alone*

They feel that nobody needs them, and they are not of use to anybody.

*Estranged feeling*
The desire for company and society is suppressed due to feelings of worthlessness and depression.

*Oversensitive*
Any kind of criticism intensifies the feeling of worthlessness. So they are very sensitive to criticism and reprimands.

*Mood swings*
Mood changes are persistent throughout the proving. They are very intense and uncontrollable. The changes of mood are also due to the intense irritation at trivial matters. One moment they are happy and another moment they can get agitated over trifles.

*Revengeful*
They feel hurt and want others to experience the same painful feeling. Past offenses are recalled with a lot of anger and resentment.

*Loss of control / Violent rage*
The frustration and anger is expressed initially in the form of sarcastic and critical remarks. If they are unable to argue or prove their point they become violent.

*Loathing for life*
They feel that others are living in misery because of them. When the frustration and worthlessness reaches a peak they feel like ending their life.

## Clinical Manifestations
Its venom contains a powerful neurotoxin, called taipoxin, causing respiratory paralysis. Taipoxin also attacks muscles, releasing myoglobin and muscle enzymes such as creatine kinase, resulting in widespread muscle damage. This causes muscle weakness, muscle tenderness, muscle movement pain, diminished deep tendon reflexes, rise in serum CK, and frank myoglobinuria [dark brown urine]. If muscle damage is severe, recovery may take weeks, although full functional recovery is possible. Severe muscle wasting may be apparent, and intensive physiotherapy is required to prevent contractures in the early stages, and to promote rapid muscle regeneration in the later stages.

The other important venom component is a direct prothrombin activator, which can rapidly cause complete defibrination, i.e. consumption of the clotting protein fibrinogen, resulting in non-coagulable blood, putting victims at risk of major and persistent bleeding from any vascular injury. As the venom is not apparently vasculotoxic, however, in the absence of vascular injury bleeding does not occur, thus in many patients the coagulopathy proves relatively benign.

Overall taipan snake venom is one of the most potent of all known snake venoms. Although taipans are a relatively minor cause of snakebites in Australia in relation to numbers of cases, they assume a far more important position due to the extreme hazard of their bites. Progressive neuromuscular flaccid paralysis [muscle weakness, respiratory failure] is the common cause of death.

SNAKES

## Nearly Always Fatal

Without appropriate antivenom treatment taipan bites will be nearly always fatal. In the era prior to specific antivenom therapy, there were only 2 reported survivors of taipan bite. The development of taipan antivenom began with the capture of a live taipan on July 26, 1950, by a 20-year old amateur herpetologist by the name of Kevin Budden at the ultimate cost of his live. After suffering a bite in the left hand at about 10:30 a.m., Budden was transported to the hospital. Dr. Benn documented the course of the fatal envenomation.

'Upon his arrival at Cairns Base Hospital at 11 a.m., the patient gave the general impression of bravado and excitement, showing greater interest in the welfare and comfort of the reptile than himself. When asked why he had not scarified the wound, he answered that in his opinion scarification "wasn't worth the trouble." He stated that he was not worried about himself, as he believed that snake victims died from fright more than from the effects of the poison.' . . .

'At 3 p.m. the patient complained of blurred vision. He had vomited yellowish fluid 3 times and developed a severe headache straight after. Examination revealed a slight ptosis and weakness of both masseter muscles. His pulse rate was 120 per minute, the pulse being of good volume, and his body temperature, taken by mouth, was 98.6°F [37°C]. The skin felt clammy. The affected hand was now red and swollen.

'At 7 p.m. the patient had vomited yellowish fluid twice. Examination revealed extension of the paralytic process; slight internal strabismus was now present, and ptosis was extreme. He was unable to move his tongue appreciably; his mouth gaped, and its floor sagged under the effects of gravity. As he was unable to swallow, it was necessary to aspirate saliva continuously. The patient was unable to phonate and had to resort to pencil and paper. The sterno-mastoid muscles were weak upon both sides and some upper intercostals paralysis was noted. The pulse was full, and the rate was 120 per minute. The body temperature was 97.2°F [36.2°C].

'Examination of the patient at 8 p.m. revealed almost complete loss of intercostals breathing, complete facial paralysis and some weakening of upper and lower limb musculature with corresponding loss of tendon reflexes. . . .

'At 8:25 p.m. respiratory distress was apparent; yet when the patient was placed in the artificial respiratory he fought strenuously against the artificial rhythm. This necessitated his removal and dependence upon the administration of oxygen and posturing into Fowler's position [position in which the head of the patient's bed is elevated 60 to 90 degrees]. When this was done the patient showed little respiratory distress. . . . During the night the patient slept normally and appeared to be capable of sufficient respiratory exchange. . . .

'Slight cyanosis was reported at 9 a.m. the next day. The patient was restless, and his temperature was 96°F [35.5°C]. . . . At 12:30 p.m. the patient became restless, respiratory movements became shallow and moderate cyanosis developed. . . . At 1:20 p.m. the patient remained cyanotic and cold, although respiratory exchange was adequate. At 1:30 p.m. the pulse failed, and no signs of life were detected.' [Benn, 1951]

## Survival & Recovery

The website of Queensland Museum, Brisbane, Australia, includes some personal accounts from survivors of taipans bite. One of them, a nurse, recounts her experience thus [summarised]:

'This might seem strange. In the weeks before I was bitten, I'd had nightmares about snakebite and drowning at sea. I couldn't do much about the latter, but I read up on snakebite procedure, checked the location of our [restrictive] bandages, and ensured everyone in the family knew where they were.

'It was 8 January 1995, after work at about 6:00 p.m. I was still "on call" and was walking on the almost bare earth crossing of Scrubby Ck. . . . Something touched me. . . . I realised I'd been bitten when I looked at the mid-calf area of my left leg. . . . Now the person "on call" for the hospital was the patient, not the nurse.

'[About 10 minutes post-bite] he symptoms started: blurred vision, like looking through perspex with water running on it; and an unbelievable headache. It took 20 minutes to reach the hospital. By then, I had awful stomach cramps and could hardly breathe. There was no pain at the bite for about 4 hours. When it began, it was awful, very intense. It lasted for 6 weeks. . . . Two and a half hours post-bite, semiconscious, I was in the Intensive Care Unit at Cairns Base Hospital. My kidneys didn't work for 3 days. After 6 days, I was discharged, still fragile, from hospital.

'The after effects of this bite have been fairly bad. My left leg below the bite is numb, not everywhere, but in a sort of jagged line, perhaps along a nerve. I get severe headaches I didn't have before. I'm also moody and I wasn't before. I'm also more driven not to put anything off till tomorrow. There are no guarantees about tomorrow. At the time of the bite, I thought I would die. And I thought: "So be it. If it were to happen, it wasn't a bad way to go."'
[www.qm.qld.gov.au/features/snakes/taipan/survivorsaw.asp]

## Overview Typical Signs & Symptoms

*Neurological and Neuromuscular*
These signs and symptoms have a high degree of variability from case to case and may come on subtly and progress rapidly.
Eyelid drooping
Blurred vision or difficulty seeing
Difficulty with speaking or swallowing
Headache
Convulsions or epileptiform seizures
Drowsiness
Sudden loss of consciousness
Flaccid paralysis
Stumbling gait [ataxia]
Respiratory arrest or dyspnoea

*Haematological and Vascular*
Profuse bleeding from bite site
Spitting or vomiting blood [haematemesis]
Coagulation defects
Hypotension
Circulatory collapse

*Renal and Urinary*
Haemoglobinuria
Myoglobinuria
Proteinuria
Acute renal failure

*General*
These symptoms may manifest very early [usually within 15–60 minutes follow-ing the bite] presenting as vague complaints.
Abdominal pain
Regional lymph node tenderness
Vomiting
Coughing
Profuse sweating
Swelling, oedema
[Davidson, University of California, Snakebite Protocols]

# PSEUDONAJA TEXTILIS

## Systematics
- Scientific name: Pseudonaja textilis [Duméril, Bibron & Duméril, 1854].
- Synonyms: Pseudoelaps superciliosus [Fischer, 1856]. Demansia annulata [Günther, 1858].
- Common names: Eastern brown snake. Common brown snake.
- Family: Elapidae.

## Biological Profile
- Medium-sized elapid, slender to moderate build. Smallish head barely distinct from neck. Body colour almost any shade of brown, ranging from near black to light tan, chestnut or burnt-orange. Head colour of dark individuals slightly paler than rest of body. Belly cream, yellow or orange, blotched with pinkish-orange, brown or grey. Scales smooth and slightly glossy. Average length 1.5 m; maximum 2.4 m.
- Range: Widespread throughout eastern Australia, from northern Queensland to South Australia.
- Habitat: Dry eucalypt forests and heaths of coastal ranges, savannah wood-lands, inner grasslands, arid scrublands farmland, and more arid areas that are intermittently flooded. Not found in rainforests or other wet areas.

- Common in farmland and on outskirts of urban areas, benefitting from agriculture due to the increased numbers of its main prey, the introduced house mouse.
- Diurnal.
- Actively hunts for prey, comprising a variety of vertebrates, incl. frogs, reptiles and reptile eggs, birds and mammals, esp. introduced rats and mice. Gives chase and subdues prey using both venom and constriction.
- Cannibalistic in captivity, esp. in overcrowded conditions.
- Shares the same shelter site over winter with small groups of other eastern brown snakes.
- Males engage in ritual combat during the mating season.
- Oviparous; 5–25 eggs per clutch. In captivity females have been observed coiling around their eggs for several hours after laying, which may be seen as a low level of maternal care, or possibly just the snake recovering from the exertions of labour.
- Uses communal nests for egg laying.
- French zoologist André Marie Constant Duméril described the eastern brown snake in 1854 as Furina textilis, in French Furine tricotée [knitted furin], from a specimen collected in October 1846 by Jules Verreaux. He remarked that the fine-meshed pattern on the snake's body reminded him of fine stockings, which was the inspiration for the name.
- Notorious for its speed and defensive displays mistaken for aggression.
- Alert, nervous species that often reacts defensively if surprised or cornered, putting on a fierce display and striking with little hesitation.

Keeping a Safe Distance
'If approached over a distance, they will usually choose to flee or else remain stationary, hoping to avoid detection. The approach distance tolerated before the snake flees is temperature dependent – snakes with a body temperature below 24°C [75.2°F] allow significantly closer approach than do snakes with a body temperature over 24°C. When confronted by an intruder, the Eastern Brown displays 1 of 2 forms of threat. In the mild threat, the snake raises the head and anterior part of the body slightly off and parallel to the ground, with the neck spread laterally and slightly hooked but the mouth closed. In this posture, the snake faces the threat side on. If issuing a strong threat, the snake raises the anterior part of the body well off the ground in an s-shaped coil and with the mouth slightly open, ready to strike – in this posture, the snake faces the threat more squarely.

'Strikes delivered from this posture are slower but more accurate that strikes delivered from other postures. The common feature of both displays is the spreading of the neck and this behaviour precedes most bites. Observations in captivity have shown that for strikes in general, no matter what the posture, there was no correlation between strike speed and ambient temperature [18°–36°C], body mass or sex. Strike speeds ranged 0.25–1.80 m/sec [mean = 1.11 m/sec]. The lack of correlation between strike speed and temperature is unexpected in an ectotherm and suggests that hot snakes are no quicker in their strike than a cool snake, contrary to the common perception.' [australianmuseum.net.au]

# MATERIA MEDICA PSEUDONAJA TEXTILIS

## Sources
1 C4-trituration proving Ulrike Fechner [Germany] performed in Byron Bay, New South Wales, Australia, 2013. Four provers, 2 females, 2 males.
2 Effects of bite; clinical manifestations.
3 Effects of bite; a fatal case.

## Mind
∞ Delusion being up alone the rest of the world.
∞ Delusion surrounding world being smaller.
∞ Feeling defenceless, at a disadvantage, weak, powerless.
∞ Cruelty, brutality. Unfeeling, hard-hearted.
∞ Self-centred.
∞ Lack of care for others.
∞ Clairvoyance.
∞ Jealousy. Rivalry issues.
∞ Absence of thought. Mind as if empty; as if not knowing anything.
∞ Sitting, staring and not thinking; as if daydreaming.
∞ Delusion radius of action being limited; feeling restricted to area.
∞ Feeling of being isolated, as if not part of the world.
∞ Dwells on past disagreeable events, sexual matters.
∞ Feeling of being something / somebody special. [General theme of Elapidae.]

## Dreams
∞ Defenceless, being.
∞ Killing a male opponent in a fair fight.
∞ Mercy, being at somebody's.
∞ Persecution.
∞ Sexual harassment.

## Generals
∞ Problems getting started in the morning.
∞ Muscular weariness.
∞ Takes frequent catnaps during daytime.
∞ Fatigue, exhaustion, indolence. No urge to move.
∞ Immobility; motionless.

## Sensations
∞ Heaviness head, as if skull part of head will sink into the body, while the skin stays in place.
∞ Eyes as if swollen.
∞ Veil before eyes.
∞ Sensation of staring.
∞ Soft part of nose as if absent.
∞ Teeth as if weak, as if hollowed out.

∞ Tip of tongue as if hot and tingling.
∞ Uterus as if being petrified.

## Locals
∞ Pressure in forehead and temples.
∞ Pressure in head with blocked nose.
∞ Photophobia for daylight.
∞ Pressure in jaws, esp. upper jaw.
∞ Cutting pain in anus.
∞ Needs to stretch neck.
∞ Heavy, tired limbs < motion.
∞ Coldness feet alternating with heat.

## Restrained Reign
'In addition to numerous general snake symptoms [muscle weakness, jealousy, rivalry, sexual themes, egocentricity, etc.], it becomes apparent that Pseudonaja textilis has a stronger connection to femininity than other snakes. She shows a restrained femininity and also sobriety. She is of ordinary brown colour, without any exciting pattern, she is beautiful, but without being obtrusive. She is present, but doesn't push herself to the fore, she is extremely dangerous but doesn't rub it in. Like all snakes she carries ancient knowledge, but she doesn't have to emphasise it. If Lachesis is the attention craving beauty queen, then Pseudonaja textilis is the averagely beautiful and modest queen, who, smiling quietly, reigns her whole kingdom through her servants and her husband while pretending to not really be important, leaving the great show to her husband.' [Fechner]

## Clinical Manifestations
The venom contains powerful presynaptic neurotoxins, procoagulants, cardio-toxins and nephrotoxins, and successful envenomation can result in progressive paralysis and uncontrollable bleeding. The initial bite is generally painless and often difficult to detect.

Clinical features of 136 patients with definite brown snake envenoming.
VICC [venom-induced consumption coagulopathy]
Complete VICC – 109 patients [80%].
Partial VICC – 27 pt.[20%].
Major haemorrhage – 5 pt. [4%].
Intracranial haemorrhage – 2 pt. [1%].
Gastrointestinal haemorrhage – 3 pt. [2%].
Bleeding at bite site – 32 pt. [24%].
Bleeding at intravenous cannula site – 43 pt. [32%].
Gum bleeding – 19 pt. [14%].
Neurotoxicity [mild] – 2 pt. [1%].
Systemic Symptoms
Nausea – 71 pt. [52%].
Vomiting – 44 pt. [32%].

Headache – 78pt. [57%].
Abdominal pain – 37 pt. [27%].
Diaphoresis – 49 pt. [36%].
Diarrhoea – 11 pt. [8%].
Cardiovascular Effects
Early collapse/hypotension – 37 pt. [27%].
Cardiac arrest – 7 pt. [5%].
Seizures – 8 pt. [6%].
Thrombotic microangiopathy – 15 pt. [11%].
Acute renal failure – 11 pt. [8%].
Abnormal creatinine – 14 pt. [10%].
[Allen, 2012]

# CASE

'A girl, aged 13 years, was bitten on the naked foot below the metatarsal joint of the great toe. An ineffective ligature was applied, and the bitten area was incised. About a quarter of an hour after the bite the patient vomited; within a further half hour she complained of headache and nausea and vomited forcibly and frequently. She was still vomiting at the end of the first hour after the bite and complaining of severe abdominal pain. This continued, and a few minutes later she was vomiting dark brown fluid and was extremely giddy. Two hours after the bite her pulse rate was 108 beats per minute, her temperature was 36.5°C [97.7°F], and her respirations numbered 22 per minute. The main symptoms were then giddiness, nausea and vomiting. Early in the fourth hour she had a high bowel wash-out and a profuse evacuation, and she had a second one half an hour later. She complained of extreme thirst. Seven and a half hours after the bite she was restless, with pains in the arms, legs and teeth. At the tenth hour she developed bilateral ptosis, with general signs of bulbar affection, incl. paralysis of the tongue. The pupils were dilated but reacted to light and accommodation. The limbs were weak and flaccid but could still be moved voluntarily. The pulse rate was 128 beats per minute, the respirations numbered 40 per minute, and the temperature was 37.2°C [99°F]. Fourteen hours after the bite the patient was sleeping but was slightly cyanosed. There was blood pigment in the urine. At this time the pulse rate was 100 beats per minute, respirations numbered 23 per minute, and the temperature was 36.5°C [97.7°F]. She exhibited strong overaction of the accessory muscles of respiration with increasing cyanosis and died 17 hours after being bitten with symptoms of cardiovascular failure and without developing complete paralysis of the limbs.' [Kellaway, 1938; in Sutherland, 1983].

# Family Hydrophiidae – Sea snakes

## Biological Profile
- There is no agreement about the classification of sea snakes; some systems place them in a family of their own, others treat them as a subfamily of Elapidae.
- Sea snakes comprise approximately 70 species, 50 of which are members of the family Hydrophiidae. Sea snakes are characterised by laterally compressed bodies and vertically flattened tails and nostrils with valve-like flaps, giving them an eel-like appearance. Their most characteristic feature is a paddle-like tail, which increases their swimming ability.
- Sea snakes like all snakes are cold-blooded creatures. Consequently, their distribution is restricted to warm waters and thus they are only found in the Indo-Pacific region, along the coasts throughout the Pacific as well as on the east coast of Africa and in the Persian Gulf. There are no sea snakes in the Atlantic Ocean, in the Caribbean, or along the North American coast north of Baja California.
- Adaptations of sea snakes for marine life include a single lung that reaches almost to the tail; gas exchange through the skin when underwater; lower metabolic rate to consume less oxygen while submerged.
- Salt glands surrounding the tongue help maintain osmotic balance in seawater.
- The nostrils of snakes in the Hydrophis group are dorsally located and can be closed with valves. Although they spend much of their time underwater, they must surface regularly to breathe.
- Except for a single genus [Laticauda] with 7 species, which come to land to lay eggs, all other sea snakes are ovoviviparous. Young can swim and feed immediately. Sea snake copulation takes place underwater and takes such a long time, the couple must come up for air. The female controls the timing of these immersions and submersions, and since the male is stuck firmly inside the female until fertilisation is finished, he must gasp for a breath when she does.
- Sea snakes are generally deemed to be non-aggressive and to have a gentle disposition. They are not thought to bite humans unless provoked and they typically do not actively pursue swimming prey. Only when taken out of their natural element, water, sea snakes have been noted to become quite aggressive, exhibiting erratic movements and striking anything near them that moves.
- Prey on fish and crustaceans.
- The classification used here, separating Elapidae and Hydrophiidae, considers the latter as a family for reasons of source-based differential diagnosis.

## Living Fast
In terms of the huge amount of energy expended while swimming, writes Fry [2015], "they are more like fish than snakes. They burn through energy like no other snake and therefore must eat almost daily. They only live 4 or 5 years due to this turbo-charged metabolism. Live fast and die young.'

## Secretiveness to Avoid Retaliation

'Only patient inquiry enabled Reid in Malaya and us in Vietnam to realise the great number of sea snake bites that occur in man. In these 2 countries, superstitions forbid fishermen to relate casualties they have witnessed. In Vietnam, the King of Snakes and Genie of the Sea are believed to rule the sea snakes. *Men who talk are liable to reprisals*, in the form of bites from one of the King's subjects.

'Fishermen readily proclaim that sea snakes are very numerous in their country and that a sea snake bite may be fatal. But when one is asked whether fatalities occur among the inhabitants of the village, he usually will answer that there are none, and sometimes may add that, in the next village, there are many. In the second village, a similar answer is given. Reid has recorded the existence in Malaya of superstitions a little different with regard to relating cases, but the result remains the same: sea snake bites are *kept secret*, above all if they have been fatal.

'When we witnessed the bite of a Vietnamese fisherman, the victim would disappear. The next day it was impossible to learn from his companions what had become of him. It was only when we were able to offer an injection of serum – always eagerly accepted – that we were able to see the patients again. They became more confiding when they knew they had a means to protect themselves against death from the venom, and maybe also against their superstitions. . . . What happens in Malaya and Vietnam doubtless happens in many other countries where Hydrophiidae are numerous.' [Bücherl & Buckley, Vol. I, 1968]

## Sea Snake Envenomation

Among this group are species with some of the most potent venoms of all snakes. Nearly 80% of sea snake bites fail to produce significant envenomation and bites may be inconspicuous, painless, and free of oedema. Usually, little or no swelling is involved, and it is rare for any nearby lymph nodes to be affected. However, sea snake venom is extremely potent, and a complete envenomation by an adult sea snake may contain enough venom to kill 3 adult people. The clinically relevant toxins in sea snake venom are *neurotoxins* and *myotoxins*.

'Sea snakes bite people who are swimming and diving, bathing, washing, wading, paddling and handling fishing nets and lines. The bite is usually painless and may pass unnoticed by a fisherman intent on his work. There may be a pricking or stinging sensation, usually transient but sometimes persistent. . . . In most of Reid's patients with sea snake bites [mostly assumed to be from *Enhydrina schistose* and *Hydrophis* species during 1957–1964] symptoms began between 30 and 60 minutes of the bite. The commonest initial symptoms were *muscle aches, pains and stiffness on movement* remote from the site of the bite. Muscle tenderness and stiffness is demonstrated by passive stretching of the limb muscle. . . . Pain and stiffness may start in the throat and jaws or at the back of the neck and prevent movement of the head.

'*Muscle aches, pains, stiffness, tenderness and weakness*. The muscles of the neck, trunk, and the proximal parts of the limbs are principally affected. *Muscles are painful on active or passive movement*. Symptoms may progress rapidly, and complete recovery may take weeks or even months.

'*Paralytic symptoms.* These may begin with blurred or double vision and ptosis and progress, as with classical elapid neurotoxicity, to external ophthalmoplegia, a "thick feeling of the tongue," slurring of speech, inability to swallow, breathlessness and respiratory muscle paralysis. The pupils become dilated and sluggishly reactive to light. Paralysis of the lower limbs affects gait. Asymmetrical lower motor neuron type paralysis has been described in the bitten limb or elsewhere and can involve the cranial nerves. More usually there is generalised flaccid paresis with the "*broken neck sign*" resulting from weakness of the neck muscles.

'*Myoglobinuria:* Usually starts within 3 to 6 hours of the bite, but may be delayed, transient or absent in some cases. Duration of myoglobinuria predicts the time needed for complete resolution of muscle symptoms.

'*Trismus* is a common clinical feature of sea snake bite. Reid described the association of trismus with generalised flaccid paresis, a clinical paradox that originally stimulated his studies of sea snake bite. He distinguished trismus in tetanus [that cannot be overcome by force, is associated with a brisk jaw jerk and represents increased tone or rigidity of the masseter muscles] from 'pseudo-trismus" in snakebite that could be "reduced by sustained pressure on the lower jaw." Pseudo-trismus [furthermore] was associated with an absent or sluggish jaw jerk and was likely to be the result of a splinting reaction of intact muscle fibres protecting injured fibres against further damage by stretching. *Inability to open the mouth* is a typical feature of elapid neurotoxicity, but the jaws are not clenched shut as in the trismus of sea snake bite.

'A variety of other symptoms has been described including nausea, retching, vomiting, a feeling of coldness, excessive sweating, drowsiness, fainting, and headache. Vomiting is a particularly consistent early feature of severe envenomation.' [Gopalakrishnakone, 1994]

## Muscle Damage
Bryan Fry got bitten by a very large horned sea snake [Hydrophis peronii], watching in slow motion both sides of the snake's head go concave as it emptied its venom into the meaty part of his left thumb.

'Sea snake venom is notorious for being very quick-acting, consistent with the snakes' need to rapidly immobilise fast-moving fish. If the fish can dart off, they're gone. . . . By the time we got to the small Weipa Hospital my face was grey and my lips were green. The world was getting very distant and my lower back was hurting something fierce: I was feeling the effects of severe neurotoxicity and my *muscles* were being severely damaged by myotoxins, which made my urine look like Coca-Cola. By then, I was also in extreme pain. [Two vials of antivenom] reversed the nerve effects and halted the muscle effects.

'But the damage was already done. Back home, for a week I could barely walk, and even short steps defeated me. If I put a backpack on, my back would sway under the load. For two weeks my body felt like I had *competed in an ironman triathlon without training*. It took me a month to be pain free. I waited another 2 weeks and then resumed swim training. On my very first lap, when doing butterfly stroke, both of the rotator cuffs in my shoulders disintegrated – they were torn halfway through. For 6 months, I could not lift either arm above my shoulder. If I moved my shoulders in certain ways, it sounded like gravel grating against more gravel.' [Fry, 2015]

## Overview of Bite Symptoms
Euphoria.
Anxiety.
Malaise.
Drowsiness or mild confusion.
Headache.
Myalgias [typically worse with movement, usually beginning in the afflicted extremity, as well as the neck, within 30–60 min after envenomation].
Arthralgias.
Bulbar paralysis.
Ptosis.
Mydriasis with sluggish reaction to light.
Ophthalmoplegia, leading to diplopia.
Failing vision [usually a terminal symptom].
Dysarthria and slurred speech.
Hypersalivation.
Trismus.
Facial paralysis.
Dysphagia.
Nausea, vomiting, abdominal pain, cramping.
Dyspnoea – Apnoea – Tachypnoea – Respiratory distress or respiratory failure.
Change in urine colour [dusky yellow to reddish brown].
Oliguria.
Thirst.
Hyporeflexia [progressing to loss of reflexes].
Cyanosis.
Cardiac arrest [secondary to hyperkalemia].
Muscle paralysis [usually ascending, may be flaccid or spastic].
Differential diagnosis: Guillain-Barré Syndrome.
[Papanagnou, 2008]


## HYDROPHIIDAE IN HOMEOPATHY

| Homeopathic name | Common name | Abbreviation | Symptoms |
|---|---|---|---|
| Hydrophis cyanocinctus | Annulated sea snake | Hydroph. | ++ |
| Laticauda colubrina | Banded sea krait | Latic-co. | + |
| Pelamis platurus[1] | Yellow-bellied sea snake | Pelam-pl. | + |

1 = Hydrophis platurus.

# HYDROPHIS CYANOCINCTUS

## Systematics
- Scientific name: Hydrophis cyanocinctus [Daudin, 1803].
- Synonyms: Leioselasma striata [Lacépède, 1804]. Hydrophis striata [Schlegel, 1837].
- Common names: Annulated sea snake. Black-tailed hydrophis.
- Family: Hydrophiidae [subfamily of Elapidae].

## Biological Profile
- Slender venomous sea snake. Head moderate and not or scarcely distinct from neck; body elongate; anterior part of body round, posterior part compressed. Body pale yellow green or greyish above, whitish below. Chin lighter; tip of tail black, except for ventral side. Dorsal pattern of alternating light and dark bands; 55–70 dark bands; black bands widest dorsally; light bands widest laterally. Average length 1.5 m, maximum 2 m.
- Range: Indo-West Pacific: from the Persian Gulf to Japan and the Indo-Australian Archipelago. Prefers warm, shallow waters over reef, sea-grass or sand. Sometimes comes out onto land.
- Diurnal and nocturnal, preys on various available fish.
- Sometimes attracted toward lights on boats or docks at night.
- Believed to sense prey not visually but through its cutaneous mechanoreceptors and/or receptors in the inner ear, which are known to detect the weak water motion such as that generated by prey.
- Ovoviviparous; 3–16 live young per brood. Breeds in estuary areas among rocks and inlets.
- Venom neurotoxic and myotoxic.

## MATERIA MEDICA HYDROPHIS CYANOCINCTUS

### Sources
1 Proving Raeside [UK], 10 provers [2 females, 8 males], 6c, 30c; 1958.
2 Clinical observations Mangialavori [Italy].
3 Degroote, Dream Repertory.
4 Synthesis Repertory Treasure Edition 2009.

### Mind
∞ Depressive, clouded mental state, weepy, especially during menopause. Disgust for life.[1]
∞ Feel as if living under a heavy dark cloud. Depressed. Disinclination to do anything. Sad thoughts, singing sad songs. No joy in life. [2 pr.].[1]
∞ Fear of waking from a dream.[4]
∞ Disgruntled, lethargy, < before menses.[1]
∞ Lack of initiative.[4]

∞ Sadness > when alone.[4]

∞ Sadness during menopause.[4]

∞ Irritable, tearful > alone, < consolation.[1]

∞ Horrible things, sad stories affect her profoundly. Oversensitive when hearing of cruelties.[2]

∞ Suspicious and mistrustful. Jealousy.[2]

∞ Forsaken feeling.[2]

∞ Thinks someone is in the room with him.[1]

∞ The theme of 'distance' is one of the most interesting issues. They need to keep their own, safe space that other people cannot enter. They need to keep their distance. It doesn't mean that there isn't a good relationship; this can be there, but it is not possible to get too close. They at least need to know that there is a space in the self where "it's just 'me' and where I can stay to recover my energy".[2]

∞ Hydrophis, Elaps and Naja [all elapids] more or less look very reserved and shy. You could confuse them with Sepia or Natrum muriaticum. They are nothing at all like Lachesis.[2]

∞ Ticklish.[3]

∞ Affectionate, returns affection.[3]

∞ Desire for black and/or rust red. Aversion to white.[3]

∞ Euphoria alternating with sadness.[3]

∞ Fear of death. Afraid to go to sleep and not wake up.[3]

∞ Boys who like to wear girls' clothes.[3]

∞ Mannish habits in girls.[3]

∞ Jealousy, interrupts others.[3]

∞ Vanity.[3]

## Dreams

∞ All or nothing, chooses to be dead instead of becoming handicapped.[3]

∞ Aquarium as big as room.[3]

∞ Being attacked.[1]

∞ Bitten in face by animal or dog.[3]

∞ Bitten in wrist by cat, dog, lizard.[3]

∞ Blamed publicly, being.[3]

∞ Boat capsizing.[3]

∞ Breasts.[3]

∞ Car with brakes not functioning.[3]

∞ Cheated by husband.[3]

∞ Conspiracy against one.[3]

∞ Eels.[1]

∞ Envy.[3]

∞ Flood.[3]

∞ Forsaken, being or feeling; not helped by anyone.[3]

∞ Guardian angel, helped by.[3]

∞ Handicap, lower limb lost.[3]

∞ Hide, desire to, from danger.[3]

∞ Insects.[1]
∞ Losing the group, due to difficulties to follow.[3]
∞ Nakedness; woman with naked upper half of body.[3]
∞ Privacy, want of; infringement of.[3]
∞ Pursued, being.[3]
∞ Swimming, can breathe underwater.[3]
∞ Threatened, feeling.[3]

## Generals
∞ Left side more affected.[1]
∞ Seashore air <.[2]
∞ Desire for chocolate; milk.[2]
∞ Desire for salmon.[3]
∞ Thirst for cold drinks.[1]
∞ Appetite increased before menses.[2]
∞ Ailments or < exposure to sun.[1,2] Sun = Heavy head, headache.[1] Sun = Erythema.[2]
∞ Morning <.[1]
∞ Faintness on stooping; on washing face.[3]
∞ Flushes of heat upward from abdomen or feet.[3]
∞ Sleeplessness > when traveling.[3]
∞ Restless sleep. Wakes 3–5 a.m.[1]
∞ Sleep disturbed by headache.[1]
∞ Daytime sleepiness.[1]
∞ Dystrophy of muscles.[4]

## Sensations
∞ Tight band/ring round head with beating in temples.[1]
∞ Pressure on eyes.[1]
∞ Salty taste in mouth.[1]
∞ Something in throat.[3]
∞ Throat as if swollen on waking.[1]
∞ Movements of foetus feel like those of a snake under the skin.[3]
∞ Chest as if dry and burning inside.[1]
∞ Chest as if in an iron armour, with dyspnoea.[3]
∞ Ribs as if compressed.[1]
∞ Suffocation < lying down.[1]
∞ Numbness finger morning on waking.[3]
∞ Heaviness legs in morning.[1]
∞ Feels as if walking in the air.[1]

## Locals
∞ Heavy head, worse on left side, > open air, < movement, sun, on waking.[1]
∞ Pain occiput when lying on back.[3]
∞ Eyes heavy in morning, cannot open them.[1]
∞ Vertical hemianopsia; vision disturbed – left side of faces disappears.[1]

∞ Deafness left ear in morning, as from air lock.[1]
∞ Cold feet and hot head during coryza.[1]
∞ Dry mouth all day and < mornings.[1]
∞ Loss of sense of taste.[1]
∞ Dryness throat < before menses.[1]
∞ Talking = sore throat.[1]
∞ Must clear throat continually.[1]
∞ Eructations and flatulence when turning in bed.[3]
∞ Nausea < smell of food.[1]
∞ Nausea on brushing teeth.[3]
∞ Violent, sharp, stinging pains with feeling of tension along colon, < morning and on left side.[1]
∞ Pain hypogastrium in act of sitting down.[3]
∞ Pain hypogastrium extending upward.[3]
∞ Constipation before menses, > during.[3]
∞ Urinary retention in presence of strangers.[3]
∞ Menses dark, scanty, too short, daytime only.[2]
∞ Menses heavy, excessive, red.[1]
∞ Difficulty breathing with belching.[3]
∞ Pain in precordial region, spreading to left hemi-thorax, < lying flat.[1]
∞ Pain heart < lying.[4]
∞ Palpitation on waking.[1]
∞ Pain armpit on raising arm.[3]
∞ Pain nape of neck/cervical region on raising arm.[3]
∞ Neuralgic pain [stitching pain in back] after herpes.[2]
∞ Pain sacroiliac joint < bending backward, > sitting erect.[3]
∞ Weakness legs.[1]
∞ Cannot have knees touch each other when lying on side.[3]
∞ Left foot hot, right foot cold.[1]

## Upper & Lower Body

'From the very clinical point of view, there is the clear division from one side of the individual and the other. This tends to be the upper and lower parts of the body. . . . From a psychological point of view, it seems clear in these 2 cases that there is a kind of separation. These 2 people would have liked to integrate the lower part of the body and clearly this process was extremely difficult. . . . For Hydrophis you get a sense of, "I wish I could put together these 2 sides of myself to become an entire person. But this is extremely difficult for me." A common way to over-compensate is to be over-active, independent, to show that you don't need other people, a kind of selfishness. . . . Massimo's cases of Hydrophis are not seductive at all. Their perception is that half of their body can be seductive, but the other half won't support this. They are strongly inhibited in the region of the genitals. The lady disliked her bottom but liked her breasts! The physical instincts are often related to the lower part of the body, but this is not integrated. In some way, it is dirty and disgusting. . . . There is a kind of frigidity, also known for Sepia and several other sea animals.' [Mangialavori]

# CASES

**Case 1**

'Female, born 1969, first seen in August 1996. Problems began in May 1995 with aches and pains and feeling tired and then pains in lower back, pins and needles and tingling, which spread to legs and to arms and hands. Also headaches, in June legs and feet swollen for 2 days. Recently the upper abdomen is swollen. Is very tired and fed up with it all, feels as though it has drained her. Is always moving around doing different things.

'After university in 1992 got a job in West Sussex; it was a very stressful job and took on a lot of responsibility. Has been thinking of training as a solicitor as she did a business studies degree.

Christmas 1995 got depressed; she had a job she was not happy with.

'Has hay fever and has had sinusitis, also bad varicose veins, which comes from the paternal side of the family. When run down gets flu; fever, aches and pains, better after sleeping for 24 hours. For a time it was difficult to walk. Polymyalgia rheumatica was suspected, had the test for it but it was negative. Was given steroids, which did not help either. Pins and needles come and go in waves throughout the body; has had pains in her feet and shooting pains in her body.

'Very angry teenager, parents split up, esp. angry with her father. Mother was ill and tried to take charge of her brothers and sisters, patient left to go and live with her father. Confident, mature, responsible as a child. At age 13 went to live with her father. At age 13 wanted to be successful, not to get married and have kids. Can never really see herself settling down. Always has a reason to move, is always moving on. Has moved many times, perhaps something she would like to change. Had a relationship with her best friend's brother in April 1993 for a year. Was angry at herself for getting involved with him. Is afraid to say to someone that she needs them. Feels she might be emotionally detached. Fears: heights [2] snakes [1].

'Is stubborn, does not like to give up battles until forced to give in. Upset by animals on TV. Loves tigers and big cats. Scuba dives and is fascinated by fish etc.

'Food: vegetarian, loves cheese and mushrooms. Finds prawns to rich. Cannot bear porridge, rice pudding and hot milk products.

'Feels she has been run down physically for some years and that this is a culmination. Wants to do employment and social law issues. Did have a bad reaction to an insect bite, soon after this started, leg was very swollen.

'8/96 Rx Hydrophis cyanocinctus 12c/twice daily. Two weeks later: Results of MRI scan were OK. She was told she was clinically depressed, which she was surprised and angry about. Feels her muscles are developing and not wasting. Is very worried about letting people down. Is worried about making up her mind, agonises over decisions. Feels she has to make changes but is worried about doing them on her own. Has felt more positive but no change in physical symptoms but is sleeping better. Rx Hydrophis cyanocinctus 30c/twice daily.

'10/96 All pains pins and needles have completely gone. Wants to go back to her diving club. Rx Hydrophis cyanocinctus 200c/3xW.

'12/96 Very well; life is starting to slot into place; is clear about making choices and saying no. Rx Hydrophis cyanocinctus 200c/1xW.

'8/97 Phoned patient; she is well and symptom free.

'Looking back over this case a year later there are rubrics I might have added and subtracted but this was not how I arrived at the successful remedy. I was familiar with the proving by Raeside of Hydrophis cyanocinctus who made the following comment: "From a toxicological point of view, an attack on the peripheral nerves can be seen, giving a symptomatological table analogous to that of poliomyelitis."

'I also noticed her desire to swim and dive! I had previously used the remedy in a patient with some success who had a serious fear of snakes, presented with a neck problem, had pains and other sensations throughout the body, and had polio at age 14 months.

'Swimming, diving, love of the water has been noted in my cases although it should be said that all snakes are good swimmers. It is indicated in neurological problems, like poliomyelitis, as is commented on in the provings by Raeside.' [Case Michael Thompson; RefWorks]

## Case 2

'B. is a 57-year old white woman whose chief complaint is left leg and ankle pain resulting from having had a rare form of polio at the age of 6. Polio destroyed the cartilage in that ankle, and her left leg never developed as well as her right. Doctors have said that there are no nerve responses in that leg. Doctors also thought that she would never walk again.

'She doesn't walk evenly, favouring the right side and not able to pick up left foot completely. She can't walk on cobblestones nor can she wear shoes with heels. She slips a lot and a few years ago fractured a bone in left lower leg. Now if she goes for a 3-mile walk, later her ankle will hurt so bad she can barely stand on it. It gives a constant ache.

'She has heart arrhythmia and a history of fibroids and ovarian cysts. She has an anaphylactic reaction to Sulfa medications. She used to have premenstrual migraines. She has intermittent sciatica on the right side. She describes herself as driven by a desire to be a part of transforming the world. She is a highly successful college professor at a prominent college and very involved with international human rights. She is a very closeted lesbian and teaches at a conservative Catholic university.

'She is extremely loquacious but strangely incoherent, talking in circles. B. loves snakes – wants to pick them up. She likes intricate patterns, such as aboriginal art with 4 snakes. Loves anything with water and snakes. She loves water and swimming and was a big water skier and a slalomer.

'She told she came out of the experience of being hospitalised at the age of 6 with "a hideous fixation of not wanting to be in a wheelchair." "I don't want that to be me."

'She became very athletic, captain of many sports teams. She never talked about her polio history, and she never used it as an excuse although she was in a great deal of pain a lot of the time as a child and young adult.

*Analysis*
'This woman presented as a very highly functioning snake: powerful, accomplished, in leadership, a go-getter. In this case we see the particular themes of physical overcompensation as well as compartmentalization. Having been told she would never walk again she nonetheless overcame her pain and disability to excel at many sports. Her life is compartmentalized, emotionally and politically. The post-polio syndrome indicated a neurotoxic snake.

Rx: Hydrophis cyanocinctus 30c.

'After a couple of months, her ankle pain went away. Now is able to walk extensively, exercise on a treadmill, and use the ankle normally. Over the course of 2 years, she took Hydrophis 200 and 1M. Her sciatica also went away. She has become less driven and more relaxed about her life, her work, and her relationship. This year, she tripped and fell on stairs in her house and she did not suffer any injury whatsoever, not to her ankle nor to any other part.' [Case Patricia Maher, Interhomeopathy, September 2009]

**Case 3**
S is a 28-year-old man whose chief complaint is leg pain. He suffers from Bilateral Compartment Syndrome, a condition of severe ischemia in the calves, typically from overexercise. He is a small man who as a youth had compensated for his small stature by overdeveloping his legs. While in the US Marines it was discovered that he had sustained nerve damage there. He has a flat affect and seems old for his age. He is incoherent and speaks in a circular fashion. He has concentration difficulties and poor memory. He complains also of stomach pain, "bubbles" in his stomach < from eating. He has issues about surviving and fears of being shot. He is a working class African-American who cleans offices for a living.

*Analysis*
The most striking things about this man were:

- "bilateral compartment syndrome," and that his legs had been developed out of proportion to the rest of his body;
- the compartmentalization of his feelings and memory;
- the themes of violence, getting shot, and survival.

Although I initially was considering a plant in the Compositae family because of his shock-y demeanor, I ultimately went for snake remedies. The survival issues are very strong – a few times he referred to the need to "stay alive". His fear of being shot seemed to be out of proportion to his actual immediate living situation – apart from the real dangers of being a young black man in the USA.

The "compartment" syndrome in his legs is about constriction and pressure. But the 'compartment' theme is carried throughout his personality. He had a very "shut down" feeling to him and he also spoke about information being buried in the "vault" of his memory.

I looked for a snake that was mild yet powerful and had issues about compartmentalization, as well as of course the nerve damage. That he had had these extremely large, overdeveloped and powerful legs as a youth led me to Hydrophis cyanocinctus.

I thought that the opposite polarity from fluidity must also be in this remedy, and this case may very well represent it. This man is the opposite of fluidity: stiff, *muscle-bound*, compressed, and compartmentalized.

Lastly, I was struck by S's description of a childhood dream of "not being able to see straight, as if he was wall-eyed". This remedy has issues about loss of vision, but particularly has extreme strabismus. Again, its opposite is contained in this case – extreme wall-eyes.

After Hydrophis 30c, his leg pain began to abate immediately. After 6 weeks, he was able to move much more freely, had a lot more energy and appeared far less shut down. After one year, his leg pain only occurs with very cold weather. [Case Patricia Maher, Interhomeopathy, September 2009]

# LATICAUDA COLUBRINA

## Systematics
- Scientific name: Laticauda colubrina [Schneider, 1799].
- Common names: Banded sea krait. Yellow-lipped sea krait.
- Family: Hydrophiidae [subfamily of Elapidae].

## Biological Profile
- Amphibious sea snake closer in its build to land snakes than to other sea snakes. Body less flattened and nostrils placed laterally rather than at tip of snout.
- Has both 'terrestrial' and 'aquatic' breathing rhythms, whereas true sea snakes have only an aquatic rhythm. The terrestrial rhythm consists of frequent relatively evenly spaced breaths, whilst the aquatic one is composed of long periods of apnoea with short bursts of rapid breathing.
- Average length 1 m, maximum 1.4 m. Females much larger than males.
- Dorsal colour light or dark bluish grey; yellow on sides and below. Scales pale at tip. 20–65 solid blackish-brown rings around body and 3 on tail, rings widest

on middle of back and narrowest on belly. Head black, snout and upper lip bright yellow.
- Range: Coast of Thailand down to south Pacific islands and New Guinea; found at depths ranging between 1–10 m in shallow water surrounding small coral islands, coral reefs and mangroves, usually with a sand or coral substrate.
- Habitat: Distinguished from other sea snakes by being amphibious [living on land and water] versus aquatic [never leaving the water]. Regularly comes ashore, usually at night, and may climb rocks to a height of 6 m or more. Moves into terrestrial habitats to digest food, drink freshwater, mate, shed its skin, and lay eggs.
- Mainly nocturnal, moving over large areas in search of food. Preys predominantly on eel and occasionally on small fish.
- Dehydrates in seawater; must drink freshwater for water balance.
- Aggregates in large groups at breeding and resting sites.
- Oviparous, lays its eggs in caves and rocky crevices; 4–20 eggs per clutch.
- Not aggressive unless subjected to *considerable provocation*. 'Completely inoffensive to humans,' according to Mark O'Shea, 'it is possible to pick up handfuls of snakes without any attempting to bite as I found when catching sea kraits in New Caledonia.'

### Head or Tail

'In a deadly game of heads or tails venomous sea snakes in the Pacific and Indian Oceans deceive their predators into believing they have 2 heads, claims research published August 5 in Marine Ecology.

The discovery, made by Rasmussen and Elmberg, showed that yellow-lipped sea kraits [Laticauda colubrina] use skin markings and behaviour patterns to fool predators into thinking their tail is a second head, complete with lethal venom. . . .

'When hunting for food sea snakes probe crevices and coral formations, temporarily forcing them to drop their guard to threats from the surrounding waters and making them highly vulnerable to attack. However, the yellow-lipped sea krait has been found to twist its tail so that the tip corresponds with the dorsal view of the head, which combined with deceptive colouring, gives the illusion of having 2 heads and 2 loads of deadly venom. . . . To build upon this discovery researchers examined 98 sea kraits. . . .

'The research confirmed that all snakes of this species had a distinctive colouration pattern, with a bright yellow horseshoe marking on the tip of the head and the tail. The yellow was deeper than the colours on the rest of the body and the black colourations were much longer than the dark bands on the rest of the body, highlighting the similarity between the head and the tail. . . .

'The reason for this mixture of behaviour and colouration results from a developed defence strategy needed when the snake is probing for prey. Despite being extremely venomous sea snakes are susceptible to attack from several predators such as sharks, large bony fishes, and even birds.

' "The value of such an adaptation is 2-fold; it may increase the chances of surviving predator attack by exposing a less 'vital' body part, but more importantly it may deter attack in the first place if attackers perceive the tail as the venomous snakes head," said Rasmussen.

'This research is the first record of a combined false-head-behaviour and false-head-camouflage defence strategy used as instinct when a snake is hunting for food.

'"It is intriguing that this discovery is observed in this species, as one of the key differences between the yellow-lipped sea krait and other sea snakes is that they spend almost equal time on land and in the sea," said Rasmussen. "They therefore live in 2 worlds where 2 very different rules of survival apply. It remains to be confirmed whether sea kraits use their sea defence tactic of motioning their tails when on land."' [Rasmussen, 2009]

## MATERIA MEDICA LATICAUDA COLUBRINA

### Sources
1 Effects of bite; clinical manifestations.

### Clinical Manifestations
Venom neurotoxic and myotoxic. Systemic effects of envenomation consist particularly of generalised muscle pain and weakness, in combination with ptosis, trismus, blurring of vision, and myoglobinuria. Respiratory failure and/or renal failure may occur.

# PELAMIS PLATURUS

### Systematics
- Scientific name: Hydrophis platurus [L., 1766].
- Synonyms: Pelamis platurus [L., 1766]. Anguis platura [L., 1766]. Hydrus bicolor [Schneider, 1799]. Pelamis bicolor [Schneider, 1799]. Hydrus platurus [Boulenger, 1896].
- Common names: Yellow-bellied sea snake. Pelagic sea snake.
- Family: Hydrophiidae [subfamily of Elapidae].

### Biological Profile
- Moderately-built sea snake with narrow head and elongated snout. Body compressed, posterior less than half the diameter of the neck. Upper half of body black to dark blueish-brown, sharply delineated from yellowish lower half. Tail paddle-shaped, yellow with dark spots or bars. Body scales small, smooth and hexagonal in shape; head scales large and regular. Average length 75 cm; maximum 1.1 m.
- Range: Widespread in tropical and subtropical parts of Pacific and Indian Oceans, incl. coasts of Africa, Asia, Australia, Mexico, Baja California and Central America. Occasionally carried by currents into temperate waters. Avoids brackish or fresh water.

- Habitat: Most pelagic of all sea snakes, occurring in open ocean well away from coasts and reefs.
- Has upper and lower thermal tolerances of 36°C [96.8°F] and 11.7°C [53.1°F]. With rapid cooling, stops feeding at 16–18°C [60.8–64.4°F]. Has a high resistance to cold temperature and can withstand 5°C [41°F] for 1 hr. Does not acclimate to 17°C [62.6°F] after 10 days' exposure and thus would not be able to survive for long periods in water this cold. [Graham, 1971]
- Preys on small surface-dwelling fish and eels. Feeds during the day and spends night on ocean bottom, occasionally rising to the surface to breathe. Capable of cutaneous breathing.
- Swim by lateral undulation of body. Can *move both forwards and backwards*. Capable of bursts of speed of up to 1m/sec when diving, fleeing and feeding. May carry head out of water when swimming rapidly. Unable to stay upright and move effectively on land because its compressed shape makes it roll onto its side. Practically helpless if washed ashore.
- Capable of spending up to 3 hours underwater without surfacing. Studies estimate it spends up to 87% of its life underwater, surfacing mainly when the seas are calm.
- Often occurs in large numbers [up to several thousand] in open ocean in association with drift lines of floating debris [consisting variously of debris, foam and scum brought together by converging water currents, creating quiet waters].
- Ovoviviparous; 2–6 live young per brood.

## Stealthy Approach & Motionless Waiting
Hunts by stealthily approaching its prey or by waiting motionless at the surface and ambushing fish that come to shelter underneath it [small fish are often attracted to inanimate objects such as floating debris]. With its mouth agape the snake makes a rapid sideways swipe to snare any fish that comes too close. This snake can even ambush small fish behind its head by smoothly swimming backwards so that the prey then comes within range of its mouth.

In captivity, the snake will feed on whole fish [both alive and dead] or pieces of fish and may also accept frogs. When feeding, the snakes will lunge and bite at anything, incl. other snakes in the tank, and is known to stick its head out of water to take prey dangled above it. [australianmuseum.net.au]

## Knotting Behaviour
Being a pelagic species the yellow-bellied sea snake has limited access to hard objects, such as coral, to rub against when the skin is due to be shed. Instead the snake uses a knotting behaviour whereby it coils and twists upon itself, sometimes for hours on end, to loosen the old skin. [Ties a knot in its body and runs the knot from one end of the body to the other.] The skin is shed frequently and in captivity may be sloughed as often as every 2 to 3 weeks. The knotting behaviour also helps to detach organisms such as algae and barnacles that adhere to the skin. [australianmuseum.net.au]

## Sources
1 Effects of bite; clinical manifestations.

## Clinical Manifestations
Venom highly toxic; contains potent neurotoxins and myotoxins. Symptoms of envenomation include muscle pain and stiffness, drooping eyelids, drowsiness and vomiting. A serious bite can lead to total paralysis and death.

# Family Viperidae, subfamily Crotalinae – Pit vipers

## Biological Profile
- Snakes of the subfamily Crotalinae within the family Viperidae are called pit vipers because they possess special heat-sensitive pit organs on their heads, located between the nostrils and the eyes. All of the best-known North American venomous snakes are pit vipers, such as the several species of rattlesnakes, cottonmouths and copperheads. The pits are supplied with a dense packing of free nerve endings from the fifth cranial nerve. They are exceedingly sensitive to radiant energy [long-wave infrared] and can distinguish temperature differences <0.003°C from a radiating surface. The pits work with heat as human eyes do with light, creating stereoscopic 'vision' and thus a fine discrimination of direction and distance. Pit vipers use the pits to track warm-blooded prey and to aim strikes, which they can make as effectively in total darkness as in daylight. Most pit vipers are nocturnal.
- S.B. Higgins in his book *Ophidians* [1873] launched the absurd idea that pit vipers are so called 'because the varieties [of the genus Crotalus] choose their dwelling place in pits and caves, most generally frequented by burrowing or small animals.'
- Pit vipers may be either slender or thick-bodied. Their heads are usually much wider than their necks. They are mostly brown with dark blotches, but some kinds are green.

  Rattlesnakes are the only pit vipers that possess a rattle at the tip of the tail. Most will try to escape without a fight when approached, but there is always a chance one will strike at a passerby. They do not always give a warning; they may strike first and rattle afterwards or not at all.
- All pit vipers are *ambush predators*: they take up a promising position and wait for suitable prey to arrive.

## Venom
Crotalid venom is a complex mixture of many different toxins. Ninety percent of the dry weight consists of protein and polypeptides. Venom components will

vary not only between species, but also within the same species depending on geography, season, age and nutritional status of the snake. Crotalid venom contains proteolytic enzymes, which cause tissue damage. Various neurotoxins, haematologic toxins, and cardiac toxins are also found.

## Turning Yellow

Dr. William Lambert de Humboldt introduced the practice of inoculation with the venom of an unspecified Mexican snake as a prophylactic against yellow fever. He came to his discovery by observing that 'galley-slaves, brought from Mexico to Vera Cruz, who had been bitten by *some viper* on the way, always had decided symptoms of yellow fever.'

He tried it first out on Mexican prisoners in 1847 and later in 1854 inoculated the Spanish troops stationed in Cuba. While the overall results were questionable, i.e. did not impart immunity against yellow fever, the large-scale Cuban experiment did produce yellowness of the skin, amongst a host of other unpleasant effects, which were regarded as representing 'a portrait of the principal and most important phenomena of the yellow fever.' Dr. Manzini, Humboldt's Cuban co-worker, claimed similarity of the effects with the symptoms elicited in Mure's provings of Crotalus cascavella and Elaps. Nothing further was heard of Humboldt's method and Humboldt never revealed the precise species of snake from which his material for inoculations was obtained. S.L. Kotar & J.E. Gessler in their book *Yellow Fever: A Worldwide History* [2017] claim to know better, asserting that it concerned a mixture of Crotalus horridus venom and a 'Mikamia-guaco' [*sic*] syrup, 'the well-known antidote for snakebites'.

In about the same period, Dr. Charles Neidhard [1809–1895] compared the symptoms produced by Crotalus with those observed in the yellow fever epidemic of 1853 in Philadelphia. Making no distinction between the haemotoxic horridus and the neurotoxic cascavella, Neidhard insisted that C. horridus in the second or third trituration gave the best results in the treatment of yellow fever.

To accentuate the soundness of his reasoning on the link between rattlesnakes and yellow skin, Neidhard brought forward 'a well-authenticated fact' that today will strike us as being equally ludicrous as it is absurd. He wrote: 'Dr. Fellger, of Philadelphia, mentioned to me, as a well-authenticated fact, that Heinrich Witte, of Northampton County, Pennsylvania, fired a shot among hundreds of rattlesnakes copulating in the forest. After quitting the place without being bitten, from the mere deadly effluvium of so many snakes he had pains in the whole body, which became swollen, and also vertigo, lasting nearly 9 months. Since then, now 10 years, every year, about the same time, he has a return of the same symptoms. His skin assumed a dirty yellow colour and has remained so ever since.'

Silly superstitions and medical misconceptions aside, the truth of the matter is that potentially *any haemotoxic* snake, i.e. most pit vipers and true vipers, can cause haemorrhaging, bleeding disorders, hepatitis, jaundice and/or liver failure, whether associated with yellow fever, liver cirrhosis, alcoholic liver disease, chronic hepatitis C, or any other severe liver disorder. When the liver is no longer able to make essential clotting substances, bleeding is a common consequence.

Linking the liver with neurotoxic snakes, such as C. cascavella and Elaps, however, would be much harder to substantiate.

## Yellow & Copperhead

Generally speaking, Neidhard's and to some degree also Humboldt's endeavours merely show us that predominantly haemotoxic snake remedies affect the liver. In Hering's Guiding Symptoms examples are given of the successful treatment of jaundice, hepatitis, and yellow fever with Lachesis. In addition, a bite by the pit viper Bothrops atrox can make you turn yellow, among others.

In this context we can readily see Calmette's point regarding the similarity between envenomation by haemotoxic snakes of the genus Bothrops and yellow fever: 'Certain symptoms, which are produced by disorders of the sympathetic, as vomiting, so constant in yellow fever, are observed likewise in snake-poisoning. Frontal headache, disturbance of vision, dilatation of pupils, regurgitations of bile, a profound depression of forces, the fear of death, are symptoms, which are observed as much in yellow fever as in snake-poisoning. The same thing is said of nose bleeding, haematuria, stomatorrhage [bleeding from the mouth], intestinal haemorrhage, jaundice, and albuminuria, which constitute the horrid picture of the last stage of yellow fever and of snake-poisoning.' [Calmette, 1908]

The following report demonstrates that it is no different with the highly haemotoxic copperhead. [Note that the informant is aware of the yellowing effects of alcohol on the liver.]

'While engaged in a hand-to-hand conflict with yellow fever last year, I received a hurried call 15 miles away to see a case of "snake-bite." My informant was a brother to the victim, and in response to my questions said: "Hain't bin doin' nuthin. Hain't no whisky on the mountain, and hit's a d. . .d copperhead, doctor."

'Now this reptile is deemed by all mountaineers the most vicious and dangerous – striking silently, swiftly, deeply, and often fatally. I had never treated a case of this character, and therefore gladly seized this opportunity of witnessing and learning something new. So, turning my yellow fever patients over to a co-labourer, I rode to the cabin of my new patient on the mountain, and arrived about 7 h. after he had received his wound. When I entered the room the pitiable, trembling victim was lying on a couch before me. He was about 21 years old, heavy built, of sanguine-lymphatic temperament. His right arm was bandaged, and his hand covered with saturated tobacco.

'Standing by his side I remarked the following symptoms: Trembling all over, rigors, hurried, laborious breathing; flushed face, eyes bloodshot and suffused with tears, great anxiety, voice tremulous and weak, extremities cold, pulse 110 to 115, small, jerky, wiry. Laying his hand over his heart, he said: "Here, doctor, I suffer the most. Hit's powerful sore. I know I'll die." Heart's action tumultuous, slight nausea, tenderness over the epigastric region, intense headache, photophobia, severe aching in back and limbs, tongue flat, spongy, with red edges; much mucus. When I had stripped off the bandages I discovered 2 small, penetrating wounds on the dorsal surface of the hand, near the knuckle of the second finger, about three-fourths of an inch apart, from which oozed a watery substance, and around which the tissues were of a greenish hue, shading off into yellow from the wound. His hand was considerably swollen, as was also the arm up to the shoulder.

'I was surprised to see in the totality of the symptoms such a *facsimile* of the train of terrible symptoms I was combating in the city. The case was a miniature mirror, reflecting, as it were, the condition of my patients in the city. With much confidence thought sped along the track of theory to conclusions; from conclusions rapidly to action, thus: First stage of blood poison; its similar, first stage of yellow fever. Decision: Acon. 1st, 1 dr. to 5 oz. water; 1 teaspoonful every 30 min. till reaction sets in and perspiration freely follows, then every hour.

'I ordered his hand plunged in as hot water as could be borne; hot bricks around and extra clothing over the patient. Result: Free perspiration in 1 hour, with great improvement in his condition. Passed night comfortably, and at 9 a.m., 24 hours from the time he was poisoned, I found him resting easy. A marked yellow tinge of the entire surface, with eyes and tongue deeply tinged; a general stiffness and soreness, with "tired feeling," took the place of the intense pain of the few hours previous; heart still painful. The next day he was up, presenting all the appearance of one who had shaken hands with "Bronze John" [yellow fever] upon short acquaintance and could not let go; a deep yellow pervaded the entire surface of his body. A month later I met the patient again. His hand was still puffy, with a general soreness upon pressure.' [D.C. Curtis, M.D., American Homeopath, Nov. 1879]

## Clinical Features of North American Pit Viper Envenomation

Most bites in the United States result from pit vipers, commonly referred to as crotalids. They include Agkistrodon [Cenchris in homeopathy] contortrix or copperhead, Agkistrodon piscivorus or cottonmouth, Crotalus horridus or timber rattlesnake, and Sistrurus miliarius or pigmy rattlesnake.

'The dry bite will present with local pain and irritation, whereas the most severe envenomations may result in coagulopathy, hypotension, shock, or even death. Pain is a generally an early and persistent feature of snakebites. . . . If envenomation does occur, tissue oedema and ecchymoses will ensue as the toxins begin to affect the microvasculature. Tissue oedema commonly progresses to involve the entire extremity. Ecchymoses may progress as well and haemorrhagic blebs commonly appear. Frank tissue necrosis may occur in later stages. Lymphadenopathy and lymphangitis may occur, and usually represent inflammation rather than secondary bacterial infection.

'Rarely compartment syndrome will occur. It is more commonly described with intramuscular injection of venom. Compartment syndrome presents with typical symptoms of pain [esp. with *passive motion*], paraesthesias, pallor, and sometimes paralysis. The clinical diagnosis of compartment syndrome can be difficult in light of ongoing pain, oedema, haemorrhage, and swelling. Elevated CK [creatine kinase] levels are expected secondary to muscle necrosis and rhabdomyolysis and may occur in the absence of compartment syndrome.

'Coagulopathy may range from mild to severe. Bleeding is usually a problem only in the most severe cases. Although true DIC [disseminated intravascular coagulation] is rare, it has been reported. Bleeding times may become prolonged and thrombocytopenia may develop. Fibrin split products may be elevated, but d-dimer, anti-thrombin III, and factor XIII levels are normal [except in true DIC].

'Fluid losses from third spacing, and sometimes vomiting, may cause hypovolemia and hypotension. Rarely, anaphylaxis may occur, particularly if the patient has been sensitized from a previous bite. Rapid cardiovascular collapse and refractory hypotension have been described for the rare case when venom is injected intravascularly.

'Renal damage may occur, usually in the form of acute tubular necrosis [ATN]. ATN is usually due either to hypoperfusion secondary to hypovolemia, or rhabdomyolysis. However, cortical necrosis has been described in severe envenomations.

'Rarely pulmonary oedema will occur, but usually represents ARDS [acute respiratory distress syndrome] rather than left ventricular failure. Bites to the face, mouth, or tongue may result in life threatening oedema and prompt, pre-emptive intubation is mandatory.

'Many patients experience various nonspecific symptoms. Nausea and vomiting are common, and diarrhoea may be a feature as well. Weakness, diaphoresis, malaise, peri-oral or digital paraesthesias may occur. Myokymia [spontaneous, fine fascicular contractions of muscle without muscular atrophy or weakness] is seen with timber rattler bites and mild fasciculations are possible with most crotalid bites. Weakness or paralysis are extremely rare and are more commonly described with the Mojave rattlesnake of the SW United States.

'These signs and symptoms generally manifest early on, and progress steadily depending upon degree of envenomation. If no clinical or laboratory evidence of venom toxicity exist 6 hours after a bite from a snake indigenous to Kentucky, then envenomation is highly unlikely. It is important to realize that significant coagulopathy and thrombocytopenia may occur without significant oedema or pain at the bite site. Possible late sequelae include persistent extremity pain and oedema, and wound infection.' [Mattingly & Bosse]

### Clinical Features of Bothrops Envenomation

Dr. Nilo Cairo da Silva [1874–1928], of Curitiba in the Brazilian state Parana, published in 1910 a materia medica of *Lachesis lanceolatus*, a name based on the 'Catalogue of the Snakes in the British Museum, Vol. III, 1896'. In the catalogue Lachesis lanceolatus is put forward incorrectly as the proper designation for *Bothrops lanceolatus*, the lance-headed viper. At the time the lance-headed viper was thought to be a single species, as becomes evident from Cairo's assertion: 'In Brazil, we name it jararaca, and, in some islands of the Antilles, it is known by the vulgar name of fer-de-lance or vipère jaune.' He further states that 'The Lachesis lanceolatus is found in Mexico and Central America and in the whole of South America; it is the most common snake in all the States of Brazil, and the one that causes also the greater number of snake-poisoning. This viper inhabits also some islands of the Antilles, as Martinique, Guadeloupe, Saint-Lucie and Bequia, where it is the only venomous species, but very numerous.'

The good doctor Cairo took 'Lachesis lanceolatus' to include *2 different* species of Bothrops [Bothrops lanceolatus and Bothrops jararaca]. However, checking the 32 [!] synonyms given by Cairo shows us that the name 'Lachesis lanceolatus' incorporated then at least *five* different Bothrops species: Bothrops asper, Bothrops atrox, Bothrops caribbaeus, Bothrops jararaca, and Bothrops lanceolatus.

Consequently, the entire pathogenesis of Lachesis lanceolatus, as provided by Dr. Cairo and proceeding 'from observations of bites in men and animals, as well as from experiments on animals with its venom,' can be taken as a *general overview of signs and symptoms of Bothrops envenomation*:

- *General Symptoms* – Weariness, restlessness, distress, inexpressible lassitude, sluggishness, staggering, falling and inability to stand or sit up. Nervous trembling, twitching, quivering. General weakness. Extreme debility. Anaemia: emaciation. Prostration. General numbness. Syncope. Muscular relaxation. Convulsions [in children; opisthotonus]. Hemiplegia with aphasia, though tongue is not paralysed. Internal heat, sometimes very intense. Congestion of internal organs. Haemorrhages, constant and intense, from every orifice of the body. Great sensibility to touch. Worse on right side. Hemiplegia of right side, with or without aphasia. Slight jaundice. Anorexia.
- *Mind* – Obstinate hypochondriasis. Confusion of mind. Delirium, more or less violent. Hardly answers questions, indifferent to all. Attacks of sudden loquacity and of frenzy and gaiety. Great sensibility to least noise: he is readily annoyed and cries and weeps at least noise.
- *Sleep* – Tendency to sleep; drowsiness; coma, more and more profound until death.
- *Fever* – General heat; at first feverish temperature, high fever or fever at 38°C.; afterwards, the temperature falls; chilliness, slight shivering, followed by very profuse cold sweat. General coldness, cold and clammy sweat, very copious. Feeling of external heat, sometimes very intense, with an ardent thirst. Feeling of external coldness with a devouring internal heat and intense thirst. Fever with pulmonary congestion or pneumonia, oppression of chest and bloody saliva more or less abundant.
- *Head* – Headache in forehead and eyes. Megrim with hypochondriasis. Giddiness, vertigo, fainting.
- *Eye* – Dimness of vision. Hemeralopia [day blindness]. Pupils dilated and insensible to light. Blindness, temporary or persisting. Eyes injected, watery, tearful, and weak. Lachrymation. Haemorrhage; extravasations of blood in conjunctiva. Upper lids heavy, half closed and sleepy. Photophobia. Purulent ophthalmia.
- *Ear* – Haemorrhages.
- *Nose* – Epistaxis.
- *Face* – Swollen and puffy, red-injected face, as if drunk; besotted expression. Face bluish-purple; deathly pale: hippocratic.

- *Mouth* – Contractions of jaws and lips; trismus. Aphasia; cannot speak, although tongue is mobile. Haemorrhages from gums and tongue. Tongue enlarged and heavy; tongue paralysed. White coated tongue. Extreme dryness of mouth; intense thirst, with a feeling of external heat or devouring internal fire.
- *Throat and Neck* – Constriction in throat, with redness and dryness; difficult swallowing, so that he cannot pass liquids. Extreme dryness in throat. Enlargement of lymphatic glands of neck. Hydrophobia.
- *Stomach* – Enlargement of stomach. Nausea. Spasmodic vomiting, at first alimentary, afterwards bilious and later bloody. Intense haematemesis. Extreme epigastric distress. Black vomiting. Vomiting very frequent. Vomiting followed by nervous trembling. Vomiting followed by cold sweats and syncope.
- *Abdomen & Rectum* – Bilious diarrhoea; colliquative diarrhoea. Bloody stools; stools black like coffee-grounds. Haemorrhage from bowels. Tenesmus. Colic; severe pains in abdomen, which extend to epigastrium and become intolerable. Abdomen painful to pressure; great sensibility of whole abdomen. Fatty degeneration of liver.
- *Urinary & Sexual Organs* – Haemorrhages from kidneys; haematuria. Nephritis. Albuminous urine. Metrorrhagia.
- *Chest & Heart* – Pains in chest. Violent pains in heart. Oppression of chest & difficult breathing; great dyspnoea; orthopnoea. Suffocation. At first accelerated and profound breathing, afterwards slow and superficial, then arrested completely. Anguish in heart. Pulmonary congestion, & acute fever, difficult breathing and bloody expectoration, more or less abundant. Haemoptysis. Pneumonia.
- *Limbs* – Speedy and painful swelling of bitten limb. The swelling of the bitten part gradually extends to a great distance from its original seat; the limb becomes triple its ordinary size, and is soft and flabby, appearing as if it distended with gas. Intolerable pains in the swelling, extending to the whole frame. Cellular and muscular tissue engorged with black blood. Very extensive suppuration. Large phlegmon, with destruction of the skin, gangrene, necrosis, fistulae; portions of cellular tissue are detached, the tendons and bones are laid bare; the joints are exposed. Cramps in bitten limb. Caries of bones. Numbness of bitten arm; soft swelling, from the fingers, hand, forearm, to the shoulder and adjacent portion of the chest, with blue spots, very painful. Intense pains in whole arm. Enormous swelling of leg: bluish colour of the skin; haemorrhagic infiltration; haemorrhagic bullae, gangrene of skin of leg; gangrene of muscles of leg. Pains in joints.
- *Skin* – Copious cold sweat at beginning and end of sickness. Skin of bitten part of a bluish colour, like an enormous bruise; skin of body a bluish colour like that of Asiatic cholera in the algid stage, or of a yellowish colour, as in yellow fever. Slight jaundice. Bluish-purple spots issuing spontaneously here and there. Ecchymosis. Haemorrhages from the skin; haemorrhages from interstices of nails. Skin of leg and abdomen completely blackened, though bite is at the foot. Bloody phlyctenae. Bloody subcutaneous or intra-muscular infiltration.

Abscess. Diffuse phlegmons. Easy suppuration. Gangrene of skin. Slow cicatrisation of wounds. Chronic or periodical ulcers. Small wounds or ulcers bleed abundantly. [Cairo da Silva, 1910]

## VIPERIDAE, SUBFAMILY CROTALINAE IN HOMEOPATHY

| Homeopathic name | Common name | Abbreviation | Symptoms |
|---|---|---|---|
| Acrochordon chocoe | = Lachesis acrochorda | Acro-c-f. | + |
| Ancistrodon piscivorus[1] | Cottonmouth | Ancis-p. | ++ |
| Bothriechis schlegelii | Eyelash pit viper | Bothri-sg. | + |
| Bothrocophias colombianus | Colombian toadh. pitviper | Bothc-hp. | + |
| Bothrops alternatus | Crossed pit viper | Both-a. | + |
| Bothrops asper | Asper | Both-as. | + |
| Bothrops atrox | Common lancehead | Both-ax. | ++ |
| Bothrops caribbaeus[2] | St. Lucia pit viper | Both-car. | + |
| Bothrops colombiensis | = Bothrops atrox | | |
| Bothrops insularis | Golden lancehead | Both-in. | − |
| Bothrops jararaca | Jararaca | Both-jara. | + |
| Bothrops jararacussu | Jararacussu | Both-jasu. | ++ |
| Bothrops lanceolatus | Fer-de-lance | Both. | ++ |
| Bothrops neuwiedi urutu | Neuwied's lancehead | Both-n-ur. | + |
| Cenchris contortrix | Copperhead | Cench. | +++ |
| Crotalus adamanteus | Eastern diamondback | Crot-ad. | + |
| Crotalus atrox | Western diamondback | Crot-atr. | + |
| Crotalus cascavella | South American rattlesnake | Crot-c. | +++ |
| Crotalus cerastes cerastes | Mojave Desert sidewinder | Crot-cer. | + |
| Crotalus enyo | Baja California rattlesnake | Crot-eny. | − |
| Crotalus horridus | Timber rattlesnake | Crot-h. | +++ |
| Crotalus lepidus | Rock rattlesnake | Crot-le. | + |
| Crotalus mitchellii | Speckled rattlensnake | Crot-mi. | + |
| Crotalus molossus | Black-tailed rattlesnake | Crot-mo. | + |
| Crotalus polystictus | Mexican lance-headed rattlesnake | Crot-po. | + |
| Crotalus viridis viridis | Prairie rattlesnake | Crot-vir. | + |
| Deinagkistrodon acutus | Sharp-nosed pit viper | Dein-ac. | + |
| Lachesis acrochorda | Chocoan bushmaster | Acro-c-f. | + |
| Lachesis muta | Bushmaster | Lach. | +++ |
| Sistrurus catenatus caten. | Eastern massasauga | Sist-cc. | − |
| Sistrurus miliarius barbouri | Dusky pygmy rattlesnake | Sist-mb. | − |
| Trimeresurus flavoviridis[3] | Habu | Trim-fl. | + |

| Trimeresurus mucrosquamatus[4] | Brown spotted pit viper | Trim-mu. | + |
| Trimeresurus puniceus | Flat-nosed pit viper | Trim-pu. | – |
| Trimeresurus purpureomaculatus | Mangrove pit viper | Trim-pur. | – |
| Trimeresurus stejnegeri | Green tree viper | Trim-st. | + |
| Trimeresurus wagleri[5] | Temple pit viper | Trim. | + |
| Vipera lachesis fel[6] | Toad-headed pit viper bile | Vip-l-f. | + |

1 Listed under 2 different names: Ancistrodon piscivorus [Ancis-p.] & Toxicophis pugnax [Toxi.]. 2 Symptoms of bites in Allen wrongly credited to Naja. 3 = Protobothrops flavoviridis. 4 = Protobothrops mucrosquamatus. 5 = Tropidolaemus wagleri. 6 = Bothrocophias colombianus.

# ACROCHORDON CHOCOE

see **Lachesis acrochorda**.

# ANCISTRODON PISCIVORUS

## Systematics
- Scientific name: Agkistrodon piscivorus [Lacépède, 1789].
- Synonyms: Ancistrodon piscivorus [Lacépède, 1789]. Ancistrodon pugnax [Baird & Girard, 1853]. Toxicophis pugnax [Baird & Girard, 1853]. Trigono-cephalus piscivorus [Lacépède, 1789]
- Common names: Cottonmouth. Water moccasin. Cottonmouth moccasin.
- Family: Viperidae, subfamily Crotalinae.

## Biological Profile
- Dark-coloured, heavy-bodied venomous semi-aquatic pit viper with large, triangular head with a dark line through the eye, elliptical pupils, and large jowls due to the venom glands. Average length 50–120 cm, maximum 1.9 m. Colouration highly variable: can be beautifully marked with dark reddish-brown crossbands on a brown and yellow ground colour or completely brown or black. Belly typically has dark and brownish-yellow blotches; underside of tail black. Top of head in front of eyes covered with large plate-like scales. Deep facial pit between nostril and eye. Keeled scales.
- Range: SE United States, incl. very southern Virginia to Florida and east to eastern Texas.
- Habitat: Along streams, springs, rivers, lakes, ponds, marshes, swamps, sloughs, reservoirs, retention pools, canals, and roadside ditches; prefers slow-moving and shallow lakes and streams. Occasionally found far from water.

- The world's only semi-aquatic viper, the cottonmouth is a strong swimmer and will even enter the sea, successfully colonising islands off both the Atlantic and Gulf coasts.
- Juvenile cottonmouths hold their bright, sulfur yellow tail erect, wiggling it like a caterpillar to lure prey within striking range. The colour fades with age and is lost by age 3 or 4.
- Preys on fish, frogs, and water snakes, but is otherwise highly varied and, uniquely, has even been reported to include carrion in its diet. Employ both ambush and active foraging strategies.
- Adults have few enemies other than alligators and humans. Juveniles are preyed on by a multitude of animals: large fish, snapping turtles, snakes, large wading birds, horned owls, hawks, eagles, raccoons, otters, cats, dogs.
- Becomes inactive at the onset of cold weather, hibernating underground over winter. Common hibernacula are on rocky wooded hillsides, in crayfish burrows, under rotting stumps and in mammal burrows.
- More tolerant to cold than most snakes and thus one of the last to enter hibernation.
- Ovoviviparous.
- Specific name derives from the Latin words *pisces*, fish, and *voro*, to eat; hence 'fish eater'. Receives its common name cottonmouth from the whiteness of the interior of its mouth that it exposes as a defensive display.
- Three recognized subspecies: the eastern, Florida, and western cottonmouths.

### Behaviour & Temperament
During the spring and fall, activity is mostly diurnal, but in summer cottonmouths are predominantly nocturnal, while basking in the sun in the morning. Because they spend much of their time in water, and water draws away heat more quickly than air, they must somehow maintain a high body temperature, particularly for their digestive metabolism. This is accomplished partly by basking.

Cottonmouths have varying temperaments. They are usually not aggressive and will not attack unless agitated. One of their unique behaviours is their ability to '*stand their ground*'. When thoroughly aroused, a cottonmouth coils its body and threatens the intruder with its mouth wide open and its fangs exposed, showing the white lining of its mouth. Given the chance, the cottonmouth usually will retreat. Its reputation for aggression is largely undeserved; its open mouth threat display has led to the widespread belief that cottonmouths are aggressive snakes. However, when first grasped or pinned down, they thrash about violently, striking at any near object, and may even bite themselves. Like many other pit vipers, male cottonmouths sometimes participate in combat dances [*see* copperhead].

Some people believe cottonmouths lie in wait on tree limbs overhanging water so they can drop into boats. These are usually cases of mistaken identity with the harmless brown water snake, which often basks on tree limbs over the water, and when frightened will escape by throwing themselves off the limb and into the water or into the boat when its attempt to flee comes too late.

Prey such as frogs, fish, and other snakes are held in the jaws for a few moments after capture to allow them to succumb to the venom. Mammals [that are likely to bite back] are struck and then instantly released. If the victim flees before the venom takes effect, the cottonmouth tracks it by scent. It then examines the carcass by touching it with its tongue to make sure that the prey is dead. It swallows the prey headfirst. Unlike non-venomous reptiles, the cottonmouth *takes its time when feeding*, perhaps because its prey is dead.

Breeding takes place during the spring. It begins with the male nudging the female's back and sides. This continues for as long as several hours, until she exposes her tail and opens her cloaca for copulation. Ovulation takes place only in alternate years. The gestation period usually lasts from 3 to 4 months. The female produces a litter of up to 12 living young. Each young is brightly patterned with a yellow tail and is relatively large, about 20 to 25 cm long and 2 cm in diameter. [Smithsonian National Zoological Park]

## Social in the Wild – Wildly Unsocial in Captivity

In the wild a 'social' snake like its near-relative the copperhead, the cottonmouth overwinters in large numbers together with rattlesnakes, copperheads, and other snakes in cracks between the ledges of limestone and sandstone hills and along bluffs overlooking large swamps.

Specimens that have been captive for many years, according to Ditmars, "never show intimations of hostility, and in fact the general demeanour of this snake when removed from a wild state is a *lazy indifference to everything but food.*"

'They live well with no other water than that contained in a small drinking dish, and usually congregate in social clusters with heads protruding in all directions. With other snakes of equal or even larger size they are generally quarrelsome. Smaller snakes of other species are usually eaten, while many young moccasins may be in the cage with the adults and escape molestation. The pugnacious attitude of the moccasin toward other snakes was illustrated by the escape from a cage in my collection of a specimen of moderate size. This reptile prowled about the "snake room" until, prompted by curiosity or seeking a place to hide, it entered, through the ventilating apparatus, the cage of a large South American anaconda. There it battled with the big constrictor, biting him in a dozen places. The catastrophe occurred during the night.

'Morning revealed the presence of the moccasin, quietly coiled in the quarters of the anaconda, and the 12-foot serpent lay contorted and dead after its struggle against the action of the formidable poison of its diminutive adversary, a snake of less than 4 feet. Captive moccasins feed upon small rabbits, rats, birds, fishes and frogs. Rabbits and large rats seem to greatly excite these snakes. They strike many times, and wildly, as if in fear of being attacked by the animals.' [Ditmars, 1937a]

## Calling the Bluff

As its old specific name 'pugnax' says, the cottonmouth is allegedly very *pugnacious* – eager and ready to fight; quarrelsome; combative. The cottonmouth shares this cantankerous, grouchy reputation with its nearest relative, the copperhead [Cenchris in homeopathy]. Both irascible ophidians are believed to actively chase offenders, humans included.

Adjunct Professor of Biological Science at Florida State University and herpetologist D. Bruce Means devotes a chapter to 'the feared cottonmouth' in his excellent book *Stalking the Plumed Serpent*, raising the question 'Is It Aggressive?' Just about everybody who lives in the southeastern United States, he says, will mention the cottonmouth when asked which snake they fear the most, because 'it is aggressive' or because 'it chases you'. Whilst being 'chased' by a cottonmouth is a behaviour Means has pooh-poohed for years as an old wives' tale, he admits that 'it is true that the cottonmouth will strike at you suddenly from a coiled position. This serves to keep you at a distance that is safe for the cottonmouth, and I suppose one could call this aggressive behaviour.'

Then, one fine day, while leading a field class of 15 people down a sandy road somewhere in Florida and stumbling upon a cottonmouth, our friend the herpetologist is forced to adjust his opinion.

'I spotted a 3½ foot long female cottonmouth stretched out in the characteristic frozen posture of a snake caught in the open. Earlier in the day I told the class, "The cottonmouth does *not* chase people." We all piled out of the van and freaked the poor snake into coiling up. When I approached closely, it struck suddenly and made me and my entourage jump back, just as the behaviour is designed to do. Frightened, the dark brown cottonmouth began vibrating its tail. It coiled up, flattened its body, threw its head back, and opened its mouth to display the white lining. I was standing between the cottonmouth and the swamp from which it had come. . . . Then an amazing thing happened. The cottonmouth raised the forward one-third of its body off the ground and crawled as fast as it could in this posture right at me! I was forced to back up at least 10 feet. I noticed that the neck and head were tilted a little sideways toward me and flattened, cobra-like, to appear larger. I shouted at the students, "Look, the cottonmouth is charging me!"

'. . . I had only a few furious moments to observe the new behaviour, to eat crow for all those people whose own similar observations I had pooh-poohed, and to relish my good fortune – for in the next few seconds I made a momentous discovery. While the cottonmouth was "chasing" me, I stepped to one side, away from the trajectory the snake seemed to be taking and noticed that the snake did not turn and follow me. It simply kept up its "cobra crawl" in the direction it had been going, which was the shortest distance necessary for it to reach safety. . . . The cottonmouth was using *bluffing behaviour* to make safe passage to where it wanted to go. . . . Over the next several summers my wife and I stimulated more than 20 other cottonmouths to display this same behaviour. We discovered that some other snakes besides the cottonmouth do the same thing.

'The behaviour is a type of bluff, designed to ward off dangerous predators while enabling the snake to escape. I call the behaviour, "*shammed aggression during blocked flight.*" . . . It was during these attempts to escape to the safety of the road shoulder that each snake rose up like a cobra, spread its jaws, sometimes struck viciously, and advanced directly towards me. Of course, I reacted just as any dog, raccoon, or other snake predator would do: I backed up rapidly or jumped to the side to get out of the way of the snake. If I backed up in front of the snake, it continued advancing and bluffing; if I jumped to one side, it paid me no more attention. In no instance when I stepped aside, did any of the fleeing cottonmouths change direction and move towards me. They simply continued straight in their intended direction. Even more intriguing is what they did if I did not move aside, In 12 episodes, the snakes simply crawled over my boot or between my legs. None of the snakes attempted to bite me. . . . I now understand why the cottonmouth is so feared. Any person, not realising he is standing in the cottonmouth's path to safety, would interpret the snake's aggressive bluffing as an attack. This conclusion would be especially likely if the person were backing up and the snake continued advancing. Who would believe that he was not being chased by the snake?' [Means, 2008]

### Venom & Clinical Manifestations

Venom primarily haemotoxic [or haemorrhagic], affecting blood cells and blood vessels, though some neurotoxic elements are included.

Symptoms of a cottonmouth bite usually appear from minutes to hours after a bite and can include:

Severe, immediate *burning, searing, excruciating* pain with rapid swelling.

Progressive swelling, erythema, petechiae, ecchymosis, and haemorrhagic blebs may develop over the next several hours.

Bitten limb may swell to twice its normal size within the first few hours.

Discolouration of the skin.

Difficult or rapid breathing.

Changes in heart rate or rhythm.

Metallic, rubbery, or minty taste in the mouth.

Numbness or tingling around mouth, tongue, scalp, feet, or the bite area.

Swelling in lymph nodes near the bite injury.

Bleeding.

Signs of shock.


# MATERIA MEDICA AGKISTRODON PISCIVORUS

### Sources

1 Proving Farokh Master [India], 16 provers [6 were given verum, 1M; 10 got placebo]; 1996; proving substance listed as Toxicophis pugnax. Unmarked symptoms.

2 Synthesis Repertory Treasure Edition 2009.

### Mind

∞ Irritability and anger over small matters, < when questioned. Abusive without cause.

∞ Argumentative [aggressive, confrontational] & desire to hit and strike someone during argument.

∞ Anger at trifles.[2]

∞ Feeling of inflicting injury on opposite person or killing myself. Desire to abuse people without respecting their age. Using bad words.
∞ Answers snappishly.
∞ Alternating periods of indecision and confidence.
∞ Oversensitive to rudeness of others; can start crying at slightest cause.
∞ Desire to be hugged and caressed, wants physical intimacy.
∞ Long periods of silence: Wanting to say so many things but unable to express self.
∞ Sadness; 'paralysing depression'; nothing seems interesting; no desire to talk to anyone.
∞ Fear of being alone in the dark.
∞ Delusion someone behind one on entering house.
∞ Delusion being criticized; impression of danger.[2]
∞ Sees frightful images on closing eyes.[2]
∞ Fear after waking in night; on waking from a dream.[2]
∞ Fear of being alone.[2]
∞ Fear of cockroaches.[2]
∞ Feeling of helplessness.[2]
∞ Indifference to life.[2]

## Dreams
∞ Holding an alligator's mouth open, cutting its tongue out and eating its flesh.
∞ Attacked by a dark blue crocodile, which eats friend.
∞ Danger to loved and dear ones; attempts to save them.
∞ Violent anger and hitting someone very hard with a stick without it having any effect.
∞ Being followed by a cat and after some by its head only.
∞ Water everywhere, a male and a female snake emerging from it, the male coiling around the female.
∞ Criticized and laughed at by friends.
∞ Travelling by sea. Visiting a mosque with many stairs.
∞ Dissecting snakes at college.
∞ Drinking lime juice with a long, crawling creature in it.
∞ Burials in a small cemetery; dead people put on top of each other in very deep graves.
∞ Preparing for marriage that is fixed.
∞ Getting married in a catholic church wearing a white dress.
∞ Arguments in family, with shouting and crying.
∞ Exposing parts of body.
∞ Visiting temples and praying for long time.
∞ Lizards, horrible and huge with large heads, coming out of all corners.
∞ Death in family; deceased person getting up and going away.
∞ Being pregnant and miserable.
∞ Being laughed at.[2]
∞ Of God.[2]

## Generals
∞ Thirst for cold water, & dryness of mouth.
∞ Unrefreshed on waking in morning, dull and listless during the day.
∞ Aversion to non-vegetarian food and eggs.
∞ Right side more affected [eye, throat to ear, jaw, breast]; left side [head, lower leg – knee, ankle].
∞ Wandering pain.[2]
∞ Periodical neuralgic pain.[2]
∞ Wounds bleeding freely.[2]

## Sensations
∞ Suffocation, as of heavy weight on chest, & desire to take deep breaths.
∞ Oppression chest > taking a deep breath and holding hands on chest.

## Locals
∞ Hair very dry and brittle; falling out.
∞ Swollen eyelids. Watering eyes. Redness eyes > cold water application. Running nose, thin, watery discharge and sneezing.
∞ Puffy swelling of upper and lower eyelids of right eye, & inability to open eye.
∞ Menses profuse, esp. on second day, offensive, with large, dark maroon clots; severe dysmenorrhoea, pain in lower back and legs as if legs would give way. Before menses: depressed, offended easily, sensitive.

# BOTHRIECHIS SCHLEGELII

## Systematics
• Scientific name: Bothriechis schlegelii [Berthold, 1846].
• Synonyms: Lachesis nitidus [Günther, 1859]. Trigonocephalus schlegelii [Berthold, 1846].
• Common names: Eyelash pit viper. Schlegel's palm viper. Horned palm viper.
• Family: Viperidae, subfamily Crotalinae.

## Biological Profile
• Small, moderately slender, arboreal pit viper, with relatively wide, triangular head and prehensile tail. Wide range of colour. Dorsal colouration usually bright green or yellow, but can also be bright yellow, brown, dark grey, green, silver and even pink. Markings variable: black or brown speckling, green, orange, pink or red markings on base colour. Some may not have any patterns.
• Body length ranges from 55 to 82 cm, with females [35 to 82 cm] typically longer and more variable in size than males [37 to 69 cm].
• Range: Central and South America.
• Habitat: Tropical moist forest, wet subtropical forest [cloud forest], and montane wet forest. Usually found in shrubs, trees, and vine tangles close to rivers and streams. Frequently reported in plantations, on the branches of coffee trees.

- Its most distinguishing feature, and origin of its common name, is the set of small, bristly, keeled scales over the eyes that look much like eyelashes.
- Primarily arboreal and nocturnal.
- Slow-moving predator, relying on camouflage to ambush their prey. Choose their habitat in accordance with their colouring: red ones inhabit red coloured bromeliads and yellow ones inhabit areas where there are a lot of bananas.
- Has well-developed binocular vision, giving it great depth perception.
- Preys mainly on arboreal lizards, frogs, and small mammals [may also hunt these same prey on the ground].
- Ovoviviparous; 2–20 live young per brood. Females invest very little time in the young once they are born as they are *fully equipped for immediate independence*.
- Characteristically coils with mouth wide open when disturbed. Usually non-aggressive, but reportedly can be quick to bite when disturbed or just brushed against.

## Courtship Behaviour
'Courtship behaviour is an important part of mating. Males participate in a "dance of the adders," which is a courtship ritual in which 2 males face one another in an upright, cobra-like stance. Through posturing, males attempt to intimidate one another, often until one is pushed away or falls to the ground. This courtship ritual typically does not harm either participant, as biting does not occur. This ritual may continue for many hours. Like most snakes, eyelash pit vipers are polygynous.' [animaldiversity.org]

## MATERIA MEDICA BOTHRIECHIS SCHLEGELII

### Sources
1 Effects of bite; clinical manifestations.

### Clinical Manifestations
Venom mainly haemotoxic.

A few humans bitten and envenomated by this species each year within its range, but fatalities [mainly of smaller children] reportedly rare. Typical serious envenomation symptoms include: *local intense pain and swelling, with mild but slowly spreading tissue necrosis, dizziness, nausea, and difficulty breathing*.

'From limited case data it appears bites can cause moderate to severe local pain, mild to severe local swelling, with the potential for fluid shifts into the bitten limb and secondary shock and blistering and oozing from fang marks can occur. Necrosis is certainly a possibility, but it is unclear how frequently it occurs, and current data suggests it may be uncommon, even rare. Similarly, if local swelling and tissue injury is severe, compartment syndrome is possible, but incidence is unknown and possibly low. Systemic effects are possible, but their incidence is unclear. Coagulopathy can occur, with bleeding from IV sites and gums, haematuria, epistaxis, and possibly elsewhere. Without treatment, the coagulopathy may persist for days. Secondary renal failure, though not well documented for this snake, is certainly possible. Neurotoxicity is not expected, but myotoxicity should be considered, based on venom research, although no clinical cases are reported.' [www.toxinology.net]

# BOTHROCOPHIAS COLOMBIANUS

## Systematics
- Scientific name: Bothrocophias colombianus [Rendahl & Vestergren, 1940].
- Synonym: Bothrops microphthalmus colombianus [Rendahl & Vestergren, 1940].
- Common names: Colombian toad-headed pit viper. Frog-headed mapana. Cabeza de sapo.
- Family: Viperidae, subfamily Crotalinae.

## Biological Profile
- Stout terrestrial pit viper with distinctly wide head and upturned snout. Length up to 120 cm [4 ft].
- Colouration dark brown to grey. Side of head slightly paler to slightly darker than top of head, and moderately to heavily mottled with very dark brown or black. Dark blotch below each eye.
- Range: W Colombia.
- Habitat: Found almost exclusively in lower montane wet forests & cloud forests of the Pacific slopes of the Andes in western Columbia, at 800–2000+ m elevation.
- Preys on centipedes, anurans, lizards and rodents.
- Ovoviviparous.
- Described by Higgins as Vipera lachesis Bufocephalus, common names: Frog-headed mapana or Cabeza de sapo.

## Toad-headed Pit Viper Bile as Antivenom Treatment
Mr. S.B. Higgins, 'honorary member of the homoeopathic institute of the United States of Colombia', resided for most of the 1860–70s in Colombia, a country very prolific in poisonous snakes.

In Hempel's Materia Medica and Therapeutics, 1880, the following is said about Mr. Higgins as the propagator of a curious method of antidoting snake-bites: 'He became acquainted with the methods adopted by the curers of snakebites, and learned that the bile of poisonous snakes entered into the composition of most of their vaunted antidotes. The idea occurred to him to try the effects of the administration of the bile of the snake that imparted the poisonous bite and this treatment he assures us he has found perfectly success-ful, and he says it has been largely adopted by the 'curers' and medical men of Colombia. His mode of preparing the antidote is to take the bile from the gall-bladder of the snake shortly after it has cast its skin, when the virtues of the bile are most developed. One drop of this bile to 10 drops of alcohol, strong wine, or spirits, is the proportion for his tincture. For the treatment of bites 5 to 10 drops of this tincture are to be mixed with a tumbler-full of water, and a table-spoonful given every 5, 10, 15, or 20 minutes. He also makes a crucial incision in the wound and bathes the limb in hot water in which are a few drops of the tincture of bile. He warns against giving too much of the bile, for though it will remove the symptoms of poisoning it may kill the patient from its own poisonous properties.'

Mr. Higgins tried the method on himself prophylactically 'by making incisions in the lower extremity of each deltoid muscle, with a preparation of the gall of the Lachesis. [Bufocephalus lachesis one-tenth, or 1 drop of pure gall to 10 drops of 95 per cent alcohol.]'

'The symptoms experienced were fugitive pains of different degrees of intensity in different parts of the head; slight epistaxis; adipsia; anorexia; dysuria; diarrhoea that lasted 4 days [for 15 days previously I had been much consti-pated]; rheumatic pains in joints and limbs; cough, soreness of throat, accom-panied with painful deglutition; accesses of erotism; great debility of body and mind; vertigo; paleness of face and skin, and inclination to fainting fits at times.

'These symptoms diminished in intensity after 6 or 8 days by intermissions, and finally ceased one by one, till after 20 days all that remained was a strange taste of the leaves of a plant [Aristolochia colombiana] upon the tongue, which was noticeable for more than a month afterwards.

'Since being inoculated, I have never seen any snake make the slightest attempt to bite me, unless provoked, and I have observed the same fact in all the Curers and every person inoculated; one is also freed, by inoculation, from the annoyance of flies, fleas, and sand-flies, which is by no means an inconsiderable relief in any tropical climate.'


## MATERIA MEDICA BOTHROCOPHIAS COLOMBIANUS [Vipera lachesis, fel]

### Sources
1 Proving Berridge [UK] on himself, with repeated doses of CM, and another man, who 'took 6 globules without knowing the name of medicine'; *c.* 1874. The second prover produced all symptoms, except for the symptom marked 'B' produced by Berridge.
2 Effects of bite; clinical manifestations.

### Identity
In some of the recent homeopathic literature this remedy is *misidentified as Bitis arietans*, the puff adder, a true viper species native to Africa and Asia. Allen clearly specifies that the bile is obtained from 'Vipera lachesis, Bufocephalus' by Higgins, who, as we have seen above, lived and worked with snakes in Colombia.

Colombia houses many different snakes but no puff adders. Higgins regarded the 'Bufocephalus' as a variety of Lachesis, differing in the shape of its head as being 'toad-like' rather than triangular-shaped ['trigonocephalus'].

The reference to the shape of the head suggests 1 of 4 species in the genus Bothrocophias, all four called toad-headed pit vipers. Of these 4, the most likely candidate for having been called 'Vipera lachesis, Bufocephalus' is Bothrocophias colombianus, synonyms: Bothrops colombianus, the Colombian toad-headed pit viper, locally known as 'mapana' and 'vibora cabeza de sapo'.

## Symptoms Berridge
∞ Bitter taste in mouth.
∞ Every day since the dose, intense bitter taste in the mouth.
∞ Lower lip, on inside, as if swollen, and there was a sore feeling as if there was a longitudinal ridge on it.
∞ Feeling in throat of choking; desire to clear throat; tongue especially at tip, as if smaller; desire to loosen clothes round throat.
∞ Woke at 5 a.m., with a dull heavy pain under left ribs [near cardiac end of stomach], which seemed to rest at one spot for a few minutes then slowly moved round to the right in an upward direction to stomach-pit;
∞ Twice during days, in open air, shooting in region of left nipple. [B]
∞ In outer side of left arm, shooting downwards, from just below shoulder to elbow.
∞ Sore painful feeling at end of right thumb [palmar surface].
∞ 2 p.m., when walking out, a dull heavy pain struck him suddenly in the right hip, in one spot; it seemed to be in the hip-bone; it only remained a few minutes, and then passed away without his noticing it.
∞ Sore pain behind right internal malleolus,
∞ During the day, tingling in toes of right foot.

## Clinical Manifestations
'Toxical effects of the poison of the Vipera lachesis bufocephalus are: Convulsions; great pain in the bitten limb; intensely feverish pulse; intense thirst; flow of a dark blood, semi-coagulated, from the nose, ears, and rectum; veins of the conjunctiva are surcharged, so that the eyes have the colour of raw beef; tremulousness and subsultus tendinum; discolouration of the bitten part; the blood is coagulated near the wound, and will only flow from it after deep incisions have been made just at or above the wound made by the fangs, and the limb has been bathed repeatedly in hot water, rubbing it down towards the bitten part so as to force out the coagulated blood. This poison causes death in from 3 hours to 3 days, according to the "condition of virulence" of the poison.' [Higgins, pp. 109–110]

# BOTHROPS ALTERNATUS

## Systematics
• Scientific name: Bothrops alternatus [Duméril, Bibron and Duméril, 1854].
• Synonyms: Lachesis alternatus [Boulenger, 1896]. Trigonocephalus alternatus [Jan. 1859].

- Common names: Crossed pit viper. Urutu.
- Family: Viperidae, subfamily Crotalinae.

## Biological Profile
- Large, heavy-bodied venomous pit viper up to 1.7 m long, maximum more than 2 m.
- Body colour variable; may be brown, tan, or grey, sometimes with an olive cast. Body usually has a series of C-shaped darker markings boldly outlined with paler scales. Belly pale whitish-grey, with a dark brown stripe [wider toward tail] from neck to tail tip..
- Range: Brazil, Paraguay, Uruguay, Argentina.
- Habitat: Low-lying swampy areas, river banks, marshes, & other humid habitats at elevations up to 700 m. Common in cultivated areas & near human habitations. Seldom found in very dry situations.
- Terrestrial and nocturnal.
- Preys on rodents, birds and lizards.
- Ovoviviparous; 1–24 live young per brood.
- Easily aroused when threatened; can be aggressive & will defend itself vigorously.
- Venom haemotoxic, cytotoxic and cardiotoxic, decreasing blood pressure, cardiac output, perfusion pressure, and stroke volume.

**Symptoms in MM** from a proving by 2 male provers in 1934. The source of the proving substance was later definitely identified as having been Bothrops *atrox* instead of B. alternatus, so that the 40–45 symptoms listed for the latter ought to be included with Bothrops atrox, as is done below.

# BOTHROPS ASPER

## Systematics
- Scientific name: Bothrops asper [Garman, 1883].
- Synonyms: Bothrops xanthogrammus [Amaral, 1930]. Lachesis xanthogrammus [Boulenger, 1896]. Trigonocephalus xanthogrammus [Cope, 1868].
- Common names: Asper. Boquidorada. Terciopelo.
- Family: Viperidae, subfamily Crotalinae.

## Biological Profile
- Large, moderately slender venomous pit viper. Head broad, flattened, lance-shaped when viewed from above and distinct from narrow neck. Snout not elevated. Dorsal scales keeled. Average length 1.5 m, maximum 2.5 m.
- Dorsal ground colour dark grey, light brown, or olive green. Characteristic series of dark triangular dorsal blotches at each side of body that resemble the letter X from a dorsal view; which is why in some localities along its distribution the species is known as "equis" [X-snake]. Belly pale yellow, cream or whitish-grey.

- The most sexually dimorphic of all snakes, the 2 sexes are born the same size, but at the age of 7 to 12 months, females begin to grow faster than males. Females then generally exceed the length of the males 2-fold and may weigh 4 to 5 times that of a male of equal age.
- Range: Central America to NW South America, from Mexico to Colombia.
- Habitat: Mainly tropical rainforest and tropical evergreen forest but is also found in dryer regions of tropical deciduous forest, frorn forest and pine savannah in near proximity to rivers, streams or lakes. Often also found in agricultural areas, plantations, and near human habitations.
- Nocturnal, solitary. Activity varies seasonally; becomes less active in colder and dryer months.
- Primarily terrestrial, but also very agile climbers and can be found resting several meters off the ground.
- Feeds mainly on small mammals but will take lizards, frogs, birds and centipedes. Typically hunts along jungle trails, lying in wait to ambush a rodent as it scampers down a jungle trail, but will not hesitate to take up a hunting site near a coffee or banana plantation.
- Ovoviviparous; 25–90 live young per brood.
- Named after Latin asper, rough, in reference to the nasty temper of the snake, or to the roughness of the keeled scales on the dorsum.
- No subspecies.

## Behaviour & Temperament

Mainly a terrestrial and nocturnal snake, spending the day hidden among roots, leaf litter or other similar locations. Fast moving snake that will defend itself vigorously if disturbed. It is regarded as being more excitable and unpredictable than Bothrops atrox and has a reputation for being aggressive. Its large size and habit of raising its head high off the ground can result in bites above the knee. It has also been observed to eject venom over a distance of at least 6 feet [1.8 m] in fine jets from the tips of its fangs.

Being considered 'a *psychotic, unpredictable* snake', reacting *explosively* when disturbed, the temperament of an asper has mythological attributes and most people fear and respect them greatly. In general, they will remain perfectly calm in a coil, until they are *touched*! Then they explode like a coil and go helter-skelter every which way.

'Aspers may strike repeatedly from anybody position, requires no fixed coil, and strikes at movement as well as heat. These snakes are extremely fast and agile. When threatened it will vibrate its tail and also expand itself to appear larger. Mostly a shy snake, it will try to escape but if it feels cornered, this nervous snake is extremely dangerous.

'Aspers are also known to ambush their pursuers . . . by initially fleeing then doing a lightning quick U-turn and waiting for the pursuer to get within striking range. I have witnessed this personally, it is quite startling, and you could be in real trouble if unprepared for this tactic. Another tactic it uses is to strike its head just past its target, then double back quickly twisting its neck to catch the prey from behind. "By my estimation, the world's most dangerous viper to catch," according to Dean Ripa.' [www.venomousreptiles.org]

Having observed aspers in Panama, Vinton [1956] brings up its inclination to *overeat* when opportunity permits. When that happens, 'it becomes so weighted down that upon being disturbed, it is unable to run. In fact, it can barely crawl under these conditions and may be encountered still hiding near the trail while it waits for its overtaxed digestive system to dispose of its overload of calories. At these times the frustrated snake is more irritable than usual and will strike anything that comes near it.'

## MATERIA MEDIA BOTHROPS ASPER

### Sources
1 Effects of bite; clinical manifestations.

### Identity
The information on this species comes from S.B. Higgins, who published in 1873 a small booklet on snakes with an astonishingly long title: 'Ophidians: Zoological Arrangement of the different genera, including varieties known in North and South America, the East Indies, South Africa, and Australia. Their Poisons and all that is known of their nature. Their Galls as antidotes to the snake venom. Pathological, toxicological, and microscopical facts; together with much interesting matter not hitherto published.'

The names used by Higgins to describe the snake include 'Boqui Dorada, Yellow-mouthed Viper, Gilded mouth, or Vipera lachesis os flavus', because 'the edges of the mouth and throat are of a golden-yellow hue, hence its name.' In many areas in Central America, locals call it *barba amarilla*, or 'yellow beard', a reference to its yellow throat, whilst it is known in Belize as yellow-jaw tommygoff. Synonyms of its scientific name, e.g. Trigonocephalus xanthogrammus and Lachesis xanthogrammus, also point to the colour, xanthos meaning yellow.

### Symptoms
'The Boqui Dorada, Yellow-mouthed Viper, or Vipera lachesis os flavus, is possessed of a very virulent poison, which causes as many deaths as that of any other variety in the valleys of the River Magdalena and its tributaries. Its poison is very deadly and its bite much feared, as the Curers [snake handlers] consider a cure of it a great test of their powers and proof of the efficacy of their secrets. They lose, however, many cases, but save their reputation by attributing the unfortunate termination of the case to a tithe [every tenth case] due to "La Suerte," their god of Chance, whose assistance they invoke upon undertaking to perform every case of cure.

'Toxicological effects are: Flow of blood from nose and mouth; evacuations of faecal matter, with clots of dark-coloured blood, or scanty, suppressed evacuations; heaviness of the head; stupor; sensation of oppression in chest and lungs;

repeated blows upon the tympanum [like those made by a hammer]; vertigo; loss of sight; intense pains in spinal column and shoulder-blades; cramps; colicky pains in abdomen; throbbing pains in the bitten part, increasing with the oedema; discharge of bloody urine; pulse has a slow, heavy beat; rheumatic pains in muscles in twinges; blue-black spots under nails of fingers and toes; lips discoloured; eyes bloodshot; chills, followed by tremors in whole body, while skin is flushed and indicates a highly feverish condition; flow of a greenish, bloody foam from mouth. This latter symptom invariably precedes death and continues for some hours after it has ensued. Death ensues in from 3 hours to 3 days.' [Higgins, 1873]

## Clinical Manifestations
Venom primarily haemotoxic and cytotoxic [necrotic].

'This species is an important cause of snakebite within its range. Together with Crotalus durissus, Bothrops asper is the leading cause of snakebite in Yucatán, Mexico. It is considered the most dangerous snake in Costa Rica, responsible for 46% of all bites and 30% of all hospitalised cases; before 1947 the fatality rate was 7%, but this has since declined to almost 0%. In the Colombian states of Antioquia and Chocó it causes 50–70% of all snakebites with a sequelae rate of 6% and a fatality rate of 5%. . . . One of the reasons so many people are bitten is because of its association with human habitation and many bites actually occur indoors. Well-known herpetologist Douglas March died after being bitten by this species.

'Bite symptoms include pain, oozing from the puncture wounds, local swelling that may increase for up to 36 hours, bruising that spreads from the bite site, blisters, numbness, mild fever, headache, bleeding from nose and gums, haemoptysis, gastrointestinal bleeding, haematuria, hypotension, nausea, vomiting, impaired consciousness and tenderness of the spleen. In untreated cases, local necrosis frequently occurs and may require amputation. In 12 fatal cases the cause of death was septicemia [5], intracranial haemorrhage [3], acute renal failure with hyperkalemia and metabolic acidosis [2] and haemorrhagic shock [1].

'It has been suggested that the venomous bite of Bothrops asper was a factor in the choice of certain Mayan settlements such as Nim Li Punit, where the thick jungle inhabited by these snakes was used as a defensive boundary.' [Wikipedia]

Causes more human deaths than any other pitviper species in the Western Hemisphere.

## A Chill of Death
Costa Rica's first academic biologist and a pioneering expert on snakebites, Clodomiro Picado, wrote in the 1930s a chilling description of the effect of the haemotoxic venom of Bothrops asper: 'Moments after being bitten, the man feels a live fire germinating in the wound, as if red-hot tongs contorted his flesh; that which was most mortified enlarges to monstrosity, and lividness invades him. The unfortunate victim witnesses his body becoming a corpse piece by piece; a *chill of death* invades all his being; and soon bloody threads fall from his gums;

and his eyes, without intending to, will also cry blood, until, beaten by suffering and anguish, he loses his sense of reality. If we then ask the unlucky man something, he may still see us through blurred eyes, but we get no response, and perhaps a final sweat of red pearls or a mouthful of blackish blood warns of impending death.' [cited in Greene, 2000]

### Surviving a Viper Bite

'On the morning of March 23 at 8.00 a.m., I hiked into the tropical forest in the Heredia province of Costa Rica with 3 other members of our production crew, a local guide named Gerhard, and a local wildlife expert named Pomipilio. We needed a solid rainforest location, and this area of Costa Rica offered amazing terrain and loads of biodiversity. . . .

'I scrambled up a 5 foot fallen tree. I paused and glanced up ahead at the 2 guides before looking down to check for anything slithering near my feet. Then I jumped off the trunk.

'Bang. It felt like I'd been stabbed in the left foot. I jumped away from the tree and looked back. I saw the writhing brown mottled outline of a snake. It looked maybe 5 or 6 feet long and as thick as my wrist. It was right up against the tree. I saw the large, distinct, arrow-shaped head of a pit viper. I knew it was venomous.

"Snake," I yelled. Pompi and Gerhard thought I'd spotted one. "I've been bitten."

They rushed 40 feet back to me. The whole time I kept my eye on the snake, so I didn't lose it. It was maybe 8 feet away from me.

'One of the guides said, "Terciopelo." I looked at Gerhard, confused. "A fer-de-lance," he said. "We call them terciopelo here."

'Within seconds, my heart started racing. I felt a painful burning sensation in my left foot. I put my weight on my right foot. I suddenly felt weak. The guys grabbed my shoulders and held me up. My knees immediately went to jelly. I was panting like a horse. "Breathe. Breathe slowly – in and out, in and out," said Derek, a cameraman. "Try not to let the venom spread too quickly."

"Easy for you to say," I said.

'Someone took off my boot. I dreaded what would be revealed. I tried to think positive. I thought, "Maybe I got lucky. Maybe it was just a warning shot. A hiking boot surely would protect me to some extent?"

'Once the boot came off, the sock said everything. A red stain was spreading across the grey fabric covering my instep. "Crap," I thought. The puncture wounds on the top of my foot were bleeding freely. The venom must have stopped the blood from clotting. There wasn't a moment to lose. Someone strapped the boot back on. Chris, a line producer, was already on the phone giving our position, organizing a car to meet us, and calling in a chopper. The crew stayed calm, organized, and disciplined. Fear and panic were running around my head. In the midst of that, I just thought, "Keep calm. Keep moving. Keep focused."

'We started hacking our way back through the undergrowth. After about 20 minutes of hiking with 2 guys holding onto my shoulders to support me, we hit a trail. The guys built a makeshift stretcher out of branches, backpacks, and ponchos. We still had a long way to go, and I became concerned about the time it would take to get to a hospital. The guys gently helped me onto the stretcher and carried me along 2 miles of trail. We came to a small house with a tin roof and a round barn near some dirt tracks. A 4 × 4 truck was waiting there to pick us up.

'The pain really started to kick in during the truck ride. I felt every bump on the dirt road. Each jostle sent a spike of pain from my foot all the way up to the top of my thigh. Waves of *searing* heat pulsed through my leg while stabbing pains, like knives shoved into my flesh, added more agony.

'After a 10-minute drive, we arrived at the lodge, where a chopper was waiting. Thirty minutes later, I was at a hospital in San Jose. All told, it took 2 hours to get from the bite site to the hospital.

'At Clinica Biblica, the medical team checked out my foot, administered antivenom, and gave me antibiotics and painkillers. Two doctors, Dr. Wu and Dr. Nunoz, checked my condition frequently. I felt safe. I thought, "What a lucky escape."

'My leg continued to swell for the next 5 or 6 days. My left foot blistered as the pain from the bite subsided. The trouble was, every time I stood up, the pain from the swelling took hold. I remember it felt like every muscle fibre in my leg was *full of pressure and about to explode*. Picture a bubbling sausage on a grill about to burst. That pressure was more painful than the pain immediately after the bite. I'd never felt anything like it. I remember leaning on my fiancé, Jackie, to use the toilet as tears just poured down my face.

'By April Fool's Day, one week after the initial bite, the blisters popped, and the resulting wounds began festering. "To be expected," said the doctors. Then Dr. Wu sniffed my foot and frowned. "We better get you to the OR," he said.

'The flesh in my foot was rotting. Nurses put me on a gurney. As they wheeled me away, I watched my foot drip a trail of pus and blood onto the hospital clean floor.

'The surgeons opened up my foot and removed the infected, liquefied flesh. They cut away any extra bits of tissue that were beginning to go bad and dressed the ankle and foot with a vacuum bag – a big polythene sack that they wrapped around my lower leg and attached to a pump. I was full of morphine, so I couldn't feel much pain, but my lower leg felt heavy and thick. It felt something like a throbbing concrete block.

'They couldn't say that the spread of dead tissue had been completely arrested. I wondered if I was going to keep my foot. The people in Costa Rica knew their stuff about treating snakebites. A lot of people at work said it was best to deal with the snakebite in Costa Rica because they dealt with so many. But the reconstructive surgery I needed would be better in the U.S, especially where I'm from – Hollywood.

'After one more cleaning operation on my foot, Clinica Biblica released me on April 5. I left San Jose around midnight on a Lear Jet kitted out like a mobile ICU. In Los Angeles, an ambulance drove me to Cedars Sinai Medical Center, where a team of new doctors took a look at me every few minutes. They performed an 8-hour operation that included taking a chunk of flesh from my left thigh and grafting it onto my foot.' [Steve Rankin, Surviving a Viper Bite; www.outsideonline.com]

# BOTHROPS ATROX

## Systematics
- Scientific name: Bothrops atrox [L., 1758].
- Synonyms: Bothrops colombiensis [Hoge, 1966]. Lachesis atrox [Boulenger, 1896].
- Common names: Common lancehead. Fer-de-lance.
- Family: Viperidae, subfamily Crotalinae.

## Biological Profile
- Moderately heavy-bodied venomous pit viper with short tail and variable colouration, from grey to olive, brown, or reddish, with dark triangles edged with light scales. Triangles are narrow at the top and wide at the bottom. Head broad, flattened, lance-shaped when viewed from above and distinct from narrow neck. Dorsal scales keeled. Average length 1.4 m, maximum 2.4 m.
- Range: Northern South America east of the Andes.
- Habitat: Tropical lowlands; flooded scrub, meadows. Frequently encountered in cultivated areas and human settlements [incl. urban fringes] in close proximity to rivers, streams or lakes.
- Nocturnal; hidden among roots, leaf litter or other similar locations during daytime.
- Primarily terrestrial, but also very agile climbers and can be found resting several meters off the ground.
- Preys on rodents and other small mammals, birds, and lizards.
- Ovoviviparous; 8–60 live young per brood.
- Fast moving; will defend itself vigorously if disturbed. Irritable disposition, ready to strike with little provocation.
- Highly dangerous snake, responsible for a high mortality rate.

## MATERIA MEDICA BOTHROPS ATROX

### Sources
1 Proving Roberts [USA], 4 provers [2 females, 2 males], 200c; 1934, 1936, 1937.
2 Effects of bite; clinical manifestations.
3 Degroote, Dream Repertory.
4 Synthesis Repertory Treasure Edition 2009.
5 Clinical observations Farokh Master [India].

## Mind

∞ Depression and exhaustion associated with the pains.[1]

∞ General feeling of depression and oppression < afternoon, in hot and oppressive weather; & feeling of apprehension which seems to start in stomach.[1]

∞ Anxiety after fright.[4]

∞ Anxiety felt in stomach, ext. to head.[4]

∞ Fear heart will cease beating unless one were constantly on the move.[4]

∞ Sadness from pain; from pain in heart.[4]

∞ Weeping from shock of a fall.[4]

## Dreams

∞ Amputation of foot.[3]

∞ Being controlled by road police.[3]

∞ Driving a car in wrong direction.[3]

∞ Falling in love with a very kind person.[3]

∞ Having anginal attacks.[1]

∞ Having too wear too narrow clothes.[3]

∞ Heart troubles in others and of having heart trouble oneself.[1]

∞ Losing one's way, going astray; being lost in a city.[3]

∞ Patients with coronary thrombosis, feeling very depressed during dream state.[3]

∞ Unsuccessful efforts.[3]

## Generals

∞ All symptoms < after eating, both general and particular.[1]

∞ Warm room >.[1]

∞ Hot and oppressive weather <.[1]

∞ Putrid odour [probably from sweat] more marked at a distance of 5 or 6 feet than close to the prover; < after unusual exertion or weariness.[1]

∞ Perspiration of painful parts.[4]

∞ Craving for green grapes.[3]

∞ Wounds bleeding freely.[4]

∞ Exhaustion and depression associated with pains, esp. anginal pain, infarction pain, gangrenous pain, and pain of ulcers. Profound effects of shock from pain.[5]

∞ Weakness from pain.[4]

∞ Internal trembling, shuddering without coldness, shuddering and feeling of apprehension in stomach at onset of menstrual flow.[5]

∞ Sexual intercourse < almost all complaints.[5]

∞ While or after eating <.[4]

∞ Lying in horizontal position >.[4]

∞ Raising affected limbs <.[4]

## Sensations

∞ Nail in right parietal bone.[1]

∞ Right ear as if full.[1]

∞ Tongue as if thick.[4]

∞ Throat as if thick, swollen.[4]
∞ Shuddering and feeling of apprehension in stomach at onset of menstrual flow.[1]
∞ Heart as if about to cease beating.[1]
∞ Persistent pressure about cardiac region, as if there were not sufficient room.[1]
∞ Distressing feeling or persistent pressure [as if there was no place for the heart to move] in cardiac region, < midnight to sunrise.[5]
∞ Feeling as if heart will cease beating unless constantly on the move.[5]
∞ Weight in left chest, most marked when lying on left side, and felt more posteriorly than anteriorly; sensation of heat internally in same region. Weight in chest causes desire to sit bent forward.[1]
∞ Oppression chest < lying on left side.[4]
∞ Heaviness in left chest, < after eating, marked < 2–5 p.m.[1]
∞ Chest as if too small.[4]
∞ Right lung as if filled with smoke.[1]
∞ Prickling as of icy mist or fine icy needle points on left forearm.[1]
∞ Heaviness left arm < lifting arm, & weight in chest.[1]

## Locals
∞ Sudden momentary giddiness & tendency to fall to left or to right; comes and goes very suddenly.[1]
∞ Giddiness on carrying a heavy package; on raising arms level with shoulders; on exertion; on turning in bed the room seems to turn around; on rising from a seat.[1]
∞ Dizziness on rising from sitting.[4]
∞ Pains in back of eyeball; seem to shoot back a short distance into head.[1]
∞ Nosebleed when menses were due, on getting up in morning, instead of menses.[1]
∞ Tip of nose reddish-purple in cold air.[4]
∞ Brown discolouration of tongue.[4]
∞ Clothing about waist and abdomen became unbearable about 8 p.m.; obliged to take them off.[1]
∞ Burning itching in vagina and urethra; constant desire to urinate, but no > from emptying bladder; no urging.[1]
∞ Dull pressing pain in region of heart extending to left axilla, waking from sleep, < 4–6 a.m.[1]
∞ Persistent pressure in heart region that extends to axilla, left arm, < severe exertion and deep inspiration.[5]
∞ Sticking pain in heart, < talking, < deep inspiration.[1]
∞ Stitching pain in heart region < slightest exertion.[4]
∞ Heart complaints accompanied by numbness upper limbs.[3]
∞ Cough with heart affections.[4]
∞ Lumbar backache < standing, > lying down.[4]
∞ Awkwardness lower limbs, stumbling when ascending or descending stairs.[4]
∞ Hands blue or bluish-white, esp. right, < when hanging down or when bearing weight on it, as leaning on the hand or carrying weight.[1]

∞ Raynaud's like phenomena in right hand; < hanging arm or carrying anything in hand.[5]

∞ Sweaty hands, clammy, cold or sticky.[4]

## Clinical Manifestations

Has a large amount of potent venom that is mainly hemotoxic with cytotoxic factors; envenomation can result in intense immediate pain, oedema, severe local tissue necrosis, systemic internal bleeding, renal failure, hypotension & shock.

# CASE

59-year-old man with hereditary cholesterolemia, a rare disease where the high cholesterol level is unrelated to the diet. There is an increased level of low-density lipoprotein [LDL] and a low level of high-density lipoprotein [HDL] and an increased level of triglycerides and cholesterol.

'Due to this particular anomaly, the patient had a lot of cardiac problems and he complained of angina pectoris. He also had problems with his vision, but the main problem was recurrent occlusion of the internal carotid artery. He was on cholesterol reducing drugs, coronary artery dilators, aspirin and vitamins. He was just recovering from his last episode of carotid artery occlusion in the hospital when I was asked to see him.

'What I gathered from the history was that with every attack of occlusion, he suffered from a mild reduction in the level of consciousness. His eyes were slightly deviated and not in the centre and in one of the episodes his speech was greatly affected. When I tried to palpate the carotid artery from the angle of the jaw on the affected side, the pulsation was weak and cardiac auscultation revealed poorly conducted heart sounds. One clear-cut symptom that was evident was a mild disturbance of vision before every episode of occlusion. The high cholesterol level affected his blood supply in the Circle of Willis [the brain's major arterial formation], which produced a certain degree of cerebral ischemia affecting mainly the anterior and middle cerebral arterial territories. Doctors had warned him that any further episode would produce a definite, permanent and severe neurological deficit, therefore he constantly lived with the fear of heart attack, major catastrophic heart illness, stroke and paralysis. He also complained of vertigo, which came whenever there was any nervous excitement or anxiety. The vertigo was sudden in onset lasting for a fraction of a second with a sensation of falling on either the left or right side.

'After every attack of carotid artery occlusion, it was strenuous for him to even talk and his speech became slow. He had a choking sensation when sipping any carbonated drink. After every sexual intercourse he would develop weakness and prostration for a few days. On examination I noticed venous stasis on lower extremities.

He was an executive in the bank. At a very young age of 10, his father died, and his mother brought him up single handedly. She did not have enough financial resources to support his education. It was really difficult for her to work, earn, run the house, look after her son and save enough money for his education. So he was sent to a boarding school. Here he felt very lonely and forsaken for a long period of time. During college, he preferred to stay in a hostel as his mother was still working and there was no one to look after him.

'When he finished his post-graduate studies, he took a job as a salesman in a multinational company. He was an ambitious, self-made man who came up in life due to hard work and sincerity. At the age of 35, he married a woman whom he loved very much. He could not express his feelings and emotions easily not even to his wife of 17 years. He hid his feelings as if wearing a mask. He still missed his childhood and youth when he saw other children with their parents. This was due to loss of his family at an early age, from death of his father and life away from home in a boarding school.

'After considering the full totality, I took the following symptoms: Forsaken feeling. Ailments from single parent syndrome. Reserved, not showing true emotions, a sort of mask. Recurrent occlusion of internal carotid artery. Hereditary high cholesterol. Characteristic vertigo. Aggravation coitus. Venous stasis in lower extremities. Speech slow.

'Over several years, his doctor had gradually increased his dosage of anti-lipid and anti-cholesterol drugs. He exhibited abnormal liver function due to the side effects of the anticholesterol drugs: Lopid 600 mg and Zevast 200 mg, i.e. atorvastatin. He was also taking Nicotinic acid, which helps increase levels of HDL and lower the levels of LDL.

'I restudied the case and confirmed that he had many features of Bothrops and yet Bothrops lanceolatus did not help him. During that time, I was preparing for my seminar on snake remedies and I came across a very nice article by Dr. H.A. Roberts on Bothrops atrox. I saw in this remedy a very strong fear of heart disease like that seen in Gelsemium and Lachesis. The reference to this remedy is found in the book The Study of Remedies by Comparison by Dr. H.A. Roberts [1941].

'In this patient, Bothrops atrox covered his fear of cardiac illness and paralysis, nervous vertigo with a tendency to fall and aggravation from coitus. It is also a very good remedy for recurrent thrombosis, especially in the large vessels. This remedy does not cover the speech element that was present in this patient. The patient had all the symptoms of Bothrops in general and other snake features, including: Forsaken feeling, industriousness and ambition to come up on his own even though he did not have many resources. So I shifted my prescription to Bothrops atrox. This was the very first time I prescribed Bothrops atrox.

'The remedy was procured from Schmidt-Nagel in Switzerland and prescribed in 30c daily in the 5 cup method for 15 days. For the very first time, the LDL levels decreased. I continued the same treatment for another 45 days and observed around 80 to 90% improvement in the symptomatology. I then reduced the dose of Zevast to 10 mg each day and kept him under observation. Instead of a daily dose of Bothrops atrox 30c, I now administered it every third day and kept him under regular observation; monitoring blood pressure and lipid levels. After 6 months I reduced the dose of Zevast to 10 mg on alternate days. In one year, I reduced the Zevast to 5 mg on alternate days. Within 2 years, I completely stopped the Zevast. He was now only on Lopid 600 mg, once a day. In 2 years, he had no recurrence of any episode of carotid artery occlusion. The cholesterol and LDL remained within the normal range and HDL levels ranged from 75 to 80mg/dl. I advised a CT scan to check for neurological deficit, but everything was normal. Digital subtraction angiography of the internal and external carotid artery system showed no new formation of blocks.

'After seeing these results, the patient was given Bothrops atrox 30c only once a month for 3 to 4 months. He was advised to check his lipid levels every 6 months and to report any change in symptomatology.' [Farokh Master, 2008]

# BOTHROPS CARIBBAEUS

## Systematics
- Scientific name: Bothrops caribbaeus [Garman, 1887].
- Synonyms: Bothrops lanceolatus caribbaeus [Garman, 1887]. Trigonocephalus caribbaeus [Garman, 1887].
- Common names: St. Lucian pit viper. St. Lucian fer-de-lance.
- Family: Viperidae, subfamily Crotalinae.

## Biological Profile
- Large, semi-arboreal venomous pit viper with broadly triangular head & slightly upturned snout. usually grey [concrete-coloured] to grey-brown; markings vary from slate grey, on the paler, concrete-coloured specimens, to chocolate on the darker ones. Belly yellow to cream-coloured, sometimes finely peppered with grey laterally but never blotched or mottled. Dull dark brown to black postorbital stripe behind each eye. Length up to 2 m.
- Range: Found only in St. Lucia, an island in the eastern Caribbean.
- Habitat: Confined mainly to coastal areas. Very often encountered in trees, at a maximum height of about 6 m.
- Preys on warm-blooded animals like birds and rats and even mongoose.
- Ovoviviparous; 20–30 live young per brood.
- Usually avoids humans but will quickly strike if disturbed even a little bit.

## Systemic Thrombotic Complications

Bites by the St. Lucian pit viper are very rare. Numeric et al. reported in 2002 'the case of a healthy 32-year-old Saint Lucian man who developed multiple cerebral infarctions following envenoming by this snake. The patient developed signs and symptoms very similar to those observed in patients envenomed by Bothrops lanceolatus, a snake found only in Martinique, the neighbour island of Saint Lucia.' In Martinique, the severity of envenoming by B. lanceolatus is due to the development of severe thrombotic complications, mainly cerebral infarctions that may appear within 7 hours to 1 week after the bite in 30 to 40% of envenomed patients.

The effects of B. caribbaeus are very similar, in the reported case resulting in 'a left hemiplegia with a left facial paralysis and a partial Wernicke's aphasia [including difficulties to repeat spoken words and to understand simple straight-forward orders]. Local signs of envenoming were severe with sterile bloody leakage at the site of the bite, extensive swelling of the right lower limb, and oedema of the abdominal wall and upper chest. . . . A 10-cm diameter area of local necrosis developed around the site of the bite, despite the use of hyperbaric oxygen chamber treatment, leading to a skin graft that was performed on February 1, 1999. He subsequently recovered with minimal neurological sequelae and went back to Saint Lucia after a 2-month hospital stay.' [Numeric, 2002].


## MATERIA MEDICA BOTHROPS CARIBBAEUS

### Sources
1 Ireland, effects of bites. Symptoms wrongly assigned to Naja in Allen's Ency-clopedia as sources "28, Ireland, effects of bite of Coluber carinatus on hand, Med.-Chir. Trans., 1813, p. 396; 29, same, second case; 30, same, third case."

### Symptoms
∞ He appeared as if much intoxicated [after 10 minutes].
∞ Torpid, senseless state [after 10 minutes].
∞ Torpor [after a few minutes].
∞ Senselessness [after a few minutes].
∞ Hand and arm of the same side began to swell and were even mottled [after a few minutes].
∞ Hand, arm, and breast of the same side were much swelled, mottled, and of a dark purple and livid colour [after 10 minutes].

### Four Cases of Bites
The symptoms in the homeopathic materia medica are from observations made more than 200 years ago on the island of St. Lucia: 'Some account of the Effects of Arsenic in counteracting the Poison of Serpents. Communicated in a letter from Mr. J.P. Ireland, Surgeon to the fourth battalion of the sixtieth regiment of foot, to Thomas Chevalier, Esq. – Read before the Medico-Chirurgical Society, June 12, 1811.' Ireland writes:

'Having heard you mention in your lectures "that the Indians were in the habit of administering arsenic in large doses, after the bites of venomous animals; and that you would strongly recommend to gentlemen who might have opportunities of trying its effects in such cases, to exhibit it, in order to ascertain its powers," I resolved to make trial of it whenever an opportunity offered; and I have great pleasure in having it in my power to acquaint you with the following important facts, which occurred under my own observation during several years residence in the West Indies.

'In some of the islands at present in our possession, venomous serpents are very numerous, and one of the deadliest in its bite is found in the island of St. Lucia; it is from 3 to 6 feet in length and appears to be the Coluber carinatus of Linnaeus. Its fangs are from 1½ to 2 inches long; and the wound inflicted by them is generally of considerable extent.

'On my arrival in the island, I was informed that an officer and several men, belonging to the 68th regiment, [then quartered there, and to which I was attached,] had died within a few months from the bites of those destructive animals; that everything had been tried by the attending medical men to no purpose as all the patients had died, some in 6, and others in about 12 hours, from the time of their receiving the wound. A case, however, soon came under my own care, and as nothing that had been done before seemed to be of any avail, I determined on trying the effects of arsenic to its full extent.

# CASES

'**Case 1.** Jacob Course, soldier in the York light infantry volunteers, was bitten in the left hand, and the middle finger was so much lacerated that I found it necessary to amputate it immediately, at the joint with the metacarpal bone. I first saw him about 10 minutes after he had received the wound, and found him in a *torpid, senseless state*: the hand, arm, and breast of the same side were much swelled, mottled, and of a dark purple and livid colour. He was vomiting and appeared as if much intoxicated. Pulse quick and hard: he felt little or no pain during the operation. [After treatment with arsenic, opium, and Mentha piperita] . . . He became more sensible when touched and from that time he gradually recovered his faculties; he took some nourishment and had several hours sleep. The next day he appeared very weak and fatigued; the fomentation and liniment were repeated. The swelling diminished gradually; the natural colour and feeling returned, and by proper dressings to the wound, and attention to the state of his bowels, he soon recovered and returned to his duty.

'**Case 2.** Dover, a black soldier in the 3rd West India regiment, was bitten in the left hand; the swelling was not so extensive as in the former case, and the discolouration was not so strongly marked. I saw him within a few minutes after he was bitten, and vomiting, senselessness and torpor had commenced. The wound inflicted was not of so large extent; I removed the torn edges of the lacerated integuments, dressed the wound, and gave him the arsenical medicine precisely as in the former case; the fomentation and liniment were also applied; the cathartic clyster given every hour and the medicine repeated every half hour for 4 hours, when purging came on and the medicine was discontinued, after which he had some hours repose. The next day he appeared less debilitated, and he soon recovered, and returned to his duty.

'**Case 3**. Thomas Rally was bitten in the calf of the right leg and brought to the hospital in nearly the same state as Jacob Course; the ragged edges of the integuments were immediately removed, the wound dressed and the arsenical medicine administered. [After treatment] . . . Next day he was still *much debilitated* and had much difficulty in voiding his urine; it was, however, drawn off with a catheter twice a day for 2 days and fomentations applied to the region of the bladder. On the third day every aggravating symptom began to abate and from that time he gradually recovered and returned to his duty.

'**Case 4**. Patrick Murphy, of the 68th regiment, was bitten in the wrist. I saw him within a few minutes after the wound had been received. The hand and arm of the same side had begun to swell and were even mottled; but vomiting had not come on. I removed the torn edges of the integuments, dressed the wound and gave him the arsenical medicine. He gradually recovered [after 2 days of treatment] and returned to his duty.

'These were the only cases I had an opportunity of seeing during my stay in St. Lucia; but some time after I went to the island of Martinique, where a venomous serpent is found of a smaller size, . . . the bite of which is as deadly as of those found in St. Lucia. I was present when a soldier belonging to the 63rd regiment received a wound in the leg from one of those serpents, and I requested the surgeon of the regiment to allow me to try the effects of arsenic; he was very glad to give me the case as he had not before seen one of the kind. The patient was treated precisely in the same manner as those in St. Lucia and when I left the island on other duty, a few days afterwards, I had the pleasure to leave him so well that I do not entertain a doubt of his having perfectly recovered.' [The arsenic as mentioned above was Fowler's solution, alias potassium arsenite, or Kali arsenicosum in homeopathic nomenclature.] [Ireland, 1813]

# BOTHROPS INSULARIS

## Systematics
- Scientific name: Bothrops insularis [Amaral, 1922].
- Synonyms: Lachesis insularis [Amaral, 1922]. Trimeresurus insularis [Hoge, 1950].
- Common names: Golden lancehead. Insular lancehead. Island jararaca.
- Family: Viperidae, subfamily Crotalinae.

## Biological Profile
- Moderately slender, medium-sized pit viper, usually 70–100 cm long. Body colour mostly pale yellowish-brown, sometimes with a series of darker irregular bands or large blotches. Head pale yellowish-brown dorsally. Belly lighter yellowish brown, sometimes speckled with small darker blotches.
- Range: Endemic to Ilha da Queimada Grande [state of Sao Paulo], an island 64 km southwest of Bahia de Santos off the southeast coast of Brazil.
- Habitat: Dry, rocky, open scrubby forests.
- Terrestrial and diurnal with strong arboreal tendencies. Tends to seek shelter under leaf litter or in rock crevices during storms or after ingesting prey.
- Preys almost exclusively on birds [there are no mammals on the island], but has been reported to eat lizards, other snakes, and even resort to cannibalism.
- Ambush predator, lies coiled with the conspicuous tail tip close to the head in order to lure lizards, frogs and birds within striking distance.
- Ovoviviparous; average 6 live young per brood.
- Relatively quiet and non-aggressive snake for a Bothrops species.
- Within the genus Bothrops, the closest living relative of the golden lancehead is B. jararaca.

## Snake Island
Ilha de Queimada Grande, nicknamed Snake Island, is home to a species of Bothrops, known as B. insularis, with one of the most powerful venoms in the world. Local legend exaggeratedly claims that there are 5 snakes to every square metre. B. insularis is the only species of snake on the island.

Bothrops venom primarily is haemotoxic and often has cytotoxic factors; envenomation can cause systemic internal bleeding and local tissue destruction. B. insularis venom reportedly is exceptionally toxic.

'Because B. insularis is only found in an area uninhabited by humans, there has never been an official report of a human being bitten by one, but other lance-heads are responsible for more human deaths than any other group of snakes in either North or South America. The mortality rate for lancehead envenomations is 0.5–3% if the patient receives treatment and 7% if the patient does not receive treatment. The effects of envenomations by lanceheads include swelling, local pain, nausea and vomiting, blood blisters, bruising, blood in the vomit and urine, intestinal bleeding, kidney failure, haemorrhage in the brain and necrosis of muscular tissue. Chemical analysis of the venom of B. insularis suggests that it is 5 times as potent as that of B. jararaca and is the fastest acting venom in the genus Bothrops.' [Wikipedia]

## Materia Medica
- No symptoms.

# BOTHROPS JARARACA

## Systematics
- Scientific name: Bothrops jararaca [Wied-Neuwied, 1824].
- Synonyms: Bothrops leucostigma [Wagler, 1824]. Bothropoides jararaca [Fenwick, 2009]. Craspedocephalus brasiliensis [Günther, 1858].
- Common names: Jararaca. Brazilian arrowhead pit viper.
- Family: Viperidae, subfamily Crotalinae.

## Biological Profile
- Medium-sized, relatively slender, terrestrial pit viper with flat, sharply ridged head. Usually 80–160 cm long. Overall dorsal colouration olive, brown, grey, tan, yellow, or maroon. Dark brown trapezoidal to subtriangular markings on both flanks, surrounded by more pale colouration. Belly nearly always lighter than dorsum. Females significantly larger and heavier than males.
- Range: South America – Brazil, Argentina, Paraguay.
- Habitat: Most common in open regions near vegetation cover at low to intermediate elevations. Occupies a diversity of habitats: tropical deciduous [broadleaf] forests and semitropical upland forests.
- Terrestrial and mainly nocturnal.
- Ambush predator equipped with intricate camouflage.
- Preys on birds and small mammals. Juveniles have a light tip on their tails, used for caudal luring of prey.
- Significant reduction in activity in colder months of year. Peak activity observed during warmer/rainier months, concurrent with breeding.
- Has refined binocular vision for depth perception, aided by vertical slits in pupils.
- Ovoviviparous; up to 20 live young per brood.
- Name derived from the Tupi words *yarará* and *ca*, meaning 'large snake'.
- Very fast and aggressive.
- In Brazil, about 75% of notified venomous snakebites are caused by Bothrops spp., about 7% by Crotalus spp., 1.5% by Lachesis, and 0.5% by Micrurus spp. [coral snakes].

## Less Inclined to Compete
'Males have been observed to mate with more than one female. Generally, male-male fighting occurs in viperids, activated by the presence of sex steroids such as androgens and oestrogens, prior to copulation. Male-male fighting, as well as any other establishment of dominance, may be less likely in this species than

other viperids, however, as females are significantly larger than males.' [animal-diversity.org]

## MATERIA MEDICA BOTHROPS JARARACA

### Sources
1 Effects of bite; clinical manifestations.

### Clinical Manifestations
Venom primarily haemotoxic, often with cytotoxic factors. Venom composition varies significantly between males and females, with male venom containing more protein diversity. Female venom is more potent for hyaluronidasic and haemorrhagic activities and is more lethal. In contrast, male venom is more potent for coagulant, phospholipasic, and myotoxic activities. Venom of juveniles has a greater anticoagulant effect than that of adults.

'It is the most well-known venomous snake in the wealthy and heavily populated areas of southeastern Brazil, where is was responsible for 52% [3,446 cases] of snakebite between 1902 and 1945 with an 0.7% mortality rate [25 deaths]. . . .

'Typical envenomation symptoms include local swelling, petechiae, bruising and blistering of the affected limb, spontaneous systemic bleeding of the gums and into the skin, sub-conjunctival haemorrhage and incoagulable blood. The systemic symptoms can potentially be fatal and may involve haemostatic disorders, intracranial haemorrhage, shock and renal failure.

'The drug, captopril, which is used for the treatment of hypertension and some types of congestive heart failure, was developed from a peptide found in the venom of this species.' [Wikipedia]

'A 39-year-old male was admitted 5 h after being bitten on the lower right leg. Physical examination revealed tense swelling, ecchymosis, hypoesthesia, and intense local pain that worsened after passive stretching, limited right foot dorsiflexion, and gingival bleeding.'

# BOTHROPS JARARACUSSU

### Systematics
- Scientific name: Bothrops jararacussu [Lacerda, 1884].
- Synonym: Lachesis jararacussu [Serié, 1915].
- Common names: Jararacussu. Surucucu tapete.
- Family: Viperidae, subfamily Crotalinae.

### Biological Profile
- Heavily built pit viper with dark brown lateral markings. Average length 1.5 m, maximum 2.2 m. Females larger than males.

- Body colour and patterns of head and body extremely variable – background colour can vary from tan or yellow to nearly black. Pattern of dark and pale scales on many specimens looks like a series of dark arches along each side [edged with white]; sometimes blotches are joined at dorsal mid-line forming narrow 'saddles' [may look like dark 'X'-es, viewed from directly above].
- Range: Brazil, southern Bolivia, Paraguay and NE Argentina.
- Habitat: Highly amphibious snake found in a wide variety of habitats, incl. tropical rainforest, tropical semi-deciduous forest, broadleaf evergreen forest, and pine forest in swampy, low-lying areas and along river margins, but usually not found far from rivers, lakes, or other bodies of water.
- Habitually nocturnal, but juveniles may forage for frogs by day on stream-banks.
- Preys on rodents and amphibians. Ambushes or lures prey, esp. frogs, by wiggling movements of its coloured tail tip.

## MATERIA MEDICA BOTHROPS JARARACUSSU

### Sources
1 Proving Brazilian Homeopathic Medical Association, 30 provers, 12c, 30c, 200c, 1M, 10M, 50M; 1996–8. [Symptoms copied from Farokh Master, 2008]
2 Effects of bite; clinical manifestations.

### Mind
∞ Aggressive, rude, agitated, critical, sarcastic.
∞ Ailments from injustice, humiliation and indignation. Fights bitterly for any injustice done to him in a very aggressive and critical manner.
∞ Altered state of consciousness, felt like she was looking at her own body from the outside.
∞ Cold and indifferent to life dramas and sufferings of others; lack of affection; or the opposite: helpful, attentive, and joyful.
∞ Helpful, attentive, and joyful.
∞ Intolerance of criticism, contradiction, noise, voices, people, traffic, etc.
∞ Irritability accompanied by anger.
∞ Lack of affection.
∞ Lack of worries and anxieties; calm with sensation of freedom and independence.
∞ Mental dullness and slowness in action. Lack of concentration and distraction, lack of memory for what one has to do or has done.
∞ Non-conformity.
∞ Pessimism.
∞ Quiet; desire to be isolated
∞ Quiet; desire to be isolated from the environment and avoid people; aversion to answer questions. Feelings of sadness, of being alone in the world with nostalgic thoughts.
∞ Mental symptoms accompanied by nausea.

- ∞ Reduced sensitivity to sensorial impressions sometimes accompanied by weeping and nostalgia.
- ∞ Sensation of apprehension followed by preoccupation and unreasonable anxiety.

### Dreams
- ∞ Erotic.
- ∞ Nostalgic.
- ∞ Thieves, chases.
- ∞ Worms, earthworms, snakes, etc.

### Generals
- ∞ Voracious appetite.
- ∞ Desire for cheese; chocolate; coffee; frozen yogurt; pepper; sweets. Aversion to meat.
- ∞ Thirst for large quantities of water or juice.
- ∞ Muscular pains as if from great physical effort. Tremors, cramps, contractions, and fasciculations [muscular twitching involving contiguous groups of muscle fibers].

### Sensations
- ∞ Liquid in face during movement.
- ∞ Genitals as if absent, as if there is nothing between one's legs; penis cold.

### Locals
- ∞ Dizziness & sensation of an empty, hollow and light head, swaying from side to side, disappearing when standing up.
- ∞ Headache pressing, nail-like, throbbing and burning.
- ∞ Eyes burning, redness, stitching, throbbing.
- ∞ Visual alterations such as luminous halos around luminous objects, foggy vision and loss of visual focus.
- ∞ Lower jaw, teeth, muscles of mastication, angle of jaw, esp. right side. Constrictive pains < pressure.
- ∞ Urgent desire for stool; stool excoriating, putrid and acrid smell.
- ∞ Menses more copious, salty smell.
- ∞ Difficulty to breathe deeply after exercise.
- ∞ Palpitation & choking sensation.
- ∞ Erratic pains in small joints < pressure.

### Guiding Symptoms
- ∞ Chronic depression that stems from constant indignation [Calc-p., Coloc., Staph.] producing a sense of dullness, indifference, lack of affection, lack of concentration, loss of memory, pessimism, and desire to be isolated from the environment.
- ∞ Fights bitterly for any injustice done to him in a very aggressive and critical manner [Caust., Falco., Foll., Staph.].

∞ Forsaken feeling from the people whom he loved and cared, but became indignant and was humiliated by their actions and behaviour [Lac-h., Mag-c., Nat-m., Puls., Sep.].

∞ Often a victim of humiliation due to social and domestic circumstances [Ambr., Bar-c., Bung-fa., Crot-c., Lac-h., Op., Sep.].

∞ Strong sensitivity to any sort of criticism [Agar., Carc., Gels., Ign., Sep., Staph.]; takes everything personally; hence intolerance to contradiction is a part of its personality [Aur., Lyc., Nux-v., Sep.]. [Farokh Master, 2008]

## Clinical Manifestations

Venom primarily haemotoxic and cytotoxic; envenomation can result in systemic internal bleeding and local tissue destruction. Loss of muscle mass consequent to poor muscle regeneration is a common result of Bothrops jararacussu envenomation.

'The jararacucu is one of the most dreaded snakes in its range. Up to 1000 mg [dry weight] of highly-lethal venom may be milked from its venom glands on a single occasion. It has accounted for 0.8% to 10% of series of snakebites in Sao Paulo State, Brazil. We examined 29 cases of proven jararacucu bites recruited over a 20-year period in 2 Sao Paulo hospitals. Severe signs of local and systemic envenoming [local necrosis, shock, spontaneous systemic bleeding, renal failure] were seen only in patients bitten by snakes longer than 50 cm; bites by shorter specimens were more likely to cause incoagulable blood. Fourteen patients developed coagulopathy, 6 local necrosis [requiring amputation in one] and 5 local abscesses. Two became shocked and 4 developed renal failure.

'Three patients, aged 3, 11 and 65 years, died 18, 27 and 83 hours after being bitten, with respiratory and circulatory failure despite large doses of specific antivenom and intensive care-unit management. In 2 patients, autopsies revealed acute renal tubular necrosis, cerebral oedema, haemorrhagic rhabdomyolysis at the site of the bite and disseminated intravascular coagulation. In one survivor with chronic renal failure, renal biopsy showed bilateral cortical necrosis; the patient remains dependent on haemodialysis. Effects of polyspecific Bothrops antivenom were not impressive, and it has been suggested that anti-Bothrops and anti-Crotalus antivenoms should be given in combination.' [Milani, 1997]

# BOTHROPS LANCEOLATUS

## Systematics

- Scientific name: Bothrops lanceolatus [Bonnaterre, 1790].
- Synonyms: Lachesis lanceolatus [Lacépède, 1789]. Trigonocephalus lanceolatus [Oppel, 1811].
- Common names: Fer-de-lance. Martinique lancehead.
- Family: Viperidae, subfamily Crotalinae.

## Biological Profile

- Venomous pit viper species endemic to the island of Martinique. Unknown on nearly all other Caribbean islands. Some reserve the name fer-de-lance for this species, while others also apply it for Bothrops atrox. No subspecies are currently recognized.
- Large, heavy-bodied pit viper. Usually 150–200 cm long; max. 298 cm. Body colour varies from grey to brown to yellowish-tan, usually with indistinct darker markings dorsally & laterally; top of head usually darker than body. Belly usually lighter yellowish-grey to greyish-brown, sometimes speckled with small darker greyish blotches.
- Mainly nocturnal & mainly terrestrial, but may be semi-arboreal; seems especially to prefer the masses of vine that form interrupted canopies along forest edges; may ascend to 20 m above ground.
- Very large and gravid females often encountered on the ground and in rock piles.
- Preys on small mammals, birds, lizards, and frogs.
- Ovoviviparous.
- Appears to never attempt tail vibration or to inflate the throat, no matter how irritated. Large females are rather lethargic, to the point of docility; males, on the other hand, are fast and aggressive. Can strike quickly when surprised or threatened.

## Always on the Alert

'"In the islands in which it is found," says Dr. Rufz de Lavison, "its presence makes itself felt even where man has built his dwelling and cultivates the soil. Because of it no one can carelessly lie down to rest in the shade of a tree; no one can walk in the woods or enter unconcernedly into the pleasures of the chase." It is especially abundant in coffee and sugar plantations and is met with from the sea level up to the summits of the highest mountains in Martinique and St. Lucia. It not infrequently makes its way into human habitations, and is not uncommon in gardens, even entering those of the town of Fort-de-France.

'It does not seek its prey by day, but remains on the alert, always ready to bite. With open mouth, and fangs projecting forwards, it strikes with the rapidity of lightning. It swims in the rivers and moves over the ground with great speed. Oviposition takes place in July, and the young are hatched forthwith, the usual number being from about 50–60.

'It feeds upon lizards and rats, but also destroys a certain number of fowls and turkeys. All the large animals are afraid of it. Its bite is extremely dangerous and causes about a hundred deaths in Martinique every year.

'In striking at its prey or at a man, the Fer-de-lance throws back its head and opens its jaws widely, with the fangs directed forwards. It drives in its poison-teeth as with the blow of a hammer, and quickly draws back again. When very excited, it resumes its position and strikes afresh. It never becomes tame but is capable of living a fairly long time in captivity. I have kept a number of specimens of it for more than 2 years, caged in my laboratory.' [Calmette, 1908]

## Fear the Lance

The shaking-snaking terror inspired by the fer-de-lance on Martinique is in vivid terms described in *Harper's New Monthly Magazine,* August 1888.

'And the fer-de-lance reigns absolute king over the mountains and the ravines; he is lord of the forests and the solitudes by day, and by night he extends his dominion over the public roads, the familiar paths, the parks, the pleasure resorts. People must remain at home after dark unless they dwell in the city itself; if you happen to be out visiting after sunset, only a mile from town, your friends will caution you anxiously not to follow the boulevard as you go back, and to keep as closely as possible to the very centre of the path. Even in the brightest noon you cannot venture to enter the woods unescorted; you cannot trust your eyes to detect danger; at any moment a seeming branch, a knot of lianas, a pink or grey root, a clump of pendent yellow fruit, may suddenly take life, writhe, swell, stretch, spring, strike.

'Then you will need aid indeed, and most quickly; for within the space of a few heart-beats the stricken flesh chills, tumefies, softens, changes colour, spots violaceously, and an icy coldness crawls through all the blood. If the physician or the *pauseur* arrives in time, and no artery or vein has been directly pierced, there is hope; but the danger is not passed when the life has been saved. Necrosis of the tissues begins; the flesh corrupts, tatters, tumbles from the bone; and the colours of its putrefaction are frightful mockeries of the hues of vegetable death, of forest decomposition, the ghastly pinks and grays and yellows of rotting trunks and roots melting back into the thick foetid clay that gave them birth.

'You moulder as the trees moulder; you crumble and dissolve as dissolves the substance of the balatas and the palms and the acomats; the Death-of-the-Woods has seized upon you! And this pestilence that walketh in darkness, this destruction that wasteth at noonday, may not be exorcised. Each female produces viviparously from 40 to 60 young at a birth. The haunts of the creature are in many cases inaccessible, inexplorable; its multiplication is prodigious; it is only the surplus of its swarming that overpours into the cane fields, and makes the high-roads perilous after sunset, yet to destroy 300 or 400 hundred thanatophidia [viz. venomous, deadly snakes] on a single small plantation during the lapse of 12 months has not been uncommon.'

Depicted as an equally dreadful scourge in *Sporting Magazine*, 1817, the author of the article *The Horse and Viper,* goes so far as proclaiming that the fer-de-lance is 'so savage, that the moment it sees any person it immediately erects itself and springs upon him. In raising itself, it rests upon 4 equal circles formed by the lower part of the body; when it springs, these circles are suddenly dissolved. After the spring, if it should miss its object, it may be attacked with advantage, but this requires considerable courage, for as soon as it can erect itself again, the assailant runs the greatest risk of being bitten. Often, too, it is so bold as to follow its enemy by leaps and bounds, instead of fleeing from him; and it does not cease the pursuit till its revenge is glutted. In its erect position it is so much the more formidable, because it is as high as a man, and can even bite a person upon horseback.'

# MATERIA MEDICA BOTHROPS LANCEOLATUS

## Sources

1 Ozanam [France], collection of cases and general observations on effects of bite, quoted from Rufz, 1859.
2 Clinical observations Mangialavori [Italy]; ReferenceWorks.
3 Clinical observations Farokh Master [India], in From Snakes to Simillimum, 2008.
4 Effects of bite; clinical manifestations.

## Mind

∞ Consecutive and long-lasting hypochondria.[1] Ideas confused.[1]
∞ Delusion he is neglected.[2]
∞ Forsaken feeling.[2]
∞ Jealousy, in children, when a new baby takes attention of family away.[2]
∞ Speech disorders that range from slow, inarticulate, confused speech to aphasia as a result of an ischemic insult to the brain. Strong premonition with an uneasy restless feeling before developing strokes or thrombosis or hypertensive episodes. This makes the person develop an uneasy sensation in head, chest and stomach; as a result the person may walk about or may develop a strong fear and sit in a corner very silently.[3]
∞ Strongly opinionated personality with stubborn obstinacy.[3]
∞ Conscientious about trifles.[3]
∞ Taciturn.[3]
∞ Dictatorial. Love of power. Sense of omnipotence.[2]
∞ Bothrops is a kind of super-Lachesis. It is more egotistic. The goal of this person's existence is to dominate. And to do this in a very, very powerful way. Sometimes in an aggressive way. "I want to reach this place." Whatever is between me and that place has to be erased or avoided.[2]
∞ Very often, because of the need to be well-considered by someone else, they will consume one relationship after another and not be able to stay in any one of these. Very often they are left or not interested in the relationship after a while. For them, it is not important to recognise someone else. They are not interested in knowing another person. They feel great if someone is adoring them, recognising their power and depending on them. But he has to control by being the most powerful and the strongest. If this is missing, Bothrops cannot stand any relationship so will have to break it off.[2]
∞ To be at the top is absolutely fundamental. It does not matter what the job or occupation is. But whatever they do, they must be the first. A common strategy, specifically in the case of Bothrops is to be unable to stand any competition. When he has the feeling that he is powerful enough, he will get closer to his hypothetical master. Then to do his best to betray him and take his position. They move to a kind of physical elimination.[2]

## Dreams

∞ Betrayal.[2]

## Generals

∞ Haemorrhages of various kinds, and esp. from wounds. Blood dark, very fluid. Very fluid black blood flows in jets at the least movement.[1]

∞ Wounds heal with difficulty.[1]

∞ Great chilliness. Profuse cold sweat.[1]

∞ Clothing too tight, > loosening it.[2]

∞ Before menses <.[2]

∞ Diagonal course of symptoms, e.g. left upper and right lower, or right upper and left lower.[3]

∞ Fullness and sensation of swelling in various parts of body, such as head, chest and abdomen; leading to persistent restlessness.[3]

∞ Right-sided affections esp. right cortex, liver, appendix, right upper and lower limb, etc.[3]

∞ Hypercholesterolemia[3] [high cholesterol levels in blood; manifesting as chest pain; small bumps on skin, usually on hands, elbows, knees, or around eyes; xanthomas, waxy cholesterol deposits in skin or tendons, often affecting the Achilles tendons and tendons in hands and fingers; small, yellow deposits of cholesterol that build up under eyes or around eyelids].

∞ Post-surgical thrombophlebitis [inflammation of a vein caused by a blood clot; typically occurring in the legs].[3]

∞ Tendency to thrombosis, thromboembolic phenomena in arteries like carotid, cerebral, coronaries, etc., producing hemiplegia, monoplegia, quadriplegia, etc.[3]

∞ Sharp, cutting, lancinating pains that make the person shiver; pains worse from motion.[3]

∞ Tendency to septicemia.[3]

∞ Weakness, tiredness and sleepiness; weakness from diarrhoea.[3]

∞ Cerebral haemorrhage leading to hemiplegia and coma.[3]

∞ Persistent high blood pressure, even after having suffered a stroke.[3]

## Locals

∞ Benign positional dizziness due to poor cerebral circulation, esp. in old people, that leads to persistent giddiness, < carrying any load on head, raising arm above shoulder, on exertion, or turning in bed; room seems to turn around.[3]

∞ Low-grade headaches of subdural haematoma and essential hypertension in old people.[3]

∞ Blindness, acute or persistent; without perceptible dilation of pupil.[1]

∞ Blindness from retinal haemorrhage.[3]

∞ Hemeralopia [inability to see clearly in bright light; opposite of night blindness] – can scarcely see her way, esp. after sunrise.[1]

∞ Boring pain in right eye [ophthalmic migraine], < after eating.[3]

∞ Epistaxis before or instead of menses, < morning on waking.[3]

∞ Face more or less dark and bluish.[1]

∞ Tongue cracked and furrowed crosswise.[3]

∞ Back part of tongue covered with heavy brown fur.[3]

∞ Can't swallow liquids due to sense of constriction.[3]

- ∞ Nausea and vomiting; vomiting followed by nervous trembling.[1]
- ∞ Abdomen all over sensitive to pressure.[1]
- ∞ Conductive system of the heart most affected, producing frequent, irregular and slow pulse.[3]
- ∞ Dull pain in heart ext. to left axilla, < 4–5 a.m.[3]
- ∞ Swelling of part bitten gradually extends to a great distance from its original seat; the limb becomes triple its ordinary size, and is soft and flabby, appearing as if distended with gas.[1]
- ∞ Almost entire inability to move right arm or right leg. Paralysis of one arm, or of one leg, only.[1]
- ∞ Extremities cold.[1]

## Clinical Manifestations

Among the Crotalinae, envenomation by Bothrops lanceolatus is unique because of the incidence of thrombotic complications, particularly cerebral, in 40% of patients not treated with specific antivenom serum.

Thromboses involve cerebral, myocardial, and pulmonary arteries, occur despite heparin therapy, and lead to death or major functional sequelae.

'Bothrops lanceolatus envenoming has been documented to produce a unique syndrome different from that of other species of Bothrops. In addition to local symptoms such as pain, swelling, bleeding at the site of the bite, ecchymosis and necrosis, which are common to most crotaline envenomings, the systemic bothropic syndrome observed in Central and South America is characterised by the development of consumption coagulopathies and spontaneous systemic bleeding, depending on venom components, which affect clotting factors, as well as haemorrhagins, which damage vascular endotheliums.

'On the other hand, apart from similar local signs, the severity of systemic envenoming by Bothrops lanceolatus in Martinique was correlated with the development of multiple *cerebral infarctions* and/or other major vessel occlusion that may appear within 8 hours to 7 days after the bite in approximately 30 to 40% of cases. Infarctions can develop in patients who present initially with signs of moderate envenoming with normal blood clotting and low serum levels of venom antigens. The infarction process can involve several small vascular territories altogether and is associated with the development of an isolated thrombocytopenia.

'Bogarin et al. [1999] demonstrated that Bothrops lanceolatus venom, obtained from 20 specimens collected at different locations in Martinique, is devoid of thrombin-like enzymes and of in vitro coagulant and defibrinating activities, and is not coagulant when added to human citrated plasma, even at concentration as high as 100 ug/mL. These data suggest that thromboses observed in human B. lanceolatus envenoming result from a toxin-linked vasculitis process rather than from a systemic pro-coagulant effect.' [Wüster et al., 2002]

# CASE

A middle-aged woman, 56 years old, developed cerebral stroke due to thrombosis of the left middle cerebral artery. She was a known case of hypertension for many years and was on irregular treatment. She was a right-handed person who developed right-sided hemiplegia due to the stroke. She had also lost her speech and was in a state of unconsciousness. At the hospital, she was given all the standard medical treatments, such as antihypertensives, anti-oedema drugs, etc., but her clinical condition did not improve. Her blood pressure persistently remained high. [Normally, after a stroke, the blood pressure always drops, but not in this case.] On the sixth day, I was asked to see the patient and following were my observations:

Darkening of the face.
History of bloody vomiting in the hospital.
Hypertension.
Loss of speech.
Right-sided hemiplegia.
Thrombosis of cerebral artery.
Varicose veins on both legs.

I tried to gather some more symptoms from her daughter. Here are the details:

She was a widow for the past 25 years having only one daughter who was 27 years old. She was a very strong-willed, duty-bound, responsible mother, who was an extrovert by nature and had good taste, for example, wearing good clothes, eating good food, etc. The greatest grief in her life was losing her husband at a very young age. She was an extremely religious-minded woman. She had a strong fascination and love for animals, esp. for dogs, cats and pigeons. She had a lot of concern for their welfare. She habitually made fun of everybody to the extent of being sarcastic at times.

Now I could add more symptoms to my totality from the above information:

Ailments from death of husband.
Desire for entertainment.
Jesting.
Loquacious.
Sarcasm.
Suppressed sexual desire.

My first prescription was Lachesis 1M, repeated every 2 hours. After 3 days of Lachesis, her clinical condition had hardly improved.

I changed the prescription to Bothrops lanceolatus 1M, 4 drops every 2 hours. This prescription reduced the blood pressure within 12 hours. On the fourth day, the corneal reflex became weakly positive. Response to oral commands was elicited and at the end of 1 month the patient was completely conscious and oriented, though a little confused and weak in memory. At this stage, I increased the potency to 10M once a day and slowly over the next 15 days, she experienced further improvement in her orientation. For the first time, she was able to sit in a chair. After 3 months of homeopathic treatment her allopathic drugs were gradually tapered down. She completely recovered in 6 months with active physiotherapy. [Farokh Master, 2008]

# BOTHROPS NEUWIEDI URUTU

## Systematics
- Scientific name: Bothrops neuwiedi [Wagler, 1824].
- Subspecies: B. n. urutu [Orejas-Miranda, 1970].
- Synonyms: Bothrops urutu [Lacerda, 1884]. Lachesis neuwiedi [Boulenger, 1896].
- Common name: Neuwied's lancehead.
- Family: Viperidae, subfamily Crotalinae.

## Biological Profile
- Small to medium-sized, moderately slender pit viper. Usually 60–70 cm long; max. 120 cm. Brown or dark-brown ground colour overlaid with dark brown or black dorso-lateral blotches edged in white and [depending on subspecies] trapezoidal, triangular, sub-triangular, or headphone-shaped and oppose each other mid-dorsally. Belly white or yellow with grey speckling. Juveniles have a white tail tip.
- Head broad, flattened, lance-shaped when viewed from above; distinct from narrow neck.
- Range: Brazil.
- Habitat: Savannah, thorn scrub, tropical and semi-tropical deciduous forest, in dry or semi-arid rocky sites.
- Terrestrial and mainly nocturnal.
- Preys mainly on rodents and other small mammals, birds, snakes, frogs and lizards..
- Oviparous.
- Urutu is one of 5 recognized subspecies [neuwiedi, goyazensis, meridionalis, paranaensis].
- A popular proverb 'Urutu when it doesn't kill, it cripples. . .' is partially true, since its poison destroys the cells of the bite area and may cause necrosis and loss of muscle mass.

## Sources
1 Effects of bite; clinical manifestations.

## Clinical Manifestations
Haemotoxic and cytotoxic; venom produces extensive tissue destruction. All of the 18 cases observed between 1975 and 1992 in Brazil presented with pain and most [83%] had oedema, but fewer had ecchymosis [50%], necrosis [17%], abscess [5%] and/or systemic blood-coagulation disorders [12%].

# CENCHRIS CONTORTRIX

## Systematics
- Scientific name: Agkistrodon contortrix [L., 1766].
- Synonyms: Cenchris contortrix [L., 1766]. Trigonocephalus cenchris [Schlegel, 1837]. Trigonocephalus contortrix [L., 1766].
- Common names: Copperhead. Highland moccasin. Chunkhead.
- Family: Viperidae, subfamily Crotalinae.

## Biological Profile
- Stout-bodied pit viper, pinkish to greyish-brown, with an orange to copper or rust-red, unpatterned head, and a series of 10–21 brown to reddish-brown, saddle-shaped bands on the body. Southern copperheads sometimes have an overall pinkish tint. Body scales keeled and contain apical pits. Top of head in front of eyes covered with large plate-like scales. Pupil elliptical, a catlike vertical slit. Deep facial pit between nostril and eye. Average length 60–90 cm, maximum 135 cm.
- Sexually dimorphic in size, males have longer tails than females and females grow to greater lengths.
- Range: SE United States, extending north to Massachusetts and west to Texas and SE Nebraska.
- Habitat: Prefers low, wet areas around swamps, streambeds, river bottoms, and damp ravines; also occurs on hillsides above wet areas, as well as in suburban neighbourhoods near people.
- Diurnal in spring [morning and afternoon] and fall [esp. in morning]; crepuscular or nocturnal during hot summer months; may be quite active in summer after an evening shower.
- Ambush predator. Preys mostly on mice but also on small birds, lizards, small snakes, amphibians and large insects, esp. cicadas and grasshoppers. May climb in low bushes or trees after prey or to bask.
- Especially gregarious at the time of hibernation.
- Ovoviviparous; 2–12 live young per brood. Some gravid females will not eat because the embryos occupy so much of the body cavity.

- No maternal care. However, captive females have been observed to become irritable, vibrating their tails and assuming a particularly menacing demeanour when their recently born young were disturbed or removed from the cages containing their mothers.
- Juvenile copperheads hold their bright, sulfur yellow tail erect, wiggling it like a caterpillar to lure prey within striking range. The colour fades with age and is lost by age 3 or 4.
- Name from Gr. *agkistron*, hook, and *odon*, tooth; contortrix means twisted or turned back.
- Three recognized subspecies [contortrix, mokasen, phaeogaster].

### The Copperhead

Go seek him: he coils in the ooze and the drip,
Like a thong idly flung from the slave-driver's whip;
But beware the false footstep, – the stumble that brings
A deadlier lash than the overseer swings.
Never arrow so true, never bullet so dread,
As the straight steady strokes of that hammer-shaped head;
Whether slave or proud planter, who braves that dull crest,
Woe to him who shall trouble the Copperhead's rest!
   Bret Harte [1836–1902]

## Behaviour & Temperament

Copperheads have a natural camouflage ability to blend in with the environment. A copperhead lying on a bed of dead leaves becomes invisible. They are rather quiet and inoffensive in disposition but will defend themselves vigorously. However, unlike other pit vipers they will often 'freeze' instead of slithering away, and as a result many bites occur from people unknowingly stepping on or near them. This tendency to freeze seems related to the extreme effectiveness of their camouflage. Southern copperheads will frequently stay still even when approached closely and will generally strike only if physical contact is made. Sometimes when touched, they emit a foul-smelling fluid from musk glands located near the cloaca.

Vulnerable to the stress of capture and confinement, wild-caught copperheads will often refuse to feed, or they may strike and kill food animals and then refuse to swallow them.

Opinions differ about the copperhead, Barringer deeming it a vicious pest. 'The rattlesnake, drop for drop of venom, is the more poisonous, but his life-habits are such as to make bites from him quite rare, while with the copperhead they are common. This arises from the difference in temperament, if I may so speak, in the 2 snakes. Observe them in captivity, and you will at once see this difference. The rattlesnake is sluggish and slow in movement. It is boldly indifferent to approach, and half the time will not take the trouble to coil when approached. At rest it lies with the head drawn down on the coil and will seldom attempt to strike except from a coil. How different with the copperhead! Ever on the *qui vive*, he coils when he hears you coming. Whether fresh or tired, he will not put his head down, but keeps it well up, ever on the alert. As his classical name signifies [Agkistrodon contortrix], he is a snake of action. He can strike under conditions where a rattlesnake would be helpless. Some of the feats that I have seen this serpent perform in this line seem incredible. I have seen him strike the sole of the foot through an opening in the floor not appreciably larger than the snake's head. This summer I knew a child bitten by a horizontal blow from under a warped plank on a barn floor. It is the vicious nature and extreme agility of this pest rather than its real poisoning power that makes it so much to be feared.' [Barringer, 1892]

## Social Snake

'This is a social snake, which may overwinter in a communal den with other copperheads or other species of snakes including timber rattlesnakes and black rat snakes. They tend to return to the same den year after year. Females with young are gregarious whereas barren females and males are solitary. Copperheads are found close to one another near denning, sunning, courting, mating, eating and drinking sites. They are believed to migrate late in the spring to reach summer feeding territories and reverse this migration in early autumn. Males are aggressive during the spring and autumn mating seasons. They will try to over-power each other and even pin the other's body to the ground. This behaviour is exhibited most often in front of females but is not always the case. These inter-actions can include elevating their bodies, swaying side to side, hooking each other's necks, eventually intertwining their entire body length. Copperheads have been reported to climb into low bushes or trees after prey or to bask in the sun. They have also been seen voluntarily entering water and swimming on numerous occasions. [Bree Herrmann, Michigan State University]

## Mating

'Mating begins in the spring after the snakes emerge from winter dens [there are some reports of autumn mating]. At this time males begin to seek out sexually active females using their tongue to detect pheromones in the air. Once he has located a female, the male will begin moving his head or rubbing his chin on the ground. Eventually, after a lot of tail movements, slow to rapid back to forth waving from the female, the male aligns his body with hers. This courtship may last for an hour or more if the female does not respond. After being sufficiently stimulated, the female lifts and arches her tail and lowers the scale that covers her cloaca. Then the male arches his body and tail, everting one of his 2 sex organs and mates with the female. Mating time varies; the range can be as much as 3.5 to 8.5 hours. The long mating time correlates with the fact that females usually only mate with one male per year. This is because during the mating period males produce a pheromone that makes the female *unattractive* to other males, who pay little or no attention to mating or just mated females. Females also have *little interest in mating* after a long successful first mating.' [Bree Herrmann, Michigan State University]

## Combat Dances
'Males sometimes engage in combat dances. After meeting, the male snakes make body contact and then almost immediately rise up facing each other to a height of 30–40% of their body lengths. Much tongue flicking occurs, and the males seem to try to outstare each other. Next both sway back and forth in unison with heads bent at a sharp angle. Sometimes their elevated bodies are parallel to each other or one snake may actually turn its back towards its opponent. One male then leans over and tries to push the other's head and neck to the ground [topping behaviour]. The attacked snake responds by entwining its aggressor and tries to pin it by pushing with the anterior body and neck. The pushing match may continue for some time [usually 20–30 minutes, but sometimes over 2 hours], but eventually one snake, usually the shorter, is pinned to the ground, breaks off contact and crawls away. Studies by Schuett [1986] indicate that male *A. contortrix* participate in these combat bouts only during the breeding season. Female defence seems to be involved, so Schuett thought male competition the major function of these encounters. However, this is not certain, as combat will occur in captivity when no female is present. Perhaps male combat is a form of food competition or territoriality involving a food source or critical space.' [Ernst, 1999]

## Clinical Manifestations
The venom, which is highly haemolytic, causes massive haemorrhaging to the copperhead's prey. As for humans, recorded symptoms include pain, swelling, weakness, giddiness, breathing difficulty, haemorrhage, either an increased or decreased pulse, nausea, vomiting, gangrene, ecchymosis, unconsciousness, stupor, fever, sweating, headache and intestinal discomfort. Pain and swelling may persist for over a week, and localised tissue destruction may ensue.

The copperhead is the cause of many snakebites yearly but they are rarely fatal. The venom is not particularly potent, and has an estimated lethal dose of around 100 mg. Since an adult snake can only produce around 70 mg, a copperhead bite is not normally life threatening to healthy adults. They can be dangerous to children or older citizens in poor health.

## A Snake Coiled Up in the Stomach
'A clergyman, about 30 years of age, of general good health, with the exception of a bronchial affection; in Sept. 1852, was bitten in the calf of the leg by a copper-headed snake. He immediately immersed the leg in black mud, after tying a handkerchief tightly around just below the knee. The first sensation of the bite was as of a scratch, or prick of a pin, or a nettle sting; followed by a burning smarting, and then a severe pain set in with the burning and smarting. The burning was like fire, and accompanying it was numb prickling all over the body, but esp. in the wounded leg. This numb prickling sensation continued for several days.

'The leg soon after the bite, began to swell and filled the boot-leg. When the limb was taken out of the mud, where it had been kept for about 1 hour; it was of a purplish colour, evidently caused by congestion of the capillary veins. On removing the handkerchief, a sensation as of a rush passed all over the body; but centered on the stomach with the most violent force, and a deathly sinking sickness. He was hardly able to lift his hand or elevate his head. When holding his head down, there was a roaring in the ears and a feeling as if the eyes would burst from their sockets. All the first night he applied slices of raw onions, frequently renewed, and took a cathartic.

'The sensation at the pit of the stomach was accompanied by vomiting and followed at each emesis by a feeling as though the snake was coiled up in the stomach, and very cold. What he vomited seemed cold. There was also salivation, which had the same coldness. Every time he thought of the snake, vomiting and gagging took place. After vomiting, there was a desire for large draughts of cold water, but dared not drink much, because vomiting would come on of water and the same coldness. Mouth parched, with a burnt feeling in it, or like a canker. Tongue felt stiff. When the fever subsided, purple spots, similar in some respects to beestings, appeared all over the surface of the body. On the way home after the bite and all the first night was very drowsy. Sleep full of horrid dreams of snakes and a dream of this snake produced the same sensations of coldness, drooping, gagging and vomiting, which were also reproduced by thinking of this snake in his waking hours.

'For 4 or 5 years afterwards, about the same season of the year in which he was bitten, the same spots made their appearance, accompanied by itching. Each spot about the size of a 50-cent piece.' [Redfield, 1854]


## MATERIA MEDICA CENCHRIS

### Sources
1 Proving Kent [USA], 5 provers [3 females, 2 males], 6c, 30c, 10M; c. 1888.
2 Clinical observations Mangialavori [Italy].
3 Clinical observations Farokh Master [India].
4 Clinical observations Louis Klein [Canada].
5 Clinical observations G.E. Dienst [USA]; ReferenceWorks.
6 Degroote, Dream Repertory.
7 Synthesis Repertory Treasure Edition 2009.
8 Effects of bite; see Clinical Manifestations and the snakebite case reported by Redfield.

### Mind
∞ Anxiety, with a feeling that she will die suddenly.[1]
∞ There is a fear of death without sufficient illness to cause this fear. The nature of this fear is of sudden death – by accident or disease – and this may so possess the mind as to make life miserable to the individual and his family.[5]
∞ Fear of death during heart symptoms. Fear of sudden death or that one will die soon.[7]
∞ Horrors of dreams of previous night seem to follow her. 'Instantly after lying down at night she was seized with a horrible, sickening anxiety, all over the

body, but most at the heart and through the chest, exclaiming, I shall die! I shall die! This soon passed into profound sleep, which was not interrupted until morning, but full of horrible dreams.'[1]

∞ Suspicious. Thinks that her family is plotting to place her in an insane asylum.[1]

∞ Angry when disturbed.[1] Anger from contradiction; from interruption.[7]

∞ Anger alternating with mildness.[7] Cheerfulness alternating with sadness.[7]

∞ Not able to rest in bed, much walk the floor to ease mind.[1]

∞ No inclination to attend to her usual duties, which are pleasant.[1]

∞ Catch myself staring into space and forget what people are saying to me, or that there is anyone in the room.[1]

∞ Dreamy, absent-minded, took wrong car without realising where was going. Misdirected letters.[1]

∞ Lack of determination and snap, has to use all reserve mental force to get up and go out. 'Time passes too slowly, seems to drag along. I am longing to go yet, I cannot tear myself out of my chair and move along. When at last I do pick up enough determination to go, I go very suddenly.'[1]

∞ Longing for the woods so intense I wandered out to the park alone.[1]

∞ Alternation of opposite moods and desires.[1]

∞ Too coquettish; strongly concerned about physical appearance, stylishness.[2]

∞ Usually Cenchris looks much milder than the other snakes. Much more seductive and like a pretty, nice person. The aggression is very inhibited. But when by chance it happens that they really cannot do anything else, you can see a real vindictiveness. All the injuries in life can come out in one moment. It is like an explosion; an atomic bomb![2]

∞ Forsaken feeling. Delusion he is neglected.[2]

∞ Curiosity in Cenchris individuals is something that I have often noticed. They love to read books or material on diverse topics.[3]

∞ Sexual intensity. Ritualistic abuse. Idealizing sexual abuser, leading to disassociation. Stalked; being stalked or stalking; sexual predator. Manipulation through sex. Making rules about sex. Great fear of homosexuality, raped or attempted rape by same sex. Ailments from lack of sex.[4]

∞ Mood swings – depression alternating with uncontrolled laughing.[4]

∞ Delusions: Being persecuted, pursued; devils, possessed by devil.[4]

∞ Sensitivity to odours; smells trigger traumatic memories.[4]

∞ Competitive, wants to be the first or the best.[6] Wants to achieve great things.[6] Wants to be challenged.[6]

∞ Child biting other children. Biting and pinching.[6] Striking.[6]

∞ Boasting, loud-mouthed but small-hearted.[6]

∞ Envious of qualities of others.[6]

∞ Fanatical about health.[6]

∞ Fear of snakes.[6] Fear arising from stomach.[6]

∞ Throws himself backward when angry.[6]

## Dreams

∞ Absent-mindedness, alights too early from bus.[6]

∞ Amputation of leg.[6]

∞ Betrayal.[2]
∞ Buried alive.[2]
∞ Being arrested while innocent.[6]
∞ Being wrongly accused.[6]
∞ Car accident.[6]
∞ Dissecting living and dead people; going up and down ditches; being in peril of engines.[1]
∞ Drunken people, dead people, naked people, robbers, indecent conduct of men and women.[1]
∞ Fire.[6]
∞ Fish.[6]
∞ Fleeing from danger.[6]
∞ Being or feeling forsaken.[6]
∞ Incest between mother and son.[6]
∞ Having all upper incisors pulled out.[1]
∞ Indecent behaviour of men and women.[6]
∞ Making love, in a car; in the countryside; seeing her parents making love.[6]
∞ Male animals following her in the field to injure her.[1]
∞ Being naked.[6]
∞ Naked people; wild animals pursuing her.[1]
∞ Plotting to fire the town or any building.[1]
∞ Rape.[1,6]
∞ Threats of rape.[6]
∞ Seeing animals copulating [2 pr.].[1]
∞ Seeing dead infants.[1]
∞ Snakes, coiled ready to strike, bitten on left hand; hand swelled, pulse went up to 160 per minute.[1]
∞ Horrid dreams of snakes.[5]
∞ Dreams vivid and horrible; make such deep impressions that they can't be shaken off during the waking hours. These dreams are often distressingly lascivious, even in virtuous people.[5]
∞ Wandering in field with cattle, with fear of being hurt.[1]

## Generals
∞ All tight clothing unbearable.[1]
∞ All symptoms < pressure.[5]
∞ Compelled to lie down [all afternoon] due to dizziness; vertigo < 4–7 p.m.[1]
∞ Sleeplessness until 1–3 a.m.[1]
∞ Sleep position: on back; with head backwards.[6] Lies motionless.[6]
∞ Typical 3 p.m. aggravation, especially fever, chill, cough, heart symptoms, urinary symptoms.[3]
∞ Left side more affected.[1] [Left-sided symptoms 44 times listed in Kent's proving; right-sided symptoms 28 times.]
∞ Great thirst for cold water in evening.[1]
∞ Desire for large draughts of cold water, after vomiting; but drinking cold water < vomiting.[8]

∞ Dislike for everything put before her to eat and finds fault with everything. No appetite for anything at breakfast.[1]
∞ Craving for salt bacon[1]; chocolate[2].
∞ Dairy <.[4]
∞ Pain throbbing.[1]
∞ Inclined to be chilly all day and more so at night, must keep wrapped warmly, even when feeling feverish. Body feels flushed, but contact of cold things is disagreeable, causing chills.[1]
∞ Chilly, yet heat = dull headache and makes one feel smothered.[1]
∞ Before menses <.[2]
∞ Sauna <.[6]

## Sensations

∞ Whole body as if enlarged to bursting.[1]
∞ Sensation of intoxication; feeling as if about to fall; unable to walk in a direct line; goes from side to side of pavement; < 4–7 p.m.[1]
∞ Head as if full; as if all the blood in the body has rushed to head.[1]
∞ Transient sensation of prickling in the scalp, like a gentle current of electricity.[1]
∞ Sensation as if eyes would burst from sockets on holding head down.[8]
∞ Roaring in ears on holding head down.[8]
∞ Tongue as if stiff.[5]
∞ Choking sensation < tight collars around neck.[4]
∞ Vomiting with sensation of snake coiled up in stomach.[5]
∞ Bottle of water as if in left hypochondrium, shaking up and down with motion of carriage.[1]
∞ Hard thump in left side of abdomen.[1]
∞ Intestines as if filled with water.[1]
∞ Warmth over region of liver.[1]
∞ Suffocating feeling after lying down in evening; must lie with head drawn back. Dyspnoea as if dying from anxiety. The thought of going to sleep brings on great anxiety.[1]
∞ Whole chest as if distended and the heart very sore.[1]
∞ Heart as if distended or swelling to fill the chest.[1]
∞ Fluttering of heart, followed by sensation as if heart fell down into abdomen.[1]
∞ Cord as if tied around hip.[1]

## Locals

∞ Violent headache in both temples in forenoon; < any warmth in room; lips dry and parched.[1]
∞ Headache in both temples on rising, passing off after breakfast.[1]
∞ Aching in frontal sinuses, nose and throat, as if having taken a severe cold, but no discharge of mucus.[1]
∞ Hard, aching pain commenced in left frontal eminence and spread down left side to teeth, then spread to right frontal eminence, then to teeth on right side.[1]

∞ Headache > coffee.[6]

∞ Swelling above eyes below brow like an overhanging bag of water. Baggy swellings above and below eyes.[1]

∞ Itching of eyes; begins in left eye and extends to right.[1]

∞ Sneezing violently on awaking in the morning.[1]

∞ Cold nose.[1]

∞ Impossible to breathe through nose.[1]

∞ Hay fever & obstruction nose while lying; & paroxysmal sneezing.[2]

∞ Besotted countenance. Purple, deep, dark red face.[1]

∞ Taste of copper in mouth.[1]

∞ Profuse saliva, running out of mouth on pillow in sleep.[1]

∞ Sore throat; empty swallowing painful, water or solid food swallowed without pain.[1]

∞ Intolerance of clothing about neck, causing a constrictive, choking feeling.[1]

∞ Nausea, > ice, water makes sick.[1]

∞ Stomach pain > chocolate.[6]

∞ Aching all around waist, at attachments of diaphragm; pain < when laughing.[1]

∞ Bands or tight clothing around waist unbearable.[1]

∞ Pain abdomen after postponing urination.[6]

∞ On waking in morning, has to hasten to closet; stool watery, dark with a black sediment like coffee grounds; stool intermits, has to sit a long time, passing small quantities every minute or 2.[1]

∞ Bladder inflammation in newly married women.[2] Bladder infection after coition.[4]

∞ Urination difficult or impossible in presence of strangers.[6]

∞ When doing mental work, frequent desire to urinate, pass large quantities of colourless urine.[1]

∞ Menstrual flow very profuse, bright red, with dark clots. Dull aching in small of back and sacral region, at night during menses.[1]

∞ Pain in right ovary[1]; before and during menses, stitching pain extending to back.[2]

∞ Coughing = dull pain in abdomen and loss of urine. Cough comes on when walking fast or walking up stairs, or at night after retiring.[1]

∞ Respiration difficult > belching; > sighing; before going to sleep before menses.[6]

∞ Stops breathing on going to sleep.[1]

∞ Can hardly find breath enough to talk, has to stop and gasp in midst of a word or short sentence.[1]

∞ Back, cannot bear draft of air on neck.[6]

∞ Dorsal backache from coughing; > raising arm high.[6]

∞ Lumbar backache; compelled to walk bent; > gentle motion; > sitting erect.[6]

# CASES

## Case 1

A 27-year-old woman came in complaining of panic attacks occurring at night which woke her from sleep. She had the following fears: war, spiders, snakes and contracting an incurable disease. Her chief fear was of men and of being raped, which had occurred when she was 18. Violated by an acquaintance in a hotel, at the time she had not registered the act as rape. She knew she did not enjoy it but said nothing to him. Later she realized it was rape and became furious wanting to take a knife to him.

Since then she feared a man coming into her bedroom at night which caused her to awake with her heart pounding fearing she would die.

A quiet person, she had few friends or social contacts. Mistrusted everyone. She refused social invitations as she feared something terrible might occur from which she could not defend herself. If she did agree to see someone she became anxious.

. . . I want to emphasize the way in which this young woman experienced her rape. She said she was violated but did not notice it. She got angry at the man afterwards when she realized that what happened was against her will and that it had not bothered him at all. Kent described something similar in New Remedies. The prover reported, "so absent minded and stupid that I tremble and shiver and my teeth chatter for some time before I begin to realize that I feel cold." This then is the same kind of delay in perception that my patient reported. In her case it had to do with being raped, in the proving it had to do with registering cold. Perhaps a delay in perception might be typical of Cenchris. [Christine Hug, A Case of Cenchris contortrix; Homeopathic Links, 1995]

## Case 2

Single woman aged: 25 years. Date first seen: June 1997.

This patient was referred by her General Practitioner. Her doctor was concerned she was exercising excessively and the patient had been complaining to her doctor about being overweight and her hair falling out.

For several years she had no menstruation unless taking contraceptive pill.

"I am very outgoing and talkative and competitive. I am very up-front. I am quite jealous. I worry more about money than I should. I worry about how I look; my weight and what people think of me. I enjoy having fun and going out. I am lazy at home after a hard day's work so I can put a lot of effort into my work. I am an estate agent. I used to run races for the county and I was champion. I am dieting a lot and I use laxatives sometimes. My sister was anorexic. I am trying to lose weight. I am very conscientious at work and I like to succeed. I am very competitive. Over the last 8 months I have really been caring too much about what people think of me. I never used to at all before. I was brash and I had loads of energy. Now I care much more about how I look – it is really important for me now to dress more fashionably and to be trendier. I am getting a lot of awards at work because I am doing so well.

"I have a real fear of dying. I have had this fear all my life and it is quite big. It is worse when I am lying in bed going off to sleep. I always think horrible things when I am going off to sleep. My cousin was murdered by the IRA when he was 22. I have a real fear of dying in a car crash or a plane crash. I am convinced I will die in a car crash. I am also really frightened of hearing that someone in my family is ill or dying. I have a real fear of quicksand. I had a dream of the family falling in it after an incident when my sister really was in quicksand once. I am frightened of snakes – well it is more of a dislike really.

"I have dreams: if ever I am going out with a bloke and I am worried about a girl who he might also like I dream of them having sex together. I dream of my sister having sex with my boyfriends – I was jealous of my sister for a while. I have a dream of my dog dying – I love my dog – I wake up crying from that dream. I talk aggressively in my sleep and swear. I have dreams of being chased by a person who keeps reappearing.

"I wear black mainly, sometimes beige and cream. I never wear skirts because I dislike hair on my legs and I am a bit of a tomboy – I like the company of boys. I have been an estate agent for 9 years therefore I have had to be one of the boys to stick up for myself. I wear flirtatious clothes when I am out – I like to be noticed. I have been colouring my hair for the last year; usually a copper colour."

She is chilly. She is very scared of anything that is slightly naughty or risky. For example her boyfriend jumping into a swimming pool. She never takes drugs because of the fear of dying. The black clothes she is wearing have buttons with her name on them.

Case analysis – Rubrics: Fear of death. Fear to go to sleep. Anxiety on going to sleep. Jealousy. Dreams of coition. Fear of misfortune.
Plan: Cenchris contortrix 1M.

*Follow up after 6 weeks:*
"I cried so much after the consultation even before I took the remedy. The fears I have had for all these years have gone. I am sleeping so much better. I have much more energy. It is amazing but my breasts have grown! I am still worried about my hair falling out and my weight but I am much less worried about what people think. I have much more energy. It is the best I have felt for a long time."

Follow-up continued for 7½ months. She required one further dose of Cenchris contortrix during this period. Overall the patient reported an improvement in general of about 90%. After 7½ months she ceased treatment.

After 17 months. Contacted by telephone at 17 months after presentation. She confirmed that she remained perfectly well in every way and volunteered that she would certainly return for treatment should she experience any relapse.

*Conclusion*
This and another case of Cenchris have some remarkable similarities:

1 Dreams of being chased.
2 Fear of dying in a plane crash / dreams of planes crashing.
3 Dressing in black and dying the hair a copper colour.
4 The patient in case 2 was a champion runner. The patient in case one dreamed of winning a marathon.
5 In case 1, the patient dreamed of terrorists. In case 2, the patient's cousin was actually killed by the IRA.

The overriding feeling transmitted by both patients was one of intensity – intense fears and a very intense experience of life. [Hardy, 2000]

# GENUS CROTALUS

## Biological Profile
Crotalus is a genus of venomous pit vipers found only in the Americas from southern Canada to northern Argentina.

There are 2 genera of rattlesnakes, the primary characteristic of which is a set of disjointed noise-making scales on the end of their tails. The genus Sistrurus contains 2 pigmy rattlesnakes and the massasauga. All other 30 rattlesnakes are in the genus Crotalus.

The greatest concentration of them is in the Southwestern United States and in Northern Mexico.

Rattlesnakes can range from 1 to 8 ft. [0.3–2.4 m]. They are thick-bodied snakes with keeled [ridged] scales in a variety of colours and patterns. Most species are patterned with dark diamonds, rhombuses or hexagons on a lighter background.

Other distinctive physical characteristics include producing venom, heat-sensing facial pits, hinged fangs and live births. These characteristics are shared with other pit vipers such as the cottonmouth and copperhead."

After the rattle, rattlesnakes' most distinctive physical feature is their triangular head. Also, they have vertical pupils, like cat's eyes.

Ratters mate in the spring and summer, depending on the species, and males may engage in combat. Mothers can store sperm for months before fertilizing the eggs and then they carry young for about 3 months. Only reproduce every 2–3 years.

Rattlesnakes' favourite foods are small rodents and lizards. They lie in wait until a victim comes along and then strike at speeds of five-tenths of a second.

The digestive process can take several days and rattlesnakes become sluggish and hide during this time. [www.livescience.com/43683-rattlesnake.html]

## Frequency of Occurrence of Symptoms in Rattlesnake Bite

- Swelling and oedema [observed in 185 cases] – swelling usually soft; pitting oedema is a common finding.
- Pain [149] – pain, usually almost instantaneous, is the most characteristic early symptom of bites by rattlers in the USA; pains are described as 'a flash of fire through the veins', most violent pain victim has ever known; burning pain; excruciating; sharp, stinging.
- Weakness [93].
- Giddiness [61].
- Respiratory difficulty [43] – characteristic of rattlers with neurotoxic venom.
- Nausea and/or vomiting [33].
- Haemorrhage [31].
- Weak pulse or heart failure [21].
- Gangrene [11].
- Ecchymosis [10].
- Paralysis [7].
- Increased pulse rate [6].
- Unconsciousness or stupor [3].
- Increased temperature [1].
- Perspiration [1].
- Nervousness [1].

On a scale of 1 to 100, Russell [1980] gives the frequency of signs and symptoms of rattlesnake bites [predominantly haemotoxic] in North America as:

Swelling and oedema [74];
weakness [72];
pain [65];
sweating and/or chill [64];
numbness or tingling of tongue and mouth or scalp or feet [63];
changes in pulse rate [60];
faintness or dizziness [57];
ecchymosis [51];
nausea, vomiting, or both [48];
blood pressure changes [46];
decreased blood platelets [42];
tingling or numbness of affected part [41];
twitchings [41];
vesiculations [40];
swelling regional lymph nodes [40];
respiratory rate changes [40];
increased blood clotting time [39];
thirst [34];
decreased haemoglobin [37];

change in body temperature [31];

necrosis [27];

abnormal electrocardiogram [26];

increased salivation [20];

glycosuria [20];

increased blood platelets [16];

cyanosis [16];

haematemesis, haematuria, or melaena [15];

unconsciousness [12];

blurring of vision [12];

muscle contractions [6];

swollen eyelids [2];

retinal haemorrhage [2];

convulsions [1].

Some rattlesnake species have venom that contains neurotoxins. Mojave, tiger, and speckled rattlesnakes are examples of rattlesnakes where either the entire species or certain populations within the species produce neurotoxins. Neurotoxins act faster than haemotoxins and attack the nervous system, causing problems with vision, difficulty swallowing and speaking, skeletal muscle weakness, difficulty breathing and respiratory failure.

### Account by Mr. J. Breintal of What he Felt after Being Bitten by a Rattlesnake. Dated Philadelphia, Feb. 10, 1746

Mr. B. walking up a stony hill, his foot slipped, and falling on his knees, he laid his hand on a broad stone to stay himself; and he supposes the snake lay on the opposite side, and might be offended by some motion of the stone, so bit his hand in an instant, without any warning or sight; then slid under the stones, and sounded his rattles. Mr. B. felt a sort of chilliness when he heard the sound; because he had a constant thought, that if ever he was bitten his life was at an end. Without stop he tore up the stones, resolving to slay his murderer; at last he found him, on which he crushed his head to pieces with a stone; then took him up in his left hand, and ran to his quarters, sucking the wound on his right hand as he went, and spitting out the poison.

This kept it easy; but his tongue and lips became stiff and numb, *as if they had been frozen*. So getting quickly home, he exclaimed, "I am bitten by a rattle-snake, and there lies my murderer!" casting him down on the threshold. The first thing applied was a fowl; its belly ripped up, and put on his hand alive, like a gantlet, and there tied fast. This drew out some of the poison; for immediately the fowl swelled, grew black, and stunk. He kept his elbow bent, and his fingers up, to keep the poison from his arm. Thus he walked about and set some of the company to make a fire on the green, which was done quickly, and there they burnt the snake.

Another got some turmeric; this they bruised well, tops and roots; so made a plaster, and bound it round the arm, to keep the poison in the hand; but night came on, or else he believed it had never gone farther than the hand; for this kept the arm secure, till midnight, or past. Nor all this while had he much pain; his hand grew cold and numb but did not swell very much; *but now puffed up on a sudden, and he grew furious*; so he slit his fingers with a razor, which gave some ease. He also slit his hand on the back, and cupped it, and drew out a quart or more of ugly poisonous slimy stuff.

But his arm swelled for all they could do; then he got it tied so fast that all communication might be stopped with the body that it seemed almost void of feeling; yet would it work, jump, writhe and twist like a snake in the skin, and change colours, and be spotted; and they would move up and down on the arm, which grew painful in the bone.

Thus was it tied 2 days, and all things applied that could be got or thought on. At last, the ashes of white-ash bark, and vinegar, made into a plaster, and laid to the bite, drew out the poison apace.

His tongue and lips swelled that night, but were not very painful, occasioned only, he supposes, by sucking the wound. The swelling of his arm being sunk till it was at least half gone, they then untied it; but in 2 hours all his right side was *turned black*, yet swelled but little; nor was there any pain went along with that change of colour. He bled at the mouth soon after, and so continued spitting blood and was feverish 4 days. The pain raged still in the arm, and the severe more violent; and by turns he was delirious for an hour or 2. This happened 3 or 4 times; and 9 days being over, the fever abated, and he began to mend; but his hand and arm were spotted like a snake, and continued so all summer.

In the autumn his arm swelled, gathered, and burst; so away went the poison, spots, and all.

But the most surprising and *tormenting were his dreams*; for in all sicknesses before, if he could but sleep and dream he was happy so long, being ever in some pleasing scenes of heaven, earth, or air. On the contrary, now if he slept, so sure he dreamed of *horrid places*, on earth only; and very often rolling among old logs. Sometimes he was a white oak cut in pieces; and frequently his feet would be growing into 2 hickories. This cast a sort of damp on his waking thoughts, to find his sleeping hours thus disturbed with the operation of that horrid poison. [The Philosophical Transactions of the Royal Society of London, Vol. 44]

## An Experiment Going Horribly Wrong
Reported by R. Whitmore Clarke in 1838, the following experiment took place in Rio de Janeiro, Brazil, and was conducted with a neurotoxic rattlesnake, most likely Crotalus durissus [aka Crotalus cascavella]. [emphasis added]

Masianno Jose Machado was bitten by a rattlesnake for the express purpose of being cured of elephantiasis and lepra. The individual who made the experiment was white man, about 50 years of age, of ordinary stature, stout, and rather athletic in form; temperament sanguineo-bilious. The kind of elephantiasis with which he was affected, was that denominated by Alibert E. leontina; it was in its second stage, and, according to the patient, no energetic measures had been employed in its treatment. Nearly all his body, as well as extremities, was insensible exteriorly; the cutaneous tissue was thickened, hard, its surface rugous, covered with tuberculous elevations, but none of them were ulcerated. Some pustules under the arms had a porriginous appearance. The characters of the disease were more apparent and better developed on the face, the features of which were swollen, giving a disagreeable aspect, without, however, rendering it altogether hideous. On the extremities the skin and nails had begun to change in appearance, and the fingers and toes were altered in form.

Whilst life and sensibility appeared almost extinct on the surface of his body, his interior yet retained the remains of his former energy, and he possessed a force of mind by no means common, and seldom found in one of his sad condition. Six years of dreadful and incurable disease and 4 of seclusion in the hospital for lepers had made him look forward to death as the only termination to his sufferings. No danger counterbalanced, in his idea, the desire he felt to be freed from his disease; he willingly risked the remainder of a life, under its continuance, for the slightest probability of recovery, and no stoic ever expired more undaunted and indifferent than he did when aware of the fatal effects of his experiment.

No opinion had the least weight against the determination he had taken; nothing intimidated, nothing deterred him. Having obtained leave to quit the Lazarus Hospital, he resolutely repaired to the house of Sen. Santos, physician to the hospital, to offer himself to the fangs of the venomous reptile, whose bite sometimes destroys life in a few instants, causing, immediately, tremors, convulsions, and the blood to issue from the different outlets of the body, and even from the pores of the skin. Having signed a declaration that the act was voluntary and that he himself was alone responsible for its results, he boldly introduced his hand into the cage of the deadly reptile; it at first appeared to avoid him; he advanced his hand towards the snake; it looked inoffensively at him and began to lick his hand. Two minutes passed in this repugnance on the part of the reptile to bite him. He now provoked the serpent and seized it in his hand forcibly and it bit him between the articulations of the ring and little fingers with the metacarpus.

The bite was inflicted at 50 minutes after 11 in the morning of the 4th September. He felt no pain when bitten, nor effects from the poison introduced into the wound; he only knew that he was bitten when it was announced by the bystanders. His hand was immediately withdrawn, from the cage; it swelled slightly, and a few drops of blood escaped from the wound, but he felt no pain. The man continued perfectly tranquil; respiration natural, and his pulse regular.

- Five minutes after the bite; a slight sensation of cold in the hand.
- 12, noon. Slight pains in the palm of the hand, which increased after some minutes.
- 17 minutes past 12, noon. The pain extended to the wrist.
- 20m. The hand swelled considerably.
- 30m. The pulse became fuller. The patient all this time conversed in a lively manner, and even laughed.
- 50m. A sensation of fullness in the course of the jugulars; *some alteration in vision*; formication in the face.

- 55m. The sensation of fullness extended to the sides and back part of the neck; the hand continued to increase in volume, and the pain extended two-thirds up the forearm,
- 59m. Numbness over the whole body.
- 1h. 20m. p.m. Tremor of the whole frame; sensible to the touch.
- 36m. Cerebral disturbance; pulse more frequent: some difficulty in the movements of the lips; somnolence; *sensation of constriction in the throat*; pain more intense and extending over the whole arm; increased intumescence of hand.
- 38m. Felt cold and covered himself.
- 48m. Pain in tongue and fauces, extending down to the belly; increased pain and swelling in hand; coldness of feet.
- 2h. 5m. *Difficulty of speech.*
- 25m. *Difficult deglutition*; anguish; copious perspiration on the chest.
- 50m. *Arms powerless*; some drops of blood from the nose; increased anguish and inquietude; pulse 96.
- 3h. 4m. General swelling; involuntary groans; *sensation of sinking*.
- 8m. Pulse 100.
- 15m. Great pain in the arms; restlessness.
- 30m. Pulse 98; flushed face; continued bleeding from the nose.
- 35m. Drank a little wine and water without difficulty; his shirt was changed, wet with perspiration; *intense redness of the whole body*; some drops of blood escaped from a pustule under the arm.
- 4h. Pulse 100; redness of surface more intense, but of a darker hue, esp. in the bitten limb; violent pains in superior extremities, preventing any rest, notwithstanding the exhaustion of which he complained; constriction of throat, and breathing embarrassed; inferior extremities, and belly as yet not exhibiting any particular phenomena.
- 50m. Pulse 101; great heat over, the whole surface of the body; salivation.
- 5h. 30m. Pulse in same state; torpor. It is remarkable that the urine has all along flowed in great abundance; saliva viscid, of a dark colour, and expectorated with difficulty; *great muscular prostration*; frequent groans, caused by pains over whole body; respiration tranquil; pulse full; skin soft; increased tumefaction of bitten hand. In this state he continued till
- 7 p.m. Some disturbed sleep, with groans; he woke and said he was free from pain in the arms, but had great pain in chest and a *feeling as of a knot in the throat*; urine copious; *deglutition very difficult*; saliva viscous and white; sanguinolent fluid running from the nostrils; offered a drink of water with rum and sugar, which he could not swallow.
- 8h. Sweating ceased; groaning not so constant.
- 30m. Passed urine.
- 9h. 10m. Passed urine; ceased to groan.
- 15m. Profound sleep.
- 10h. Administered the infusion of guaco [Mikania sp.]; dose 3 tablespoonfuls, with one of eau-de-luce, which patient refused, and took the simple infusion; sanguinolent secretion from the nose stopped; pulse regular; diminution of the

tubercular elevations of both arms and face, presenting an appearance of erysipelatous redness.

- 20m. Patient passed about 2 ounces of tolerably perfect urine; remains more tranquil, and sleeps at intervals without groaning.
- 40m. Pains in chest diminished; pains in legs and feet, in which, until this time, there had been a *sensation of death-like cold*; pulse regular, 108; thirst; patient drinks water without difficulty.
- 11h. Takes 4 tablespoonfuls of infusion of guaco.
- 45m. Emission of urine high coloured; drinks water easily by spoonfuls; pulse 119; the wounded hand and arm inflamed, and very painful; restlessness. Midnight. Slept soundly, interrupted by eructations; pulse 112; passed urine.
- 30 minutes past 12. Patient very restless; his cries distressing; *calls for religious consolation*; refuses medicine.
- 40m. Again passed urine; pulse 116; *sensation of great heat in the legs*; desires the coverlet to be removed.
- 1h. Patient takes his medicine again; asks to be uncovered; passes urine; becomes more quiet.
- 15m. Passes urine; pulse 100.
- 40m. Takes a dose of infusion of guaco.
- 2h. Drinks 3 spoonfuls of water; sits up in his bed; every time he drinks, pain and restlessness increase.
- 10m. Passes urine.
- 30m. Takes his medicine; becomes more tranquil.
- 3h. Passes' urine; the lower lip, which had been much swollen and inflamed, returns to its natural state; salivation ceases.
- 55m. Passes urine; is more tranquil; takes his medicine; pulse 110; involuntary movements of right thumb and left leg.
- 4h. Passed urine.
- 45m. Takes a spoonful of medicine; pulse 100; patient tranquil and sits up.
- 5h. Passes urine.
- 30m. Passes urine; patient declares himself in great agony.
- 6h. Pulse 100; respiration free; frequent groans.
- 10m. Passed urine.
- 9h. 15m. Great prostration; *convulsive movements of the lower jaw, as also of the lower extremities*; urine bloody.
- 10h. Pulse accelerated and intermitting; *increase of convulsions*; diminution of swelling of limbs and redness of skin; deglutition extremely difficult; respiration anxious. Applied blisters to the thighs; gave a spoonful of infusion of guaco.
- 50m. Convulsions diminished; administered enema of brandy.
- 55m. Cessation of convulsions.
- 11h. Remains in same state. Gave an ounce of oil of Laga, which he swallowed with difficulty.
- 30m. The patient expired.
- In a few hours the corpse became livid and more swollen; at 10 the following morning, 11 hours after death, the body was enormously increased in volume

and covered with red and livid spots, exhaling, a foetor so insupportable as to preclude the possibility of an autopsy as we desired. [Clarke, 1838]

# CROTALUS ADAMANTEUS

## Systematics
- Scientific name: Crotalus adamanteus [Palisot de Beauvois, 1799].
- Synonyms: Crotalus rhombiferus [Brickell, 1805]. Crotalus giganteus [Brattstrom, 1954].
- Common name: Eastern diamondback rattlesnake.
- Family: Viperidae, subfamily Crotalinae.

## Biological Profile
- Venomous neurotoxic and haemotoxic pit viper, heaviest, largest and most dangerous venomous snake in North America. Largest rattlesnake; average length 1.8 m, maximum 2.5 m. Weight up to 12 kg.
- Ground colour dark olive or olive-brown overlaid with bold pattern of chain of symmetrical blackish rhombs with light centres, or 'diamonds', edged with a paler hue. Posteriorly the diamond shapes become more like cross-bands and are followed by 5–10 bands around the tail. Belly yellowish or cream-coloured with diffused dark mottling along sides. Dark band beneath eye, bordered on each side with narrow band of bright yellow.
- Range: SE USA.
- Habitat: Scrub palmetto, low brush, short-leaf pine forests, sand hammocks, salt marshes, coastal areas.
- Shelters and/or hibernates [in cooler climates] in gopher tortoise and armadillo burrows, stump holes, root channels, under palmetto thickets, and other underground cavities.
- Ambush predator, using its natural body camouflage to blend in with its surroundings and sitting silently until prey comes within striking distance. Occasionally actively foraging.
- Preys on small mammals, rodents, particularly rabbits, and birds [quails]. Prey is struck and released, after which it follows the scent trail left by the dying prey.
- Needs very little caloric intake; can survive on 3 to 4 big meals per year.
- Can strike up to 2/3 its body length; a 6-foot [1.8 m] individual may strike 4 ft [1.2 m].
- Most commonly seen in evening or early morning, when rabbits are active.
- Males engage in combat dances.
- Ovoviviparous; 12–24 live young per brood. No parental care. Young leave birth site as soon as they shed their first skin.
- Hibernates singly, not in groups as other rattlesnake species do.
- No recognized subspecies.

## Behaviour & Temperament – A Most Courageous Gentleman

'This huge rattlesnake with its bright and symmetrical markings is a beautiful and a terrible creature. Ever bold and alert, retaining its wild nature when captive, there is awe-inspiring grandeur about the coil of this reptile: the glittering black eyes, the slowly wavering tongue, and the incessant rasping note of the rattle. All dignity, the diamondback scorns to flee when surprised. . . . The vibration of a step throws the creature upon guard. Taking a deep inhalation, the snake inflates the rough, scaly body to the tune of a low, rushing sound of air. Shifting the coils to uncover the rattle, this is "sprung" with the abruptness of an electric bell. There is no hysterical striking, but careful watching, and if the opportunity to effect a blow with the long fangs is presented, the result may be mortal.

'To observe a large specimen, taken unawares, literally *fling itself into fighting position*, is to see determination and courage that exists among few reptiles. Occasionally, though rarely, a diamondback will glide for cover if disturbed. This is the case when a hiding place is immediately adjacent. This serpent may be justly rated as the *most courageous* of the North American snakes.

'As a captive, the diamondback differs from most snakes in display of a *persistently sullen disposition*. Few specimens become enough accustomed to captivity to refrain from using their rattles vigorously upon the slightest disturbance. While rattlesnakes of other species may lie silently all about them and yet be fresher captives, the rattles of the diamondbacks are seldom quiet if an observer is near. It is not necessary for these snakes to see a human form to display annoyance. So *sensitive* are they *to vibration* that a footfall starts their rattles, which continue buzzing for some time, then gradually settle to a monotonous chick-chick – chick-chick – chick-chick – chick – chick – chick – and cease to sound. Morose and hostile lie these sullen coils for month after month, never taming, but ready to fight and sound the tireless rattles.

'Taking thus unkindly to captivity, the diamondback is indifferent in feeding habits. Some specimens refuse to partake of food at all and starve themselves to death, while others feed so sparingly that they ultimately meet the same fate.' [Ditmars, 1937a] [emphasis added]

Individual disposition appears to vary significantly, with some diamondbacks allowing close approach while remaining silent, and others starting to rattle at a distance of 6–9 m. In accordance with Ditmars, Klauber [1982] put the western diamondback [*C. atrox*], followed closely by the eastern diamondback, 'at the top of the list of rattlers quick to anger.' On the other hand, some display such a mild temperament for a rattlesnake that Snellings referred to the eastern diamondback as 'the gentleman of snakes'.

Bruce Means [2008] is of the same opinion; the approximately 1,000 captures of eastern diamondbacks he has made helped him 'to discover that the eastern diamondback is actually a non-aggressive animal with a gentle nature that rarely moves or even rattles when approached by humans.' However, when threatened, many will stand their ground and may strike repeatedly, resisting violently and trashing wildly when handled or pinned down. All in all, eastern diamondbacks are extremely dangerous and should be let alone.

## MATERIA MEDICA CROTALUS ADAMANTEUS

### Sources
1 Degroote, Dream Repertory.
2 Effects of bites.

### Dreams
∞ All people dressed half in white and half in black.[1]
∞ Contrast of an old man in a young eccentric outfit.[1]
∞ Impending danger, child will be run over by wild running animals.[1]
∞ Being or feeling forsaken.[1]
∞ Being powerless to deal with one's students.[1]
∞ Danger of being squeezed [in car] by bus moving backward.[1]
∞ Being suspicious of workmen in house.[1]

### Generals
∞ Sleep position on abdomen.[1]
∞ Waking from sleep due to coldness feet.[1]

### Locals
∞ Dryness mouth from nervousness.[1]
∞ Chattering teeth from chilliness.[1]
∞ Urging to urinate from cold feet.[1]
∞ Menses copious, more at night.[1]
∞ Cramps in fingers.[1]

### Laming Rattlers
Although rattlesnakes are generally considered to be non-neurotoxic, a number of species can induce at least some paralytic effects, which vary from local effects, usually involving cranial nerves [ptosis, facial weakness, etc.], to major generalised flaccid paralysis. Neurotoxic effects are most likely after bites by Crotalus scutulatus [Mojave rattlesnake], Crotalus cascavella and Crotalus adamanteus. The following first-hand experience gives us a good idea of the serious consequences of neurotoxic envenomation. It concerns a bite by Crotalus adamanteus.

'My hand recoils as if I have touched a hot skillet. . . . I feel a little sting from the puncture wound. More alarmingly, only seconds after the bite, the tops of my forearms and the backs of both hands begin tingling. . . . I quell a couple seconds' worth of rage in which I feel like thrashing the poor snake to death. My predicament is grave. . . . I am all alone on a barrier island with no one to assist me. . . . Emotionally, I am a wreck. I want to cry out in anguish for my stupidity. I feel panicky because I know that, against all medical recommendations to lie still so the venom won't be more rapidly pumped through my body, I must exercise vigorously to get off this island and save my life. . . . I do what anyone must do in such a circumstance. I decide to steel my mind and body to survive no matter what.

SNAKES

'I suppress my fear and anxiety and use the most determined force of will I can muster to get myself into the hands of help. . . . The walk *seems like an eternity*, but I reach the kayak exactly 10 minutes after the bite. My arms and legs tingle strongly, with numbness coming over them, and my legs are now very shaky. My forehead, mouth and temples also are tingling and going numb. Oddly, my finger is neither swollen nor in pain. In fact, the bite itself is no more distressing than any puncture wound. . . . [In the kayak] . . . the tingling numbness in my hands, arms, legs, and feet increases to a *buzzing* feeling. Somewhat dehydrated, I take a drink of water and notice that the roots of my teeth and my tongue also tingle. So far I have no grogginess or loss of mental acuity. My breathing also is not affected by the venom, but I have to keep fighting hard to suppress panic.

'[When arriving on the beach 21 minutes after the bite] . . . I do not get a chance to feel relief, because I cannot get out of the kayak. When I try to move my legs I get nothing but spastic jerks. I cannot lift myself using my arms on the gunwales. So I roll the kayak to my right and fall sideways into the water. I pull myself out using my arms and crawl onto the dry beach where I try with all my effort to stand up. . . . My *legs are rubber*. On the second try I make it to my full height, then crash down on the ground in a twisted jumble. My legs are completely paralysed. I have no control over them. . . . The crawl to the car is scary. I am so uncoordinated that when I feel sandspurs [grass with spiny fruits] pricking my palms, I do not try to remove them because I can't pick them from one hand using the other. I fight off visions of dying in the sand and desperate urges to lie down grief-stricken. . . . My heart is racing wildly.

'[In the car] . . . I use my arms to position my legs and feet, and I push with my arm to help my leg depress the clutch. The car starts, but I have difficulty crossing my arms over one another while turning the steering wheel sharply I gun the engine and crash through roadside brush. . . . When I reach my destination, I clumsily fall out of the driver's seat down onto the pavement. On all fours, I am too wobbly to move across the parking lot, but I discover I can roll. . . . My recovery requires 26 units of antivenin and a 2-day initial stay in the hospital.' [Means, 2008]

## Twitching Spasmodically

Klauber [1982] cites a 1952 account of a C. adamanteus bite in the side of the leg, near the kneecap. 'Twenty-five minutes after the bite the victim could not walk and it was difficult to breathe. Every muscle in his body jumped and twitched spasmodically, due to the neurotoxic effect of the venom. This continued for 5 days and was the most dreadful and exhausting experience of any of his many injuries. The haemolytic effect of the venom caused his right leg to swell and turn black from the ankle to hip. During the fourth and fifth days, which the doctor said were the most critical, he was too weak to talk. . . . Tingling of the hands, chest, and face, with numbness of the upper lip, were experienced soon after the bite. . . . Some of the symptoms were still present when the patient left the hospital 22 days later. The pain, normally prominent in bites by this species, was apparently deadened by the large dose of venom, so that initially no pain was felt. Muscle twitching began 5 minutes after the accident. Paralysis of legs prevented walking within half an hour. One peculiar symptom was that everything appeared yellow to the victim. This symptom has been observed in other bites by the eastern diamondback.'

## A Protracted Convalescence
Boy, 15-years-old, bitten by an eastern diamondback in the ankle, in April 1864.
After receiving the bite, he ran about 400 yards, and fell, in a convulsive tremor.
Dark grumous blood flowed freely from the bite wound.
Very weak; pulse depressed, subsultus continuing.
Appearance of patient: great agitation, stupor, tremor, and prostration of vital powers.
Leg and thigh quite swollen.
Pulse 130, small in caliber.
Great thirst; skin cool.
Twitching of muscles quite subsided, with exception of some trembling of muscles of thigh.
Great pain in region of wound and along course of nerves of leg and thigh.
Skin harsh and dry.
Restless night.
[Day 2] feverish; pulse 120 and contracted; countenance anxious.
Stupor continues, accompanied with depression of nervous energies.
Sensation of coldness over whole body.
Calls frequently for water and rejects all nourishment.
Slight twitching of limb.
Ordered chicken broth; he swallowed a half-cupful with difficulty.
Leg and thigh much swollen up to hip joint.
Bloody fluid escaping from wound and smaller incisions.
[Day 3] Limb much swollen and sensitive to touch.
Constitutional symptoms somewhat improved; stupor less; pulse more regular, slightly tremulous.
Nothing passing his bowels from date of injury.
Countenance, towards close of day, looks better; pallor, shrinking of features, and sinking of eyes, improved; notices his dog; took some nourishment, the first he has taken since the bite, except the chicken broth.
[Day 4] General appearances better; constitutional excitement abated, pulse nearly natural, little above the normal standard; swelling of limb subsiding; perfectly conscious; yellowish serous fluid still oozing from wound; appetite returned, relished his food.
He had a protracted convalescence, his recovery not being complete until the month of September.
This case presented an unusual symptom, as he would swell to such a degree, at stated periods, that his natural appearance was hardly recognisable; this quickly disappeared under simple treatment.
Discharged, perfectly cured, the middle of September 1864.
[Mitchell, 1873]

# CROTALUS ATROX

## Synonyms
- Scientific name: Crotalus atrox [Baird & Girard, 1853].
- Synonym: Crotalus adamanteus var. atrox [Jan 1859].
- Common names: Western diamondback rattlesnake. Texas rattlesnake.
- Family: Viperidae, subfamily Crotalinae.

## Biological Profile
- Large, heavy-bodied, terrestrial pit viper with broad triangular head. Average length 1.5 m, maximum 2.4 m. Largest rattlesnake in its range, surpassed in length and bulk only by its eastern cousin Crotalus adamanteus.
- Body usually grey-brown and dusty-looking; may be pinkish, yellowish, red, or chalky-white [resembling colours of local soils]; 24–45 dorsal dark grey-brown to brown blotches [diamond-like toward tail]. Belly pale, whitish, cream, or pink. Tail pale with 2–8 [usually 4–6] black bands.
- Range: From central and western Texas through southern New Mexico and Arizona, and into southern California. Extends well into central Mexico.
- Habitat: Most common in seasonally dry to semi-arid lowlands; other habitats include deserts, steep rocky hillsides, thorn forest, and tropical deciduous forest in the south. Found up to 2,450 m, but most common below 1,500 m elevation.
- Activity more temperature-dependent than light-dependent; mainly nocturnal during warmer periods, diurnal during cooler periods [spring and fall]. In the spring males move an average of 102.4 m per day, and females 82.4. In the summer and fall males average 61.2 and 54.3 m, while females make average daily movements of 46.1 and 46.3 m respectively.
- Winter is spent in hibernation, most often down a rock crevice or in a cave located on a south-facing slope, but also sometimes in animal burrows.
- Preys mainly on available small to medium-sized mammals, birds, etc.
- Toward the end of summer, males will begin making large straight-line movements in search of females with which to mate. After a female has been located, a male may protect his claim from other suitors. *He may even coil directly on top of her in order to hide her from other males.*
- Males engage in combat bouts.
- Ovoviviparous; 10 live young on average per brood. Newborns will stay very near, or even on top of their mother for several days.
- Accomplished swimmer; has been seen swimming at sea about 32 km from land.
- 'Social snake'. One of the U.S. rattlesnake species that regularly congregates at specific dens for overwintering. Such dens may serve over rattlesnakes, and other species of snakes and mammals may occasionally join them. May make annual migrations of from 0.7 to 3.5 km to and from winter dens.
- Very dangerous due to its great size and aggressive nature.

### Experimental Use of Rattlesnake Venom to Treat Epilepsy

'Snake Venom as a Promising Remedy. . . . Quite recently, partly through accident and partly through scientific research, the venom of the Crotalus atrox, or the American rattlesnake, was brought to the notice of the medical profession as a cure for epilepsy. It seems that an epileptic, sorely tried and greatly worried from the fact that he was the victim of frequent severe seizures, wandered into a valley of the Southwest and there was severely bitten by a rattlesnake. A party of hunters, among whom was a physician, heard the cries of this unfortunate and immediately went to his rescue. When the man fully recovered from the snakebite, he subsequently discovered that he had been made free from his epileptic attacks, of which he had been the victim for years. These facts led to an investigation of different venoms, with special reference to the treatment of this dread malady. . . .

'After the venom has been carefully evaporated to dryness, it forms a scaly substance of amber colour, readily soluble in glycerin and in normal salt solution; and it is now ready for commercial purposes. . . .The size of the dose to be injected must be determined for each individual, the usual minimum quantity being 1/200 of a grain of the scaled venom. . . . It is customary to inject this solution deeply into the muscles of the arm or the leg. . . . After injection there is a feeling of burning, stinging pain, and swelling occurs at the point of injection and in the surrounding tissues. The pain is of a short duration and of only moderate severity. The swelling seems to commence shortly after the introduction of the venom into the muscles, and sometimes becomes quite extensive. However, within from 24 to 30 hours the swelling seems gradually to subside, so that in 3 or 4 days the part has returned to normal. . . .

'In 3 of our 14 cases [8 males, 6 females], improvement was observable from the very first dose; in others, no improvement was shown until after repeated injections; while a majority of the patients treated have given no evidence of improvement. Where any improvement at all has been noticed, it has been in the men. . . . All of these cases were idiopathic epilepsy; all were cases of grand mal; and all had been for a longer or shorter period on the classical treatment, including bromides. . . .

'It has been shown by Dr. John Turner, in The Journal of Mental Sciences, that the average rate of coagulation of the blood is increased in epileptics, and that just preceding a seizure the coagulation rate is higher. This has been confirmed by other investigators, who are convinced that there obtains a rapid coagulability of the blood for many hours preceding a major attack. Mitchell and Reichart express the opinion that snake venoms lessen the rate of coagulability of the blood. It would appear, therefore, that, if the coagulability of the blood is increased during an epileptic fit, and that the venoms prevent and retard coagulation, this fact may in a measure explain the results obtained. We also have noticed that during an attack of fever the epileptic generally is free from seizures. As to this, it is asserted by other observers that the coagulability of the blood during fevers generally is retarded. . . .

'In one of our cases, the patient immediately after the first injection of venom became almost maniacal, with pupils dilated, quickened pulse, a very slight rise in temperature, and a slight increase in respiration. This condition remained this way for about 12 hours, when the subject returned to normal, and has had no recurrence of these symptoms from subsequent injections.

'In another case, symptoms of mania, with increased temperature and pulse, occurred after the second injection; the patient remaining in this condition for several days. It has been noticed in several cases that immediately after the beginning of the use of snake venom the number of convulsions have increased for a short time. However, at no time have any of the patients under this treatment been in any serious physical condition. . . .

'Hence, the severity of the local reaction and the unpleasantness due to the general reaction, coupled with the results obtained from its use, and, aside from the fact of the possibility of infection, would suggest to our minds the discontinuance of snake venom as a routine method in the treatment of epilepsy.' [Keatley, 1914]

*Note:* Pure rattlesnake venom used medicinally went under the pharmaceutical name *crotalin*. Dependent upon whether the manufacturer resided in the east or the west of the USA, crotalin was produced from venom of Crotalus horridus or Crotalus atrox, respectively. One author mentions Crotalus adamanteus as the source of crotalin. Crotalin therapy was widely popular in the 1910s, promoted by Philadelphia-based physicians such as Mays and Spangler. Mays was responsible for its introduction as epilepsy therapy, after initially having experimented with the use of rattlesnake venom in the treatment of tuberculosis.

The proposed underlying principle of crotalin's action as thinning the blood in epileptics, who supposedly have thicker blood at the time of an epileptic attack, was adopted in allopathic circles and also by Boericke: 'A crotalin injection decreases the rate of coagulation of the blood. In epilepsy the average rate is far greater than in normal conditions.'

## MATERIA MEDICA CROTALUS ATROX

### Sources
1 Effects of bite; clinical manifestations.

### Clinical Manifestations
Venom primarily haemotoxic; venom also has potent necrotic and myotoxic factors.

C. atrox is responsible for more human deaths in northern Mexico than any other snake as well as for most snakebite casualties annually in North America.

Symptoms reported resulting from bites by C. atrox include: *intense burning* pain, swelling, discolouration of tissues, oedema, ecchymosis, haemorrhage, necrosis, haematemesis, haemolytic anaemia, *lowered blood pressure*, lowered heart rate, increased heart rate, fever, sweating, weakness, giddiness, nausea, vomiting, breathing difficulties, and secondary gangrene infection.

Colonel M.L. Crimmins of Texas, who had extensive experience with C. atrox in the 1920s, sums up the essential features of envenomation thus:

1 Fiery pain.
2 Profuse bleeding at site of bite.
3 Rapid swelling, beginning at site of bite.
4 Discolouration of tissues.
5 Rapid pulse, sometimes double normal, followed by very low blood pressure.
6 Neurotoxic symptoms, nausea, and vomiting.

The Western diamondback rattlesnake, Crotalus atrox, is responsible for the majority of snakebites in Sonora, Mexico. Cruz and Garcia reported 19 cases of children who were attacked by these snakes. Most of the rattlesnake attacks occurred in rural areas during the summer. The lower extremities, esp. the legs, were most often bitten. The signs and symptoms presented by these patients included: pain, oedema, limitation of motion, ecchymosis, bleeding and necrosis in the area of the bite, epistaxis, haematuria, and vomiting. The observed complications on envenomations included: haemolysis, local necrosis, coagulation disorders, paraesthesia, somnolence, and acute renal failure. One death occurred from disseminated intravascular coagulation. [Pediatric Emergency Care, Feb. 1994, Vol. 10, Issue 1]

## Symptoms
'One *atrox* case, that of Mrs. Grace Olive Wiley, who was bitten 4 times in the left hand while endeavouring to give water to an *atrox*, has been fully reported by Ehrlich in 1928. The symptoms, with their times of onset, were as follows, with the treatment in parentheses:
Immediate: Intense, sharp, localised burning pain; profuse bleeding from the fang wounds; bluish discolouration with localised swelling. [A tourniquet was applied above the elbow.]
After 5 minutes: Nausea and weakness; increasing localised pain, radiating in all directions.
At 20 minutes [and arrival at the hospital]: Tingling and numbness in the opposite hand; thirst; an aggravation of the previous symptoms; temperature 99° F., pulse 120, respiration 26.
[At 25 minutes, novocaine was injected, and incision and suction were applied.]
At 30 minutes: Vomiting; cold perspiration; a feeling of suffocation; increased swelling and pain.
At 35 minutes: Generalised urticaria with itching and burning; swelling reached the elbow.
At 45 minutes: Further increased swelling and pain; spasms of the respiratory muscles with *feeling of impending death*.
[At 48 minutes a 10-cc dose of antivenin was given intramuscularly, followed by 20 cc at 63 minutes; also 1 cc of adrenalin.]
At 120 minutes: Vomiting at intervals; thirst; chill. The subsequent symptoms are not given in detail.

The patient was improving at the end of 24 hours and was discharged on the twelfth day. By that time only localised sloughing at the bite was in evidence.' [cited in Klauber]

A man with over 10 years of experience with poisonous snakes and 8 years with rattlesnakes was bitten on the right index finger by a large C. atrox. Here is his account:
'Everything happened so fast, I only felt the powerful force and didn't even catch a glimpse of the action. The fang marks were on my right index finger between the knuckle connecting my finger to my hand and the first knuckle of the digit [see gross photos below]. Instantly I heard a "you're screwed" voice in my head over and over.'
9:05 p.m. time of bite.
Minute 1: Lots of blood from the puncture wound and lacerations. Tremendous pain.
Minute 2: Sharp metallic taste in mouth. Pain subsides a bit.
Minutes 3–5: *Feet feel very heavy and entire body very sensitive. Slow motion and wavy feeling*, as from drinking a bottle of tequila. Collapse. Shake and *convulse* violently for several seconds. Repeat 3 times [according to wife] I was out of it.
Minutes 6–12: Wake up feeling fine. Drink 2 bottles of water [dry throat and tongue]. Finger still hurting. Some swelling. Calm and alert while waiting for ambulance.
Minute 20: Vomiting of 2 bottles of water along with lots of blood.
The next 2 hours or so are very cloudy, *slipping in and out of reality*, accompanied by dry heaving, droopy eyes, extreme tiredness, and slurred speech.
Next morning, feeling fine other than a severely swollen hand and lack of sleep. Some clotting problems, which all disappear later the same evening.
[Summarised from message posted on FieldHerpForum.com]

## Nearly dead

'You have heard of the phrase biting the big one. Well how about the big one biting you? . . . I have caught over 200 large atrox well over 6 feet with very little problems, but this one was different. He was right out of hibernation, hungry, grouchy, and I found him in the middle of the day. I usually see the monsters at night during breeding season, so this was totally different.

[After being bitten on top of the left hand.] 'Within seconds my hand doubled in size and colour. The fingers were taking on a grotesque figure, like the wicked witch of the west or something. My hand was still bleeding very hard, and I was feeling sick to my stomach. I happened to look into the rearview mirror and noticed my eyes were yellow. I mentioned this to my wife, who at this point told me most of my skin was turning yellow too. Pain, Pain, and more Pain, but I kept silent for the most part, and the nausea was really kicking in now. So far I had suppressed going into shock, but I felt I would go into it any time now.

[After arriving at the hospital] . . . 'I'm not sure how I did it, but under my own power I got out of the truck and walked into the emergency room. By this time *certain motions became extremely difficult, like speech and walking*. Right off the bat this hospital had no antivenin. My first thought was, "Great I'm dead. But okay now what?" . . . vitals were taken and my blood pressure was at 60/38 and I was going into respiratory failure. So I was intubated. . . . Now we are off to the next hospital, only 15 minutes away. Keep in mind that during a bite of this magnitude, seconds count. . . . Some 30 hours later I woke with a tube in my mouth, a catheter, and IV lines in just about all major veins. I was pretty *sure I had died and went to hell.* My new doctor was a trauma specialist and had seen snakebites before, just not one like this. . . . My doctor says he has no idea how I survived the initial part of the bite, but I speculate that having been bitten before has a lot to do with it. . . . No one has ever seen an atrox bite cause the eyes and skin to turn yellow. I have lost most of the use of my left hand, but I've still got it!' [Bret Welch, Being Bit By the Big One; www.venomousreptiles.org]

# CROTALUS CASCAVELLA

### Systematics
- Scientific name: Crotalus durissus [L., 1758].
- Subspecies: C. d. terrificus [Laurenti, 1768].
- Synonyms: Crotalus durissus [L., 1758]. Crotalus durissus cascavella [Wagler, 1824]. Crotalus cascavella [Wagler, 1824].
- Common names: Cascavel. South American rattlesnake. Neotropical rattle-snake.
- Family: Viperidae, subfamily Crotalinae.

### Biological Profile
- Venomous neurotoxic pit viper. Average length 1.2 m, maximum 1.8 m.
- Body robust, head relatively small and not well differentiated from body, round snout and spinal ridge, at least in anterior third of body. Dorsal scales heavily keeled and protuberant. Ground colour light or dark chestnut brown, yellowish in lighter specimens. A series of almost diamond shaped, dark chestnut brown spots, in the form of a rosary covers the spine.
- Range: Central and South America, from Mexico to Northern Argentina.
- Habitat: Savannah, dry shrub-land, thorny scrub, sandy areas, and particularly sugarcane fields [cane toads!].
- Preys on birds, small mammals, amphibians and reptiles.
- Eight recognized subspecies. The subspecies previously known as Crotalus durissus collilineatus and Crotalus durissus cascavella were moved to the synonymy of Crotalus durissus terrificus following the publication of a paper by Wüster et al. in 2005. The common name of terrificus is Cascavel.

### Venom & Clinical Manifestations
Neotropical rattlesnake venom is overwhelmingly neurotoxic and the bite pathology is representative of this.

Bites are almost devoid of localised symptoms and instead follow the pattern more expected from the bite of an elapid with potential blindness, paralysis and inhibition of respiration.

'Bite symptoms are very different from those of Nearctic species due to the presence of neurotoxins [crotoxin and crotamine] that cause *progressive paralysis*. Bites from Crotalus durissus terrificus in particular can result in impaired vision or complete blindness, auditory disorders, ptosis, *paralysis of the peripheral muscles, esp. of the neck, which becomes so limp as to appear broken*, and eventually life-threatening respiratory paralysis.

'The ocular disturbances, which according to Alvaro [1939] occur in some 60% of terrificus cases, are sometimes followed by permanent blindness. Phospholipase A2 neurotoxins also cause damage to skeletal muscles and possibly the heart, causing general aches, pain and tenderness throughout the body. Myoglobin released into the blood results in dark urine. Other serious complications may result from systemic disorders [incoagulable blood and general spontaneous bleeding], hypotension and shock. Haemorrhagins may be present in the venom, but any corresponding effects are completely overshadowed by the startling and serious neurotoxic symptoms.' [Wikipedia]

'Pain, often *stinging* in character, is a consistent complaint following the bite of this snake. The pain may be followed by a feeling of numbness over the affected part. Oedema rarely develops, and ecchymosis, if it occurs, is limited to the area of the bite. Bleb formation does not occur. Visual disturbances develop within 1 hour of the bite, and ophthalmoplegia and blepharoplegia develop soon after, in some cases. Pupillary reflexes are usually intact. Rosenfeld noted the presence of "the neurotoxic facies" [*uni- or bilateral ptosis and paralysis of facial muscles*], which is diagnostic of *C. d. terrificus* bites. Muscle pain and weakness may develop.

'Paresis may be most notable in the muscles of the back of the neck. In the 2 cases seen by the author, fine muscle fasciculations were observed in the neck and face, although they were most notable over the tongue. In severe poisoning, there may be vomiting, decreased deep reflexes, prostration, and coma. Methaemoglobinuria may occur within 6 hours of the bite and is often followed by anuria in the more severe envenomations. Pulse and blood pressure may be normal until late in the course of the poisoning.' [Russell, 1980]

### Bitten in the Finger
∞ Swelling of hand.
∞ Pain in palm of hand, extending up wrist.
∞ [1 h. after bite] Hand exceedingly swollen, accompanied by a sensation of coldness, which is also felt in the lower limbs.
∞ Jugular veins as if full; same sensation soon felt in sides of throat and nape of neck.
∞ Blurred vision.
∞ Crawling sensation in face.
∞ [1 h. 30 min. after bite] Pain and swelling extend from hand up to elbow.
∞ Whole body as if filling itself up.

∞ Visible trembling all over body.

∞ Difficult to move lips.

∞ Drowsiness.

∞ Throat as if constricted.

∞ [1 h. 38 min. after bite] Cold and wants to cover himself.

∞ [1 h. 48 min. after bite] Pain in oesophagus extending to stomach and abdomen.

∞ Cold feet.

∞ [2 h. 5 min. after bite] Difficulty speaking.

∞ [2 h. 25 min. after bite] Difficulty swallowing.

∞ Copious perspiration on chest.

∞ [2 h. 50 min. after bite] Increasing restlessness and anxiety.

∞ [3 h. 4 min. after bite] Sweating all over.

∞ Feeling exceedingly downcast.

∞ [3 h. 30 min. after bite] Face much flushed.

∞ Epistaxis.

∞ Whole body flushed and red.

∞ Bleeding pustule in armpit.

∞ [4 h. after bite] Body dark red.

∞ Unbearable pain in thorax; patient excessively prostrated.

∞ Constriction throat; respiration difficult.

∞ [5 h. 30 min. after bite] Feeling of stupidity.

∞ Abundant urination.

∞ Saliva thick, dark-coloured, viscid; spits with difficulty.

∞ Muscular prostration.

∞ [7 h. after bite] Sensation of a knot in throat.

∞ Copious urination.

∞ Swallowing difficult.

∞ Bloody serous fluid from nostrils.

∞ [9 h. 15 min. after bite] Profound sleep.

[Higgins, Ophidians, 1873]

## An Array of Complications

'Snakebites represent a serious public health problem in developing countries due to their high incidence, severity and sequelae. In Brazil, fatal cases of bites involving Crotalus durissus terrificus are high, corresponding to 72% of cases not submitted to specific serum treatment and to 11% of cases submitted to specific treatment. Between 1992 and 1995, 172 annual cases of snakebites were reported by the Health Secretary Office of Ceará State.

'Crotalus venom produces neurotoxicity, coagulation disorders, systemic myotoxicity and acute renal failure, with possible additional heart and liver damage. This venom contains enzymes, toxins [crotoxin, crotamine, gyroxin, convulxin] and several peptides. Crotoxin, the major component of Crotalus durissus terrificus venom, is a neurotoxin composed of 2 subunits, crotapotin and phospholipase A2. In addition to being neurotoxic, crotoxin also exerts nephrotoxic effects when inoculated into laboratory animals.

'Acute renal failure is a frequent complication observed in victims of snake-bites. The pathogenesis of acute renal failure after viper bites appears to be multi-factorial. A direct toxic effect of the venom on tubular cells has been suspected. Rhabdomyolysis is also associated with acute renal failure among victims of Crotalus durissus terrificus bites.' [Monteiro, 2001]

## Principal Constituents of Venom & their Effects

'The Crotalus durissus complex, comprising the South American tropical rattlesnakes, is responsible for approximately 10% of cases of envenoming by snakes in Brazil; the majority of these are caused by the cascavel, Crotalus durissus terrificus. The venom of this species possesses neurotoxic, myotoxic and thrombin-like activities. The high toxicity of the whole venom is attributable to crotoxin, a phospholipase A2 complex, which is the principal component of the venom.

'Experimentally, crotoxin in combination with crotamine exerts a neurotoxic effect on peripheral nerves and a myonecrotic effect on muscle. The crotamine content of C. durissus venoms varies between different populations of snakes in Brazil and Argentina. Crotamine was absent from populations in north and eastern Brazil, present in north-western São Paulo State and adjacent areas of Paraná and Minas Gerais, and in Ceará there were mixed populations, some secreting crotamine and some not.' [Note: Mure obtained the venom used for his proving from a specimen found in Ceará.]

'An intriguing possible clinical correlation with the presence of crotamine is the *broken neck* sign resulting from paralysis of the cervical flexor muscles, possibly through direct action of crotamine. This feature has been reported from various parts of Latin America. Convulxin causes convulsions and respiratory and circulatory disturbances in mice, dogs, cats and guinea pigs; it also causes in vitro platelet aggregation in the platelet rich plasma of many mammalian species. Gyroxin, when injected intravenously, induces episodes of opisthotonos and rotation of the animal's body in the longitudinal axis. These signs are not observed in human victims.

'A thrombin-like enzyme . . . is responsible for the coagulant action of the venom. . . . Local symptoms at the site of the bite include pain, paraesthesias such as formication or anaesthesia, but little or no swelling and no local necrosis. Rosenfeld denied erythema, but we have observed this in at least 2 patients. There is a similar lack of effect when the venom is injected subcutaneously, intra-muscularly or intradermally in experimental animals. This contrasts with bites by many Crotalus species in North and Central America, which commonly cause severe local necrosis.

'Systemic envenoming usually starts with the development of symmetrical ptosis, external ophthalmoplegia and facial weakness, resulting in the character-istic myopathic/neurotoxic facies. Paresis of the pupils may impair visual accom-modation [responsible for patients' complaints of difficulties with vision], loss of pupillary reflexes and mydriasis. Rosenfeld regarded mydriasis as a fatal prog-nostic sign. Rarely, respiratory muscle involvement may lead to respiratory failure. The venom induces generalised rhabdomyolysis, causing myalgias, a massive rise in serum myoglobin and creatine kinase [CK] levels, accompanied by myoglobinuria.

'Pain throughout the whole body, possibly explained by rhabdomyolysis, was the main symptom remembered by one of the first recorded victims of cascavel bite. Father Luis Rodrigues was bitten near Bahia in north-eastern Brazil at Christmas-time in 1560. He suffered terrible symptoms for the next 20 days.

'Blood coagulation disturbances have been described in about 50% of patients. . . . Spontaneous bleeding has only been rarely observed in human patients. . . . The venom of C. durissus includes a powerful myotoxin which causes rhabdomyolysis in patients and damages the microvasculature of smooth muscle, especially that of endothelial cells lining the capillaries and arterioles. . . . Venom-induced systemic haemorrhage is rarely reported following envenoming by C. durissus terrificus; slight bleeding at the site of the bite is usual. According to Jorge and Ribeiro, about 4.8% [12 of 249] patients had systemic bleeding; gingival haemorrhage, epistaxis, and vaginal bleeding.' [Sano-Martins et al., 2001]

## Effects in Children
From January 1984 to March 1999, 31 children under 15 years old [ages 1–14 years, median 8 years] were admitted after being bitten by rattlesnakes [Crotalus durissus ssp]. One patient was classified as 'dry-bite', 3 as mild envenoming, 9 as moderate envenoming and 18 as severe envenoming. Most patients had neuromuscular manifestations, such as palpebral ptosis [27/31], myalgia [23/31] and weakness [20/31].

*The main features in 31 children bitten included:*
Oedema [at bite site] – 20 of 31 children.
Erythema [at bite site] – 19 of 31.
Pain – 15 of 31.
Paraesthesia – 3 of 31.

*Systemic Manifestations*
Ptosis – 27 of 31
Prostration – 23
Myalgia – 23
Tachycardia – 20
Weakness – 20
Dark urine – 17
Mydriasis – 17
Incoagulable blood – 17
Vomiting – 13
Diplopia – 11
Superficial breathing – 6
Diaphoresis – 5
Acute renal failure – 3
Unequal size of pupils – 2
Excessive contraction of pupils – 1

Bleeding – 1
Tetany – 1
[Bucaretchi, 2002]


## MATERIA MEDICA CROTALUS CASCAVELLA

### Sources
1 Proving Mure [France-Brazil], 1 male prover and 1 female patient [see below]; no further details; 1843.
2 Self-experimentation Nilo Cairo da Silva with 3x trit. and recording of effects of bite; 1909.
3 Effects of a bite on the finger.
4 Clinical observations Mangialavori [Italy].
5 Proving Rajan Sankaran [India], 12 provers, 30c; 1995.
6 Clinical observations Louis Klein [Canada].
7 Degroote, Dream Repertory.
8 Synthesis Repertory Treasure Edition 2009.

### Mind
∞ Delusion hearing someone walking behind him.[1]
∞ Delusion people whom he had offended would gang up and attack him.[5]
∞ 'While in a clairvoyant state, he speaks to somebody who does not answer him.'[1]
∞ Dread, nocturnal fear. Fright at night about indefinite things. Horror of being alone. Fear of death.[2]
∞ Cries distressingly and calls for religious consolation.[2]
∞ Pursued by the idea of death, esp. when alone; can only think of death, & great depression.[1]
∞ Aversion to talking; sensitive mood. Desire to move about. Answers all questions with 'no'.[1]
∞ Magnetic state. [Clinical case, see below Mure's female patient]
∞ Delusion not being appreciated; being neglected. Self-pity, desire to show being sick.[4]
∞ Excessive admiration of and looking up to someone.[7] Need of confirmation.[7]
∞ Egotism, self-esteem. Narcissistic.[4] Desire for company.[4]
∞ Forsaken feeling. Jealousy. Irritability before menses.[4]
∞ Anger from indecent behaviour of self.[5]
∞ Anger with absent persons.[7]
∞ Desire to cut, mutilate, slit others with a sharp knife. Sudden impulse to kill those who disturb him. Deceitful maliciousness. Destructiveness # fear of being harmed.[5]
∞ Fears: being caught; being forsaken; making mistakes; divine punishment; rape.[5]
∞ Constant focus on death; constant dwelling on death of loved one. Ailments or grief after sudden death [especially violent] of someone known.[6]

∞ Delusion of body falling apart, at night in bed.[7]
∞ Demanding, complaining patient alternating with over-friendliness. Pre-menses anger and violence, > flow. Sudden violence. Passionate and insightful. Gossiping. Jealousy, betrayed feeling.[6]
∞ Avarice, envy, materialism. Wants to be taken care of financially. Feels ripped off with resentment. Anxiety about financial well-being. Despair, lamenting with financial situation. Selfish.[6]
∞ Fear of spiders. Delusions spiders.[6]
∞ Self-focused mother. Lack of feeling for offspring yet many children. Overbearing parent. Frightening children into obedience.[6]
∞ Very attached to family.[7] Anxiety about family.[8] Full of cares about others.[8]
∞ High sexuality. Seductive sexually. Experimental sex. Threesomes. Aggressive sexuality.[6]
∞ Can't look at blood.[7]
∞ Desire for the colour black.[7]
∞ Inner conflict between obligations and having an own life.[7]
∞ Antagonism with oneself.[8]
∞ Aphasia after apoplexy.[8]
∞ Delusions: being attacked; being deceived; hearing footsteps behind him; being forced; being a great person; being insulted and looked down upon; having neglected one's duty; someone behind him; of grandeur, superiority; being tall.[8]
∞ Fears: being attacked; someone behind him; crossing a bridge or place; falling; high places; being injured; divine punishment; losing self-control.[8]
∞ Suspicious of one's best friends.[8]

## Dreams
∞ Abortion, threatening.[7]
∞ Accused falsely of adultery.[7]
∞ Animals copulating – dogs, frogs, horses.[7]
∞ Apocalypse, world on fire; world will collapse.[7]
∞ Arrogance; being criticized of being very arrogant.[7]
∞ Attacked by snakes.[5]
∞ Attacked with a knife.[7]
∞ Bad news, getting; of people or loved ones having died [accident or disease].[7]
∞ Being not believed about impending danger.[7]
∞ Betrayed by friends. Neglected by friends.[5]
∞ Betrayed and left by partner; of teeth falling out; jealousy.[4]
∞ Bitten by dog or snake.[7]
∞ Blamed publicly.[7]
∞ Bloody battles with swords and knives.[7]
∞ Cares, worries about anticipating negative events.[7]
∞ Coffins.[7]
∞ Being conscious during dreaming.[7]
∞ Danger, impending – airplane crash; bomb; building collapse; fire; fleeing.[7]
∞ Dead people and ghosts.[1]

∞ Death of relatives.[7]

∞ Enormous shaggy spiders walking towards one and attempting to crawl over one's person.[1]

∞ Escaping from danger of fire.[7]

∞ Falling from high place due to being pushed off from behind.[5]

∞ Fleeing to escape danger.[7]

∞ Forsaken, being or feeling; excluded; outcast.[7]

∞ Hiding, going into; seeking cover.[7]

∞ Locked up in room or house.[7]

∞ Looking for a toilet.[7]

∞ Lost, having – group; husband; wife.[7]

∞ Naked people.[7]

∞ Parties with illuminations; quarrels, battles.[1]

∞ Passed over.[7]

∞ Pursued, being.[7]

∞ Shot, being.[7]

∞ Skeletons, alive.[7]

∞ Stealing, being caught for.[7]

∞ Superstitious dreams – witches, black cats, gypsies, etc.[6]

∞ Teeth breaking off or falling out.[7]

∞ Threatened by a jealous man.[7]

∞ Urinating.[7]

## Generals

∞ Cold and clammy sweat. Perspiration and weakness after eating.[2]

∞ General coldness, despite being well covered. Feels cold and covers himself. Shivering with desire to be covered. Coldness of limbs. Ice-cold feet.[2]

∞ Chilliness all over, not > in bed. Hands cold, feet icy-cold.[1,3] Coldness tip of nose and fingertips.[6]

∞ Muscular prostration. Inability to stand or sit up. Total loss of movement and power.[2]

∞ General spasms, convulsions of limbs, esp. of arms.[2]

∞ Great sensibility to touch over whole body. Throat, stomach and abdomen sensitive to touch; cannot bear bedclothes, which cause uneasiness.[2]

∞ All symptoms < after sleeping and at night. Alarming symptoms more threatening on awaking.[2]

∞ Sleeplessness with restless startings during sleep.[2]

∞ Food displeases, above all beef. Intense thirst.[2]

∞ Restlessness and general pains < drinking.[2]

∞ Smell all day like that of the crotalus, insipid, nauseous, like the odour perceived in a hospital.[1]

∞ Sensation of constriction as by a strangling knot in neck, as by an iron armour in chest, as by a band in waist, and as by an iron helmet in head.[1]

∞ Great desire for food, suddenly passing off at the sight of it. Aversion to meat.[1]

∞ Aversion to beef[6]; sweets[4]; vinegar[4].

∞ Red wine <.[4] Bread <; cheese <.[5] Food additives <.[6]

∞ Before menses <.[4]
∞ Sleep position on back with legs crossed.[7]
∞ Lies motionless when sleeping.[7]

## Sensations
∞ Even while awake one feels as if one were falling out of bed.[1]
∞ Frontal headache, as if forehead would split, with weight above eyes, especially at night.[1]
∞ Head and thorax as if pressed by an iron armour.[1]
∞ Something alive as if walking about in a circle in head.[1]
∞ Brain pressed on by an iron helmet.[1]
∞ Red-hot iron as if sticking in vertex.[1]
∞ Bruised sensation in occiput.[2]
∞ Heaviness head after wine.[4]
∞ Right eye as if being drawn out. Left eye as if drawn towards temple by a thread.[1]
∞ Eyes as if falling out.[1]
∞ Eyeball as if cut out with a pen-knife.[1]
∞ Grains of sand in outer canthi of eyes.[1]
∞ Blue dazzling light before eyes.[1]
∞ Buzzing in ears while going downstairs.[2]
∞ Tip of nose as if drawn up by a string fastened to a central point on forehead.[1]
∞ Formication in skin of face.[2]
∞ Salty or putrid taste in mouth.[2]
∞ Taste of onions in mouth.[1]
∞ Lower gums as if touched by a red-hot iron.[1]
∞ Dust in throat.[1]
∞ Lump in throat; throat as if constricted; difficult speech, difficult swallowing.[3]
∞ Strangling knot in throat, on awaking.[2]
∞ Ball or foreign body in throat, & sensation of suffocation, on awaking. Ball and foreign body cannot be swallowed.[2]
∞ Thyroid as if constricted, as if strung together with a string.[1]
∞ Stomach as if cold after eating.[1]
∞ Excessive weight at diaphragm.[1]
∞ Bands around abdomen.[1]
∞ Heavy weight and excessive sensitiveness in hypogastrium.[2]
∞ Pain across umbilical region, with alternate sensation of spreading out and pinching together.[1]
∞ Peg sticking in middle portion of liver.[1]
∞ Cough as from dust.[8]
∞ Chest as if constricted.[2]
∞ Water in chest; heart as if floating in liquid.[1]
∞ Heart as if beating from above downwards.[1]
∞ Struck from behind on nape of neck.[2]
∞ Coldness in spinal cord.[2]
∞ Nerves of arms as if tied in a knot.[1]

SNAKES

∞ Last phalanges as if broken.[1]
∞ Sand in knees.[7]
∞ Right leg as if shorter.[1]
∞ Death-like coldness in feet.[2]

## Locals

∞ Dizziness on looking at moving objects. Dizziness when crossing running water.[5]
∞ Headache, nosebleed, and excited feeling due to having been roused from sleep suddenly.[1]
∞ Headache > clenching teeth[5]; < clothing around neck[8].
∞ Headache in whole head, beginning in forehead. Headache < at night.[2]
∞ Hair falling out, alopecia, after diseases, after mononucleosis.[4]
∞ Lachrymation; eyes bloodshot; paralysis of eyelids, lids immovable, half closed. Tearful and deadened expression. Blurred vision.[2]
∞ Noises in ears when swallowing.[7]
∞ Earache < noise; on entering warm room from cold air.[7]
∞ Epistaxis, & headache and great excitement, caused by starting out of sleep.[2]
∞ Sneezing < overeating.[4]
∞ Sensitivity to smell of ammonia.[4]
∞ Face flushed and hot, resembling erysipelatous redness.[2]
∞ Difficulty moving lips. Difficulty swallowing, even of liquids.[2]
∞ Salty taste in mouth that cannot be removed by drinking sugar water.[1]
∞ Sensitive to odour of ammonia.[4]
∞ Throatache on swallowing, from draft of air, at night, from cold things, > warm drinks.[5]
∞ Pulling pain on sides of neck in turning head.[1]
∞ Indigestion > small amount of food.[4]
∞ Each mouthful of food falls suddenly into stomach, like a stone, & pain even felt in the back.[2]
∞ Nausea on brushing teeth; on cleaning ear.[7]
∞ Epigastrium sensitive to pressure of clothing.[1]
∞ Hiccough from excessive laughing.[7]
∞ Pains in lower parts of belly when taking a cold drink.[1]
∞ Frequent urination[3,4], after drinking wine[4].
∞ Cystitis < chemical [food] additives.[6]
∞ Acute cystitis from cold feet.[7]
∞ Urinary incontinence, loss of urine, from excitement; before menses, when sneezing.[7]
∞ Polyuria – urine copious and frequent, of a clear or deep colour, rarely haemorrhagic, but always albuminous.[2]
∞ Uterine pains < bath of cold or hot water.[2]
∞ Speech difficult and confused; voice becomes a whisper. What he says is not understood.[2]
∞ Asthmatic respiration after exertion, < laughing; hay asthma or from dog hair.[4]
∞ Asthma from dogs and cats; & hives.[6]

∞ Continual contusive pain between scapulae, sometimes slow and measured lancinations when inclining backwards, as if a vertebra had been fractured.[1]
∞ Lumbar backache > sitting erect.[7]
∞ Stiffness fingers in morning.[8]
∞ Restless legs before menses.[4]

## Mure's Female Patient

Included in Mure's 'proving' is the treatment of a woman suffering from a type of manic psychosis in relation to an off schedule [intermenstrual?] uterine bleeding – 'She feels uncomfortable in consequence of having her courses and is out of humour on account of having them.' In this connection it should be noted that Mure was well aware of the use of Lachesis. He expected that his Crotalus would work even better than Lachesis, presumably in such cases as this one, given his remark that 'The Crotalus will become a useful adjunct to the Lachesis proved by Doctor Hering; it is my belief that it affects the organism longer and more thoroughly than the latter, and will effect many cures that had to remain incomplete under the use of Lachesis.'

Since Mure recorded all symptoms in order of appearance, we can piece them together to get the following story: 'Vermillion-coloured metrorrhagia. Paralysis of the tongue. She stands for 10 minutes on the windowsill, and she is arrested when on the point of precipitating herself out of the window. She rises suddenly at 3 a.m., uttering 2 shrill cries and throwing herself forward. The vermillion-coloured metrorrhagia, with which she had been affected since the morning, disappears suddenly. Profuse flow of tears. The hands are cold.

'The hands tremble. Loss of memory. Second attack at 6 a.m., after which she seats herself in an armchair. Weeping. She plays with her fingers like a child. The suffocative oppression increases. Magnetic state, she hears nothing, and again sees the phantom of death, an immense, black, fleshless skeleton; her tears and mania increase. Vacant stare. She exclaims several times: he is in the lions' den, but they will not bite him.

'At 6 p.m., another fit of mania. Magnetic state, during which she does not answer any questions but hears a strange voice on her left side and behind her; she follows it, and tilts against the doors which had been closed and which she scratches with her nails. Three very nearly similar attacks succeed each other; they are occasionally interrupted by silly laughter and always end with a flood of tears. She exclaims again: he is in the den, but the lions will not eat him. . . . Another attack of mental alienation, she hears voices which she follows, and sheds a flood of tears. Her head feels heavy, with stupor. . . .

'Intermittent metrorrhagia twice a day and alternating with the paroxysms of mania. . . . The metrorrhagia ceases. She cannot bear seeing anyone on her right side, without experiencing palpitation of the heart and a real fatigue from pleasure. . . . She feels as though her eyes were falling out. . . . She feels uncomfortable in consequence of having her courses and is out of humor on account of having them. Aversion to talking; sensitive mood. Desire to move about. She answers all questions with "no." . . . Lancinations, as if stabbed with a knife, in the uterus and anus, especially while washing herself with cold water.'

# CASE

'A lady aged 35 years consulted me for obesity, pain in the legs and acidity on September 1994. She says she gets the acidity because of eating food outside her home, in hotels. "I eat anything that I get at a hotel." Adding further she says: "I am very fond of eating and especially spicy food and sweet things. I also like to travel and if we are supposed to go for a trip and for any reason if it gets cancelled, I am very much upset."

'What do you mean by upset?

"When a trip is planned, most of the planning is done by me and when it gets cancelled I feel as if somebody has interfered and therefore the trip has got cancelled. Another thing is that I cannot tolerate is any interference in my work in any way, I like to do it my way and if somebody interferes I get angry and shout at the person, but later on there are no ill-feelings towards that person. . . . Even later I do not forget it for a few days and do not speak to the concerned person. Even when I am driving I do not like interference, especially if somebody overtakes me, that person has had it. Come what may I will overtake him. Even though I have learned driving recently I am not scared and drive very fast and rough, in fact I love to drive fast."

'Anything else you can tell me about yourself?

"During my second pregnancy I had lot of problems and especially one particular fear. During the whole pregnancy, since the first month, I had a fear that something would happen to me. That I would lose my child and these thoughts were persistent throughout the whole pregnancy."

'What do you mean by something?

"I do not know what but I felt that I would lose my baby and because of the thoughts I couldn't sleep at night. When I delivered I had severe and heavy bleeding and in order to save me, hysterectomy was performed. It was as if my death certificate was filled and it only remained to be signed. At that time I felt as if a big load was on my chest and, somebody dressed in black was trying to strangle me. Even now very often I feel somebody is coming to throttle me and I feel suffocated at that time. When I feel like this I cannot move and cannot even speak or call out to anybody and then my body turn cold."

'Somebody means who?

"It is somebody whom I do not recognise but they are all dressed in black and they surround me. Also, since childhood, I have a fear and after the second pregnancy it has become worse. It is a fear of being alone and especially at night I feel that somebody will try to do me harm. It is worse at night, especially after 7 p.m. If I have to go out after 7 p.m. I cannot go alone and need somebody with me. When my husband is out of town the fear is terrible at that time. I lock the house and shut all the windows and then sleep with my children."

'What kind of dreams do you get?

"I see that somebody, dressed in black, is chasing me up a hill, but he never catches me."

'Why is he chasing you?

"To rape me. Another dream is that I am flying in the sky. I also see a lot of temples in my dream. I am very religious and I like to see them. I also see a lot of black snakes in my dreams."

'How do you feel about that?

"I am very scared of them and I cannot even see them on the television. You never know what will happen next if a snake is near you."

'Anything else about yourself or any other dreams?

"One more thing is that my hobby is talking and if I do not talk I feel I will die. Even if I meet anybody whom I know on the road, I will talk for almost an hour."

'Which weather do you tolerate best?

"I cannot tolerate summer I feel very suffocated and especially in summer I cannot wear anything tight around my neck but even otherwise I cannot wear tight clothes but in summer it is very bad."

'*Assessment:* After the remedy Crotalus cascavella in a 1MK potency, she developed rhinitis which was better with sac lac. All the other complaints also reduced. Initially she used to bring somebody with her but after 6 months she started coming alone to my clinic. Now her fears are not there anymore and she feels much better. The acidity was markedly reduced too. Then there was no follow-up for almost a year, but 2 months back the complaint recurred and then subsided with another dose of the remedy in a 1MK potency.

The remedy was selected because of the following Mind rubrics: Sees death as of a gigantic black skeleton. Fancies that someone walks behind him. Frightened at night. Delusion someone is behind him. Fear of being alone. Fear at night. Fear somebody is behind him. Loquacity.

'The most evident feature of the case was the intense fear experienced by the patient even at the age of 55 years. She was afraid of the things usually a child is afraid of. But mostly a child, as it grows up, will overcome the fears. The other aspect associated with fear is the fear of being alone. If we look up the rubric Mind, Fear of being alone, then we come across 2 snake remedies. Crotalus cascavella and Elaps.

'Crotalus cascavella was selected because the fear was present since childhood and it became more prominent after the second pregnancy when she was suffering from post-partum haemorrhage. During that time she had visions of people in black trying to strangulate her, therefore the rubric:

'Mind, Spectres, sees ghosts, spirits. Death appears as a gigantic black skeleton. The only remedy listed is Crotalus cascavella.

'The most striking feature was the reaction of the patient towards snakes. The fear was so extreme that she could not tolerate them even on television.

SNAKES

In addition to this there were other features suffusing a snake remedy like: Loquacity, could not tolerate heat, could not wear anything around the neck.

'After the remedy she even developed a discharge in the form of a rhinitis and was better thereafter.' [Shukla, 1999]

# CROTALUS CERASTES CERASTES

## Systematics
- Scientific name: Crotalus cerastes [Hallowell, 1854].
- Subspecies: C. d. cerastes [Hallowell, 1854].
- Synonym: Aechmophrys cerastes [Hoser, 2009].
- Common names: Mojave desert sidewinder. Horned rattlesnake.
- Family: Viperidae, subfamily Crotalinae.

## Biological Profile
- Small but heavy-bodied venomous pit viper with large triangular head, raised supraocular scales above its eyes, and thin neck. Ranges from 43 to 82 cm in length. Females larger than males. The scales may help protect the eyes as the snake moves through burrows or could act as shades against the intense desert sun.
- Ground colour cream, buff, yellowish-brown, pink, or ash grey, overlaid with 28–47 dorsal blotches subrhombic or subelliptical in shape. Belly white.
- Dorsal colour usually closely matches soil surface allowing snake to blend in with background.
- Capable of displaying different colouration depending on the temperature.
- Range: E California, W Nevada, SW Utah, NW Arizona.
- Habitat: Areas of wind-blown sands, esp. where sand hummocks are topped with vegetation. Also found in hardpan, open flats, rocky hillsides, and other desert areas, esp. those grown with creosote bush, where the terrain is open, not obstructed by rocks or vegetation, allowing the broad sidewinding loco-motion.
- Reported to climb >30 cm up into creosote bushes.
- Primarily nocturnal and crepuscular during periods of excessive daytime heat, but also active during daylight when temperature is more moderate. Not active during cooler periods in winter. [www.californiaherps.com]
- Ambush predator. Preys on rodents and desert reptiles. Eats carrion and scavenges road kill rodents.
- Craters by shuffling into the sand while coiled and using its head and neck to pull sand atop its coils. Partially concealed, a cratered sidewinder is well poised to ambush lizards or rodents that happen by. Sidewinders are often found cratered into the sand in the morning.
- Solitary.

- Inactive for 5–10 days after consuming prey and 3–5 days prior to moulting.
- Juveniles use their tails to attract lizard prey; a behaviour termed 'caudal luring'. They appear to mimic both life stages of lepidopterans [butterflies and moths] in their luring motions. Their fast luring motions resemble the fluttering of a moth, and their slower tail movements resemble a caterpillar. Both movements have been observed to attract prey lizards.
- Ovoviviparous; 2–18 live young per brood.
- Usually inoffensive, but if threatened, with no escape route, usually will coil with head and neck thrown back in a horizontal S-shaped loop, hiss, rattle, and if further provoked, strikes quickly and repeatedly.
- 'This small snake can be surprisingly aggressive and a particularly peeved sidewinder may pursue a human that harasses it.' [tucsonherpsociety.org]
- Rather pugnacious; will strike readily. Will often turn and bite when restrained.
- Three recognized subspecies [cerastes, cercobombus, laterorepens].

## Avoiding Full-Body Contact

'The common name sidewinder alludes to its unusual form of locomotion, which is thought to give it traction on windblown desert sand, but this peculiar locomotor specialization is used on any substrate over which the sidewinder can move rapidly. As its body progresses over loose sand, it forms a letter J-shaped impression, with the tip of the hook pointing in the direction of travel. Sidewinding is also the primary mode of locomotion in other desert sand dwellers, such as the horned adder [Bitis caudalis] and Peringuey's adder [Bitis peringueyi], but many other snakes can assume this form of locomotion when on slick substrates [e.g. mud flats]. Sidewinder rattlesnakes can use sidewinding to ascend sandy slopes by increasing the portion of the body in contact with the sand to match the reduced yielding force of the inclined sand, allowing them to ascend up to the maximum possible sand slope without slip.' [Wikipedia]

'Males typically have a larger home range than females because they travel greater distances over mating season. Average distance traveled in a 24-h block averaged 185.4 m for males and 122.9 m for females across all ages. Subadult males traveled the farthest, on average, 223 m per day. They can travel via their namesake, sidewinding, but also have been observed using rectilinear motions and lateral undulations. The sidewinding motions minimize their contact with the hot sands. Sidewinders, esp. males during mating season, are constantly on the move for new territories. To optimize movement throughout home range, males and female will typically move in straight lines to cover more distance, but this type of movement is energetically costly for sidewinders if they cannot find a mate.' [animaldiversity.org]

'Instead of slithering lengthwise by contracting its scales as other snakes do, the sidewinder undulates in such a way that only a small part of its body touches the ground, and it uses the point of contact to lever its body sideways. The movement pattern of the sidewinder snake has the added benefit of avoiding full-body contact with the hot desert sand. The motion is analogous to that of a human being running across a hot surface on tiptoes to minimize contact. In the desert, any strategy that keeps the body cooler is a good one, and the sidewinding action of Crotalus cerastes helps accomplish that.' [sciencing.com]

## Reproduction
'Male sidewinders show annual sexual motivation regardless of ambient temperature. Female sidewinders' reproduction is contingent on the temperature of the region. The distribution of females throughout the geographic range forces males to enhance their locomotion by searching for females by straight-line paths through the desert. Males feed more often during the reproductive season, as the demands for energy are high when distances traveled to females is high. Upon finding a mate, by distinguishing scents via the vomeronasal organ and tactile efforts, the two will reproduce after courtship. Temporal distribution of females causes local polygyny, and *females will fight for males to mate*. Sidewinder males can mate up to 3 times a year, while females are dependent on warm temperatures to determine if they are suitable for mating. Female sidewinders continuously feed during vitellogenesis [the beginning of their reproductive cycle] but show a tendency to lower their consumption during gestation [which typically last 4–5 months in rattlesnakes]. This early feeding by females helps prepare them for the energetic demands for gestation and parturition. However, males increase food consumption to meet energetic needs for movement to find potential partners.' [animaldiversity.org]

## Keeping Warm
'Neonatal sidewinders engage in a remarkable behavioural homeothermy [thermoregulation that maintains a stable internal body temperature regardless of external influence] that has not been observed in any other type of snake. Following birth, the neonates mass together in their natal burrow. Most often, gravid females select an east-facing, small-diameter rodent burrow for giving birth. For the first week or so of their lives, neonatal sidewinders literally plug the entrance to this burrow during daylight hours, forming a dynamic multiple-individual mass that takes advantage of the hot exterior environment and the cool interior of the burrow to maintain an average aggregate temperature of 32°C/89.6°F [the optimal temperature for shedding]. The dynamic mass of neonates modifies the thermal environment at the burrow entrance such that the young can occupy a location that would ordinarily become lethally hot for an individual neonate [or even an adult]. Because of the constant movements of the neonates, the aggregate assumes stable temperature properties reminiscent of a homeothermic organism [i.e. maintains tight temperature tolerance ±2°C].' [Wikipedia]


## MATERIA MEDICA CROTALUS CERASTES

### Sources
1 Effects of bite; clinical manifestations.

## Clinical Manifestations

'Clinical effects following envenomation are generally similar to, although possibly less severe than those occurring after envenomation by other North American rattlesnake species. Effects may include local pain, swelling, thrombocytopenia, and coagulopathy. Neurotoxic findings after Sidewinder envenomation have not been reported previously.

'In North America, the rattlesnake best known for its neurotoxic venom is the Mojave rattlesnake, Crotalus scutulatus. Envenomation may lead to paraesthesias, weakness, fasciculations, cranial nerve paresis, and respiratory paralysis. However, fasciculations, in some cases severe enough to lead to respiratory failure, have also been reported following envenomation by other rattlesnake species, including the timber rattlesnake [Crotalus horridus], western diamondback [Crotalus atrox], southern pacific [Crotalus oreganus halleri], and midget faded rattlesnake [Crotalus oreganus concolor].

'Neurotoxicity following envenomation by the sidewinder rattlesnake, Crotalus cerastes, has not previously been reported. We describe such a case.

'A 56-year-old healthy man, without previous history of snakebite, was working in southwestern Arizona when he felt something bite him on his right foot through his leather boot. He saw a rattlesnake, which he described as a 3-foot-long sidewinder [C. cerastes], possessing "horns" and moving as if taking sideways steps. The snake was captured by a co-worker and photographed, and the photograph was forwarded to 2 independent herpetologists who confirmed the species to be a sidewinder.

'The patient immediately developed *burning* pain in his foot along with numbness of the foot and toes distal to the bite site. Within minutes, the pain spread proximally to the knee. The patient then developed nausea and dyspnoea, which resolved prior to helicopter transport from the scene 60 min after the envenomation.

'The patient arrived in the emergency department 2 h after the snakebite reporting 8/10 pain in his right foot and leg. Vital signs on arrival included a blood pressure of 125/76 mmHg, heart rate of 72 bpm, oxygen saturation 97% on room air, and afebrile. Notable findings on physical examination included a general ill appearance, a small ecchymotic lesion on the dorsal lateral aspect of the right foot without swelling, weakness of the right toes, decreased sensation of the distal half of the right foot including the toes, and pronounced fasciculations of the anterior thigh musculature. The remainder of the physical examination was benign. A puncture through the skin was not visible at the bite site. Initial laboratory values including prothrombin time, fibrinogen, platelet count, and creatinine phosphokinase were in the normal range.

'In the emergency department, the patient received a total of 8 mg of intravenous morphine for acute pain, without resolution. The patient did not receive antivenom. The decision to withhold antivenom was based on normal platelets and coagulation studies, lack of swelling, and lack of evidence to support resolution of venom-induced fasciculations with antivenom. The patient was admitted for observation and laboratory monitoring. On day 2 of hospitalization, the patient had progression of his symptoms with *burning and tingling pain of the entire right lower extremity up to the groin*, 4/5 weakness of the right upper and lower extremity, and involuntary contractions of different muscle groups of the right thigh. The patient was nauseated, anorexic, and unable to ambulate without assistance. He developed bilateral conjunctival injection and ptosis.

'He was moved to a telemetry unit for closer monitoring along with serial negative inspiratory force [NIF] measurements, as there was concern for progression of weakness to include muscles of respiration. On day 3 of hospitalization, the patient's NIF decreased to –50 cmH2O. It returned to normal within 12 h. Respiratory failure never developed. Over the next day, muscle contractions and fasciculations continued, but with diminishing frequency and intensity, and paraesthesias improved. The patient further improved on day 4 of hospitalization; although he *continued to have poor appetite and required a walker to ambulate.* On day 5, he was discharged home with *persistent right upper and lower extremity weakness*, distal right foot numbness, and improving paraesthesias. He never developed coagulopathy or thrombocytopenia.

'The patient was seen in our follow-up clinic 10 days post-envenomation. He reported intermittent epigastric pain resulting in poor oral intake, atypical chest pain, and persistent mild paraesthesias. His right-sided weakness had improved but required a cane to assist with ambulation. He did not return for further scheduled electromyography or follow-up visits.' [Bosak, 2014]

Bite victims usually experience relatively mild symptoms that include pain, swelling, itching, discolouration, weakness, dizziness, and necrosis at the site of the bite; however, fatalities have occurred. [tucsonherpsociety.org]

# CROTALUS ENYO

## Synonyms
- Scientific name: Crotalus enyo [Cope, 1861].
- Common names: Baja California rattlesnake. Lower California rattlesnake.
- Family: Viperidae, subfamily Crotalinae.

## Biological Profile
- Medium-sized, terrestrial venomous pit viper. Adults usually 70–80 cm long, maximum 90 cm.
- Head relatively small and narrow with rather large eyes. Colour and pattern variable, usually punctuated with grey and blending in well with local soil colours. Dark-brown, tan, grey-brown, or silvery-brown [paler toward tail], with 28–42 reddish to yellow-brown dorsal blotches [black-edged]. Belly cream or buff, mottled with darker grey or brown.
- Range: Western Mexico, mainly the Baja California peninsula and nearby islands.
- Habitat: Found most commonly in desert areas; mainly in rocky terrain sparsely covered with brush and cacti,
- Mainly nocturnal.

- Ovoviviparous; up to 7 live young per brood.
- Preys on lizards [mainly juveniles], small mice [mainly adults], and invertebrates [e.g. centipedes].
- If threatened and with no ready escape route, will coil with head and neck thrown back in a horizontal S-shaped loop, hiss, rattle, and if further provoked, will strike.
- The name enyo [Greek] refers to the 'goddess of war', the mother of Ares, in late Greek mythology.
- Three recognized subspecies [cerralvensis, furvus, enyo].

### Venom & Clinical Manifestations

Venom not much known; probably mainly haemotoxic but with tissue-necrotic factors. May be very painful at the bite site with rapid progression of local and systemic symptoms if envenomation occurred. Bites and significant envenomations of humans occur occasionally, but no well-documented human deaths due to this species.

### Materia Medica

- No symptoms.

# CROTALUS HORRIDUS

### Synonyms

- Scientific name: Crotalus horridus [L., 1758].
- Common names: Timber rattlesnake. Banded rattlesnake. Canebrake rattlesnake.
- Family: Viperidae, subfamily Crotalinae.

### Biological Profile

- Venomous pit viper; body elongated, tapering toward head and tail, neck slender, and head broad, triangular, flattened above. Snout blunt. Back portion of head forward to inter-orbital region covered with small keeled or tuberculated scales. Eyes small. Average length 1.5 m, maximum 1.9 m.
- Ground colour above cream yellow to yellowish brown, and even black. Dark spots dorsally, nearly black around borders and paler in centres. Posteriorly the spots coalesce, forming zigzag, dark-edged, transverse bands. All spots and bands are bordered with sulphur yellow. Belly yellow, with some mottlings and sprinklings of black. Upper lip sulphur yellow; lower lip paler.
- Range: Eastern United States.
- Habitat: Upland wooded areas, usually nearby rocky ledges or rock slides.
- Largely nocturnal in summer, less so in spring or fall. [Rattlesnakes are not universally diurnal as is commonly believed nor are they exclusively or even essentially nocturnal. Rattlers can be found abroad at all times of the day, depending on the season and temperature, and do *not* turn in for the night when darkness falls.]

- Inactive when cold or in cold weather.
- Reputed for being quarrelsome in the summer, probably due to their resentment at being disturbed, when found resting or sleeping in some cool spot in the daytime.
- Emits a foetid musk-like odour when irritated and during excessive heat.
- Ovoviviparous; 3–19, but mostly 6–10 live young per brood. Gives birth in birthing rookeries; stays with the young for 7 to 10 days after birth. At that point the young disperse and become independent.
- Sit-and-wait ambusher. Prefers warm-blooded prey – mammals [bats, shrews, moles, mice, rats, gophers, chipmunks, squirrels, rabbits, weasels, skunks] and birds; but will also take lizards, frogs, toads, insects, and other snakes. Climbs trees to catch birds and squirrels.
- No subspecies.

### Behaviour & Temperament
'In its free state this species appears to inhabit wooded districts, although it may probably sometimes be found on prairies. It especially delights in taking up its abode where there are rocks and debris among which it can find at short notice a safe retreat. Its movements of locomotion are rather slow. When surprised it will often seek to escape, without inflicting injury on its enemy. When, however, it is pressed, or there is no time for retreat, it delivers a blow with such rapidity that the motion can hardly be followed. The mouth is held open, the fangs directed forward and if possible they are buried in the victim. At the same time the poison gland is squeezed by the proper muscles, so that the poison is injected deep into the wound.

'If the amount of poison is large it may be quickly fatal to even large animals. Small animals, as birds and mice, almost immediately succumb to the deadly influence. It is usual for the rattlesnake to sound its rattle when it has been disturbed by some animal, which it has reason to fear. The use of this alarm has been much discussed. Some have regarded it as an imitation of grasshoppers in order to allure birds within its reach. Others have thought it a sexual call. Still others think it a providential arrangement to prevent injury to innocent animals and man. It is doubtless of use to warn off animals that might do injury to the snake itself, or at least compel it to use up its store of poison and its fangs, all of which it needs to procure its food.

'Dr. A.R. Wallace has suggested in his recently published "Darwinism" that the creature has acquired the structure and habit in order to warn off buzzards and other snake-eaters that might pounce on it as it lies on naked rocks. It is a warning note, saying, "Look out for yourself! Your life if you injure me."' [Hay, 1892]

### Aggregating & Assembling
Like copperheads and cottonmouths, rattlesnakes are 'social' snakes.

'Without doubt it is the rattlesnake's acute sense of smell that enables it to follow its fellows – the leaders must have some homing instinct – to a general gathering place for winter hibernation, and to find a mate in the spring. . . . One of the most interesting features of rattlesnake life is their practice of assembling at particular points – dens, they are called – for their winter hibernation. Rattlesnakes are by no means the only snakes that gather into restricted refuges from widespread summer ranges for the purpose of hibernation; yet the great numbers involved and their prominence, as they lie about the den entrances in the last sunny days of autumn or first warm days of spring – which I have termed the "lying-out" periods – have resulted in a marked focus of attention on the practice.

'These denning proclivities are more conspicuous in northern areas, or at higher altitudes, for here fully protective refuges are more necessary and population concentrations are greater. In the south, where a shorter season of hibernation prevails, or where it may even be interrupted by occasional warm spells, the snakes take advantage of any convenient hole or rock crevice. In these more makeshift situations only a few rattlers may gather together for the winter; or they may even seek separate shelters.

'The denning urge in rattlesnakes seems to be entirely predicated on temperature, a fall of temperature in the autumn starting them toward the dens. . . . Where rocky formations are available, the snakes seek deep caverns or crevices; but in the plains areas they are forced to use the holes of mammals, particularly those of the gregarious prairie dogs. The degree of cold reached in any area not only affects the duration of hibernation but also the nature – the depth, particularly – of the refuge. . . .

'Safe in their retreat below the frost line, the snakes are found to lie torpid and virtually motionless in groups of masses – "balls" as they are often termed – until aroused by the spring warmth. . . . Not only are rattlesnakes peacefully gregarious, other genera of snakes may join them in their winter seclusion. Some of the snakes reported denning with rattlers are bull snakes, gopher snakes, milk snakes, racers, garter snakes, and copperheads.

'From the somewhat inadequate data available, it appears that rattlesnakes probably have home ranges, or at least favourite refuges to which they habitually or occasionally repair, but that they do not have a defended territory, from which other rattlers are driven away.' [Klauber, 1982]

## Social Life
'Perhaps the most impressive aspect of the reproductive cycle is its communal nature. Like the denning areas, a good basking area is a prize find. In spring and summer, piles of gravid females can be found lounging in the sun together, black and yellow coils piled up in intricate mounds. These females give birth together at sites that biologists have termed "birthing rookeries." The rudimentary protective crèche they form with their entwined bodies probably makes a basking area the safest place for newborn snakes.

'Are such groupings merely chance meetings at an ideal locale, or do they constitute gatherings of more subtle and sophisticated social groups? Vertebrate biologists have long taken it almost for granted that snakes in general are asocial animals, leading simplistic lives of solitude filled only with basic instinctual drives toward food and sex. My research, in which, among other techniques, I radio-tag individual snakes and follow them around in the field, has led me to think otherwise.

'Timber rattlesnakes live as long as 30 years in the wild, and they *seem to live as stable, cooperative community members*. They appear to form lasting relationships with other individuals, follow similar paths through the woods, bask together before shedding their skins under the same fallen log, and sometimes follow each other from one den to another. Young timber snakes have demonstrated a tendency to trail older ones. A recent genetic study has demonstrated that snakes sharing a den are closely related.

'Other research on a similar species, the prairie rattlesnake [Crotalus viridis], has shown that the species can mobilise a *group defense*, mediated, in part, by alarm pheromones. Add to those findings the clear concern of mother snakes for their young, and you have to wonder whether the social lives of rattlesnakes are really so simplistic after all.' [Clark, 2005]

## Living in Captivity

'It is well known that rattlesnakes can live for long periods in captivity without food of any kind. They will last longer if they have water to drink; also they will survive longer in humid than under dry conditions, and at low temperatures rather than high, for under such circumstances life processes are slowed down and tissue and fat consumption are reduced. There is little doubt that under the more favourable conditions of a lower temperature some individuals would survive for 2 years; and most specimens, if starting in good condition, would have no difficulty in fasting for 1 year.

'Much has been written about the intense fear shown by any animal that may be put in a cage with 1 or more live rattlesnakes. Our San Diego observations have been quite the reverse. Before we learned the advantages of feeding with dead animals or found that patience and a proper cage temperature were more important than the simulation of conditions met in the wild, we were accustomed to place live creatures in the cages, including rats, mice, rabbits, birds, young chickens, and lizards.

'None of these showed any fear of the snakes, unless alarmed by some sudden movement of a rattler or the buzz of a rattle, should some snake be frightened into sounding it off. On the contrary, they ran or hopped unconcernedly around or on the snakes, much more worried by their new surroundings than by the strange co-occupants of the cages. One writer saw a rattler about to strike a chicken. The chicken pecked the snake on the nose, whereupon it withdrew and left the chicken victorious. Another observed that birds repeatedly lit on the backs of captive snakes and paid no more attention to them than if they had been inanimate objects.' [Klauber, 1982]

## Loss of Colour Vision Except for Yellow

The former subspecies Crotalus horridus atricaudatus, often referred to as the canebrake rattlesnake, is currently considered invalid. Based on an analysis of geographic variation, Pisani et al. concluded that no subspecies should be recognized; thus the timber rattlesnake and the canebrake are both one and the same

Crotalus horridus. The only distinction are colour variations and some changes in venom composition, canebrakes producing a larger percentage of neurotoxins.

Brian Fry, of the Australian Venom Research Unit, University of Melbourne, Australia, got bitten once by 'one of the neurotoxic populations of the canebrake colour form of Crotalus horridus,' experiencing: 'Over the next 30 minutes there was a lack of the pain and swelling at the bite site that are the hallmarks of a rattlesnake envenomation. So we came to the hopeful conclusion it was a dry bite and I proceeded to commence the drive home. The first indication that maybe I hadn't got away scot-free happened 10 minutes into the drive, when a strange metallic taste developed in my mouth. It wasn't long after that something much more dramatic occurred. I lost my ability to see red, blue, green or any colour other than yellow. It was a monochromatic world ranging from white to black with only shades of yellow in between. . . . Reality retreated. Shapes swirled. Sounds distorted, some bursts echoing like the reverb distortion for electric guitar often overused in 80s glam metal to cover a pathetic lack of skill. . . . [On the question whether the snake was venomous or not] My answer came in the form of me doing the "full exorcist": projectile vomiting. . . . My eyes rolled up into my head and I collapsed into a convulsing heap on the black and white chequer-patterned dusty linoleum floor.' [Fry, 2015]

## I Should be Dead

Almost instantly after being bitten in his left hand by a female black timber rattlesnake on August 12, 2007, Peter Jenkins knew he was in serious trouble:

'I could already feel a numbing in my lips, head, and arms and each step I took got clumsier and clumsier. . . . My dog eagerly licked my face as I washed the bite under the cool water and tried to press as much of the cocktail from my hand as possible. It was 6 in the morning on a Sunday. . . . My wife looked pale – a colour that I had taken on as well but would soon turn green . . . literally. In an effort to conceal my agony, I cracked a joke "the venom is making my balls tingle." Minutes later I lost all sense of humour and began to feel a *heaviness in my chest*, metallic tasting saliva, and a tingle that took on such violence that I felt like I was laying on a cheap motel *vibrating* bed. Swallowing became a challenge. My vision distorted, making the world look as if I were viewing it from behind a dusty windshield. I eagerly awaited my arrival at the hospital. . . .

'When we arrived at the hospital, the staff was ready with a wheelchair, which they rapidly produced on my arrival. When I tried to get out of the car under my own power, and was unable to do so, I just knew I was in trouble. Blake had to pick me up and place me into the wheelchair. I was as helpless as an infant. Sweat had been dripping down my face and the rapid ride in the wheelchair produced a pleasant breeze. I remember people smiling at me like in one of those bad dreams where you are naked and about to deliver a book report at school. *I thought they were laughing and ogling me*. My vision was fuzzy or dusty like the windshield of a truck driving rapidly through desert. . . .

'My temperature was taken it was 103°F [39.4°C], and I felt even hotter. . . . An obnoxiously loud and arrogant doctor came in and proclaimed that he suspected a "dry bite." I began to try to scream and protest but was later told no one could understand my mumbling. . . . I looked at him and then spewed blood and vomit all over his feet. . . . I continued to vomit a chemical tasting thick red fluid. . . . All manner of people held me down as I tried to sit up and *rip my clothes off in an attempt to breathe better*. They commenced disrobing me until I was naked and despite the natural bitter cold of a hospital, I continued to feel quite warm. . . . The events that followed were: surgery to close my arm and lots of physical therapy and pain medications. I was relieved to have survived and anxious to get home to the new recliner my wife had bought for me. As I write this on Oct 20, 2007, my left hand is still swollen and at times very sore. I was sick for nearly a week after leaving the hospital.' [Peter Jenkins, 'I Should Be Dead'; www.venomousreptiles.org/articles/345]

## Replacing the Mind on her Native Throne

John Redman Coxe [1773–1864], physician and professor at the University of Pennsylvania, began issuing his American Dispensatory in 1806. Largely based upon the Edinburgh New Dispensatory, Coxe's alphabetized compendium was the only domestic publication of its kind, making it popular among the era's most progressive and informed apothecaries and physicians. In the 1830 edition of the Dispensatory a peculiar contribution appeared by one Mr. Wallace, of Virginia, which also made it into Allen's Encyclopedia [reference 15] as one of the authorities for the materia medica of Crotalus horridus:

'I made myself *et alia* subjects of experiment with the poison of the rattlesnake. [*Crotalus horridus*.] My moral views of men, principles and things, forbade me pushing these experiments on others whose safety is my professional study [not the will play of philosophic fancy], so far as I extend them on myself. This animal substance is the true Samson of the materia medica, and I anticipate the time when rattlesnakes will be reared for medicinal purposes, as the poppy and palma-Christi are now.

'The effects of this [rattlesnake] poison are wonderful, as ethereal delights of long continuance, say for days, whereas the effects of opium soon fade away; it reddens the blood and makes the faded cheek to glow with the rose of youthful health; it is a great corrector of morbid resin of bile [whatever that is]: it drives away typhus and replaces the mind on her native throne, to administer beauties of creation and inspire the soul with physico-theology.

'[N. B. I mixed by friction in a glass mortar and pestle, the bags, venom and all, taken from 2 teeth of a large and vigorous rattlesnake with some cheese and then divided the mass into 100 pills, of which I took 1, 2, 3 or 4 pills a day. General dropsy succeeded the first state of heavenly sensations, which has not yet gone off, being March 1827, subject to swellings in the evening.]

'The diseases of the lymphatic and arterial systems are never benefitted by the use of rattlesnake poison, but the nervous and muscular systems are speedily aroused into action; palsy is much benefitted. Old rheumatisms are removed or relieved and passions of the mind are wonderfully excited; deliriums in typhus fever attended with muttering [typho-mania] is almost immediately cured and a serene mind and expressions of pleasure follows. Melancholy is quickly changed into gay anticipation. Old sores are injured. An idiot becomes improved in intellect.'

## MATERIA MEDICA CROTALUS HORRIDUS

### Sources
1 Proving Hering, 4 male provers, 1st and 2nd trits.; *c.* 1836.
2 Proving Hayward [UK] on self and 4 females, 1x, 1c, 3c; 1872, 1874, 1881, 1882.
3 Self-experimentation 35-year-old woman under guidance of Stokes [UK], 3x and 4x dils.; 1852.
4 Self-experimentation Hayward [UK] by rubbing a mixture of crotalus venom and glycerin into a small spot of denuded skin near left wrist; 1882.
5 Clinical observation Neidhard [USA], 1860.
6 Effects of bite; 20 cases in Hughes & Dake.
7 Clinical observations, in Hering.
8 Clinical observations Kent [USA].
9 Clinical observations Tyler [UK].
10 Clinical observations Mangialavori [Italy].
11 Clinical observations Farokh Master [India].
12 Clinical observations Annemarie Monahan [USA], 1990s.
13 Degroote, Dream Repertory.
14 Synthesis Repertory Treasure Edition 2009.

### Mind
∞ Excessively sensitive as to anything touching [heart-rending] in what he reads, moved to tears.[1]
∞ Depression and indifference to everything; as if only half alive.[1]
∞ Sensitive to noise and alarmed by it, e.g. crumpling up of paper or slamming of a door.[2]
∞ Mistakes in spelling familiar words.[1,4]
∞ Stupid: cannot express herself. Makes ridiculous mistakes.[9]
∞ Stupid, cannot add figures, makes mistakes in writing, transposes sentences, in words transposes letters. Unable to take care of own accounts, can't add up things that are at all particular.[8]
∞ Weakness of memory for words; word hunting.[10] Forgetful of words while speaking.[14]
∞ Weakness of memory for dates; expressing oneself; persons; places; proper names.[14]
∞ Torpid: sluggish: incoherent: hesitating.[9] Dullness with sleepiness.[14]
∞ Awaking in night struggling with imaginary foes; imagines himself surrounded by enemies or hideous animals.[7]
∞ Taking antipathies to members of family.[7]
∞ Ailments from grief; quarrels; quarrels in family.[10] Full of worries about relatives.[10]

∞ Delusions: Neglected; pursued by enemies.[10]
∞ Delusion everyone is an enemy[13]; surrounded by enemies[14].
∞ Forsaken feeling. Jealousy. Suspicion.[10]
∞ Strong ego-related issues with great aversion to family members. Cannot trust society; feels that family members are out to get him; feels betrayed or victimised by family. Does not have the security of home or family as they shun their family members. In some cases there may be a strong emotional bonding with members of the family. They are so attached to their mother or father that they cannot connect with their partner [Mother complex].[11]
∞ Dreadfully irritable and cross, so that least annoyance sends her into a fury.[2]
∞ Irritable, cross, infuriated by least annoyance.[8]
∞ Nervous: excitable: discontented with himself. Fits of rage, despair, cursing maledictions.[9]
∞ Snappish temper.[9]
∞ Bad temper, blows up, explodes; flaring quickly, calming down quickly; can be nasty behind people's back, but doesn't attack them directly.[12]
∞ Fear of going over bridges; afraid of going to fly off into the air.[12]
∞ Fear of losing one's hands; nightmares of having them cut off.[12]
∞ Irritability and discontentment 3–4 days before menses.[12]
∞ Claustrophobic in closed rooms; must have window open.[12]
∞ Ambition, striving for recognition.[13]
∞ Sadness > eating.[13]
∞ Fears: high places; males; rain; riding.[13]
∞ Everybody must hurry.[13]
∞ Jealousy, interrupts others.[13]
∞ Aversion being laughed at.[13]
∞ Monologue, speaks alone, does all the talking; one-man show.[13]
∞ Anxiety driving from place to place; with pale face; with cold sweat on face; with faintness.[14]
∞ Aphasia after apoplexy.[14] Muttering, in apoplexy.[14]
∞ Speech confused, disconnected, plaintive.[14]
∞ Aversion to family members in incipient stage of dementia.[14] Dementia senilis.[14] Forgetfulness of old people.[14]
∞ Confusion of mind, in morning.[14] Weeping when questioned.[14]
∞ Delusions: brain intoxicated by degraded blood; being an outcast; someone behind him; being persecuted.[14]
∞ Fears: hearing bad news; evil; faces looking at him; failure; misfortune; open spaces; people; walking across busy streets.[14]

## Dreams
∞ Attack is the best form of defence, verbally.[13]
∞ Baby murdered before mother's eyes.[2]
∞ Bad news, getting; of people or loved ones having died [accident, disease or murder].[13]
∞ Being a white hawk cut into pieces.[5]
∞ Betrayal.[13]

∞ Bleeding.[13]
∞ Car driving backward; in wrong direction.[13]
∞ Cares, worries, anticipating negative events.[13]
∞ Caught, being.[13]
∞ Clothes ill-fitting, too wide or too tight.[13]
∞ Communicating with a dead relative.[13]
∞ Danger, impending.[13]
∞ Death of relatives.[13]
∞ Digging graves.[13]
∞ Disease – cancer; myocardial infarction; paralysis; pustules.[13]
∞ Domination.[13]
∞ Envy.[13]
∞ Escaping from danger, of being beaten; of being killed.[13]
∞ Falling, backward; from a height; into a deep pit; into water.[13]
∞ Feet growing into 2 hickories.[5]
∞ Being or feeling forsaken; feeling of being excluded; being repudiated.[7]
∞ Funeral procession, coffin being carried.[13]
∞ Furiously angry.[13]
∞ Having broken with his father, who would no longer recognise him as his son.[1]
∞ Hiding; seeking cover, behind bushes, escapes in crowd, behind someone, under stairs.[13]
∞ Horrible dreams of murder, death, dead bodies and dead people, associating with the dead and with corpses, being in graveyards; even the smell of the cadaver is dreamed of.[8]
∞ Horrid places, of rolling amongst old rocks.[5]
∞ Injustice, being unjustly treated.[13]
∞ Looking for a toilet to urinate.[13]
∞ Nakedness.[13]
∞ One leg alive, the other dead.[13]
∞ Pursued, being; by police; to be killed; for kidnap; for rape.[13]
∞ Quarreling and fighting.[1]
∞ Remembering having forgotten something.[13]
∞ Self or family members exposed to difficulties and dangers.[2]
∞ Sexual obtrusiveness.[13]
∞ Threat of rape.[13]
∞ Threatened, being or feeling; animals; gun; knives; man.[13]
∞ Traveling about all over the world.[1]

## Generals
∞ Sleep alternates with long and tedious periods of wakefulness.[8]
∞ Sleep position on back with knees bent; with head backwards; sheet must touch chin.[13] Lies motionless.[13]
∞ Constant thirst for cold water.[5]
∞ Insatiable thirst; drinking cold water every few minutes.[6]
∞ Craving for stimulants, esp. wine[4]; fat, pork[7]; ice cream, meat[10]; brandy, pungent, spicy, sugar[7]; red meat[12].

∞ Red wine <.[6] Coffee >.[7]
∞ Profound prostration; can hardly raise himself from bed.[6]
∞ Easily tired by slight exertion.[3] Fatigued by standing up; tremulous weakness all over, as if some evil were apprehended.[3]
∞ Pleasure in exertion.[4]
∞ Swelling all over; eyes almost closed with swelling of face; tongue swollen, swallowing and talking difficult.[6]
∞ Intense restlessness, cannot sit, lie or stand, only pace up and down the house.[6]
∞ Pains burning.[6]
∞ Great chilliness; cold skin; cold sweat.[6]
∞ Very warm; sleeps naked with window open in winter.[12]
∞ Disturbed by any change to warm weather.[8]
∞ Clothing as if too tight, > loosening it.[10]
∞ Before menses <.[10]
∞ Sexual excitement during daytime only, although without any erection.[1]
∞ Sepsis. Felons, pemphigus, pustules, boils, carbuncle, furuncle, gangrene, abscesses, etc., when fever is low, parts bluish, discharges scanty, tarry or dark fluid, unhealthy.[9]
∞ Boils, carbuncles and eruptions surrounded by a purplish condition of skin – mottled – blue – or marbled. With burning and violent pains: the peculiar feature is the doughy centre. Around the boil or carbuncle for many inches, oedema, pitting on pressure.[8]
∞ Ailments from chemotherapy.[13]
∞ Flushes of heat upward from abdomen.[13]
∞ Giving blood, as blood donor >.[13]
∞ Prolonged bleeding after injuries.[14]

## Sensations
∞ Beaten all over in morning on awaking; can hardly muster up courage to rise.[1]
∞ Brain as if drawn together and lying loose within skull, falling about on moving head.[2]
∞ Attacks of lightheadedness, with sensation as if falling over a precipice.[5]
∞ Pain in eyeballs on moving eyes, as if orbits were dry inside.[1]
∞ Pressure in eyes as if eyes would be pushed out from head.[8]
∞ Letters as if double, horizontally.[2]
∞ Right ear as if stopped up.[1]
∞ Drawing in ears as if earwax were passing through Eustachian tubes into mouth.[1]
∞ Soft palate as if stiff and too long and fauces as if lined with mucus.[2]
∞ Tongue as if thick.[14]
∞ Left jaw as if paralysed.[1]
∞ Right lower jaw and teeth as if crushed.[1]
∞ Plug in throat; sensation of contraction or choking.[7]
∞ Weight on stomach and chest; breakfast lies heavy all day.[3]
∞ Stomach as if empty, during menopause.[14]
∞ Quivering in epigastrium, & nausea.[4]

∞ Coldness as from a piece of ice in stomach or abdomen.[8]

∞ Chest as if encaged.[13]

∞ Heart as if tumbling about, & flushing of heat throughout body, and heat and itching of palms.[2]

∞ Heart as if jumping out or tumbling over, & general feeling of weakness.[2]

∞ Muscles from right shoulder to nape of neck as if stretched and torn out, < moving arm backwards.[1]

∞ Weight in arms and legs, as if bones were made of heavy wood.[1]

∞ Arms, fingers and legs as if paralysed.[1]

∞ Numbness arms in morning.[3]

∞ Numbness and tingling of legs when sitting.[3]

∞ Tendons in right leg as if drawn up from sole through leg, drawing foot up.[1]

∞ Leaden weight in right foot.[1]

∞ Pain in sole near heel as if having trodden on something sharp with bare feet.[1]

## Locals

∞ Dizziness with tinnitus; pale face; headache; dilated pupils; staggering; vomiting.[14]

∞ Dizziness after fright; from lightning; must lie down; during menopause; < motion; with nausea; occipital; < sitting; > walking in open air.[14] Ménière's disease.[14]

∞ Headache above eyes and in temples, worse on right side, & nausea, vomiting of bile, and constipation; must lie down; > walking in open air.[1]

∞ Headache with surging in waves and excited by motion or jar, by turning over in bed, by rising up in bed, or by lying down. Change of position will cause this surging.[8]

∞ Dull frontal headache > nosebleed.[5]

∞ Headache with confusion, unable to collect one's senses.[14]

∞ Headache < fasting; < jar; > walking on tips of toes.[14]

∞ Congestion/heaviness head < before menses; < mental exertion.[14]

∞ Tension and pressure on top of head ext. to ears.[5]

∞ Pressing pain in vertex, with heat and flushing if face.[3]

∞ Pressing pain in eyes < motion of eyes.[14]

∞ Fading of eyesight by reading.[1,2]

∞ Eyelids swollen in morning.[14]

∞ Dimness vision, esp. for distant objects; 'could scarcely recognise face of friends across street'.[2] Vision blurred/dim during headache; < wet weather.[14]

∞ Loss of vision from exertion; from grief; < reading; from retinal haemorrhage; < wet weather.[14]

∞ Noises in ears from belching; < lying on ear.[13]

∞ Internal ears sensitive to wind.[13]

∞ Much sneezing and catarrhal irritation in nose & faint, sinking feeling in epigastrium.[4]

∞ Epistaxis < blowing nose; during headache.[14]

∞ Epistaxis during coryza or when having a temper tantrum.[12]

∞ Paralysis of tongue after apoplexy.[14] Speech wanting from paralysis of organs.[14]

∞ Choking on going to sleep.[14]

∞ Throatache < cold air; < empty swallowing; on waking.[14]

∞ Sour, acrid eructations after white bread.[1]

∞ Nausea on brushing teeth; < lying on right side.[14]

∞ Vomiting on least exertion.[6] Vomiting freely, incessantly.[6]

∞ Vomiting, vomitus black, blood, like coffee grounds, dark green.[14]

∞ Intolerance of clothing round stomach and below right hypochondrium.[1]

∞ Hiccough from laughing.[13]

∞ Pain abdomen > lying on abdomen.[13]

∞ Diarrhoea from septic conditions.[14]

∞ Urinary incontinence, loss of urine while vomiting.[14]

∞ Menses [one week] too early, preceded by weight in head and ears.[3]

∞ Aching pain in centre of chest to back, shooting to arms and back of head, and whole spine.[5]

∞ Soreness heart on turning to lie on left side.[2,4]

∞ Pain heart during painful menses.[14]

∞ Heart palpitations before and during menses; during menopause.[14]

∞ Respiration difficult, with or from dryness of mouth; from laughing; when sitting[13]; when falling asleep[14].

∞ Cough from excitement.[13]

∞ Bruised pain in scapulae on moving arms backwards.[1]

∞ Lumbar backache compelling to walk bent.[13]

∞ Oedematous swelling limbs.[14]

∞ Trembling hands on moving them.[8]

∞ Pain in bones of legs, < night.[5]

∞ Quick numbness legs on crossing them.[1]

## Dull & Stupid

Experimenting in the same way as he had done on himself, Hayward applied on a Sunday afternoon a tiny amount of a mixture of rattlesnake venom and glycerin to a denuded spot near the wrist of a young woman, who: 'Slept as usual, and awoke on Monday without either giddiness or heaviness of head, but after breakfast noticed that I could not think, comprehend, or remember distinctly; could not as usual hold my mind to a subject; and all forenoon could not as usual comprehend or follow conversation; indeed, appeared so dull and stupid that my sister laughed at me; perception appeared clouded, so that on walking in the street I would have been run over but for my sister's watchfulness; memory was so affected that after getting into a shop I found I had forgotten what I had gone for.' [cited in Hughes]

# CROTALUS LEPIDUS

## Synonyms

- Scientific name: Crotalus lepidus [Kennicott, 1861].
- Synonym: Crotalus semicornutus [Taylor, 1944].

- Common names: Rock rattlesnake. Green rattlesnake. Blue rattlesnake.
- Family: Viperidae, subfamily Crotalinae.

## Biological Profile
- Small to medium-sized, fairly stout-bodied, venomous pit viper with broad, triangular head on slender neck. Average length 50–70 cm, maximum 85 cm.
- Body colours and patterns extremely variable; body usually greenish, olive, reddish-brown, light brown, grey or pinkish-grey; dorsal pattern usually has dark, laterally expanded blotches [often white-edged] that may form complete cross-bands. Belly lighter, usually with various amounts of darker grey mottling. Tail bright yellow in juveniles and salmon or peach in adults.
- Range: Found from SE Arizona, southern New Mexico to the Edwards plateau in central Texas, then south to south-central Mexico [Jalisco].
- Habitat: Variable; incl. pine-oak forest, scrub and cactus grasslands, and Chihuahuan desert, often associated with mountains and rugged broken terrain in the vicinity of rocky outcroppings and slides. In forests, usually found in open or barren rocky areas subject to intense sunlight.
- Terrestrial. Primarily diurnal but can be active at any time of the day or night when conditions are favourable.
- Ovoviviparous; 3–9 live young per brood.
- Preys on a wide variety of available arthropods [grasshoppers, caterpillars], lizards, small mammals, and birds.
- Males participate in ritualised combat, described as 'a form of aggression for social communication'.
- Easily excited and nervous, this snake can quickly assume a defensive posture and will strike if molested or stepped on.
- Three recognized subspecies [klauberi, lepidus, maculosus].
- Two subspecies, Crotalus lepidus lepidus and Crotalus lepidus klauberi, are frequently available in the exotic animal trade and are well represented in zoos around the world. They are sought after for their wide array of potential colourations, and typically docile nature. The other subspecies is not often found in captivity outside of Mexico.


## MATERIA MEDICA CROTALUS LEPIDUS

### Sources
1 Effects of bite; clinical manifestations.

### Clinical Manifestations
Venom mainly haemotoxic, also with presynaptically acting neurotoxins.

Serious human envenomations and deaths have been reported. Envenomation symptoms may include: intense burning pain at bite site with rapid progression of pain, swelling and discolouration up the bitten limb, nausea, blistering, malaise, dizziness, and sometimes heart or breathing problems.

## Searing Pain

Bitten by a juvenile female Crotalus lepidus klauberi [banded rock rattlesnake].

∞ Pain escalates to a constant, searing pain.

∞ Bite area feels as though it is submerged in boiling oil, there is NO relief from the pain. Pain constant and intense.

∞ Numbness, on lying down, as if entire body were 'falling asleep', from head to toe.

∞ Dyspnoea; inability to pass air into lungs, as if a 200 pound weight were placed on the chest.

∞ Black out in bath. Believes he is 'not going to make it,' followed by loss of bowel control.

∞ Loss of consciousness.

∞ Blood pressure 60/40.

∞ Extreme pain from thumb engulfing hand and extending upward to rest of arm.

∞ Arm swollen to 3 times its normal size.

∞ Freezing cold [96°F–35.5°C] and very, very weak.

∞ Fears death is soon to happen.

∞ Despite being wrapped in 2 heating blankets to stop the violent shaking, insists the room is freezing cold.

∞ Thumb black, discoloured, starting to rot. Eventually fingernail falls off, as well as an area of dead tissue.

∞ Sequelae: Severe allergy to rattlesnake musk – eyes swelling shut, nose running profusely.

∞ Spontaneous bruises on body, several months after incident.

[Bear, 2008]

# CROTALUS MITCHELLII

## Synonyms
- Scientific name: Crotalus mitchellii [Cope, 1861].
- Synonym: Crotalus aureus [Kallert, 1927].
- Common names: Speckled rattlesnake. Bleached rattlesnake.
- Family: Viperidae, subfamily Crotalinae.

## Biological Profile
- Medium-large, fairly stout venomous pit viper. Average length 90–100 cm, maximum 1.3 m.
- Body colours and pattern extremely variable, usually brownish to greenish-brown, with 23–46 irregular [often interrupted] darker cross-bands, rather than blotches. Colour often matches the earth tones of the rocks and soil it inhabits. Belly lighter with darker mottling. Tail with 3–9 widely-spaced dark cross-bands, each band widest dorsally, basal rattle segment black.
- Range: Southwestern USA and NW Mexico.

- Habitat: Found most commonly inhabiting rocky hillsides, rock ledges and canyons; in desert scrub, Joshua tree, and pinon-juniper woodlands. It also occurs in low shrub areas, tropical deciduous forest, and pine-oak forest in the northern part of its range. Found up to 2,400 m elevation.
- Mainly terrestrial and like many other snakes, diurnal in cool weather, in spring and fall, and nocturnal when it gets hot. Activity peaks during late summer rainy season. Hibernates during cold months of late fall and winter.
- While usually solitary in summer, speckled rattlesnakes often congregate at suitable hibernation dens, which may contain as many as 20 to 180 snakes.
- Ovoviviparous; 1–8 live young per brood.
- Preys on lizards, small mammals, and occasionally on birds.
- Very nervous and quick to strike if disturbed even slightly.
- No subspecies.


## MATERIA MEDICA CROTALUS MITCHELLII

### Sources
1 Effects of bite; clinical manifestations.

### Clinical Manifestations
Venom mainly haemotoxic with potent tissue-necrotic factors, but lacking significant haemorrhagic activity.


# CROTALUS MOLOSSUS

### Synonyms
- Scientific name: Crotalus molossus [Baird & Girard, 1853].
- Common names: Black-tailed rattlesnake. Western blacktail rattlesnake.
- Family: Viperidae, subfamily Crotalinae.

### Biological Profile
- Large, heavy-bodied venomous pit viper. Average length 80–100 cm, maximum 1.4 m.
- Body colour and pattern extremely variable; dorsal body usually tan, brownish-olive or greyish-brown with 24–34 dark-brown diamond-like blotches, yellowish-edged [rarely all black, dorsally]. Belly cream to pale yellow with lateral dark mottling. Tail entirely black.
- Range: SW USA and Mexico.
- Found mainly in pine-oak forest, tropical deciduous forest, grassy hillsides, scrub and cactus areas, and upland Sonoran desert; often associated with rocky areas such as cliffs and rock slides along streams. Occurs from sea level to 2,930 m elevation.
- Mainly nocturnal, but also active at dusk and dawn.

- Semi-arboreal, often climbs into low bushes and trees up to height of several metres.
- Able swimmer.
- After mating occurs, the male remains with the female to guard her from other prospective mates. This species appears to have a monogamous mating system.
- Ovoviviparous; 3–16 live young per brood.
- Preys predominantly on lizards [incl. Gila monsters], mammals and birds.
- Temperament variable but considered by Greene [1997] as 'unusually mild-mannered as far as rattlesnakes go.' If threatened, and with no ready escape route, usually coils with head and neck thrown back in a horizontal S-shaped loop, hisses, rattles, and strikes if further molested.
- Three recognized subspecies [molossus, nigrescens, oaxacus].

## MATERIA MEDICA CROTALUS MOLOSSUS

### Sources
1 Effects of bite; clinical manifestations.

### Clinical Manifestations
Not well known, large venom yield, but no human deaths have been reported, so far. Venom mainly haemotoxic; may also have potent necrotic factors. Can be very painful at bite site with swelling and necrosis.

# CROTALUS POLYSTICTUS

### Synonyms
- Scientific name: Crotalus polystictus [Cope, 1865].
- Common name: Mexican lance-headed rattlesnake.
- Family: Viperidae, subfamily Crotalinae.

### Biological Profile
- Small to medium-sized, heavy-bodied venomous pit viper. Average length 70–80 cm, maximum 1 m.
- Body usually pale [grey, buff, tan, or light brown] with 30–47 closely spaced dark-brown rounded-elongated dorsal blotches; looks "giraffe-like". Head unusually slender. Belly white at front, stippled with dark-brown at middle of each ventral scale, darker toward tail. Tail yellowish with 4–7 dark brown dorsal cross-bands and brownish ventral spots.
- A sexually dimorphic species, males tend to have a larger head, which correlates to their preference for preying upon larger mammals. Smaller-headed females tend to seek out smaller prey.
- Range: Central Mexico.
- Habitat: Broad valleys, plains, and meadows at 1450–2600 m elevation. Prefers rocky situations with an abundance of tall grass.

- Mainly terrestrial; occupies rodent burrows.
- Reportedly swims readily and very well, which has earned it the name 'aquatic rattlesnake'.
- Preys on amphibians, small mammals and lizards.
- Ovoviviparous; average of 8 live young per brood.
- No subspecies.
- Specific epithet polystictus means 'many spots'.

## Behaviour & Temperament
'Crotalus polystictus is found rather commonly in late spring when summer rains have not yet been sufficiently heavy to contribute to growth of grass cover. During this period, they become somewhat nocturnal, active individuals having been recorded as late as 10 p.m. In late spring, C. polystictus displays a rather *mild disposition* and is usually quite *inoffensive*. Some specimens have been observed attempting to hide their heads beneath a coil of their body. During the summer, this species becomes much more *aggressive* and will generally not retreat when approached. We observed an individual, which upon discovery opened its mouth in a threatening pose similar to the behaviour exhibited by Agkistrodon piscivorus. Lampropeltis triangulum, a harmless colubrid snake, is common in the vicinity of the Nevado de Colima, and may be an important predator upon these rattlesnakes.' [Armstrong & Murphy, 1979]

## Postpartum Cannibalism
Cannibalism is a common phenomenon and has been reported from diverse animal species. Maternal cannibalism involves the consumption of offspring by the female parent and can be further categorised as either the consumption of non-viable offspring [eggs, undeveloped ova or stillborn neonates] or of living offspring.

Maternal cannibalism has been described from a number of animal species, incl. numerous reptiles. A Mexican-American research team produced the first quantitative description of cannibalism among female Crotalus polystictus rattlesnakes after monitoring 190 reptiles with 239 litters over a period of 4 years. The study demonstrates that 68% of post-parturient females ingested some or all of the non-viable offspring available to them. Most snakes [83%] consumed all non-viable offspring available; snakes consumed a mean of 92% of the available mass.

The consumption of non-viable offspring by female rattlesnakes may be important in allowing a rapid recuperation of some of the considerable energetic and physiological costs of reproduction. According to the scientists, cannibalism is "not an aberrant behaviour, and is not an attack on the progeny," since it does not involve live elements. It simply recovers some of what the snake invested in the reproduction process and prepares it to reproduce once again.

Whereas the consumption of non-viable offspring may be a simple outgrowth of normal rattlesnake feeding behaviour, i.e. consumption of carrion, the study provides strong support for the primacy of the maternal recovery hypothesis.

'Reproduction imposes high energetic costs on female snakes, especially in viviparous species. Rapid replenishment of energy stores may be particularly important to annually reproducing snakes. Furthermore, recycling energy invested in non-viable offspring allows females to accelerate recovery from the structural and functional losses induced by reproduction. Snakes were most likely to cannibalise when litters contained large proportions of non-viable offspring, as predicted. In addition, snakes that gave birth later in the year were more likely to cannibalise offspring than were snakes that gave birth earlier.' [Mocino-Deloya, 2009]

## MATERIA MEDICA CROTALUS POLYSTICTUS

### Sources
1 Effects of bite; clinical manifestations.

### Clinical Manifestations
Venom mainly haemotoxic and probably with necrotic factors. Envenomation results in severe symptoms. Local effects consist of swelling, ecchymosis and pain; other effects main include muscle twitching, numbness, and blebs. Thrombocytopenia, hypofibrinogenemia [deficiency of blood clotting factor], and necrosis have been observed.

# CROTALUS VIRIDIS

### Systematics
- Scientific name: Crotalus viridis [Rafinesque, 1818].
- Subspecies: C. v. viridis [Rafinesque, 1818].
- Common names: Prairie rattlesnake. Great Plains rattlesnake.
- Family: Viperidae, subfamily Crotalinae.

### Biological Profile
- Large, heavy-bodied, terrestrial venomous pit viper with large, triangular head on relatively thin neck. Average length 1 m, maximum 1.6 m; island populations mostly less than 70 cm long.
- Body variable: pale tan, dark brown, pinkish or greenish; with 33–57 dark brown mid-dorsal blotches [lighter in centre] and smaller lateral blotches. Head with 2 thin white lateral lines, upper one extends through the eye, or from the eye rearward. Belly nearly all whitish to pale grey.
- Range: From southern Canada, over much of the Great Plains of the USA and into northern Mexico.
- Habitat: Found in widely variable habitats, mainly in mesquite and brush covered grasslands and deserts; also pine-oak forest. Often found in brush-covered rocky canyons, rocky crevices, and sandy fields along the coast. May shelter in vegetation clumps and animal burrows. Often found near human habitations. Found up to 2,500 m elevation.

- Diurnal in spring and fall, prowling in morning and in late afternoon or evening; nocturnal during summer, but populations at higher altitudes seem also to be more active during daytime in the summer.
- Preys on small mammals, ground nesting birds and their eggs, toads and lizards; may sometimes be cannibalistic.
- May migrate long distances to and from the winter den in the spring and fall; radio-tagged males and post-gravid females have been found to travel up to 24 km from their dens.
- Congregates at hibernation sites for overwintering.
- Female snakes considered monogamous during a single season but will seek out a different mate the following season.
- Ovoviviparous; 3–21 live young per brood.
- Males take part in combat dominance bouts.
- Pugnacious; coils and strikes with *little provocation*. If threatened, and with no ready escape route, will usually coil with head and neck thrown back in S-shaped loop, and may strike if further molested. If forcibly restrained, a prairie rattlesnake bites, rattles, and discharges the cloacal scent glands in a fine spray.
- The previously recognized 9 subspecies have been reduced to 2 due to taxonomic revision of the species. Crotalus viridis has now 2 subspecies, while the remaining 7 subspecies are all part of Crotalus oreganus, with the common name Western rattlesnake. An even more drastic revision in 2007 suggests elevating all 7 subspecies of C. oreganus to species level.

## Social Life

Gravid females aggregate in communal birthing rookeries [maternity colonies] until parturition. Following parturition, females and neonates remain together at the rookery for several days before dispersing. It has been suggested that these postpartum aggregations allow neonates to recognise con-specific odours that are later used for finding their ancestral winter dens. Both newborn timber rattlesnakes and prairie rattlesnakes are able to follow con-specific odour trails.

Social life in snakes has not been studied extensively, but recent research indicates that complex social systems might be rather widespread in snakes. At least 3 Crotalinae species display well-developed maternal attendance and togetherness, dispelling the stereotype of snakes as antisocial, cold-blooded loners. These species include Crotalus horridus, Crotalus viridis, and Agkistrodon [Cenchris] contortrix. Females of these species seem to bond more than males. Such closeness particularly occurs in connection with pregnancy and birth. Aside from sharing maternity colonies and basking together, prairie rattlesnakes have also been shown to mobilise a group defense, mediated, in part, by alarm pheromones.

*See* Crotalus horridus, Social life.

## Sources
1 Effects of bite; clinical manifestations.

## Clinical Manifestations
Venom haemotoxic with potent necrotic factors; reportedly also has pre-synaptically acting neurotoxins.

A potent platelet aggregation inhibitor [anticoagulant], named crotavirin, has been purified from the venom. Envenomation symptoms usually include intense pain at the bite site with rapid progression of local swelling, discolouration and tissue necrosis; may also cause nausea, disorientation and cardiac or respiratory problems. Neurological symptoms may be paralytic in nature, although not as severe as those resulting from bites by the Mojave rattlesnake, Crotalus scutulatus, or the South American rattlesnake C. durissus.

Russell [1980] reported that the bite produces pronounced changes in consciousness, profuse weakness, sweating, respiratory difficulties, and tingling or numbness over the bitten area and over the tongue, mouth, and scalp.

## Aphasia & Alesia
Marvin Cole, MD, reported the case of a 43-year-old white man who was admitted to the hospital following 2 generalised convulsions. There was no history of cardiac disease. Two days prior to the convulsions he was bitten by a prairie rattlesnake, Crotalus viridis viridis.

He had Wernicke aphasia, alexia [loss of ability to read, also called word blindness], right inferior quadrantanopia [loss of vision in a quarter section of the visual field], right central facial weakness, and weakness of his right lower extremity. There were no bruits or any other neurological findings. [Cole, 1996]

*Wernicke's aphasia,* also known as reflective aphasia, fluent aphasia, or sensory aphasia, is characterised by: 'Speech is preserved, but language content is incorrect. This may vary from the insertion of a few incorrect or non-existent words to a profuse outpouring of jargon. Grammar, syntax, rate, intonation and stress are normal. Substitutions of one word for another [paraphasias, e.g. "telephone" for "television"] are common. Comprehension and repetition are poor. Patients who recover from Wernicke's aphasia report that, while aphasic, they found the speech of others to be unintelligible and, despite being cognizant of that fact that they were speaking, they could neither stop themselves nor understand their own words.' [Wikipedia]

# DEINAGKISTRODON ACUTUS

## Synonyms
- Scientific name: Deinagkistrodon acutus [Günther, 1888].
- Synonym: Agkistrodon acutus [Namiye, 1908].

- Common names: Sharp-nosed pit viper. Hundred-pace pit viper. Chinese moccasin.
- Family: Viperidae, subfamily Crotalinae.

## Biological Profile
- Medium-sized, fairly stout-bodied, venomous pit viper. Average length 1 m, maximum 1.5 m.
- Ground colour greyish or reddish brown, overlaid with a series of brown or reddish brown lateral triangles with grey or beige centres. Pointed tops of 2 opposite triangles join mid-dorsally, creating an effect of alternating triangles of different colours. Head dark brown on top, beige or pinkish on the sides. Snout ends in an upturned pointed appendage with large shields on the crown.
- Range: Taiwan, China, northern Vietnam.
- Habitat: Forested mountain slopes, rock-strewn hillsides; often found on rocks in mountain streams.
- Very active in evening and on rainy or cloudy days. Hides on warm days coiled in sheltering rock ledges, among fallen leaves or bracken, in hollow logs and other places where its colour pattern keeps it camouflaged.
- Preys on small mammals, birds, and amphibians.
- Oviparous; up to 24 eggs per clutch. Female guards and incubates eggs, abandoning her young about 24–30 days after they hatch.

## Creation Myth
The Paiwan people, an aboriginal tribe of Taiwan [known formerly as Formosa] call themselves the 'descendants of the paipushe snake'. The paipushe, meaning 'one hundred paces', is the sacred animal that played a central role in their creation myth. The myth holds that the Paiwan people were hatched from 2 eggs laid by the sun and kept in a ceramic pot guarded by the paipushe. The snake is revered and protected despite its lethality. The snake, it is believed, protects the Paiwan from difficulties, sufferings, and misfortune. A totem revered and worshipped; the snake becomes their spiritual faith. The Paiwan neither eat snakes nor injure them. According to Paiwan beliefs, the only way human beings can live safely on this earth is in a long-term relationship of friendship, mutual sacrifice and mutual support with the paipushe snake.

Paipushe motifs are carved or painted on houses, ancestors' spirit posts, weapons, and various kinds of utensils. When facing or using them, any form of disrespect or vulgarity in behaviour or speech is taboo.

Mark Cherrington, editor of Cultural Survival Quarterly, reports that 'Every Paiwan household has one of these large ceramic pots; it is used to hold sacred items and is seen as the embodiment of the culture and the repository of its history. There are male and female versions of the pots, with female pots having 2 protruding nipples and male pots featuring an inscribed image of the viper. When a child leaves the household to be married, the mother will break off a piece of the pot's mouth and give it to child to keep in his or her home. Then, when the first grandchild is born, the child returns the pot fragment to the mother, who glues it back in place to symbolically integrate the new generation into the family and the tribe.' [Cultural Survival Quarterly, Winter 2008]

## Sign of Distinction

Discussing Paiwan aesthetics and performances in Taiwan, Hu Tai-li writes that 'the hundred-pace snake is often considered the ancestor of the chief's family. Originally *'vetsik'* referred to the triangular design on the body of the hundred-pace snake. From the study of Tingrwei Ho we know that in the past only the members of a chief's family had the right to wear tattoos, that is, to impose the designs [*vetsik*] of the hundred-pace snake and sometimes of ancestral heads on the back of the hands [for females], the arm, chest and back [for males]. In other words, the chief's family identify with their ancestral hundred-pace snake by putting simplified designs of the snake on their bodies. The emphasis on dressing in splendid costumes and decorations is an extension of imposing the *'vetsik'* on the body.

'The Paiwan people, especially of chieftain families, wish to be filmed with *'vetsik'* on their clothes and head ornaments. In the legends, the hundred-pace snake transforms into a Hodgson's hawk eagle, which has the same triangular design [vetsik] on the feathers of its wings. The 4 feathers with clearest *vetsik* on each wing of the Hodgson's hawk eagle are exclusively used as head ornaments of the chief. When members of the chief's family wear splendid clothes with *vetsik*, they are more closely identified with the gods and ancestors. When people see the *vetsik* on clothes, they immediately think of the sacred origin of the chief's family, and the emotion of thoughtful sorrow reconfirms the chief's ritual authority. . . . The Paiwan people not only imitate the designs [*vetsik*] but also the "sound" of the hundred-pace snake, Both designs and sounds catalyze the emotions and aesthetics of thoughtful sorrow. . . . "Becoming a hundred-pace snake" is the core metaphor of Paiwan aesthetics.' [Stewart & Strathern, 2005]

'To mark the advent of the Year of the Snake, Taiuan Publishing invited the Taiwanese public to vote for native animals to represent the 12 creatures of the Chinese zodiac. Although Taiwan has over 50 snake species, by far the most popular choice for the snake was the hundred-pace viper. . . .

'Other Taiwanese aboriginal peoples with a close relationship to the hundred-pacer are the Bunun and the Rukai. The Bunun call the snake *kaviiad*, meaning "friend." According to Bunun lore, if one meets a hundred-pacer one need only wave a red cloth at it and it will go away. . . .

'However, among the Han Chinese, the hundred-pace viper is seen merely as a first-rate tonic medicine to boost male sexual powers. Paiwan poet Monaneng has written: "The hundred-pacer is dead; / They've put it in a big transparent medicine jar / With 'aphrodisiac' on the label, / To tempt men wandering among back street red lights. / The hundred-pacer of our fairytales is dead; / We Paiwan worshipped its eggs as our ancestors, / But now they've put it in a medicine jar / As a tool to excite urban lust." . . .

'One mountain lover who often encounters snakes on his hiking expeditions describes the hundred-pacer as "cool, calm and collected," and people who have kept or observed hundred-pacers also say they "don't lash out blindly." Hu Tai-li describes them as "really the chieftain among snakes – they have a serene, tolerant nature, and are not apt to attack people wantonly." Perhaps it is because of this regal temperament that they are revered as ancestral spirits by the Paiwan. . . .

'Perhaps in this Year of the Snake, the hundred-pacer, just like the Paiwan people who also still live in close communion with nature, is singing us some long-forgotten songs of life-if only you are willing to listen with your soul.' [Chang Chin-ju, King of Taiwan's Snakes: The Hundred-Pace Viper; www.taiwan-panorama.com]

## Food & Medicine
Used in Vietnam and China for food and in traditional medicine. In China it is believed that liquor infused with hundred-pace vipers can detoxify the body and strengthen the kidneys. Hundred-pace viper spirits are used to remedy impotence, bronchitis, and various skin complaints.


## MATERIA MEDICA DEINAGKISTRODON ACUTUS

### Sources
1 Effects of bite; clinical manifestations.

### Clinical Manifestations
Potent haemotoxin; strongly haemorrhagic. Envenomation symptoms include severe local pain and bleeding, which may begin almost immediately, followed by serious swelling, blistering, necrosis, and ulceration. Systemic symptoms may occur early and suddenly, and often include heart palpitations. Variable non-specific effects which may include headache, nausea, vomiting, abdominal pain, diarrhoea, dizziness, collapse or convulsions The popular name 'hundred pacer' refers to a local belief that, after being bitten, the victim will only be able to walk 100 paces before expiring. In areas where the snake is regarded as even more venomous, it has been called the 'fifty pacer'.

Swelling subsides in about 12 days, but necrosis may take months to heal. In 8% of cases necrosis requires amputation of digits or limbs. Local bruising, initially around the site of the bite, may extend up the bitten limb in 60% of cases with development of large haematomas in severe cases. Spontaneous systemic bleeding is common; sites of bleeding include nose, gums, urinary tract, old wounds, and bite sites. Persistent bleeding has resulted in severe anaemia. Petechiae have been described on the limbs, face, and oral mucosa.

Acuthrombin-B, a thrombin-like enzyme from the venom, has been used clinically in China for the treatment of *acute cerebral infarction*.

# LACHESIS ACROCHORDA

## Systematics
- Scientific name: Lachesis acrochorda [Garcia, 1896].
- Synonym: Bothrops achrochordus [Garcia, 1896].
- Common names: Chocoan bushmaster. Verrugosa. Diamante. Mapana rayo. Verrugosa del Choco. Pudridora
- Family: Viperidae, subfamily Crotalinae.

## Biological Profile
- Very large, relatively slender, big-headed terrestrial pit viper, usually 1.8–2.3 m long, with a pronounced mid-dorsal ridge and a yellowish-brown to reddish-tan body. Dorsal scales heavily keeled and protuberant. Head reddish or brown with dark spots; belly white or cream with small darker blotches along sides.
- Range: Found on both Atlantic & Pacific slopes of eastern Panama and western Colombia, then south along the pacific slope into northwestern Ecuador.
- Habitat: Found predominantly in tropical wet and moist forests with annual rainfall of 2.5–6.0 m.
- Mainly nocturnal, inactive during day. Usually hides under logs, in rodent burrows or rock crevices.
- Preys mainly on small mammals and birds.
- Males engage in ritual combat during the mating season.
- Oviparous, females often remain coiled around or on their clutch [up to 10 eggs].
- Four species of Lachesis are currently recognized: Lachesis muta, from the Amazon Basin, the Guianas and the Brazilian Atlantic forest; Lachesis melanocephala, from the southern Pacific versant of Costa Rica; Lachesis stenophrys, from the Atlantic versant of Costa Rica, western Panama and southern Nicaragua; and Lachesis acrochorda, from eastern Panama and the northwestern parts of South America [W. Colombia incl. Magdalena and Cauca Valleys and the forests of Chocó].

## Identity
The sparse information we have about this snake comes from S.B. Higgins, whose quasi-scientific work *Ophidians* [1873] served as an important reference for snake remedies in the days of Hering and Allen. [*See* also Bothrops asper and Vipera Lachesis fel.]

Unfortunately, Higgins' understanding of the rules of nomenclature was problematic and confused, resulting in a curious mingling of pretentious but invalid Latin names and local lingo. Some of these names cannot be traced back; for example, what to think of 'Vipera Calamaris venenosus rubrum'? Other names are easier to trace. Higgins' description of 'Vipera lachesis niger' as being blackish dorsally and on the upper surface of the head, helps us to understand that he refers to *Lachesis melanocephala*, black-headed bushmaster.

The powerful haemotoxic properties of Lachesis venom in general moreover are in keeping with Higgins' observation that 'The poison of Vipera lachesis niger always produces a shock, which throws down the person bitten with great violence; an immediate and violent flow of blood ensues from eyes, mouth, nostrils, urinary canal, and from under the nails of the fingers and toes; veins of the conjunctiva are intensely injected; suspension of the urine ensues, followed by violent fugitive pains in the bitten limb, and intense cephalalgia. Death ensues in from 1 to 12 hours.'

What may be safely assumed to be yet another bushmaster – Lachesis acrochorda – receives in Higgins' *Ophidians* the name 'Acrochordon chocoe, Verrugosa'. The names Acrochordon and verrugosa both allude to the warty look of the scales. Incidentally, all 4 Lachesis species are known as verrugosa, warty, in their native areas. Rather than being flat or smooth like the scales of most other snakes, each dorsal scale of the bushmasters is raised to a knobby point, making the skin very bumpy.

Confusing specific and generic names, Higgins places this snake in the *genus* Acrochordon, mixing it up with Acrochordus, a small Asian genus with 3 aquatic, non-venomous species called wart snakes. Higgins' slip-up becomes quickly apparent when the harmless Asian wart snakes are depicted as occurring 'in great abundance in the forests of the River Atrato in the United States of Colombia. Its poison is known to be very deadly.'

Higgins lived at the time in Colombia, which since 1863 called itself 'United States of Colombia' to become in 1886 'Republic of Colombia', under which name it is still known today. Name and place must have baffled Dr. C.F. Nichols, of Boston, who published a short article titled *Acrochordon chocoe – Characteristics* in the September issue of 1881 of the Homeopathic Physician. The opening line of his article exemplifies the sheer confusion: 'Verrugosa Acrochordon Chocoe is a wart-snake of the province of Choco in British Columbia.' Dr. Nichols correctly attributes the symptoms to the bite of the snake as recorded in Higgins' *Ophidians*, but incorrectly asserts that 'Dr. Swan potentised the gall of the snake and made provings, which confirmed Higgins' indications.' Not so. Swan did not conduct a proving with the snake gall he obtained from Higgins, but instead merely listed it in his *Catalogue of Morbific Products, Nosodes, and other Remedies*, 1886, in the process distorting its name to 'Achrocordon Chococ' – 'South American Serpent. Inveterate ulcers and sores; pains in scrofulous patients.'

The domino effect of inaccuracies leading to slip-ups leading to glaring errors has resulted in the remedy being advertised as a *nosode* in some of today's homeopathic literature.

## Confusion of Identity

'The population in question is endemic to the Pacific and Caribbean slopes of eastern Panama and northwestern South America – often called the *Choco* after its indigenous inhabitants. This is an area of great biological interest for its unique and often shared fauna with Central America. Authorities were divided as to which species the Choco snake represented.

Some South American scientists [e.g. Hoge and Romano-Hoge, 1981; Martínez and Bolaños, 1982] catalogued it with Daudin's [1803b] Lachesis mutus [muta] [acknowledging Taylor's trinominal, Lachesis muta muta], presumably on the basis of its locality in South America. The North American museums buried it in a different hole, with the American Cope's [1875] Lachesis stenophrys [and the American Taylor's subspecies Lachesis muta stenophrys].

On the basis of morphology, I concluded that the Chocoan snake was neither one nor the other of the 2 species in question [Lachesis muta muta or Lachesis stenophrys], but an entirely novel form, one with its own status and meaning. The Chocoan bushmaster was, in my vocabulary, a distinct species.' [Ripa, 2004]

## MATERIA MEDICA LACHESIS ACROCHORDA

### Sources
1 Higgins, effects of bite [c. 1873]; symptoms taken from van Zandvoort's Millennium Repertory.

### Mind
∞ Dullness, sluggishness, difficulty of thinking and comprehending.

### Generals
∞ Extreme thirst.
∞ Bloody sweat.
∞ Swelling. Oedematous swelling. Trembling.

### Locals
∞ Tearing headache.
∞ Falling of hair, alopecia.
∞ Conjunctivitis.
∞ Face distorted.
∞ Ichorous vesicular eruptions on limbs.
∞ Ulcerating vesicles lower and upper limbs.
∞ Watery vesicles upper and lower limbs.
∞ Pulsating, throbbing pain in limbs.
∞ Chronic ulcers on legs. Ulcers deep, funnel-shaped, phagedenic.
∞ Vesicular eruptions with thin, watery discharge. Vesicles fine; small.
∞ Skin ulcers cancerous; deep; discharge corrosive, ichorous, purulent, sloughing, watery, yellow.
∞ Skin ulcers painful, burning, pulsating.

### Clinical Manifestations
• Venom includes factors that are proteolytic, haemorrhagic, myotoxic, clotting inhibitors and possibly neurotoxic. The sheer volume that can potentially be injected in 1 bite make these snakes [esp. adults] very dangerous.
• Higgins provides the following information about the snake and the effects of its bite:
'This serpent is the most feared by the natives of all those found in the Choco region; the "Curers" [snake charmers] say that its bite produces death,

frequently in from 2 to 3 hours; and that the first symptoms that the poison develops are lethargy, trembling of the muscles in the whole body, a flow of blood from the pores of the skin, eyes bloodshot, and loosening of the hair, followed by a distortion of the features. What effects the poison does actually produce can only be determined by experiment. Some of its effects, in cases of bites, are the following: Soon after the introduction of the poison into the blood, the skin of the surface of the bitten limb is thickly covered with small vesicles, filled with an ichorous liquid; when these have attained the size of a grain of barley they burst, leaving a small sore, which soon increases in size, preserving its funnel shape; these continue sloughing away, until they unite one with another and thus destroy all the fleshy substance down to the bone. This is accompanied with intense throbbing pains up the limb. In cases where the poison does not cause death, on account of its deadly principle not being fully developed, it almost invariably produces these funnel-shaped ulcers.'

Evident from this account is the extensive tissue necrosis, a characteristic feature of the venom of Lachesis as well as Bothrops spp. Rather fantastical and without any foundation, however, is Higgins's assertion that, 'Immediately after the death of the snake, a thick milk-white fluid exudes from the warts, which, applied to the skin of man or beast, produces a well-nigh incurable ulcer.'

### Lachesis Syndrome

Notwithstanding minor qualitative and quantitative differences, the venom arsenals of Lachesis melanocephala and Lachesis acrochorda are broadly similar between themselves and also closely mirror those of adult Lachesis stenophrys and Lachesis muta venoms. The high conservation of the overall composition of Central and South American bushmaster venoms provides the ground for rationalizing the 'Lachesis syndrome', characterized by vagal symptomatology, sensorial disorders, haematologic, and cardiovascular manifestations.

The envenomation caused by snakes of the genus Lachesis represents 4.5% of all registered snakebites in Brazil and is characterized by the so-called 'Lachesis Syndrome'. Within the first few minutes after the bite, the victim is affected by agonizing burning throbbing local pain and oedema, followed by intense inflammation, bleeding disorders, clotting disorders, kidney malfunction, myotoxicity and autonomic syndrome evidenced by sweating, nausea, vomiting, abdominal cramps, diarrhoea, hypotension and bradycardia.

# CASE

'Man, aet. 50. Ulcers and sores on legs are hereditary [syphilitic]; his mother and other maternal relative having inveterate ulcers.

'Nov. 17. 1876. On both calves irregular-shaped sores; 6 in all, the largest, 2 by 1½ inches across, bleeding easily, having an odourless, dirty brown ichorous discharge, and indolently granulating surface, with blue edges; blue, shining skin of the whole leg; burning, stinging, itching, in the sores; ulcers may be developed anywhere on the legs where rubbed or pressed; they tend to work downward; grinding pain in legs; vertigo when stooping; feet sweat [warm, offensive]; emaciated, weak; despondent, sad, has recently lost a child; diarrhoea, with colic, occasionally. During the 6 months following, he took *Sil.* 200, *Sulph.* 200, and *Lach.* 200, of each 4 doses in water, lastly, *Lach.* 17M [Fincke], dry.

'June 24. Pain, deafness, and purulent discharge from the right ear, which he had had 15 years ago; the ulcers were larger; several more had appeared, their discharge thin, offensive, sanguineous, the neighboring skin copper-hued, erysipelatous; there were flushes, sweats, nausea and poor appetite, no medicine, until July 24. *Ars.* 200, dry.

'Sept. 6 *Phos.* CM, dry. Oct. 4 *Syph.* CM, dry. Nov. 3 *Syph.* DM, dry. Dec. 3 *Syph.* CMM, dry.

Jan. 3, 1878 *Ulcerine* CM, 3 doses in water. Jan. 28 *Ulcerine* DM, 3 doses in water. March 4 *Glanderine* DM, dry. March 21 *Lyc.* DM, dry. July 19 *Puls.* DM, dry. Aug. 17 *Calc-fl.* 12, 5 doses in water, 3 days apart. Sept. 6 *Merc-sol.* CM, 4 doses in water. Oct. 31 same.

'Feb. 7, 1879. After slight improvement under *Syph.*, the ulcers had grown worse, sloughing, enlarging, increasing in numbers. [The varicosities disappeared as the sores increased]. *Achroc. choc.* CM, 8 doses in water, were given. Improvement gradually took place without repetition of the prescription and progressed until the legs had become free from ulcers. Varicosities did not return. The patient ate considerable fruit. No change was made in his position, seated leg-bent at shoemaking. June 1880. He is well, with rough legs.'

[C.F. Nichols, Ulcers on leg; Achroc. choc., etc.; Medical Advance, Dec. 1880]

# LACHESIS MUTA

## Systematics
- Scientific name: Lachesis muta [Schinz, 1822].
- Synonyms: Crotalus mutus [L.,1766]. Lachesis mutus [Daudin, 1803].
- Common names: Bushmaster. Surucucu.
- Family: Viperidae, subfamily Crotalinae.

## Biological Profile
- Very large, rather slender, big-headed terrestrial pit viper, adults usually 2–3 m, maximum 3.7 m; longest poisonous snake in the Americas.
- Body reddish-brown, yellowish-tan, or pinkish-tan, with dark brown or black diamond-shaped dorsal blotches [often edged with yellow or cream]. Prominent mid-dorsal ridge, esp. on the front half of body. Belly white or ivory.

Scales extremely rough. Dorsal scales raised to knobby points, making the skin very bumpy.
- Range: NE South America. Lives in remote and isolated habitats and is largely nocturnal in its feeding habits.
- Habitat: Mainly found in tropical rainforests and lower montane wet forests that get 2.0–4.0 m annual rainfall; may occur along rivers in drier regions. Often found near large, buttressed trees or fallen logs, from near sea level up to 1,000 m elevation.
- Highly active frequent feeder on small prey; preys mainly on small mammals.
- Mainly terrestrial and nocturnal, most likely to respond quickly to disturbance near dawn.
- Displays recognisably social behaviour among its own species and even a commensal relationship with the large rodents that construct its underground refuge. [Dean Ripa]
- In courtship, the male bushmaster uses its dorsal ridge and rasp-like scales to stimulate the female, inverting his body on top of hers and, using fiddling motions, literally 'sawing' himself against her.
- Oviparous; 5–18 eggs per clutch. Females brood their eggs until hatching.
- Large adult captive specimens reportedly occasionally emit a long 'whistling' sound.

### Heat Strike

Pit vipers use their thermal [infrared] receptors to help locate prey, guide the predatory strike, and as anti-predator devices. Bushmasters use their *heat pits* almost exclusively in striking, whilst conversely relying greatly on vision in courting and male-male combating.

When confronted with an edible but non-moving target, e.g. a rodent too scared to move, bushmasters sometimes 'bob' their heads rapidly in order to thermally 'sight' the prey. In Dean Ripa's view this lends credence to the idea that pit viper pits act as a kind of imaging device rather than as simple thermal receptors: the prey object [or else the receptor itself] must 'move' or the object cannot be accurately targeted.

Bushmasters are sensitive to stress and typically die rapidly in captivity once subjected to the stress of venom extraction. Captive bushmasters produce less potent venoms, which results in the low laboratory toxicity of bushmasters vis-à-vis high mortality in persons bitten.

Striking first, asking questions later, bushmasters have the tendency to *strike-hold*, i.e. to hold on tighter and inject more venom when resistance is offered. In contrast to snakes that strike and release, bushmasters don't release their grip. Bushmasters require heat and not chemical cues to provoke strike-hold. They will rarely bite anything [even in a defence strike] unless it is warm.

Flashlights produce both light and enough heat to induce bushmasters to strike. 'Persons walking with a flashlight through jungle at night can be in for a startling experience, if a bushmaster is lying close-by. In a mild sequence, the snake merely raises its head up to considerable height in order to investigate the unusual phenomenon. But when the light is very bright, sudden and close-by, the startled snake attacks the light frenziedly, hurling itself at the "hot" object in a series of maddened, rapid strikes, one after another.

'This can be disconcerting in a snake that can strike 4 feet high! The strikes may be so violent as to propel the snake's entire body toward the intruder. The sudden appearance of heat appears to cause of sort of sensory overload, and the snake literally goes berserk. Native hunters who had been searching for small game at night using various kinds of torch lights [electric, carbon, gas, etc.] have told me tales of bushmasters "rising up out of nowhere" to strike light out of their hands [after which the terrified hunters fled the scene, abandoning the torch light behind them]. The sudden ignition of a match flame can have the same effect, as smokers visiting my facility have observed when an alarmed bushmaster [demonstrating the possible health hazards of cigarettes], made an unexpected lunge to bite them in the face – the glass front of the enclosure, however, protecting them from harm. Native tales of bushmasters being *attracted to fires* built in the jungle probably have a factual basis; if a bushmaster were nearby when the fire was being built, one could almost expect it to come over to investigate. In my travels I was intrigued at the extreme caution with which some native persons approached the task of building a cook-fire while we were hunting bushmasters in remote areas at night.' [Data and citations from Ripa, 2001, and Ripa, 2015]

## Maternal Protection

'While other vipers are, or may be, born outside on open ground, bushmasters hatch in a secure hideaway, probably an animal burrow. . . . Egg-laying requires that the female sped about 60 to 75 days out of each breeding year completely underground while guarding the eggs.

'Sexual pairs occupy the burrow together during the 1–3 month breeding period, but the male departs before the eggs are laid. Indeed, once the male has left the burrow for whatever reason [to eat, drink or shed the skin] the female will often not let him return. During the later stages of her pregnancy she becomes aggressive to all intruders, incl. other bushmasters. Using a language of threat signals, she confronts the mail intruder and begins displaying. This display consists of gular inflation, a strongly elevated head and stiffened, arched neck, body blocking and tail rattling. The male seems literate to this language and obligingly departs – there need not be any physical confrontation or contact.

'I have observed this ritual repeatedly in our large enclosures: the male, watchful, as though daunted by her displays and afraid to come closer; the female, tense with the enactment of her performance, her head elevated to as much as one-third body length, her stiffened anterior portion undulating slightly. Not only will she chase away the male, she will herself forcefully against any other object or person that comes near the nest site. The burrow, once selected by the female for egg-laying, is ceded by the male to her needs.

'The female will use these signal-displays toward humans as well. Lying watchfully at the mouth of her burrow, she appears cued to any signs of movement. Even a shadow projected through a glass door from more than 4 m away will sometimes inspire her to adopt an aggressive-signaling response. Tales of aggressiveness in bushmasters no doubt have much of their foundation in this nest-defending habit of females. Upon occasion I have been chased out of the enclosure by such displaying females, who bore down ominously after me with a slow, steady speed, and literally 'bossed' me away from the vicinity. One female pursued me for a distance of more than 4 m before turning back.' [Ripa, 2002]

## Venom & Clinical Manifestations - One Who Strikes Repeatedly

Venom is both haemotoxic and neurotoxic ['cobra-like']. Venom contains potent proteolysins, protein dissolving enzymes. Envenomation causes intense pain, swelling, and necrosis [often extensive] at the bite site, sometimes followed by gangrene.

'Proven Lachesis-inflicted accidents are rare in scientific literature while, on the other hand, the genus is given almost mythological status by common folk. According to the Villas-Boas brothers [indigenists and field men, who dedicated most of their lives to making first contact with previously unknown Indian tribes in the Amazon where "white man" had never set foot before in the late 1940s], "[Lachesis] is the only venomous snake of Brazil that might actually attack a human being." In ancient Tupi-Guarani Indian language, "surucucu" stands for "one who strikes repeatedly." Exploratory expeditions to South America such as those carried on by Von Spix and Von Martius [1817–1820] brought back to Europe weird, exaggerated accounts of huge snakes attacking campfires.

'Those who actually deal with Lachesis on a daily basis, find it of "calm disposition and delicate constitution." However, when cornered, wounded, thermally disoriented or guarding eggs, the genus may react in a very particular way. In the words of the experienced Rob Carmichael [pers. com.]: "As far as safety goes, I never work with these snakes unless I am 100% focused and alert. I keep many elapids [including king cobras], bothrops, crotalines, etc. but nothing strikes more concern in me than these bushmasters. I fully know that a bite could end my life, which is why when I work with the bushmasters, I don't work with any other snake that day. . . . I want to make sure that I am ready, focused, relaxed and ready for anything. So far, I have found the bushmasters to be amazingly calm and wonderful animals, however, I also have experienced first-hand the full wrath of this species. . . . Even a 16 ft king cobra coming full steam at me didn't scare me as much as an 8 ft bushmaster in full "I want to kill you" mode did a year ago. It made me completely re-think my strategies and safety procedures when working with them. But, for the most part, they have been very easy going and I think staying calm, deliberate and keeping movements slow and always working on the bushmaster's terms is the best course of action."

'This dauntless behaviour, its almost mythical status and even religious associations with "the evil one" fuel the ongoing slaughter of the species. In the case of the Atlantic Bushmasters [Lachesis muta rhombeata], the destruction of 93% of its natural habitat makes it a highly endangered species, classified as "Vulnerable" by the "International Union for the Conservation of Nature".' [de Souza, 2007]

**Bitten**

'Confirmed snakebite accidents involving Lachesis vipers ["surucucu"] are rare in the literature. We present 2 cases that occurred recently in the southern region of Bahia State, Brazil. These 2 cases were singled out of a series of 9 accidents. Both presented intense local pain, oedema, mild local ecchymosis, local haemorrhage and dramatic systemic alterations within the first 30 minutes after the bite: hypotension, vomiting and diarrhoea, sinus bradycardia configuring a pre-chock state. Both received Bothropic-Lachetic Antivenom, and both recovered fully.

'If there is venom inoculation, the first 60 minutes of these accidents are always dramatic and similar to the evolution of hypovolemic shock: severe hypotension may occur within 20 minutes, along with hypothermia as low as 35°C, vomiting, diarrhoea, abdominal pain, difficulty to swallow, sensorial disorientation, sinus bradycardia, and eventually shock and cardiac arrest. Although these signs and symptoms are the norm in our experience, while reviewing the literature we found out that there is no general agreement around the onset of such signs and symptoms, something that could be explained at least in part by the difficulty in determining the genus that actually caused the accident, esp. in the Amazon area where large Bothrops atrox are commonly confused with [small] Lachesis specimens.'

# CASE

Case 1: 23-year old male, bitten on top of his head by a 2-m long male Lachesis at 11.40 a.m.
[11.45] Severe local pain. [11.50] Pain in entire face, throat, and neck. [11.55] Profuse sweating, upper abdominal pain, vomiting. [12.00] Hypotension, weak pulse, sinus bradycardia, pale, profuse sweating, pre-shock. Drowsy, vision, hearing and speech alterations, hyper-salivation and great difficulty to swallow. [12.20] Not rousable, carried to the ICU of Regional Hospital. Watery diarrhoea. Blood pressure upon admission 60 × 40 mmHg. [12.25] Antivenom, promethazine, hydrocortisone. [12.40] Intense pain. [13.40] End of antivenom treatment. Drowsy. Profuse bleeding at wound site. [14.00] Recovering consciousness. [14.07] Intense, diffuse head pain. Diarrhoea, drowsiness, vomiting. [14.52] Profuse local bleeding persists. [60 hours later] Stable with normal kidney function. [de Souza, 2007]

**Quickly Reduced to a State of Exhaustion & Helplessness**

'And yet what is most striking about bushmaster bite cannot be photographed. The third and most serious of my own 4 bushmaster envenomings is a case in point.

'At 10 minutes [post bite]: Dizziness, loss of coordination and inability to stand; temporary losses of consciousness; altered sensorium [visions of hallucinogenic colour patterns, sense of enlarged surrounding space]; drowsiness with feelings of euphoria.

'15 minutes: Nausea, sweating and cool skin; feeling of swollen tongue [making speech difficult]; numbing of lips; uncontrollable drooling alternating with dry mouth and difficulty swallowing; lymphadenitis; rapid pulse [rising to above 110].

'20 minutes: Projectile vomiting; explosive diarrhoea; increasingly rapid pulse [to 125]; lowered blood pressure [91/54].

'25 minutes: Chills; intense stabbing pains in upper abdomen/lower chest; intense burning pain in kidneys [lower back] and violent cramping in muscles of the lower back; hyperpnoea [abnormally rapid breathing]; falling blood pressure [67/51]; rising pulse [130].

'30 minutes: Continued upper abdominal/lower chest and lower back pain [becoming more severe]; continued vomiting and diarrhoea; cold ashen skin; laboured breathing; blood pressure continuing to fall [48/35].

'35 minutes: Blood pressure nearly undetectable; pulse nearly undetectable; respiratory distress; acrocyanosis [cyanosis of the feet]; red spots on face, neck and chest; general body numbness; inability to sit up or stand; speech difficult. . . .

'40 minutes: No detectable blood pressure, absent pulse. Conscious, but disinterested in fate.'

'Bushmaster bite may be compared to being struck by a car: one is too weak to accomplish even simple tasks. Violent abdominal/lower chest pain [as though being pounded in the stomach], dizziness, weakness, nausea, explosive vomiting and diarrhoea – to say nothing of the agonized extremity – quickly the victim to a state of exhaustion and helplessness. Space seems altered and objects may appear disproportionately far away. However, the mind remains clear and one is at all times aware of his fate.' [Ripa, 2002]

- Dean Ripa: "Each snakebite is its own secret education. After 6 bushmaster bites, I had learned my bed of nails – the hard way. . . . This was the death bite, the bite I would probably not be coming back from. . . . I knew it because I had collected gobs of venom from bushmasters in strike sequences that mirrored this bite identically. I knew it in the devouring, pressure-boiling pain I felt within seconds of the injection. I knew it in the strange stiffness invading my back and limbs and a sudden, not unpleasant weakness, as though I had just stood up after having had too many cocktails. I knew it in a cold feeling coming all over me, as though I had been bathed with death's own hands. I knew it when my skin turned bright green. I knew it when I flopped down in the floor and couldn't get up again – the feeling of my limbs turning to wood."

## MATERIA MEDICA LACHESIS

### Sources

1 Self-experimentation Hering [USA], 1st and 2nd trit., including effects observed during trituration, 1828, and some symptoms seen in patients.

2 Proving Hering, 17 male provers and 3–4 female patients, 30th dil.; *c.* 1834–35.
3 Self-experimentation with Lachesis 10M [Fincke] by a "very nervous little woman" under guidance of Kent, 1887.
4 Clinical observations, in Hering.
5 Clinical observations Mangialavori [Italy].
6 Degroote, Dream Repertory.
7 Synthesis Repertory Treasure Edition 2009.

For effects of bite; clinical manifestations; see above.

## Mind

∞ 'A kind of ecstasy, as after sublime impressions or excessive joy, throughout day, he constantly wishes to talk and do much, and even more seems to be at his command. Great sensitivity, soothing poetry moved him to immoderate weeping, was obliged to cry for joy.'[1]

∞ In evening, unable to sleep, talks a great deal, wishes to tell stories, constantly goes from one thing to another, distorting and mixing things up, correcting himself, then repeating the same mistakes.[1]

∞ Great inclination to be communicative, extraordinarily vivid imagination, & extreme impatience at tedious and dry things; the more cause for fretfulness, the greater inclination for humour, jest, satire, and humorous fancies.[1] Desire for amusement, laughs about his own lively fancies.[2]

∞ Lively, social, and unusually communicative, despite disagreeable feeling of fulness.[2]

∞ Increased power of originality in all mental work, increased activity of fancy, scenes and occurrences gather and crowd in his mind in an unusual amount; no sooner does one idea occur to him than a number of others follow in quick succession while he is writing it down.[1]

∞ Mistrustful and evil thoughts; towards evening almost crazy jealousy, as foolish as it is irresistible.[1]

∞ Mistrustful, believes himself intentionally injured by all about him, and attaches the most hateful significance to the most innocent occurrences.[1]

∞ Great inclination for mental labour when controlling strongly increased sexual desire.[1]

∞ Wants to accomplish much, begins many things.[1] Very active, but not the least perseverance.[2]

∞ Must do everything very rapidly, bolts down his food, and can't remain sitting at table.[2]

∞ Unusually contentious and obstinate, quarrels with everything about him; so quarrelsome that he disputes with a mother about the age of her daughters and affirms the younger to be the elder.[2]

∞ Delusion she is somebody else and in the hands of a stronger power; under superhuman control.[4]

∞ Delusion she is dead and preparations are made for funeral, or that she is nearly dead and wishes someone would help her off.[4]

∞ Delusions: pursued by enemies; medicine is poison; robbers in house, wants to jump out of window; followed by enemies who are trying to harm him; being clear animal right through, whilst all mental power is dormant; as if charmed and unable to break the spell; everybody conspires to kill him.[4]

∞ Delusion possessed by a demon, impossible to be satisfied, perfectly insatiable. [Fincke]

∞ Delusions: conspiracies against him; having committed a crime; criticized; doomed; friendless, in morning on waking; hated; lost; spied upon.[7]

∞ Religious monomania, fear of being damned.[4]

∞ Afraid to go to sleep after retiring; put hand on heart to watch its beating.[3]

∞ Inability to speak/talk due to palpitations.[3]

∞ Physical and spiritual will not harmonize. Longing to break the tie that binds the spiritual to the physical. The influence of evil is uppermost. Morbid tendency to decide that wrong is right. Realize this only after it is committed, then feel crushed. Cannot rise above it. When alone the mortification of such mistakes nearly drives me wild. Cry for help and receive mockery.[3]

∞ Grief at committing actions that at the time seem proper, but afterward seem improper.[3]

∞ Self-consciousness that cannot be overcome.[3]

∞ Remorse followed by tears.[3]

∞ Easily angered by small provocations; quickly repents.[6]

∞ Craves attention.[6] Desires flattery.[6] Need of recognition.[6] Wants to be famous.[7]

∞ Aversion to people who speak slowly.[6] Impatience when others are talking.[6]

∞ Loud-mouthed but small-hearted.[6]

∞ Censorious due to jealousy, can't help oneself.[6] Jealousy, interrupts others.[6]

∞ Abusive, insulting; children insulting parents.[7]

∞ Anxiety: morning on waking; during menses; from pressure on chest; on going to sleep; before traveling.[7]

∞ Desire for the colour blue[7]; white[7]; red[6]. Aversion to green; orange.[7]

∞ Cunning.[7]

∞ Fears: in night on waking; apoplexy; someone behind him; betrayal; damnation; death, after falling asleep; contagious disease; heart disease; getting old; suffering.[7]

∞ Forgetful during menopause; from mental exertion; of words while speaking.[7]

∞ Weakness of memory – for past facts; recent facts; orthography; proper names; time; words. Weakness of memory after sunstroke.[7]

∞ Loves to mock/ridicule others.[7]

## Dreams

∞ Abyss, walking near an.[6]

∞ Accusations.[6]

∞ Bad news, getting; of people or loved ones having died.[6]

∞ Beating someone or oneself.[6]

∞ Being accused of stealing.[2]

∞ Bitten by cat, crocodile, dog, snake, vampire.[6]

∞ Blamed or blaming publicly.[6]

∞ Car accidents, running over somebody or being run over.[6]

∞ Clothed/dressed in black, people.[6]

∞ Coffins.[6]

∞ Complot to kill.[6]

∞ Conspiracies.[6]

∞ Control, controlling others or being controlled.[6]

∞ Death of person very dear to him.[2]

∞ Defiance.[6]

∞ Difficulties to move, progress, run.[6]

∞ Dying of dropsy from kidney disease; water collecting about heart.[3]

∞ Envy.[6]

∞ Falling into abyss, deep pit, water.[6]

∞ Fire.[6]

∞ Flying like a bird, like superman.[6]

∞ Forsaken, being or feeling disgraced, excluded or repudiated.[6]

∞ Funeral, own; nobody of the family is present.[6]

∞ Good and bad.[6]

∞ Home, & anxious feeling as if something bad had happened to him.[2]

∞ Hurry, being hurried, to be on time.[6]

∞ Ignored by everyone.[6]

∞ Intruder, intruding someone's house.[6]

∞ Joyous, humorous, or poetic full of inventions.[1]

∞ Laughed or mocked at.[6]

∞ Left by partner.[5]

∞ Locked up in basement, bedroom, building, closet.[6]

∞ Losing way, going astray.[6]

∞ Misjudgment of people, situations or time.[6]

∞ Naked people.[6]

∞ Nobody listens to one's protests.[6]

∞ Obtrusiveness; sexual harassment.[6]

∞ Planning revenge on a haughty earl, having knives ready at hand in case his behaviour is insolent.[2]

∞ Poisoned, being.[6]

∞ Praying or preaching.[6]

∞ Privacy, infringed or lacking.[6]

∞ Pursued, being; by animals; to be killed; by witches.[6]

∞ Riding in a strong wind taking one's breath away.[3]

∞ Riding on horseback.[3]

∞ Saving people.[6]

∞ Shot at by pursuer or sniper.[6]

∞ Slander, jealous.[6]

∞ Snakes.[5]

∞ Teeth falling out.[5]

∞ Threatened, being or feeling.

∞ Tied down with ropes.[6]

∞ Time, passing too quickly or standing still.[6]

## Generals

∞ Desire for beer, wine[1,2]; oysters[2]; coffee [which > dysmenorrhoea][4]; mushrooms[5]. Fruit >.[4]

∞ Aversion to bread and rolls[2]; vinegar[5]. Wine = flushes of heat.[5]

∞ Acids = vertigo & dazzling before eyes[2]; pressure in throat[2]; diarrhoea[1,2,4]; pain in lumbar region[2]; constriction heart[2]; pain in bones of arms[2]; burning in skin[2]; hunger[4].

∞ Sensitive to smell of coffee during menopause.[7]

∞ Evening > or <.[1,2]

∞ Restless sleep, frequent waking all through night, yet awakes early and rises refreshed.[1]

∞ Complaints < after sleeping.[1]

∞ Sleepiness, exhaustion before and after eating.[1,2]

∞ Sleep position on left side, with hand upon heart.[3]

∞ Sleep position, with head backwards; on left side. Lies motionless.[6]

∞ Pains burning[1,2]; stitching[2].

∞ Left side more affected.[1,2]

∞ Allergy, metal dermatitis for gold, nickel, silver.[5]

## Sensations

∞ String as if drawn from nape of neck above ears internally to eyes, on coughing.[1]

∞ Water in skull.[2]

∞ Lead in occiput, can scarcely raise head from pillow in morning.[2]

∞ Ball rising up or rolling in head.[7]

∞ Bubbling in head.[7] Swashing.[7]

∞ Wavelike upward motion in head.[7]

∞ Eyes as if stiff and full of dust.[2]

∞ Eyes as if larger, orbits as if too small.[2]

∞ Eyes feel as if they had been taken out and squeezed, and then put back again.[4]

∞ Eyes as if forced out when throat is pressed.[4]

∞ Eyes as if loose.[7]

∞ Eyes as if smaller.[7]

∞ Flickering before eyes as from threads or sunrays.[2]

∞ Bluish-grey ring with fiery rays around light source.[2]

∞ Whirring as from insects in ears, extending back into head.[2]

∞ Left half of face as if burnt by exposure to sun heat.[2]

∞ Two large lumps as if coming together in throat.[1]

∞ Throat as if drawn up to palate by tendons.[2]

∞ Plug in throat after acids.[2]

∞ Crumb of bread as if sticking in throat.[2]

∞ Fishbone as if stuck or sponge as if hanging in throat.[4]

∞ Grasped by the throat by someone, = suffocation.[4]

∞ Throat as if squeezed.[7]

∞ Throat as if swollen on swallowing.[2]

∞ Nausea & feeling as if poisoned.[2]

∞ Stone in stomach and upper abdomen, which seems to fall down lest he steps carefully.[1]
∞ Stomach as if cold inside.[2]
∞ Stomach as if empty at night, despite evening meal.[2]
∞ Inner parts or ligaments of stomach as if being stretched, < slightest pressure.[2]
∞ Something in stomach and intestines as if drawn up into a ball.[2]
∞ Stomach as if turning.[7]
∞ Ball as if rolling from ride side of abdomen towards stomach.[4]
∞ Faeces as if ascending to chest.[4]
∞ Bladder as if cold.[7]
∞ Ball rolling through urethra.[7]
∞ Labour-like pains as if extending up into breasts.[2]
∞ Mouth of uterus as if open.[4]
∞ Cannot lie on r. side due to feeling something were rolling over to that side, & left-sided ovaritis.[4]
∞ Trachea as if narrowed, after midday nap.[1]
∞ Suffocative feeling, must loosen clothes about neck.[2]
∞ Suffocative feeling and palpitation in a crowd.[3]
∞ Pressure upon chest as if it were full of air, > eructations.[1]
∞ Bubbles in chest.[2]
∞ Chest as if excoriated or raw.[7]
∞ Great dyspnoea, lungs as if being pressed up into throat, or as if cord were tightly tied around neck.[4]
∞ Drawing sensation around heart when lying on right side.[3]
∞ Weakness and sinking sensation from heart to stomach.[3]
∞ Heart as if constricted, after acids.[2]
∞ Heart as if squeezed.[7]
∞ Heart as if turning over and ceasing to beat for a moment, then starting again with increased force.[4]
∞ Heart as if too large for its space.[4] Heart as if swollen.[7]
∞ Heart as if hanging or swinging by a thread, and every heartbeat would tear it off.[7]
∞ Tendons in left arm as if too short.[1]
∞ Aching in left arm ext. upward to shoulder, as if arm would drop out.[3]
∞ Left arm as if pulled.[3]
∞ Heavy ache in both thighs, as if they would come off or break.[3]
∞ Knee joints as if paralysed, > walking.[2]
∞ Hot air going through knee joints.[4]
∞ Feet so cold as if walking on ice.[3]
∞ Toenails right foot as if pushed up.[2]

## Locals
∞ Dizziness on looking up or on looking at any object closely.[4]
∞ Dizziness < closing eyes, with nausea; on reaching up with hands; < turning in bed; from suppressed menses; > menses.[7]
∞ Hair loss from grief; during pregnancy.[7]

∞ Pressing outward pain in eyes when pressing or touching throat.[7]
∞ Noises in ears/tinnitus on blowing nose; during inspiration.[6]
∞ Itching in nose when eating.[1]
∞ Tongue heavy and difficult to move or protrude; speech difficult.[7]
∞ Pain in throat on empty swallowing, not on swallowing food; throat very sensitive to slightest external pressure, so that everything about throat is distressing, no position is comfortable.[1,2]
∞ Pain in throat with pain in nape of neck.[6]
∞ Pain in throat, making opening mouth difficult.[7]
∞ Pain in throat < putting out tongue.[7]
∞ Cannot swallow sweet or acrid things.[4]
∞ Liquids cause more difficulty in swallowing than solid food.[2]
∞ Indigestion [heartburn, nausea, belching, etc.] from smoking, > tea.[1]
∞ Nausea from smoking.[1,2] Nausea from milk.[2]
∞ Nausea from anything tight on throat.[2]
∞ Sour and bitter eructations from meat fried in butter.[2]
∞ Pain stomach > lying on abdomen; > passing flatus.[6]
∞ Heat abdomen, wants to uncover abdomen.[6]
∞ Pain abdomen as if menses would appear, during pregnancy.[6]
∞ Diarrhoea from acids or fruit.[1]
∞ Urging to urinate on hearing water running.[6]
∞ Before menses: desire for open air; vertigo; nosebleed; labour-like pains, < in 1. ovarian region; bruised feeling in hips; > when flow begins.[4] The smaller the discharge, the greater the pain.[4]
∞ Respiration difficult > bending forward or holding arms away from body.[7]
∞ Respiration difficult < covering nose or mouth; < exertion of arms; < laughing; < raising arms; as from smoke; after talking or < talking; < touch of larynx.[7]
∞ Aching in heart region, raises and lowers left shoulder to get relief.[3]
∞ Palpitation and sense of suffocation in a crowd.[3]
∞ Palpitations extending to pit of throat.[6]
∞ Palpitations < warmth [bathing, drinks, room].[7]
∞ Oppression chest < clothing; < before menses; < talking; < walking.[7]
∞ Chest pain < bending forward; < pressure of clothes.[7]
∞ Attacks of palpitation & hacking cough.[3]
∞ Garlic smell to axillary sweat.[2]
∞ Cannot bear draft of air on nape of neck.[6]
∞ Pain nape of neck/cervical region < or > bending head backward.[6]
∞ Pain lumbar region on bending head forward; > sitting erect.[6]
∞ Aching in left arm < hanging arm down.[3]
∞ Veins in hands so distended; must hold them up to get relief.[3]
∞ Aching in left leg > resting leg on chair and taking off shoe.[3]
∞ Must move feet to prevent them jerking/twitching upward uncontrollably.[2]

## Frightened by a Snake

'Crawls upon floor, laughs and is very cross by turns; attacks last from half an hour to an hour; child acts strangely, will not play with other children; exhibits no love for mother; seems to hate her mother and friends, hides; runs away from strangers, looks at them through her fingers; bites and spits at other children; 6 years ago was frightened by a snake.' [Hering]

# SISTRURUS CATENATUS CATENATUS

## Systematics
- Scientific name: Sistrurus catenatus [Rafinesque, 1818].
- Subspecies: S. c. catenatus [Rafinesque, 1818].
- Synonyms: Crotalinus catenatus [Rafinesque, 1818]. Crotalus messasaugus [Kirtland, 1838].
- Common names: Eastern massasauga. Black rattler. Black snapper.
- Family: Viperidae, subfamily Crotalinae.

## Biological Profile
- Relatively small, heavy-bodied venomous pit viper. Average length 70 cm, maximum 1 m.
- Body grey to grey-brown, distinctively marked with a row of large black or dark brown hourglass-shaped markings along the back and 3 rows of smaller dark spots on each side. Belly white or cream with dark grey or brownish blotches along sides. Tail ends in series of paired 'rattles'. Head diamond-shaped with white stripes along jaw.
- Range: North America, from central New York and southern Ontario [Canada] west to the prairies of Iowa and Missouri.
- Habitat: Wetland habitats, incl. bogs, fens, shrub swamps, wet meadows, marshes, moist grasslands, wet prairies and floodplain forests. Migrates in summer to drier, upland sites, ranging from forest openings to old fields, agricultural lands and prairies.
- Mainly terrestrial and nocturnal.
- Preys on small mammals, lizards, and occasionally invertebrates.
- Does not hibernate in a group like other snake species. Looks for a place to hide alone. Hibernation sites are located below the frost line, often close to groundwater level. The presence of water that does not freeze is critical for suitable hibernaculum.
- Males engage in dominance [combat] bouts.
- Ovoviviparous; 4–20 live young per brood.
- Three subspecies recognized, of which S. catenatus catenatus, the eastern massasauga, occurs in the U.S. from SE Minnesota, eastern Iowa, and NE Missouri east to southern Ontario, western New York, and NW Pennsylvania.
- 'Massasauga' translates to 'great river-mouth' and probably refers to the snake's preference for wet habitats, incl. riverine bottomlands.

## Behaviour & Temperament
'Having kept these snakes now for several years – in fact I may say that they have been a hobby with me – I have had considerable opportunity of studying them

and their ways. Harmless snakes I had often made pets of both here and in Europe, but without much regard to scientific data; and my first massasauga soon showed me that the habits of the one were very different from those of the other.

'In disposition, I have found the massasauga particularly docile. For a dog they appear to have a special antipathy. One of these has only to sniff around the cages to set the whole colony rattling. Their sense of smell appears to be particularly acute and they will detect a dog at the back of the cage directly. For a cat they do not seem to entertain the same dislike.

'On the approach of a thunderstorm they always become restless and noisy and are excellent barometers in this respect. . . . I would say here that when a snake strikes a mouse it releases it at once; when it strikes a bird it holds on till it is dead, the reason for which is not hard to see.' [Selous, 1900]

## Materia Medica
- No symptoms.

# SISTRURUS MILIARIUS BARBOURI ▬▬▬

### Systematics
- Scientific name: Sistrurus miliarius [L., 1766].
- Subspecies: S. m. barbouri [Gloyd, 1935].
- Common names: Dusky pygmy rattlesnake. Ground rattler.
- Family: Viperidae, subfamily Crotalinae.

### Biological Profile
- Small but thick-bodied venomous pit viper with triangular head topped by 9 large scales. Average length 30–60 cm, maximum 79 cm.
- Ground colour light to dark grey to nearly black, with 1 or 2 rows of lateral spots. Row of black to brownish red mid-dorsal spots. Belly heavily mottled with black and white.
- Range: SE USA; throughout Florida, north to eastern North Carolina and west to eastern Texas and southern Missouri.
- Habitat: Lowland pine flatwoods, prairies, around lakes and ponds, and along the borders of many freshwater marshes and cypress swamps.
- Ambush predator preying on lizards, frogs, small mammals, and insects as well as centipedes.
- Small territory, primarily made up of the burrow or log that it inhabits.
- Spends most of its time well-hidden among leaf litter in the vicinity of its burrow or log. Can be very hard to spot.
- Most active in warm weather. Covers itself in debris or takes refuge in its burrow when temperatures dip to freezing or below.
- Solitary.
- Rattle has no free rattle segment and only produces a slight buzzing sound when rattled.
- Tip of tail of juveniles sulphur yellow and used for caudal luring.

- Ovoviviparous; 2–12 live young per brood. Young stay near their mother for 7–10 days for protection, leaving after their first moult.
- Three recognized subspecies [barbouri, miliarius, streckeri].

## Guarding the Female

'Pygmy rattlesnakes are monogamous, with only one male successfully fertilizing a female. Males are not aggressive towards each other during mating seasons and many males will pursue one female without conflict. Multiple males will compete to mate with one female and will continue their attempts to mate until one male successfully fertilizes the female. Once a male fertilizes a female, all other males cease their mating attempts with the female snake. This occurs because the male leaves a gelatinous plug in the female after she has been fertilized, closing up the cloaca [the opening for the reproductive tract] and preventing the female from mating with other snakes. The male will continue to remain in close proximity to the fertilized female for most of her pregnancy. The male will "mate guard" the female and they can sometimes be found coiled around one another. This guarding will continue for an extended period of time, sometimes for days, weeks, or even months at a time. The snakes often can be found coiled up together during this period of time. Males typically leave the females before the young are born.' [animaldiversity.org]

## Behaviour & Temperament

'Their small size and moderately mild venom keeps them from being a serious threat to human life, but the bite is still extremely painful. One man I know was bitten severely enough by a large pygmy that he was hospitalized, and very nearly died. Despite their diminutive size, I have yet to meet one that didn't act like it was 12 feet long and ready to take on anything. If you give the snake half of an opportunity to bite you, it will happen. Don't count on hearing the rattle, as it is very slender and does not produce much noise.' [Greg (Snakeman) Longhurst, Venomous Snakes of Florida]

'Because of its very small size for a rattlesnake the tail rattle does not make a very loud noise. This means that pigmy rattlesnakes are especially dangerous because a person can be nearly on top of one before they realize they are about to step on the snake. Pygmy rattlesnakes are also known to be exceptionally aggressive towards humans. When one feels threatened it can bite a human multiple times, delivering a small amount of venom. . . . The venom produced by pigmy rattlesnakes is typically not enough to kill a human, but it should still be taken seriously. The [haemotoxic] venom causes intense bleeding at the site of the wound, and the pygmy rattlesnake bite is the most common cause of snake envenomation in many areas.' [www.snake-removal.com]

## Materia Medica

- No symptoms.

# TRIMERESURUS FLAVOVIRIDIS

## Systematics
- Scientific name: Protobothrops flavoviridis [Hallowell, 1861].
- Synonyms: Bothrops flavoviridis [Hallowell, 1861]. Lachesis flavoviridis [Boulenger, 1896]. Trimeresurus flavoviridis [Hallowell, 1861].
- Common names: Habu. Okinawa habu. Yellow-green pit viper.
- Family: Viperidae, subfamily Crotalinae.

## Biological Profile
- Slender, gracefully proportioned venomous pit viper with broad triangular head. Average length 1.3 m, maximum 2.3 m. Largest member of genus.
- Ground colour light olive or brown, overlaid with elongated dark green or brownish blotches with yellow edges, sometimes containing yellow spots, and frequently fusing to produce wavy stripes. Belly whitish with dark colouring along edges.
- Range: Japan – Amami and Okinawa groups in Ryukyu Islands.
- Habitat: Rock walls and in old tombs and caves in transition zone between palm forest and cultivated fields.
- Oviparous; up to 18 eggs per clutch.
- Mostly nocturnal; often enters homes and other structures in search of rats and mice.
- Often climbs trees.
- One specimen survived 3 years and 3 months without food in an experiment in Naze City, Japan, in the 1970s, putting the habu snake in the record books as having the longest fast of any vertebrate animal.
- Bold and irritable, it can strike quickly and has a long reach. Most aggressive during the rainy season.
- No subspecies.

## Snake in a Bottle
'Habushu is an awamori-based [rice] liqueur made in Okinawa, Japan. The awamori is first mixed with various herbs and honey giving the clear liquid a yellow hue. A pit viper is then inserted into the liquid and stored until consumed. The viper is believed by some to have medicinal properties. Some brands of habushu come with the snake still inside the bottle. There are 2 methods of inserting the snake into the alcohol. The maker may choose to simply submerge the snake in the alcohol and seal the bottle, thus drowning the snake. Alternatively, the snake may be put on ice until it passes out, at which point it is then gutted, bled and sewed up. The viper is then thawed and is then quickly drowned in the sealed habushu bottle. Removing the intestines of the snake, as in the second method, is thought to decrease the drink's particularly unpleasant smell.' [Wikipedia]

The drink is said to have health benefits, which range from improving stamina and sexual performance to alleviating back pain and arthritic symptoms. Some believe that it removes toxins from the body.

## Sources
1 Effects of bite; clinical manifestations

## Clinical Manifestations
Venom haemorrhagic, haemolytic and necrotic. Envenomation results in strong, throbbing pain; blood oozing from bite site; marked swelling; bluish discolouration around bite site; nausea and vomiting; disorientation; low blood pressure; shock; irregular breathing.

'The region of the bite is of a dark, purple colour and shows great swelling, accompanied by a severe burning pain, the latter being characteristic of habu venom intoxication. The lymph glands near the bite also become enlarged and sensitive to pressure. Loss of appetite and vomiting with colic and trouble in the thorax occur in chronic cases, the face is pale; the pulse feeble and rapid [90 to 120]. In most instances respiration remains normal. A slight fever is not infrequent. The pupils are neither dilated nor contracted. A cold sweat ending in death finally sets in. The end is also preceded by coldness of the extremities and dyspnoea. Blood in the urine or in the faeces has been observed. Sensory or motor disturbances, which persists after recovery from acute symptoms, are usually due to secondary infections or improper treatment.' [Kitajima, 1908]

# TRIMERESURUS MUCROSQUAMATUS

## Systematics
- Scientific name: Protobothrops mucrosquamatus [Hoge & Romano-Hoge, 1983].
- Synonyms: Lachesis mucrosquamatus [Boulenger, 1896]. Trigonocephalus mucrosquamatus [Cantor, 1839]. Trimeresurus mucrosquamatus [Cantor, 1839].
- Common names: Brown-spotted pit viper. Taiwan habu. Chinese habu.
- Family: Viperidae, subfamily Crotalinae.

## Biological Profile
- Relatively slender venomous pit viper with broad, flattened, distinctly triangular head and thin neck. Average length 1 m, maximum 1.3 m.
- Ground colour light brown, greyish brown or brown above with a vertebral row of large purplish-brown or chocolate coloured spots sometimes edged with a pale yellow line, and dark circular blotches laterally. Belly whitish with brownish dots.
- Range: Asia from northeast of India [Assam] to Taiwan and Vietnam; introduced in Japan.
- Habitat: Farmlands, orchards, riversides and woods, up to 2000 m elevation.
- Nocturnal. Preys on frogs, lizards, birds, mice or bats..
- Oviparous; 3–15 eggs per clutch.

- Can be aggressive, attacking shadows and moving objects.
- No subspecies.

## MATERIA MEDICA TRIMERESURUS MUCROSQUAMATUS

### Sources
1 Effects of bite; clinical manifestations

### Clinical Manifestations
Venom haemotoxic/haemorrhagic by destroying fibrinogen in circulating blood. A sticky, fibrous coagulant playing a key role in blood clotting, fibrinogen is considered a powerful predictor of stroke – including fatal and nonfatal strokes, first time strokes, and haemorrhagic and ischemic strokes.

Envenomation usually causes severe local pain and swelling, may involve entire bitten limb with tender enlargement of regional lymph nodes. Systemic symptoms may include nausea, vomiting, epigastric pain, fever, and shock, sometimes causing impaired consciousness or even generalised convulsions.

# TRIMERESURUS PUNICEUS

### Systematics
- Scientific name: Trimeresurus puniceus [Boie, 1827].
- Synonyms: Atropos puniceus [Wagler, 1830]. Lachesis puniceus [Boulenger, 1896]. Vipera punicea [Boie, 1827].
- Common names: Flat-nosed pit viper. Ashy pit viper. Bornean pit viper.
- Family: Viperidae, subfamily Crotalinae.

### Biological Profile
- Small, stout-bodied, venomous pit viper with very large, triangular head distinct from neck. Average length 40–50 cm, maximum 64 cm.
- Usually uniformly light reddish-brown above, with irregular darker blotches; usually slightly darker grey-brown below. Light, dark-edged streak behind each eye. Tail and belly mottled with brown. Flattened, slightly upturned snout, with an elevated ridge from each eye to snout.
- Range: Southern Thailand, Malaysia, Indonesia.
- Habitat: Lowland forest, from near sea level to 1450 m elevation.
- Semi-arboreal. Found as high as 20 m above ground level in primary lowland forest; will descend to the ground in search of prey. Preys on small mammals and birds; occasionally lizards and frogs.
- Ambush predator active at night or after rain. Very sluggish in daytime, not aggressive, but will defend itself if molested. Rarely encountered by humans.
- Oviparous; 7–14 eggs per clutch. It has been reported that the females would coil up around their clutches and keep this position until their young eventually hatch.

- Venom haemotoxic. Envenomation causes immediate burning pain, swelling, and limited local discolouration.

## Materia Medica
- No symptoms.


# TRIMERESURUS PURPUREOMACULATUS

## Systematics
- Scientific name: Trimeresurus purpureomaculatus [Gray, 1832].
- Synonyms: Lachesis purpureomaculatus [Boulenger, 1896]. Cryptelytrops purpureomaculatus [Gray, 1832].
- Common names: Mangrove pit viper. Shore pit viper. Purple-spotted pit viper.
- Family: Viperidae, subfamily Crotalinae.

## Biological Profile
- Medium-sized, fairly stout-bodied pit viper. Average length 70–80 cm, maximum 1 m.
- Body colour highly variable, above olive, greyish, to dark purplish brown; below whitish, greenish or brown, uniform or spotted with brown. May have a white dotted line low down on each side of its body. Females larger than males.
- Range: India [Assam, Andaman Islands], Bangladesh, Burma, Thailand, West Malaysia, Singapore and Indonesia [Sumatra and Java].
- Habitat: Rocky coastal areas in mangrove and coastal swampy forests.
- Predominantly nocturnal, may also be active during day.
- Terrestrial, but commonly encountered in low bushes.
- Readily enters and swims in salt water; often moves to and from near-shore islands.
- Ovoviviparous; 7–14 live young per brood.
- Very aggressive; strikes with little provocation. "Bad-tempered snake. Once they get going they are slow to calm down."
- No subspecies.
- Potent haemotoxin. Envenomation may cause severe pain, local swelling involving entire bitten limb, tender enlargement of local lymph nodes, local necrosis, and incoagulable blood. Bites common. Human deaths reported but not very common.

## Materia Medica
- No symptoms.

# TRIMERESURUS STEJNEGERI

## Systematics
- Scientific name: Trimeresurus stejnegeri [Schmidt, 1925].
- Synonym: Trimeresurus gramineus [Stejneger, 1907]. Viridovipera stejnegeri [Schmidt, 1925].
- Common names: Green tree viper. Bamboo viper. Chinese tree viper.
- Family: Viperidae, subfamily Crotalinae.

## Biological Profile
- Medium-sized, fairly stout, arboreal venomous pit viper with triangular head and red eyes. Average length 60–70 cm, maximum 1 m.
- Body uniformly leaf-green to chartreuse-green; no markings except thin white, yellowish-white, or red and white [red below, white above] stripe along each side. Belly pale green, prehensile tail terracotta or rust-coloured above.
- Range: S Asia from India [Assam] to China and Taiwan.
- Habitat: Mainly found in montane forest areas, usually in bamboo thickets, bushes, and trees along water courses; found more frequently on hillsides than on level terrain, often in edges of agricultural areas. Occurs up to 2845 m elevation.
- Mainly nocturnal; sluggish by day. Preys on small frogs, lizards and small mammals.
- Ovoviviparous; 3–10 live young per brood.
- Usually calm disposition but strikes quickly if surprised or brushed against while resting in arboreal shelters. When threatened while on the ground, may coil & rapidly vibrate tail as a warning.
- Two recognized subspecies [chenbihuii, stejnegeri].

## MATERIA MEDICA TRIMERESURUS STEJNEGERI

### Sources
1 Effects of bite; clinical manifestations.

### Clinical Manifestations
Venom chiefly haemotoxic.

Envenomation symptoms include severe local pain, oozing from fang marks, extensive local swelling, bruising, nausea, and vomiting. Many bites of humans in agricultural areas, or people who walk along narrow bamboo forest trails. Human fatalities recorded but not common.

'The wound usually feels extremely painful, as if it had been branded with a hot iron, and the pain does not subside until about 24 hours after being bitten.' [Wikipedia]

# TRIMERESURUS WAGLERI

## Systematics
- Scientific name: Tropidolaemus wagleri [Boie, 1827].
- Synonyms: Bothrops wagleri [Müller, 1882]. Lachesis wagleri [Boulenger, 1896]. Trimeresurus maculatus [Gray, 1842]. Trimeresurus wagleri [Günther, 1864].
- Common names: Temple pit viper. Wagler's pit viper. Bamboo snake.
- Family: Viperidae, subfamily Crotalinae.

## Biological Profile
- Venomous long-fanged pit viper with large, triangular head and prehensile tail. Head covered with distinctly keeled small scales. Males light green with red and white post-auricular stripes, as well as red and white spots on the dorsum. Females black or dark green with yellow cross-banding. Average length 60 cm, maximum 1 m. Females bulky, much larger than slender males.
- Range: Malaysian Peninsula and Archipelago, Indonesia, Borneo, Philippines, Ryukyu Islands.
- Habitat: Dense rain forests, but often found near human settlements. Mainly found in lowland forests and swamps, but also found at higher elevations if conditions are moist enough; often found in low shrubs and bushes, and small trees, up to 600 m elevation.
- Nocturnal and arboreal.
- Ambush predator; appears quite sluggish as it remains motionless for long periods of time – days to weeks – waiting for prey to pass by. Can strike quickly when prey does pass by or if disturbed.
- Preys on rodents, birds, and lizards.
- Ovoviviparous.
- No subspecies.

## Temple
The name 'temple viper' comes from the famous Temple of the Azure Cloud, also known as The Snake Temple, a 150-year-old temple located now in a bustling city on the island of Penang, off of peninsular Malaysia. The vipers are seen as holy representatives of the deity Chor Soo Kong. Large numbers of T. wagleri are kept on plants and statues in and around the temple and are handled freely and freehandedly by the temple keepers. The snakes are said to have inhabited the temple naturally and are reported by the keepers not to bite, possibly due to thick clouds of incense burned inside the temple, which is said to calm the already mostly lethargic snakes. The temple was built in honour of Chor Soo Kong, a Buddhist monk who had moved to Penang. Legend has it that Chor Soo Kong, who was also a healer, gave shelter to snakes when he lived in the jungle. Snakes entered the temple to pay respect to Chor Soo Kong.

## Behaviour & Temperament

'Tropidolaemus wagleri are usually lethargic animals. In captivity, they some-times go without noticeable movement for days or even months – the trait of an ambusher. Without rain they become dormant, waiting for the inevitable tropical weather to stimulate animation. They are able to withstand weeks of water scarcity by lying still, yet survival in captivity depends on adequate hydration, and adequate hydration depends on the stimulation that is usually provided by rain. They also appear to be highly territorial, and because of this – extremely dangerous [though only observed by me in captive housing en-closures]. Do not enter their strike range while they are on their roost! Interest-ingly, during manipulation their demeanor totally changes to a placid, apparently curious snake, but as with all venomous snakes: never let your guard down and always work cautiously with them.

'. . . One of the tricks used to elicit a feeding response in a temperamental T. wagleri is to irritate or anger the snake by using long tweezers or forceps and tapping the snake on the tail with a mouse and then the snout if needed. Manipulation of the snake can also anger it enough to strike. If a strike occurs with a fickle feeder, stay still, or exit the animal's field of vision. Once the animal has grabbed the prey item they will typically swallow it, but movement may startle the animal and cause it to lose interest. Evenings are the best times to try to feed.

'T. wagleri are not social animals. Give them enough room to establish their own territory if housed with others. Plants or other forms of dividers should be used to obstruct the view of other Waglers. Over a period of time they will establish their own territory in the enclosure and defend it vigorously. Once removed from their territory they will become more placid. If introducing a new viper into an enclosure of a long term captive, it's best to remove the long term specimen for a day or 2 and rearrange the caging materials before introducing them both. Failure to do so has resulted in extremely aggressive behaviour from the long term specimen, and harm to both specimens is both possible and probable.' [Lacina, 2000]

## Captivity

'There are various attributes and statements that have been used to describe Wagler's viper in captivity: docile snake, lethargic, beautiful but difficult to keep and feed, problems with lung infection, constipation etc.

'All of these potential problems may arise, or not, depending on how one generally approaches husbandry of this snake. This snake, with exception to adult females, is primarily a lizard eater. Those who have ever experienced the speed with which this viper strikes at geckos [even following the prey if necessary] know its true nature.

'Wagler's viper reacts very sensitive to alterations of climatic conditions. Tropi-dolaemus wagleri requires high humidity, 80% and up. . . . This snake needs to drink water regularly. Drinking here means not just some drops at the wall of the container but providing water as long as the animal wants to drink [by spraying droplets on the body and let the snake drink it or applying water directly to the mouth using a pipette]. . . . Not doing so will result in digestive problems, ultimately clogging the intestine by dehydrated and hardened undigested matter. In the worst case, the intestinal tissue can stick to the faecal pellet. Wagler's viper needs a lot of water to discharge uric acid effectively.

'Lots of fresh air, for instance by means of small electric fans [like the ones used to cool computers] installed in a large container, or by continuous operation of an air-pump [as used for the aquarium] in a small container. Negligence of these facts results, sooner or later, to lung infections, which are often due to the common soil bacterium Pseudomonas aeruginosa.

'As T. wagleri is a lowland tropical rainforest inhabitant, temperatures of 28–32°C during the day are fine and dropping down to 24–25°C at night. . . . A healthy T. wagleri is usually recognized by an S-shaped resting position, being highly alert during night to movements or changes in temperature which are detected with its heat sensors hidden in the loreal pits.

'Rainfall stimulates the animals to drink. They turn their heads towards the body and start drinking water droplets attached to it. . . . Healthy adult females are usually good rodent eaters but tend to become overfed. . . . Females can keep faeces for months [up to 6 months may be possible]. Then, certain measures should be taken to stimulate defecation. . . . The size of the container also influences the constipation problem: Waglers should be given ample space, meaning that once these rarely moving snakes actually become active they like to wander around which often triggers defecation. Males behave differently, as they usually defecate after each meal.' [Thomas Jaekel; ophiotropics.com]

## MATERIA MEDICA TRIMERESURUS WAGLERI

### Sources
1 Effects of bite; clinical manifestations.

### Clinical Manifestations
Venom haemotoxic, causing cell and tissue destruction.

Bites by Wagler's pit viper are often minor, but may cause local effects, varying from minor pain and swelling, to severe pain, extensive swelling, oozing, numbness, even necrosis, but significant systemic effects do not appear to occur.

Symptom in Synthesis Repertory 2009:

∞ Generals, Pulse, weak.

# VIPERA LACHESIS FEL

*see* **Bothrocophias colombianus.**

# Family Viperidae, subfamily Viperinae
# – True vipers

## Biological Profile
- The viperinae, or true vipers, usually have short, robust bodies and spade-shaped heads that are broad to accommodate large venom glands and much wider than their necks. There are many different sizes, markings and colourations. True vipers lack facial heat-sensing pits. Dorsal scales keeled and apically pitted.
- Primarily terrestrial, sometimes arboreal [e.g. bush vipers of genus Atheris].
- Occupying diverse habitats, the heat-retaining heavy body shape enables true vipers to live in many habitats over a wide geographic range. Many species are designed for life in deserts and mountains.
- Most are ovoviviparous, but egg laying occurs in Causus [night adders] and some other genera.
- 'Thermal, visual and chemical cues guide the strike, with warm targets being struck more frequently than cold targets. Thermal detections may involve scale organs, microscopic organs near the mouth, or highly developed regions of free nerve endings beneath a thinned layer of epidermis.' [Mallow, 2003]
- The group of true vipers is comprised of approximately 14 genera and 85 species, all of which are restricted to the Old World.

## Venom & Clinical Manifestations
- Viper venom is usually haemotoxic, with some cytotoxic factors. The most common clinical manifestation of viper bite is incoagulable blood, resulting in prolonged oozing of blood from fang punctures and haemorrhage from mouth, nose, stomach, intestines and other organs.
- 'Perhaps the most characteristic traits are the bite and the venom delivery system. Vipers can strike, deliver a lethal dose of venom and resume a defensive posture very quickly. This *ability to kill with minimal contact* is advantageous, esp. when dealing with large and potentially dangerous prey. After striking, vipers follow a scent trail to their prey. Some vipers hold specific prey items from initial strike through swallowing, suggesting a discriminatory mechanism. Factors such as prey size, activity and resistance to immobilisation determine whether prey are held or released during envenomation. The venom apparatus includes a pair of retractable folding front fangs. Each viper fang is capable of being moved independently.' [Mallow, 2003]

| Homeopathic name | Common name | Abbreviation | Symptoms |
|---|---|---|---|
| Atheris squamigera | African bush viper | Ather-sq. | + |
| Bitis arietans | Puff adder | Bit-ar. | ++ |
| Bitis atropos | Berg adder | Bit-atr. | ++ |
| Bitis caudalis | Horned adder | Bit-ca. | + |
| Bitis gabonica | Gaboon viper | Bit-ga. | ++ |
| Bitis nasicornis | Rhinoceros viper | Bit-nas. | + |
| Cerastes cerastes | Horned viper | Ceras-ce. | ++ |
| Daboia russelii | Russell's viper | Vip-d. | + |
| Daboia siamensis | Eastern Russell's viper | Vip-ds. | + |
| Echis carinatus | Saw-scaled viper | Echis-ca. | ++ |
| Proatheris superciliaris | Swamp viper | Proa-su. | + |
| Vipera ammodytes merid. | Eastern nose-horned viper | Vip-am-m. | + |
| Vipera aspis | Asp viper | Vip-a. | ++ |
| Vipera berus | Common European viper | Vip. | +++ |
| Vipera daboia | = Daboia russelii | Vip-d. | |
| Vipera lebetina[1] | Blunt-nosed viper | Vip-ll. | + |
| Vipera palaestinae[2] | Palestine viper | Vip-pal. | + |
| Vipera redi | Central Italian asp viper | Vip-r. | + |
| Vipera torva | = Vipera berus | Vip. | |
| Vipera xanthina[3] | Ottoman viper | Vip-x. | + |

1 = Macrovipera lebetina. 2 = Daboia palaestinae. 3 = Montivipera xanthina.

# ATHERIS SQUAMIGERA

## Systematics
- Scientific name: Atheris squamigera [Hallowell, 1856].
- Synonyms: Echis squamigera [Hallowell, 1856]. Toxicoa squamigera [Cope, 1860].
- Common names: African bush viper. Rough-scale bush viper. Variable bush viper.
- Family: Viperidae, subfamily Viperinae.

## Biological Profile
- Arboreal true viper with broad triangular head, distinct from narrow neck, and strongly keeled scales. Varying in colours, exhibiting polymorphism incl. shades of light greens to darker olive, brown and rust colours as well as in reds, blues, yellows and greys. Colouration consistent in some populations, variable in others. Belly some shade of yellow or green, often with black markings.

Snout broad; mouth unusually large. Average length 45–50 cm; females much larger than males and may reach a length of 82 cm.
- Tail prehensile, used for grasping branches, or hanging from them to ambush unsuspecting prey. Tail tips usually yellow or cream coloured and used for caudal luring by juveniles.
- Range: Central Africa.
- Habitat: Primarily rainforest; also open woodland bordering rainforests and swamps.
- Ovoviviparous; 5–9 live young per brood.
- Nocturnal. Descends at night through the foliage to hang just above the ground in order to ambush prey. From this position it strikes small mammals passing underneath. It also manages to drink while hanging from vegetation by ingesting condensing water running downward on the body.
- 'Atheris squamigera is able to move quickly when necessity dictates, but in general this taxon is *inactive to the point of lethargy*. They will find a quiet elevated perch in their terrarium, coil, and may remain, barely moving, for several days. But, if disturbed, they can and will strike quickly and accurately.' [reptilesmagazine.com]
- Preys on small rodents, amphibians and lizards.
- In captivity, many bush vipers will feed to obesity, esp. females readily enjoy being fed.

### Behaviour & Temperament
Active nocturnally, during the day it basks in the sun above foliage. A very alert and irritable snake, it strikes violently when molested. It is not, however, aggressive when not disturbed. Deliberate in its climbing movements. When disturbed in vegetation it freezes. If the disturbance continues it may drop in a 'free fall' through the foliage. [Mallow, 2003]


## MATERIA MEDICA ATHERIS SQUAMIGERA

### Sources
1 Effects of bite; clinical manifestations.
2 Effects of bite to left pinky finger.

### Clinical Manifestations
Venom haemotoxic. Full specifics of venom yield, toxicity and content are not known; this is likely the case simply because humans have little contact with this highly arboreal snake of dense forest habitats.

# CASE

*Case reports found in the literature:*
A 34-year-old male bitten by an adult Atheris squamigera developed symptoms of nausea, vomiting, diarrhoea, which were followed by drowsiness and impaired breathing. Local haemorrhage, oedema and pain at the bite site occurred, but no systemic bleeding or haemorrhagic diathesis developed. All clinical and laboratory parameters were in the normal range except for afibrinogenemia, thrombocytopenia and slight proteinuria. Replacement therapy [fibrinogen and platelet concentrates] and treatment of shock stabilized the patient within 2 days and coagulation returned to normal. [Mebs, 1998]

Knoepffler described a bite which he experienced himself. His forearm was bitten by a captive animal identified as 'probably *A. squamigera*. The snake was small, about 30 cm. There was severe pain, swelling of the forearm, dizziness, chills, severe nausea, regional swelling of lymph nodes, interference with vision and pain on breathing. His rectal temperature peaked after 12 hours at 38.5°C [101.3°F]. No specific therapy was employed, aspirin was taken for pain and recovery was complete. [Mallow, 2003]

The African bush viper's bite is not deadly but can be extremely painful. 'To an adult, it would be like suffering several bee stings,' said Van Wallach, a curatorial assistant with Harvard University's Museum of Comparative Zoology. 'They're very painful at first – it's *excruciating* pain. There's a burning sensation that's immediate. [The worst one] felt like somebody had a *blowtorch* and was burning you inside your arm. . . . It went on for 3 straight days before I had any relief.' The last bite he suffered, which blasted him with an unusually large dose of venom, caused him to become delirious for 3 days. The swelling and discolouration on his hand eventually spread to his arm, chest and stomach, lasting for about a month.

## Atheris squamigera Male Bite to Left Pinky Finger

'Immediate burning pain and it feels like the tip of my finger is *on fire*. . . . It hurts *worse when I hold the hand down*, so I am keeping it elevated – the tip of the finger is very sensitive.

'10 minutes – serious pain and it's swelling immediately. Two bruises at tip where fangs punctured skin.

'20 minutes – finger is swelling and getting stiff. I can't and don't want to use that finger for anything. Throbbing pain with my heartbeat.

'4 hours – finger swollen and thick. Half of the back of that hand is swelling and I can't see the veins in it any longer. No other symptoms at this time.

'12 hours – wow, I think it's a tad better already! Didn't sleep well last night due to throbbing pain in the finger. Took some aspirin so I could sleep, but it didn't help.

'24 hours – it's definitely getting better and has stopped hurting already. I can bend the finger just a tad and that was impossible this morning. Swelling is down.

'Essentially a total recovery in 72 hours.' [Morgan, 2009]

# BITIS ARIETANS

## Systematics
- Scientific name: Bitis arietans [Merrem, 1820].
- Synonyms: Vipera arietans [Schlegel, 1837]. Clotho arietans [Gray, 1842]. Bitis lachesis [Mertens, 1953].
- Common name: Puff adder.
- Family: Viperidae, subfamily Viperinae.

## Biological Profile
- Heavy-bodied true viper with large, flattened, triangular head, much wider than neck, and large nostrils that point vertically upwards. Body yellowish, light brown or orange with chevron-shaped dark brown or black bars. Belly yellowish-white to grey with black blotches. Scales small, keeled, overlapping. Average length 1.2 m, maximum 1.9 m. Weight up to 6 kg. Males longer than females.
- Range: Most of Africa, Saudi Arabia and neighbouring countries of SW Asia.
- Habitat: Encountered almost anywhere in Africa, at both low and high elevations, except for rain forests and extreme desert conditions. Found mainly in savannah or open grassland incl. areas with scattered scrubby bushes, from sea level to 3,500 m elevation. Common around human settlements and in agricultural areas due to the abundance of rats and chickens.
- Largely nocturnal, often basks in early morning or late afternoon.
- Terrestrial but may climb sturdy bushes to bask.
- Often lie on roads at night to absorb heat during cooler weather.
- Sit-and-wait predator, lying camouflaged along rodent runs. Preys on small rodents, birds, amphibians and sometimes other snakes.
- Hibernates and does not feed during winter. Feeds ravenously during warm months to build fat reserves to last through hibernation. Death of puff adders from *gluttony* has been reported.
- Does not move like other serpents; moves in a rectilinear motion or in a straight line similar to the way a caterpillar moves.
- Excellent swimmer and capable climber [if need be].
- Males engage in combat dances.
- Ovoviviparous; 20–40 live young per brood. Gravid females do not feed, spend considerable time basking and become increasingly aggressive.
- Two recognized subspecies [arietans and somalica].

## Behaviour & Temperament

The second largest of the dangerous vipers, the puff adder is one of the most common snakes in Africa. Largely nocturnal, foraging at night and seeking shelter during day's heat. Generally sluggish; relies on cryptic colouration to avoid notice and escape detection. Not shy when approached. Draws head close to coils, makes a loud hissing sound and is quick to strike any intruder but does not hold on. Bad-tempered and excitable. The specific epithet arietans means 'to strike violently' and strike it will. Strikes vigorously and quickly in all directions. Able to lash out sideways without warning or withdrawing its head like other snakes do. Quickly recoils after a bite, ready to strike again.

## Taming of the Puffing Shrew

Snake man Ionides gave it his best to tame female puff adders, trying 3 times and failing 3 times. The second female puff adder Ionides attempted to tame is quite easy going at first, but 'she began to get bad tempered till eventually she would start puffing and hissing the moment anyone went near her box. To get her to strike you had merely to wave a handkerchief in front, if you were wise at the end of a stick, and the next thing you would suddenly see was a gaping mouth hit the wire then go back again so fast it was difficult for the eye to follow the movement.' He releases this 'exceptionally bad tempered' female in the bush, recalling it didn't go any better the first time he attempted to tame one.

This first one initially didn't object to being picked up and put in his lap while he was reading a book. 'With great affection I called her Fatuma. I think our relationship first became strained when I found she would not feed . . . so I fed her forcibly by pouring raw eggs into her through a funnel. That led to her getting *surly and puffy* whenever I picked her up and she would go on puffing for quite a good while after she had been put down. She was the one, fickle bint, who in the end repaid my kindness with a nasty haemotoxic jab. . . . Shortly after that Fatuma and I parted company – she too was decanted into the bush. I subsequently made one further attempt to tame a puff adder. This was another female I named Nagi, but that affair too wound up with the lady being left in the bush. Since then, and it has been a long time, I have never taken the risk with a puff adder.' [Ionides, 1969]

## MATERIA MEDICA BITIS ARIETANS

### Sources

1 Proving Craig Wright [South Africa], 15 provers [9 females, 6 males], 30c; 1998.
2 Proving Farokh Master [India], 5 provers [3 females, 2 males], 30c; 2003.
3 Clinical observations Farokh Master.
4 Degroote, Dream Repertory.
5 Synthesis Repertory Treasure Edition 2009.
6 Effects of bite; clinical manifestations.
7 Effects of bite; case reports.

## Mind

∞ Spacey feeling, as if drunk with difficulty concentrating. Removed from reality. Conversations seem to be unreal. Feeling of floatiness; almost fatigue-like with mixing up of words and ideas.[1]

∞ Difficulty concentrating during conversations. 'Hears without hearing'. Not taking in the information.[1]

∞ Feeling 'not-all-there'.[1]

∞ Craving company, but with little tolerance of people. Conversation and concentration difficult; mind wandering off in middle of conversations.[1]

∞ Difficulty remembering simple words, conveying ideas or expressing oneself. Feeling foolish. Mouth as if disconnected from brain.[1]

∞ Mind goes blank when trying to think.[1]

∞ Dullness in morning on waking.[5]

∞ Feeling isolated and estranged from people due to having cynical points of view.[1]

∞ Boundaries expanding, almost as if one can see through the physicality of the world.[1]

∞ Feeling very sentimental. Listening to old songs and feeling emotional and melancholy; looking back over the past few years of one's life.[1]

∞ Desire to be outdoors for gardening or to be outside in nature, in the mountains.[1]

∞ Suspicious; fears to be robbed, abused, attacked.[2]

∞ Fear of own impulses to do violence, loss of self-control from anger, hitting others. Active attempts to mask anger. Quarrelsome during menses.[2]

∞ Abusive and out of control anger.[2]

∞ Shouts/screams loudly when angry; can't discuss or argue without shouting.[2]

∞ Irrational irritability.[1]

∞ Too irritated to deal with crowds.[1]

∞ Irritability in morning.[4]

∞ Increased activity at night.[1,2]

∞ Forsaken feeling. Delusion of being alone, separated from the world.[1]

∞ Delusion being neglected and excluded.[1]

∞ Delusion body is enlarged, feeling fat.[5]

∞ Delusions: being alone; being far off; forsaken; everything seems unreal.[5]

∞ Nothing seems to please. Everything seems boring.[2]

∞ Nervous and palpitations on waking from nap or sleep.[2]

∞ Envy.[4]

∞ Fear of contagion.[4]

∞ Fear of undertaking new things.[4]

∞ Bashful timidity about being naked or undressing oneself.[4]

∞ Hurry with slow execution.[5]

∞ Laziness followed by mania for work.[5]

∞ Loquacity, changing quickly from one subject to another.[5]

∞ Mental power increased.[5]

## Dreams

∞ Abused/scolded, being.[4]
∞ Accused, falsely, of murder.[4]
∞ Aggressive.[4]
∞ Ambiguous sexuality.[1]
∞ Attacked by horses.[4]
∞ Bitten, being.[4]
∞ Black marble coffin.[4]
∞ Black snake biting people.[2]
∞ Buried alive.[4]
∞ Burying loved ones.[2]
∞ Car brakes not working.[4]
∞ Cheated, being.[4]
∞ Criticized, being.[4]
∞ Cut into pieces, dead body.[4]
∞ Danger, impending, flood or landslide.[4]
∞ Dead bodies.[1]
∞ Dead bodies on railway tracks.[2]
∞ Detached and helpless.[1]
∞ Embarrassment, standing naked in front of many people.[2]
∞ Enemies, friends behave like.[4]
∞ Enemies, surrounded by.[4]
∞ Escape, attempting or unable to.[4]
∞ Exploited, being.[4]
∞ Failing final year examination.[2]
∞ Fighting.[4]
∞ Fighting a gang of roughnecks with serrated weapons.[2]
∞ Fire.[4]
∞ Fire, arson, riots.[2]
∞ Funeral, person to be buried is still alive.[4]
∞ Gambling and getting things not really yours.[1]
∞ Getting married.[2]
∞ Guns, shooting, murder, violence.[1]
∞ Hanging in the air in an elevator.[2]
∞ Hide, desire to.[4]
∞ Homosexual relations.[4]
∞ Ignored, being.[4]
∞ Lured into a trap.[4]
∞ Mothers, children and violence.[1]
∞ Naked in the street.[4]
∞ Parturition, painless.[4]
∞ Privacy, lack of.[4]
∞ Pursued, being.[1,2]
∞ Pursued by a bull.[4]
∞ Rage from being hit or punched, striking back.[2]
∞ Running for one's life from men brandishing swords.[2]

∞ Running from policeman.[2]
∞ Shooting, pursuit, impending danger.[1]
∞ Threatened to be killed.[4]
∞ Throwing away old shoes.[2]
∞ Tortured, being.[4]
∞ Unable to hold urine.[2]
∞ Water, waves and sea.[1,4]
∞ Wearing see-through dress and exposing breasts.[2]

## Generals
∞ Drowsiness in afternoon.[2]
∞ Fatigue, lethargy, tiredness.[1]
∞ Weariness > exertion; < during menses.[5]
∞ Anaemia after haemorrhage.[1]
∞ Wounds bleeding freely.[1]
∞ Blackness of external parts.[1]
∞ Great chilliness; lack of vital heat, warm covering does not >.[1]
∞ Can't control hunger.[2]
∞ Wants to eat at small intervals.[2]
∞ Desire for coffee; cold drinks; ice-cream; meat; peanut butter; salty; spices; sweets; warm drinks.[1]
∞ Desire for bread; cheese; milk; potatoes.[2]
∞ Desire for honey; meat; tomatoes.[4]
∞ Aversion to cooked food; fried food; lentils; rice.[2]
∞ Aversion to mushrooms; green vegetables.[4]
∞ Venous swelling; venous thrombosis, varicose veins, cellulitis. Pyoderma; furunculosis.[3]
∞ Rubbing >.[1]
∞ Magnetism >.[4]
∞ Movement <.[1]

## Sensations
∞ Body as if shaking inside; as if vibrating.[1]
∞ Everything stagnated, no flow in body.[1]
∞ Layer of heat around body.[1]
∞ Veil between mind and reality.[1]
∞ Dizziness as if being turned around.[2]
∞ Head as if filled with cotton wool; as if congested, foggy, heavy [5 pr.].[1]
∞ Head heavy as a concrete block.[1]
∞ Band across forehead > squeezing face tight, making faces.[1]
∞ Eyes as if moving slower than head.[1]
∞ Seeing the world only through the right eye.[1]
∞ Noises echoing and louder as if right next to one, or the reverse: sounds as if distant.[1]
∞ Fullness root of nose.[5]
∞ Left side of face as if paralyzed.[4]

∞ Tongue or lower lip as if cold.[5]
∞ Tongue or tip of tongue as if burned.[1]
∞ Lump in throat, as if being choked.[2]
∞ Difficulty in swallowing with a tight, constricted feeling around throat and larynx, as if very tense and constricting neck muscles.[1]
∞ Entire contents of abdomen as if falling out, & dysmenorrhoea.[1]
∞ Coldness in airways and lungs.[1]
∞ Lungs as if squeezed.[1]
∞ Weight on chest; chest as if closed, tight.[1]
∞ Heaviness on left side of chest.[2]
∞ Heart as if constricted, with pain in 4th intercostal space.[2]
∞ Heart as if pulled toward the left, with sudden palpitations.[2]
∞ Arms as if heavy.[1]
∞ Lower limbs as if heavy.[1]
∞ Ankles as if sprained, > motion.[5]

## Locals
∞ Giddiness when turning around or turning the head.[1]
∞ Dizziness and unsteadiness on closing eyes [2 pr.].[1]
∞ Off balance when leaning forward with head down.[1]
∞ Dizziness with tendency to fall to left; while sitting; when looking intently at an object.[2]
∞ Dull temporal headache, > stretching neck. Neck and trapezius muscles feel very tight.[1]
∞ Headache from cold drinks or cold food; from exertion; from fasting; from loss of sleep; when lying on back or on left side.[2]
∞ Pain occiput extending down back of neck.[5]
∞ Eyes dry, burning, blurry, tired, strained, & desire to blink or close eyes.[1]
∞ Dryness nose < dust and in morning on waking.[2]
∞ Hay fever with asthmatic breathing.[5]
∞ Persistent dryness of mouth and throat, drinking water does not >.[1]
∞ Dryness mouth returns after drinking.[4]
∞ Clenching teeth in anger.[2]
∞ Clenching teeth during sleep.[5]
∞ Dryness lips and mouth & thirstlessness.[2]
∞ Throat pain, central, at level of lower oro-pharynx or upper larynx; > swallowing, empty swallowing or warm or cold drinks.[1]
∞ Vomiting and heaviness abdomen after eating cheese.[2]
∞ Abdominal bloating after eating cheese.[2]
∞ Abdominal bloating [4 pr.], < eating anything; & urging for stool.[1]
∞ Abdominal cramp before menses.[5]
∞ Abdominal cramp < passing flatus, running, sitting, standing; > lying on back.[5]
∞ Intolerance of tight clothes around abdomen.[2]
∞ Pain lower abdomen when controlling urge to urinate.[2]
∞ Difficulty in passing stool; desire to pass stool but cannot; ineffectual urging.[1,2]
∞ Diarrhoea after anticipation.[5]

∞ Urinary retention in presence of strangers.[4]

∞ Menses early, sudden onset and very heavy. Dark blood with many dark red/black clots.[1]

∞ Asthma attack; sudden onset of high pitched expiratory wheeze at 23:00; need for cold fresh air, must sit up; < pressure on chest and lying down; > company and slow, deep breathing; & itching of soft palate, nose blocked and stuffed up, anxiety.[1]

∞ Asthmatic respiration & itching.[5]

∞ Asthmatic respiration & obstruction of nose.[5]

∞ Asthmatic respiration > company.[5]

∞ Difficult respiration, wants to be fanned.[5]

∞ Cough < talking.[4]

∞ Sudden electric shock-like pain behind sternum and in area of 4th and 5th left intercostal space, extending to external throat; < rest and pressure, > motion.[2]

∞ Pain nape of neck/cervical region on bending head forwards.[2]

∞ Pain nape of neck/cervical region > lying on back with head high.[4]

∞ Stiffness neck and/or shoulders [6 pr.].[1]

∞ Stiffness all over; in morning on waking.[1] Desire to stretch.[1]

∞ Muscle stiffness and tenderness extreme for amount of exercise done. Gluteal muscles, quadriceps femoris and extensor muscles of forearm mainly affected.[1]

∞ Extreme muscular pain in hips/buttocks, < movement and & stiffness everywhere.[1]

∞ Weakness ankles < walking.[5]

## Split

'Woke up naturally and 'dream' the following: I feel suspended between sleep and wakefulness with a semi-conscious awareness of daytime, light and noises. I feel also an amazing split in me. I feel split between 2 images. As I lie in bed, my body is split longitudinally. Superimposed on the left side is a grainy black-and-white image of a woman; on the right hand side is a grainy black-and-white image of a man. Both images are equal in size and have indistinct features. I feel a physical pull between the 2 halves. I am aware of a conflict between the 2 – the one wants something from the other, but what it is, I am not sure.' [prover 7]

## Synopsis of South African Proving

- Notable effects were seen in the mind, abdomen, rectum, respiratory system and the musculoskeletal system, as well as the female sexual system.
- Most characteristic is spaciness or spaced-out feeling also described as being intoxicated with alcohol or Cannabis. Spacey feeling, as if disconnected, detached or removed from reality – separated from environment or from body, feeling of being left out of group. This is accompanied by a depleted, energyless state.

  Slothful, sluggish, lazy and dull. Mistakes in speech and writing. Conversation and reading difficult. Difficulty in concentrating and studying; absent-minded and forgetful. Depressed and overwhelmed – feeling of inability to cope. Nostalgia and homesickness. Desire to be out of doors.

Alternatively, very energized and full of life, happy, talkative and speaking fast. Feeling capable of doing many things especially cleaning and tidying and may have difficulty sleeping when in this state.

- A split or division is a theme that runs through the snake venoms. In Bitis, some of the divisions may be between being present or absent, in the body or out of the body, between the individual and the group – included or excluded; between the real and unreal, near or distant. There appears to be a split between the left and right brains possibly indicating an influence on the corpus callosum [cf. 'Cannot find the correct words or names for people or objects and struggling to express myself.']
- Tiredness, lethargy, fatigue, exhaustion were characteristic features. The puff adder is known to be a slow, slothful animal and is responsible for many snakebites simply because it does not get out of the way. The laziness experienced by the provers has reference here and this seems to be more from the physical energy-depleted state than from a mental causation.

However, once the puff adder is roused, it is an exceptionally fast striker – so fast in fact that it has given rise to the myth that the snake can strike backwards. A similar theme seems to appear in the proving, where provers let things build up [such as housework] and then in a flurry of activity would clean up. This energised, 'manic' state also appeared in a number of provers.
- Stiffness occurred in many provers in a generalised form and seems to be a characteristic of this remedy.
- Few prominent food cravings or aversions were caused, however, the desire for ice cream and peanut butter was fairly strong.
- Appetite was predominantly diminished and thirst was predominantly increased.
- The remedy seems to be cold sensitive and chilly and this symptom is confirmed in a case of envenomation, where the patient was cold and sweating. Coldness also occurred in the upper and lower limbs and cold sensations occurred in the mouth and airways.
- Heaviness occurred in head, neck and upper torso, eyelids, arms, thighs and as a general sensation. One prover described a sensation of being 'heavy in my being'.
- Dryness occurred in mouth, lips, throat, eyes, stool and cough. Increased thirst could be grouped together with these symptoms.
- Only 2 clear modalities were discovered on analysis: Rubbing > [3 separate particulars] and Movement < [4 separate particulars].
- Clear symptoms of bronchial asthma were produced with expiratory wheeze, tightness in chest and fine rattling of secretions. There was concomitant hay fever, itching and sneezing which would point to an allergic basis to the asthma. Attacks were at night. Congested or weight sensations were produced in the chest. [Craig Wright; RefWorks]

## Clinical Manifestations

Puff adder venom has strong haemotoxic activity. The primary mode of action is extensive haemorrhage due to blood and capillary breakdown, causing suffusion of blood into tissues. Blood is sometimes found in the sputum, urine, faeces, and vomitus after 18 hours and small petechial haemorrhages may be observed under mucus membranes and skin. Suffusion of blood into the tissues is accompanied by profound swelling, extreme pain and nausea, leading eventually to death by sheer exhaustion.

'The symptoms and signs of puff adder bite are very similar to those of rattlesnake bites: pain, swelling, ecchymosis, bleb formation, lymphadenitis, and lymphangitis. Tissue necrosis may develop, and nausea and vomiting have been reported, as has thrombophlebitis.' [Russell, 1980]

'Red and purple discolouration around the wound, which changes to blue-black; pain and enlargement of regional lymph nodes and profound swelling which is hot and painful to touch. After several days, swelling usually subsides, except for the area immediately around the wound. . . . Necrotic skin, subcutaneous tissue and muscle separate from healthy tissue and eventually slough with serous exudate. The slough may be superficial or deep, sometimes exposing bone. Gangrene is common and may result in appendage loss. Secondary infection may further complicate healing. Despite prompt treatment, complete healing of the sloughed region may take an extended period and some victims are permanently disabled with stiffness. In human victims, hypotension with accompanying dizziness, weakness and periods of semi- or unconsciousness is reported. . . . If untreated, death may ensue within several days due to cerebral haemorrhage leading to convulsions, kidney failure, and complications caused by extensive swelling.' [Mallow, 2003]

## Case Reports

'An 18-year-old Hausa man trod on a snake during the night and was bitten on the right calf. On admission 3 hours later his leg was tender and swollen to up the knee. He brought the 82-cm Bitis arietans. No antivenom was available. Eighteen hours after the bite he complained of abdominal pain, was cold and sweating, and had a blood pressure of 100/70 mmHg and a pulse rate of 110/min. During the next hour his blood pressure fell to 84/40 mmHg and his pulse rose to 132/min. The electrocardiogram was normal. The foot of the bed was raised, 1 litre of dextrosesaline was infused intravenously, and the blood pressure returned to normal. The swelling extended to the groin, and blisters appeared on the ankle 25 hrs after the bite, later coalescing to mid-calf level. Two days after the bite the limb was cold, anaesthetic, and pulseless below the knee.

'On the 4th day after the bite the patient had 2 epistaxes. He was *severely anaemic* with a haemoglobin of 3–6g/dl, and there was a leucocytosis of 11–4 × $10^9/1$. Poikilocytes and schistocytes were seen in the blood film, suggesting microangiopathic haemolysis. The blood was coagulable and clot quality was normal. One unit of fresh blood was transfused without reaction. Although the limb had become frankly gangrenous, amputation was vigorously opposed by his relatives. On the 7th day pitting oedema extended up to the chest wall.

Haemoglobin had risen slightly and his platelet count was 278 × 109/l but he had further arterial epistaxis and became jaundiced. Two units of blood were transfused. By the 12th day his blood urea was 35–5 mmol/l [214 mg/100 ml]. On the 23rd day his relatives agreed to amputation. Postoperatively he developed paralytic ileus; plasma potassium and urea concentrations continued to rise and he died in ventricular fibrillation 24 days after being bitten.'

'Clinical – Local pain and swelling were noticed by all 10 patients within 20 minutes of being bitten. Three vomited, but one had taken an herbal emetic. . . . Local swelling was maximal 1 or 2 days after the bite and took 5 days to 3 weeks to resolve. Local blistering was seen in 5 cases and necrosis in 3. Popliteal artery thrombosis was a complication in case 2. Spontaneous systemic bleeding occurred in 3 patients – one bled from healthy gums 4 hours after the bite [and into the aortic adventitia, found at necropsy], and 2 had epistaxes, one on the 4th, 9th and 10th days, and the other on the 4th day. In cases 3 and 4 the patients developed ecchymoses in the bitten limb. No blood was found in vomitus, stool, or urine. Five patients had fever on admission, reaching 38.7°–40.5°C [101.7°–104.9°F] [mean 39.3°C; 102.7°F] up to 8 days after the bite. Although 4 patients were drowsy on admission, all were fully rousable, and no other neurological abnormalities were found. Hypotension was observed in case 2; in case 1, in which the blood pressure fell before death [ECG was normal 13 hours earlier]; and in case 3, in which the patient had a blood pressure of 90/50 mmHg and a bradycardia of 52/min on admission. In cases 2 and 3 the patients became jaundiced on the ninth and fourth days respectively.' [Warrell, 1975]

# BITIS ATROPOS

## Systematics
- Scientific name: Bitis atropos [L., 1758].
- Synonyms: Coluber atropos [L., 1758]. Vipera montana [Smith, 1826].
- Common name: Berg adder. Mountain adder.
- Family: Viperidae, subfamily Viperinae.

## Biological Profile
- Small heavy-bodied true viper with triangular head distinct from neck. Colour variable, ranging from dark grey, greyish-brown, brown to red. Paired, triangular blotches with a pale line bordering the blotches. Belly grey or brown, spotted with darker. Average length 30–40 cm; maximum 60 cm.
- Range: SE Africa.
- Habitat: Mountain ranges, higher escarpment areas, highlands.
- Diurnal.
- Hides under rocks and in rodent burrows to escape the winter snows.
- Preys on frogs, lizards and rodents.
- Ovoviviparous; 4–15 live young per brood.

- Bad-tempered; hisses loudly, twists convulsively, strikes without undue provocation.
- 'Berg' is Afrikaans/Dutch for 'mountain'.

## MATERIA MEDICA BITIS ATROPOS

### Sources
1 Proving Victoria-Leigh Schönfeld & Shraddha Brijnath [South Africa], 22 provers [16 females, 6 males], 30c; 2013.
2 Effects of bite; clinical manifestations.

### Mind
∞ Absent-minded, confused, dazed; confusion in conversations, losing train of thought.
∞ Misunderstands words and meanings.
∞ Great irritability [8 pr.].
∞ Snappish, angry, wants to scream, be aggressive and strangle someone.
∞ Anger from indignation.
∞ Quarrelsome [4 pr.].
∞ Enraged and extremely annoyed; wants to attack annoying people.
∞ Distrustful, suspicious, careful, guarded.
∞ Wants to shed one's 'good boy persona' and become 'liberated', giving oneself over to promiscuity, sexual self-indulgence, the dark side.
∞ Libertinism [3 pr.].
∞ Dwells on own hidden urges and darker inner world.
∞ Stuck in rut and routine.
∞ Feels 'like an old woman with a teenage girl stuck inside'.
∞ Craves attention; wants to shine, take the spotlight and be noticed.
∞ Intrusive, judgmental, unscrupulous.
∞ Undermines others in order to lift up oneself.
∞ Fears: Heights; falling down the stairs; thieves.
∞ Delusion flying in the clouds, lost in space.
∞ Delusions: criticized; injured; robbed; trapped.

### Dreams
∞ Benevolence; people helping each other.
∞ Chased, being.
∞ Coffin with dead girl.
∞ Company of friends.
∞ Criticized, being.
∞ Good and evil.
∞ Inappropriate behaviour, sexually [5 pr.].
∞ Mountain, going up and down.
∞ Nakedness.
∞ Performing, singing and dancing.

∞ Pursued, being.
∞ Salvation.
∞ Searching for a wise man.
∞ Seeking comfort and refuge.
∞ Sexual.
∞ Sexual acts with strangers.
∞ Snake, massive.
∞ Wedding.

## Generals
∞ Muscle tension < at night.
∞ Tired, flat, exhausted [10 pr.].
∞ Excess of energy [5 pr.].
∞ Appetite decreased or lost [7 pr.]; increased or excessive [5 pr.].
∞ Great thirst [6 pr.].
∞ Sleep restless, fitful, interrupted [12 pr.].
∞ Desire for chocolate [3 pr.]; coffee [2 pr.]; salt [2 pr.]; tea [2 pr.]; water [2 pr.].
∞ Coffee > [2 pr.].
∞ Sweets < – throat, stomach, cough.

## Sensations
∞ Floating sensation, light-headedness, < movement, > standing still, sitting down.
∞ Forehead as if bulging, as if full of warm water.
∞ Left side of face and neck as if paralyzed, hanging down, loose, heavy.
∞ Tightness left temple.
∞ Eyes as if bruised, < sun and direct light.
∞ Eyes as if loose, smaller, sunken, swollen, or wide open.
∞ Ice stuck in right nostril, < breathing cold air.
∞ Nervous feeling in back of throat and heart.
∞ Food stuck in throat.
∞ Ball of air stuck in throat.
∞ Bone stuck at back of throat.
∞ Sharp splinters in throat.
∞ Small pins poking in stomach.
∞ Lump in stomach.
∞ Something alive in abdomen.
∞ Lump in rectum.
∞ Something warm behind sternum.
∞ Heart as if knocking on rib cage.
∞ Heart as if beating throughout chest.
∞ Cervical region as if crushed.
∞ Weight pressing on cervical region/nape of neck.
∞ Back muscles as if contracted, > stretching.
∞ Lumbar spine as if dislocated from rest of spine, > bending, stretching, standing.
∞ Hips as if loose.

## Locals

∞ Dizziness < walking [2 pr.].

∞ Headache [10 pr.], & pain or stiffness nape of neck [2 pr.]; dull pain [4 pr.].

∞ Headache > sun exposure [2 pr.].

∞ Frontal headache, extending to back of head when standing, & dizziness.

∞ Frontal headache and pressure behind eyes < stooping, > pressure.

∞ Occipital headache & dizziness.

∞ Ear pain < opening mouth.

∞ Sneezing [8 pr.].

∞ Sharp, cutting throat pain < swallowing, > water, clearing throat.

∞ Sore throat < sweets, scarf around throat, > warm drinks, fruits.

∞ Throat pain < talking.

∞ Fullness stomach < coffee.

∞ Heartburn < drinking, > eating.

∞ Nausea < rich food, putrid smells.

∞ Nausea < sweets.

∞ Abdomen sensitive to clothing; > loosening clothes.

∞ Increased urination [4 pr.].

∞ Cough < sweets.

∞ Cramping pain in left intercostal muscles, < breathing, > standing erect.

∞ Palpitations & pulsating in throat; extending to eyes.

∞ Palpitations in morning on waking.

∞ Aching knee joints and crampy aching calves, < walking down stairs.

## Clinical Manifestations

• Berg adder envenomation causes a unique syndrome of cytotoxic and neuro-toxic symptoms and signs. Local effects include initial pain in the region of the bite mark and swelling. Systemic effects include paraesthesias of the tongue and lips, ophthalmoplegia characterised by visual disturbances, ptosis, fixed dilated pupils and loss of eye movements and accommodation, as well as loss of the sense of smell [anosmia] and taste. The dilated pupils and loss of the sense of smell and taste may take weeks to months to resolve. Late-onset respiratory failure is a complication 6–36 hours after the bite, often at a stage when it is not anticipated or expected. Hyponatremia, which may lead to con-vulsions, often develops 2–3 days after the bite and should not be interpreted as a syndrome of inappropriate antidiuretic hormone secretion. Hyponatremia is probably the result of a natriuretic peptide in the venom that induces renal sodium loss. [Wium, 2017]

• 'This observational series of 14 cases documents features of berg adder enven-oming over a period of 16 years [1987–2003]. Clinical features of envenomed patients: All 14 patients developed local cytotoxic effects. Thirteen patients developed systemic effects manifesting and documented in varying degrees. These include [1] prominent vomiting; [2] disturbances in cranial nerve function [anosmia and altered taste, an ophthalmological triad of ptosis, mydriasis and visual disturbances incl. loss of accommodation, and dysphagia]; [3] a global decrease in motor power where mechanical ventilation was often required for respiratory failure and [4] hyponatremia [lowest value recorded 111 mmol/L], sometimes with associated convulsions.' [van der Walt, 2018]

# BITIS CAUDALIS

## Systematics
- Scientific name: Bitis caudalis [Smith, 1839].
- Synonyms: Vipera ocellata [Smith, 1838]. Vipera caudalis [Smith, 1838]. Cerastes caudalis [Gray, 1842].
- Common names: Horned adder. Horned puff adder.
- Family: Viperidae, subfamily Viperinae.

## Biological Profile
- Small, stocky true viper with triangular head, strongly keeled dorsal scales and short tail. Average length 46 cm, maximum 51 cm. Females larger than males.
- Body colouration sandy grey, puff to pinkish, reddish or dark brown; males may be vivid with blues, reds, greys and yellows; females generally sandy or reddish orange with little or no pattern. Dorsal row of quadrangular dark markings with pale edges. Broad V-shaped to hourglass-shaped dark mark on top of head. Belly uniform creamy to yellowish-white.
- Range: Southern Africa.
- Habitat: Desert; found mostly in sparsely vegetated sandy or stony arid scrub. Habitats in central Namibia incl. gravel plains, loose sandy soils, wooded alluvial soils and rocky outcrops.
- Preys primarily on lizards, particularly geckos, skinks and lacertids, and occasionally on small rodents and amphibians. Skinks and lacertids are taken by day, mostly by caudal luring. Geckos, small rodents and amphibians are captured when the snake forages at night.
- Basks in early morning sun, burying itself in the sand as air and surface temperature increase. Needs 5–15 seconds to bury itself completely and remains so during the day, leaving only the eyes exposed under the small sand mounds created by its horns.
- Males engage in combat bouts.
- Ovoviviparous; 4–16 live young per brood.
- Name derived from the single hornlike scale over each eye.

## Behaviour & Temperament
Predators are avoided by flattening and remaining quiet. Along with disruptive colouration, 'freezing' renders this snake highly cryptic. Hisses loudly if severely molested, at the same time forcibly inflating and deflating its body while curling into tight curves. The head is drawn back into the coils for a strike.

Irascible when disturbed, the horned adder will strike with little provocation. The strike is initiated with a loud expulsion of air and may be so forceful that the entire body is lifted as it lunges forward. At the strike midpoint, the snake may be completely suspended 5 or more centimeters above ground. Similar jumping and throwing itself in the air antics are observed during frantic escape efforts.

'Aggressive courting males approach other males in a jerky rapid manner with the anterior third of the body raised to crawl on top. Non-courting males either flee or engage in combat. During combat, males attempt to force the opponent's head down while simultaneously twisting the body around in a corkscrew fashion. The courting male may strike with closed mouth while lashing its body from side to side. Males may chase after several males while courting a female. Males moult prior to combat. Unlike combat in male gaboon vipers, *B. caudalis* combat is prompted by factor others than sexual rivalry. Competition for food, sexual domination and territorial defense may prompt aggression. Males guard only their immediate surroundings with movement by other males with 1 m eliciting an immediate combat response.' [Mallow, 2003]

## MATERIA MEDICA BITIS CAUDALIS

### Sources
1 Effects of bite; clinical manifestations.

### Clinical Manifestations
Venom cytotoxic and possibly neurotoxic, containing a presynaptic protein called caudotoxin similar to bungarotoxin. Envenomation causes swelling, severe pain, nausea, vomiting and shock. Blisters followed by necrotic ulcers may form at the bite site.

Mallow [2003] reports the case of a 24-year-old male bitten on the right middle finger by a 30-cm female horned adder. Within 30 seconds the man complained of intense pain at the bite site, some minutes later followed by transient nausea during transfer to a hospital. Twelve minutes after the bite there was a dull ache in the finger, hand and forearm with pain extending to the armpit. Blood pressure and pulse were slightly elevated. The dorsum of the hand was swollen and tender. Five hours after the bite the patient experienced extreme apprehension and pain. White blood cell count was in the range of a mild immune response, similar to getting a cold; all other haematological and urinary parameters were normal. At discharge from the hospital 7 days after the bite the white blood cell count was 6800 [normal range 4300–10800] while all other factors were normal.

# BITIS GABONICA

### Systematics
• Scientific name: Bitis gabonica [Duméril, Bibron & Duméril, 1854].
• Synonyms: Cerastes nasicornis [Hallowell, 1847]. Bitis arietans gabonica [Mertens, 1951].

- Common names: Gaboon viper. Forest puff adder. Gaboon.
- Family: Viperidae, subfamily Viperinae.

## Biological Profile
- Largest and heaviest of all true vipers, weighing up to 10 kg, with large triangular head and very heavy body, connected by a greatly narrowed neck almost one-third of the head diameter, giving an appearance of great fragility. Body pink to brown with a vertebral series of elongated yellowish or light brown spots connected by hourglass-shaped markings on each side. Dark brown stripe behind each eye. Average length 1.2 m, maximum 2 m.
- Range: Most of Africa, but particularly along the equatorial belt, which consists mainly of tropical rain forests.
- Habitat: Dense rain forests, secondary thickets, cashew, coffee, and cacao plantations. Common in farmed areas near forested country and on roads at night. Occasionally found in open country.
- Small pair of horns between raised nostrils – much smaller than in Bitis [gabonica] rhinoceros. Eyes large and moveable, set well forward and surrounded by 15–21 circumorbital scales.
- Parry [1975] describes how this species has a wider range of eye movement than other snakes. Along a horizontal plane, eye movement can be maintained even if the head is rotated up or down to an angle of up to 45°. If the head is rotated 360°, one eye will tilt up and the other down, depending on the direction of rotation. Also, if one eye looks forwards the other looks back, as if both are connected to a fixed position on an axis between them. In general, the eyes often flick back and forth in a rapid and jerky manner. When asleep, there is no eye movement and the pupils are strongly contracted. The pupils dilate suddenly and eye movement resumes when the animal wakes up. [cited in Wikipedia]
- Withdraws to abandoned mammal burrows, holes, and cavities in ant-hills during dry months, lying dormant until the first rains, usually in November.
- Preys on a variety of birds and mammals. Appetite voracious.
- Males engage in combat dances during periods of peak sexual activity.
- Ovoviviparous; 8–43 live young per brood. Neonates are reported to be vigorously active and aggressive, puffing and hissing at each other as they collide, while the mother remains placid throughout.
- Prone to defecate only after long periods of time, constipation is a frequent cause of death of captive gaboons.

## Behaviour & Temperament
- This dangerous viper is almost invisible on the forest floor due to their colour pattern. This effect is enhanced because they like to 'dig themselves in' so that they become virtually invisible.

    Primarily nocturnal, it comes out at dusk to feed. It has been known to hunt actively, mostly during the first 6 hours of the night, but usually it will hunt by ambush. Spending most of its time motionless in the direct neighbourhood of the paths where prey animals are likely to pass by, it strikes with a speed and fierceness unexpected for such a seemingly sluggish and placid snake when a prey animal comes within striking range. The speed used to strike is unsurpassed and not to be followed with the naked eye. The Gaboon viper does not let go of its prey after it has struck, but hangs on to it, rather than letting it go and waiting for it to die. Prey is also lifted off the ground to prevent it getting hold of anything. This behaviour is different from the behaviour of other species of vipers.

It is not aggressive, but it will stand its ground if approached, remaining motionless and hissing loudly as a warning at first, striking with great force when severely molested or stepped on. Fast as lightning the gaboon viper is able to strike in all directions, be it sideways, forwards, backwards or upwards. It *goes from immobile to explosive in a split second*. One snake handler describes 'a really motivated gaboon as an exploding snake grenade; their physical capabilities are greater, and where a rattlesnake or a cobra cannot turn around and reach you, a gaboon really can and with absolutely no warning.'

Its fangs are enormous, often measuring 5 cm long, the longest of any venomous snake. It injects a large amount of venom when it strikes. Although their venom is not as toxic as many other African snakes, this species has enormous venom glands and the longest fangs of any snake in the world.

- In stark contrast to this stands the test method of snake man C.J.P. Ionides, who believed gaboon vipers could be tread on with bare feet and, if unhurt, they would do little more than hiss and try to get away. Having 'taken over 1200 gaboon vipers with my bare hands', Ionides wrote in his autobiography, *Mambas and Man-Eaters*: 'There are quite a number of snake people with the idea that having anything to do with the gaboon viper is tantamount to dicing with death. This, of course, sounds highly dramatic and may look good on the sort of blurb they put on the notice outside a snake's cage in a zoo, but I am sorry to have to say that the gaboon viper is such a charming and good-natured snake it very seldom bites anybody. You might get the odd one that takes a cut at you, but they always make a noise about it by hissing loudly and you are warned right away.'

Elsewhere he describes a capture method further attesting to the docility of this snake. 'He first lightly touched the top of the head with a pair of tongs to test the reaction. Unless anger was displayed, which was rare, tongs were laid aside. The neck was then calmly but firmly grasped with one hand while the body was grasped and lifted with the other. He stated that the snakes seldom struggled. He would also stroke them before catching them. In some parts of Africa, native children drag live gaboon vipers by the tail to their villages before killing them for food.' [Mallow, 2003]

## MATERIA MEDICA BITIS GABONICA

### Sources
1 Proving Bruce Thomson [South Africa], 15 provers [11 females, 4 males], 30c; c. 2004.

2 Effects of bite; clinical manifestations.
3 Effects of bite; blood coagulation.
4 Effects of bite; struggling to breathe & live.

## Mind
∞ Feeling alone, friendless, isolated from companions and loved ones, on the outside. Self-pity.
∞ Panic attacks in night or early morning, waking disoriented and terrified, suddenly feeling alone or in the company of strangers.
∞ Sadness < nightfall.
∞ Overwhelmed by people, noise, and activity. Drained, unsettled, irritable, vulnerable.

## Dreams
∞ Chased by bear.
∞ Embarrassment, being laughed at.
∞ Intimidated by parents.
∞ Paralysis.
∞ Rejection, isolation, shut out.
∞ Threatened and hurried.

## Generals
∞ Cold drinks/cold food = headache.
∞ Great thirst, desperately hungry and huge appetite.
∞ Waking too early and tired.
∞ Craving for chocolate; coffee [3 pr.]; sweets [2 pr.].

## Sensations
∞ Dizziness as if falling from a height.
∞ Left eye as if swollen and larger than right eye, < at night.
∞ Eyeballs as if dry.
∞ Lump in throat when swallowing.
∞ Cold air in throat.
∞ Knot in stomach.
∞ Wave of nausea in intestines.
∞ Uterus as if grabbed and twisted/wrung.
∞ Great weight on chest [cardiac area].

## Locals
∞ Light-headed dizziness on computer, > sitting, closing eyes.
∞ Frontal headache < heat, thinking of it, > distraction, rest.
∞ Pressing occipital headache from anything around neck.
∞ Dimness vision, as if looking through mist, during headache like pressure sideways on eyes.
∞ Runny nose, thick, clear discharge, & sneezing, < cold, > eating.
∞ Dryness throat in morning on waking.

∞ Painful coition [in female]. Desire present but pleasure absent. Insensible. Bruised sensation.

∞ Sweaty hands and armpits, very dry feet.

## Clinical Manifestations

Bitis gabonica venom exerts a number of cytotoxic and cardiovascular effects: cytotoxic effects include widespread haemorrhage, caused by the presence of 2 haemorrhagic proteins. Mild 'neurotoxic' features have been reported, but not classic ptosis or major paralysis.

Serotonin is an important constituent of many non-snake venoms, such as hornets, wasps, toads, sea anemones, jellyfish, cone snails, scorpions, and plants like Urtica and Mucuna. Bitis gabonica is the only snake with relatively high [5 mg/gram] concentrations. A histamine-like substance in the venom has also been reported.

Local effects: Pain and swelling: onset almost immediately after bite. Blistering, bleb formation. Haemorrhagic oedema. Tissue necrosis: onset usually days after bite. Ecchymosis.

Cardiovascular: Severe hypotension: onset immediately. Cardiac arrhythmias. Tachycardia. Prolonged QT intervals. Supra-ventricular tachycardia. Cardiac arrest.

Haematological: Coagulation defects. Spontaneous bleeding. Mucosal bleeding. Haematemesis. Epistaxis. Ecchymoses/petechiae. Gastrointestinal bleeding. Internal haemorrhage. Haemolysis.

Pulmonary: Pulmonary oedema. Tachypnoea. Dyspnoea.

Renal/Urinary: Haematuria. Haemoglobinuria. Myoglobinuria. Renal failure.

General: Nausea/vomiting. Fever. Abdominal pain. Regional lymphadenopathy.

[Davidson, University of California, Snakebite Protocols]

## Blood Coagulation

'Gaboon viper venom is both coagulant and anti-coagulant. In some cases these contrasting effects may result from variations in protein concentration and venom preparation and storage.... Addition of [gaboon viper] venom in a 1:10,000 dilution shortened coagulation time in human haemophiliac blood from 25 to 11 minutes. *Bitis arietans* venom increased haemophiliac blood coagulation to 1 hour at similar dilutions. Normal human blood, having a coagulation time of 5 minutes, coagulated in 3 minutes.' [Mallow, 2003]

## Struggling to Breathe & Live

Famed American zoologist and reptile curator Richard Marlin Perkins [1905–1986] was bitten by a captive gaboon at 9:50 a.m. on December 31, 1928, on the dorsal surface of the index finger of the left hand. He went through a terrifying near-death experience and later said it felt like his insides were on fire. A massive blood transfusion saved his life. His 1986 obituary touted him as 'one of only a handful of people to survive the bite of a West African gaboon viper'.

The following impressive case report, summarised from the treating physician dr. Staley's report, delineates Perkins's developing symptoms.

Immediately, felt excruciating pain in the finger, followed in a few seconds by similar pain in the hand.

[After making an incision at the bite site and sucking the wound] He then started to walk to his office which was 60 feet away, becoming dizzy on the way, and nearly fainting.

He sat down in a chair, feeling extremely giddy.

[First antivenom treatment at 10 a.m.] At 10:05 the entire arm was paining him greatly and there were shooting pains in the left side of the chest radiating towards the heart.

He also complained of severe headache, limited to the top of the head.

The finger began to swell immediately after the bite and to show a dark discolouration. The swelling rapidly progressed to the hand and up the forearm and arm.

10:10 Mr. Perkins looks very pale and blood oozes freely from the end of the finger where the incision had been made. His pulse was 80, and very weak.

On admission to the hospital [between 10:25 and 10:30] he was extremely pale, but quite rational and conversed freely about his injury, although complaining of great pain in the finger, hand and arm, also of the pain previously described in the left side of his chest. He was already passing into shock.

10:30 Said he was having difficulty in getting his breath and described his condition as though the chest wall would not expand, and as though a heavy weight were pressing downward on his chest. This difficulty in breathing gradually became more marked.

Blood is flowing freely from the wound on the finger.

10:40 Pulse 70 per minute. Temperature 97.4°F [36.3°C]. Respiration 20 per minute, going up to 28. [Normal average breathing rate is 8–14 per minute.]

The pulse rate continued to get weaker and slower and at 10:50 the rate had dropped to 64.

At 10:55 the patient was breathing with great difficulty and began to complain of additional pain, severe in character, in the back over the region of the kidneys. At this time he voided urine highly coloured with blood and was seized with further great pain along the entire course of the urinary tract.

Pulse dropped quickly to 50, was very weak, and by 10:58 had become imperceptible.

Respirations now rapid, laboured, and of short excursion.

Patient looked very bad, deathly pale and bathed in a cold sweat.

At 11:00 he became unconscious. Pulse could not be felt. Pupils widely dilated, non-reactive to light.

It was thought he was dying.

[Antivenom treatment combined with caffeine sodium benzoate and strychnine sulphate.] Respirations soon after treatment began to quiet down, although the pulse was still imperceptible.

11:20 Incisions were made on the greatly swollen arm to relieve the tremendous swelling; the left upper extremity being swollen to at least twice its natural size. The index finger was nearly black. This discolouration extended to the back of the hand, which was very dark blue. The bluish and purplish discolouration extended up the arm, and, on the inner side of the arm extending upward into the armpit, the discolouration was almost black.

11:30 Both eyes extremely bloodshot. Pupils only moderately dilated, the right pupil being more dilated than the left. Lips and ears less pale.

11:45 The patient showed signs of consciousness and asked for water. The pupils were of normal size and equal.

12:02 p.m. Patient complained of headache, but said he felt a little better.

12:11 Patient having a severe chill, shaking.

12:17 still chill.

12:30 Pulse weak, rate 112 per minute; respirations 28 per minute; colour cyanotic; patient still cold, but not chilly.

13:00 Patient having another chill; still cyanotic; pulse 120; pupils normal size and equal.

13:30 Temperature 101°F [38.3°C]; pulse 116; respirations 28; patient perspiring freely; urine very bloody, in fact consisting of almost pure blood. Wounds oozing and bleeding freely.

13:50 to 14:30 Patient resting, taking fluids freely, but still complaining of great pain in the affected arm; still very pale and cyanotic; pulse very weak.

Owing to patient's marked anaemia, general weakness and resultant shock, a blood transfusion was given at 16:45. As the transfusion was going on patient began to look better and to feel much better. His lip and cheeks gradually became pink, losing their pallor.

On January 20th Mr. Perkins was discharged from hospital. [Ditmars, 1937b]

# BITIS NASICORNIS

### Systematics
- Scientific name: Bitis nasicornis [Shaw, 1792].
- Synonyms: Vipera nasicornis [Daudin, 1803]. Clotho nasicornis [Gray, 1842]. Cerastes nasicornis [Wagler, 1857].
- Common names: Rhinoceros viper. River jack. Horned puff adder. Nose-horned viper.
- Family: Viperidae, subfamily Viperinae.

### Biological Profile
- Extremely heavy-bodied true viper with narrow, flat, triangular head, small relative to body, and partially prehensile tail. Nostrils directed upward and outward. Large pair of curved horns of 3–4 keeled scales upon snout, sometimes several smaller ones at their base. Average length 60–90 cm, maximum 1.2 m. Females larger than males.
- Ground body colour varying through various shades of blue, pink, purple and green. Body pattern very complex, usually made up of a vertebral series of 15–18 paired, yellow-edged blue blotches, with a lateral series of light-edged

dark triangles extending up from the belly. Top of head blue, with a vivid black arrow-shaped mark pointing forward.

- Remains virtually invisible among leaf litter and spotty lighting on forest floor despite its brilliant colours. Often considered one of the most beautiful of all snakes.
- Body scales strongly keeled, to the extent of being likened to 'miniature shark fins'. Scales also so sharp as to inflict cuts on handlers when the snake struggles.
- Range: Central West Africa.
- Habitat: Swamps, riverbanks and other moist habitats throughout tropical rain forest regions.
- Nocturnal sit-and-wait predator catching prey via ambush while lying hidden among leaf litter. Preys on small mammals, frogs, toads, and even fish.
- Terrestrial, but able to climb into trees and thickets.
- Found sometimes in shallow pools; believed to be a good swimmer.
- Ovoviviparous; 6–38 live young per brood.

## Behaviour & Temperament

Conflicting opinions exist regarding river jack's disposition. Mallow et al. studied the literature and quote some workers as saying that B. nasicornis is 'peculiarly placid and inoffensive in disposition, and most reluctant to bite'. Seldom known to strike, even huge specimens could be kept as a pet and 'handled with ease'. Others hold the reverse to be true, deeming them as much less placid than gaboon vipers and 'to be handled with extreme caution at all times'. It is declared that they are 'placid in temperament but can be aggressive if aroused or molested,' hissing loudly [louder than any other African snake] and puffing if approached, often announcing their presence before they are even seen.


# MATERIA MEDICA BITIS NASICORNIS

## Sources
1 Effects of bite; clinical manifestations.

## Clinical Manifestations

Little is known about envenomation by B. nasicornis as accidents are rare in its natural environment due to its sedentary and nocturnal lifestyle. Based on a few detailed reports of human envenomation, the venom of the rhinoceros viper appears to be haemotoxic and cytotoxic. Massive swelling occurs, followed sometimes by necrosis. The venom reportedly also contains myocardiotoxins affecting cardiac function and blood pressure, thus it can readily provoke arrhythmia, cardiac-mediated hypotension and myocardial damage.

Postmortem examination of mice shows haemorrhage in the diaphragm, with trace signs of haemorrhage elsewhere in the abdominal cavity and local punctate haemorrhages in kidneys and lungs. In rats as well as in rabbits the venom, intravenously injected, causes a profound drop in arterial blood pressure.

# CERASTES CERASTES

## Systematics
- Scientific name: Cerastes cerastes [L., 1758].
- Synonyms: Vipera cerastes [Böttger, 1880]. Cerastes cornutus [Boulenger, 1896]. Aspis cerastes [Schmidt, 1939].
- Common names: Horned viper. Horned desert viper. Sahara horned viper.
- Family: Viperidae, subfamily Viperinae.

## Biological Profile
- Medium-sized, moderately stout-bodied true viper with broad, flat head, distinctive supraorbital horns, narrow neck, thick midsection and tapering tail. Ranges in colour from yellowish, pale grey, pinkish to pale brown [always matching the colour of the habitat] with dark semi-rectangular dorsal blotches dorsally. Belly whitish. Average length 55 cm, maximum 90 cm. Females larger than males.
- Range: Most of northern Africa and the Middle East.
- Habitat: Mainly deserts with rocky outcroppings and fine sand, often in very arid places, but may also be found near oases.
- Mainly nocturnal and terrestrial [burrowing].
- Feeds primarily on rodents, birds, and lizards [with the exception of skinks].
- Oviparous; 8–23 eggs per clutch.
- Two recognized subspecies [cerastes and hoofieni].

## Behaviour & Temperament
Can make itself almost invisible by wriggling down into loose sand. The sinking into sand process begins posteriorly, extending anteriorly until the entire head is buried with just the eyes and nostrils exposed. Often hides in rodent holes and under stones.

Fairly placid snake; when disturbed it either retreats to a hiding place or remains still. Sometimes when angered, assumes a C-shaped posture and rubs the inflated loops of body together to make a 'rasping hiss,' similar to saw-scaled vipers, genus *Echis*. Can strike quickly if disturbed.

## Sliding & Winding
Sidewinding is the primary method of locomotion for C. cerastes and the majority of desert snakes. This type of movement allows the snake to move quickly across the desert sands by lifting a loop of the body and moving it forward, while the rest of the body follows the moving loop. This also assists in preventing the snake from overheating, as minimum contact between the belly and the ground is maintained throughout the movement. In its sidewinding journey, the snake "looks something like a rolling spring and faces at an angle to its actual direction of travel: it appears to be headed in one direction while it is actually going in another," according to Cogger [2003]. Its unconventional method of locomotion notwithstanding, the desert horned viper "moves randomly over a large area," says Bauchot [2006].

## Vibration Detection

'As specialized semi-fossorial snakes, all members of the genus Cerastes exhibit predatory launch strikes from partially buried positions in the Saharan sands. As such, the majority of the communication and perception techniques demonstrated by these snakes incorporate multiple environmental stimuli in order to enhance prey localization and acquisition. Through multiple studies and experiments, it has been found that foraging by vibration detection is particularly significant in C. cerastes, as well as other members of the genus. Additionally, visual capabilities are pertinent in strike accuracy and distance, although the snake is still quite capable of capturing prey with hindered vision. Interestingly, prey capture behaviour does not seem to be limited by olfactory senses, and in contrast to common belief, chemosensory reliance in Cerastes during foraging is nearly negligible, as visual stimuli act as primary determinants of prey apprehension.

'When communicating with other members of its own species, Sahara horned vipers rely mostly upon chemical signals in the form of pheromones. This is used particularly during the mating season, as it acts to locate members of the opposite sex. Also, C. cerastes makes use of vibrational stimuli and the ability to sense heat from other organisms in the environment from its pit organs in order to locate prey. Located just behind the nostrils, the pit organs in these snakes allow them to detect warm-blooded animals, even in the dark.' [animaldiversity.org]


## MATERIA MEDICA CERASTES CERASTES

### Sources
1 Proving Uta Santos [Austria], 9 provers [6 females, 3 males], 12c, c. 2000
2 Effects of bite; clinical manifestations.
3 Effects of bite; ischemic stroke.

### Mind
∞ Soft, gentle, devoted, accommodating. Modest humble feeling, without need for expression. Happiness and gentleness replacing resistance and rebellion.
∞ Joy and gentleness become blind accommodation and weak-willed indifference.
∞ Irritable, impatient, inflexible. Depressed and disheartened.
∞ Urge to do housework.
∞ Fear from heart symptoms.

### Dreams
∞ Beautiful and powerful women. Importance and beauty of clothes. Shoes and shopping.
∞ Dressed provocatively and arousing envy and hatred of other women, but also admiration by men.
∞ Fear of heights.

∞ Lovely flowers, tender beauty and complete happiness.
∞ Man buried up to his neck.
∞ Pregnancy.
∞ Sexuality. Rage and sexual jealousy of mother. Shame and anger around sexuality.

## Generals
∞ Right side more affected.
∞ Afternoon [1–3 p.m.] < [tiredness]. Night < [gastrointestinal].
∞ Morning > [feeling refreshed in morning].
∞ Decreased urge to smoke. Desire for orange juice; sweets.
∞ Pains burning.
∞ Chilliness – icy cold hands and feet.
∞ Light sleep, waking often. Waking at 4 a.m.

## Sensations
∞ Head pain as if being knocked out with a pan.
∞ Facial features stiff, as if paralysed.
∞ Smell of dog shit before nose.
∞ Electric shocks originating in solar plexus.
∞ Heart as if gently squeezed by a hand, before falling asleep.
∞ Stitching in chest on inhaling, as from small needles.
∞ Oppression, pressure chest.

## Locals
∞ Dizziness and nausea on moving head quickly.
∞ Stitching pain in forehead and neck when cold. Stabbing pain over left eye.
∞ Difficulty focussing, vision fades to infinity.
∞ Twitching of right eye.
∞ High pitched tone in left ear, hissing or buzzing.
∞ Burning in nose before sleep. Burning with clear discharge. Right nostril stuffed up. Congestion alternating with clear coryza. Sneezing lasting 30 minutes.
∞ Tongue painful with impression of teeth on right side.
∞ Intense vomiting at night. Stomach pain at night. Watery diarrhoea at night.
∞ Tachycardia as from drinking strong coffee or palpitation & nausea.

## Clinical Manifestations
Venom is haemotoxic, causing severe damage to blood cells and tissue. Local symptoms include oedema, redness, internal haemorrhage, and areas of gangrene. Venom has coagulant activities at low concentrations, anticoagulant activities at high concentrations. Fatalities are rare but have been documented.

'Severe and even fatal envenoming by C. cerastes was reported in the 19th century. Chavasse [1891] provided what is probably the only account of a fatal bite by this species. A 28-year-old man was bitten twice on the index finger by a horned viper near Laghouat oasis, 400 km south of Algiers. After 4 days of traditional treatment, he presented with vomiting, sweats, severe headache, epistaxis and red urine. He was febrile, jaundiced and collapsed with tachypnoea, tachycardia, swelling of the entire bitten arm and painful enlargement of lymph nodes. Over the next few days, the bitten finger became gangrenous with a purulent discharge; the patient experienced persistent diarrhoea and died 1 week after the bite.

'Corkill reviewed snakes and snake bites in Iraq [1932] and the Sudan [1935]. He mentioned 2 anecdotal fatalities from Dohuk and Baghdad, in one of which the patient died 24 h after the bite with massive swelling of the bitten arm. The usual symptoms were marked swelling and necrosis followed by indolent sepsis in the neighbourhood of the bite, but with a notable absence of the haemorrhagic symptoms typical of viperine envenoming. Guyon [1862] described 2 cases in Laghouat, Algeria treated by local incisions and instillation and ingestion of ammoniacals. One man, bitten on the foot, had been subjected to a traditional remedy of having the bitten part placed inside the abdomen of a freshly killed dog. He developed local swelling up to the knee and, 4 days later, hemiparesis and difficulty speaking, attributable to a stroke. The other, who was bitten on the buttock while sleeping in his tent, coughed up blood a few hours later. . . .

'A number of cases of C. cerastes envenoming have been described in Israel. Efrati [1979] noted that the clinical features in 7 cases were similar to mild envenoming by Vipera palaestinae. One patient developed necrosis requiring amputation of a finger. Systemic symptoms were mild, comprising nausea and vomiting in most patients, with skin haemorrhages and haematuria in 4. . . .

'Shargil et al. [1973] described 6 cases of C. cerastes bite admitted to hospital in Tel Aviv. Most of the patients had applied tourniquets, and 3 developed necrosis of bitten fingers, requiring amputation in one. Common systemic symptoms were nausea, abdominal pain and sweating. Haematemesis was recorded in 1 and haematuria in 4 cases. . . . A 17-year-old man bitten on the finger was admitted to hospital in Beer-Sheva, with local swelling, haemorrhagic blister and necrosis, which required skin grafting. There was upper abdominal pain and vomiting.' [Schneemann, 2004]

## Ischemic Stroke

'We discuss 3 authenticated reports of acute ischemic cerebrovascular accidents after 3 typical severe envenomations by Cerastes cerastes vipers. The 3 patients developed extensive local swelling and life-threatening systemic envenomation characterized by disseminated intravascular coagulopathy, increased fibrinolysis, thrombocytopenia, microangiopathic haemolytic anemia and acute renal failure. This clinical picture involved atypical neurological manifestations. These patients had either low Glasgow Coma Scale [GCS] or hemiparesis within hours to 4 days after being bitten and they were found to have computed tomographic evidence of single or multiple ischemic [non-haemorrhagic] strokes of small- to large-vessel territories of the brain. One patient had good clinical recovery without neurological deficits. Thrombotic complications occurred an average of 36 hours after being bitten and their importance depends on the degree of envenomation. The possible mechanisms for cerebral infarction in these cases include generalized prothrombotic action of the venom

[consumptive coagulopathy], toxin-induced vasculitis and endothelial damage.'
[Rehabi, 2014]

# DABOIA RUSSELII

## Systematics
- Scientific name: Daboia russelii [Shaw & Nodder, 1797].
- Synonyms: Vipera daboya [Daudin, 1803]. Vipera elegans [Daudin, 1803]. Vipera russelii [Gray, 1831].
- Common name: Russell's viper.
- Family: Viperidae, subfamily Viperinae.

## Biological Profile
- Highly venomous, heavy-bodied true viper with large, triangular head and strongly keeled scales. Dorsal colour light brown with 3 longitudinal series of large black-margined brown spots or blotches. Vertebral series often merging to form a chain-like longitudinal stripe. Belly yellowish-white, occasionally with dark brown markings. Average length 1 m, maximum 1.6 m.
- Head very distinct from neck, above covered by small, keeled, imbricate scales; nostrils large, in large nasal shield; eyes with vertically elliptic pupil, surrounded by 10–15 small scales.
- Range: Pakistan, India, Nepal, Sri Lanka, Bangladesh.
- Habitat: Primarily fairly open areas with grassy, scrubby or bushy vegetation. Commonly found around human settlements, in rice fields and other agricultural areas.
- Terrestrial.
- Primarily nocturnal, esp. during hot weather; may be active during day in cool weather.
- Preys on rodents, esp. rats and mice, but will eat just about anything, incl. squirrels, domestic cats, land crabs, scorpions and other arthropods.
- Ovoviviparous; prolific breeder, 20–40 live young per brood.
- Named in honour of Dr. Patrick Russell [1726–1805], who had earlier described this animal, and the genus after the Hindi name for it, *daboia*, which means *'that lies hidden'*, or *'the lurker.'*
- The former subspecies Daboia russelii siamensis, eastern Russell's viper, was elevated to species status in 2007. [See Daboia siamensis]

## Behaviour & Temperament
This dangerous species is abundant over its entire range. It is responsible for more human fatalities than any other venomous snake. It is irritable. When threatened, it coils tightly, hisses, and lunges forward with great determination, striking with such speed that its victim has little chance of escaping.

'Adults are reported to be persistently slow and sluggish unless pushed beyond a certain limit, after which they becomes fierce and aggressive. Juveniles, on the other hand, are generally more active and will bite with minimal provocation.

When threatened they form a series of S-loops, raise the first third of the body and produce a hiss that is supposedly louder than that of any other snake. When striking from this position, they can exert so much force that even a large individual can lift most of its body off the ground in the process.

'These are difficult snakes to handle: they are strong and agile and react violently to being picked up. The bite may be a snap, or, they may hang on for many seconds. Although this genus does not have the heat-sensitive pit organs common to the Crotalinae, it is one of a number of viperines that are apparently able to react to thermal cues, further supporting the notion that they too possess a heat-sensitive organ. The identity of this sensor is not certain, but the nerve endings in the supranasal sac of these snakes resemble those found in other heat-sensitive organs.' [Wikipedia]

## Medicinal Use of Venom

The use of snake venoms as homeostatic agents [homeostasis = balance between 2 opposing forces: clot formation and dissolution] is based upon early observations of the potent coagulative properties of snake venoms, the Russell's viper in particular gaining early use as a treatment of haemophilia. In 1934, R.G. MacFarlane, a British pathologist, discovered that Russell's viper venom helped haemophiliac blood to clot. Commercial production of 'Stypen' for haemophilia treatment began soon afterwards. The mechanism of action of D. russelii venom is in the activation of the factors V, X, IX, as well as Protein C. While D. russelii venom is no longer used as a therapeutic agent, it still is used as a diagnostic agent to determine deficiencies in clotting factor X.

## MATERIA MEDICA DABOIA RUSSELII

### Sources
1 Degroote, Dream Repertory.
2 Synthesis Repertory Treasure Edition 2009.
3 Effects of bite; clinical manifestations.
4 Effects of bite; bleeding, paralysis, renal dysfunction & abdominal pain.
5 Effects of bite; complications.
6 Effects of bite; overview.

### Dreams
∞ Calming down an aggressive big pet.[1]
∞ Deceased relatives.[1]
∞ Embarrassment about improper behaviour of spouse.[1]
∞ Faithless husband.[1]
∞ Forbidden area, being in a.[1]
∞ Threatened and pursued by a fox.[1]

### Generals
∞ Desire for pickled collared herring.[1]

∞ Desire for lemon.[1]
∞ Puffy, oedematous swelling.[2]
∞ Wounds bleeding freely.[2]

## Sensations
∞ Lips so swollen as to covering whole face.[1]
∞ Heart region as if cold.[1]

## Locals
∞ Must have stool every day; uneasy when stool stays out for one day.[1]
∞ Pain lumbar region in morning on rising from bed.[1]
∞ Pain lumbar region on rising after long sitting.[1]

## Clinical Manifestations
Venom neurotoxic and haemotoxic. Powerful coagulant, damaging tissue and blood cells.

'A man, aged 40, was bitten on the finger by a Daboia. The bitten part was excised soon after and stimulants given. The hand and arm became much swollen, and on the same day he passed blood by the rectum and bloody urine. The next day he was sick and still passing blood from both channels. In this state he remained 8 days, constantly losing blood, and died on the ninth day.' [Indian Med. Gaz.; June 1872]

'Envenomation symptoms begin with pain at the site of the bite, immediately followed by swelling of the affected extremity. Bleeding is a common symptom, especially from the gums, and sputum may show signs of blood within 20 minutes post-bite. There is a drop in blood pressure and the heart rate falls. Blistering occurs at the site of the bite, developing along the affected limb in severe cases. Necrosis is usually superficial and limited to the muscles near the bite but may be severe in extreme cases. Vomiting and facial swelling occurs in about one-third of all cases.

'Severe pain may last for 2–4 weeks. Locally, it may persist depending on the level of tissue damage. Often, local swelling peaks within 48–72 hours, involving both the affected limb and the trunk. If swelling up to the trunk occurs within 1–2 hours, massive envenomation is likely. Discolouration may occur through-out the swollen area as red blood cells and plasma leak into muscle tissue. Death from septicaemia, respiratory or cardiac failure may occur 1 to 14 days post-bite or even later.' [Wikipedia]

'Twenty-two patients who had been bitten by a Russell's viper were studied. Neurological manifestations and generalized myalgia were observed, respectively, in 86.4% and 72.7%. Renal failure did not occur in 3 patients who received antivenin within 5 hours of the bite, and it is suggested that administration of antivenin within the first few hours following the bite could prevent renal failure. Of 19 patients who were in acute renal failure, 7 responded to conserva-tive management while 12 needed peritoneal dialysis. Nine patients developed pulmonary oedema and 4 had grand mal seizures. Five patients died. Autopsy revealed massive pulmonary oedema, thought to be the immediate cause of death, in 4 of them and extensive cortical and tubular necrosis in 3.' [Jeyarajah, 1984]

Causes of death include shock, pituitary and intracranial haemorrhage, massive gastrointestinal haemorrhage and acute tubular necrosis or bilateral renal cortical necrosis.

## Bleeding, Paralysis, Renal Dysfunction & Abdominal Pain

There are 37,000 snakebite admissions to Sri Lankan hospitals every year. The Russell's viper is responsible for 30–40% of the snake bites and to the greatest number of severe envenoming and fatalities compared to other snakes in Sri Lanka. Sri Lankans have been well aware of the aggressive nature and the lethality of the Russell's viper over many generations. In 1910, Abercromby noted ". . .they [native Sri Lankans] consider the Russell's viper [Tic Polonga] as a personification of the devil." Bites by Russell's vipers commonly occur in paddy [rice] fields and on footpaths at dusk and at dawn, affecting a large number of agricultural workers and so considered an occupational hazard in Sri Lanka.

Coagulopathy, characterized by prolonged clotting time and spontaneous bleeding, is the commonest clinical manifestation of systemic envenoming. Coagulopathy and acute kidney injury have been the major life threatening systemic manifestations of bites by this snake in Sri Lanka. Neuromuscular paralysis, characterized by opthalmoplegia, ptosis and *neck muscle weakness*, has been commonly observed in these with rare occurrence of respiratory muscle paralysis. Rhabdomyolysis, chronic renal failure, myocardial infarction and secondary hypopituitarism have also been reported in Russell's viper bite patients in Sri Lanka. Although generally not severe, local swelling has been a common feature seen in this country.

In Russell's viper bite, the reported incidence of dry bite has been low, with most bites resulting in significant envenoming. At the same time there were situations where, in proven cases of Russell's viper bite, *acute renal failure* was the sole manifestation of envenoming developing many hours after the bite. . . . At present there is no early sign or symptom that has been identified in Russell's viper bite that could be considered a clinical predictor of significant systemic envenoming. *Abdominal pain* has been documented as a clinical feature in some studies of Russell's viper envenoming. But abdominal pain is also a known clinical feature of envenoming by other snakes, particularly by the common krait [Bungarus caeruleus]. However, epidemiology of common krait bite is unique that it happens exclusively at night when victims are in sleep causing neuro-muscular paralysis. Nevertheless, many practicing clinicians believe that abdominal pain is a feature of systemic envenoming in Russell's viper bite. This observation is strengthened by the fact that in a comparative study of the patients of Russell's viper and Hump-nosed pit viper [Hypnale spp.] bites, abdominal pain was present only among the Russell's viper bite patients.

*Abdominal pain* was observed in 31 [79.5%] of the proven Russell's viper bite victims with systemic envenoming and in only 3 [25%] of those who had only local envenoming. The pain had developed 5 to 240 minutes [mean 71 minutes] after the bite and lasted up to the 2nd [40.7%] or 3rd day [18.2%], post bite. It was generalized in 52% of the patients, or localized to the umbilical [21%], epigastric [13%], supra-pubic [9%], right inguinal fossa [2.6%] or right lumbar [1.3%] region in others. The pain was described as colicky [60%], aching [32%], or burning [8%] in nature.

Abdominal pain co-existed with coagulopathy, neuromuscular paralysis and renal dysfunction in 78.9%, 80% and 60% of patients respectively.

Systemic involvement in Russell's viper envenoming seen in our study in rank order of frequency was as follows: coagulopathy and neurotoxicity; coagulopathy alone; coagulopathy and nephropathy; coagulopathy, neurotoxicity and nephropathy; neurotoxicity and nephropathy. [Kularatne, 2014].

## Complications

A total of 38 [11%] patients developed complications: profuse persistent spontaneous bleeding, thrombocytopenia and multiorgan dysfunction suggestive of severe disseminated intravascular coagulation [DIC] in 7 patients; hypercatabolic hyperkalemia in 9 patients; acute renal failure in 14 patients; intracranial bleeding leading to coma in 2 patients; hemiplegia in one; acute respiratory distress syndrome [ARDS] in association with DIC in 2 patients; hepatic failure in 4 patients and surgical emphysema in one patient. Patients with hepatic dysfunction developed icterus with tender hepatomegaly and elevated ALT, AST, alkaline phosphatase and bilirubin levels. All of them developed early encephalopathy but recovered with appropriate treatment.

In the years 1996/1997 respectively, 6 [4%] and 3 [1.6%] patients died. Five patients died due to acute severe DIC leading to multiorgan failure, 2 patients died due to cardiac arrest because of silent hyperkalemia and 2 died due to intracranial bleeding. The duration of hospital stay of the patients ranged from 1 to more than 5 days [mode 4 days] and 79% of the patients were able to leave the hospital before 6 days. [Kularatne, 2003]

## Overview of Effects of Bite

*Signs and symptoms* that manifest *earliest*, usually within 5 hours of envenomation, include:
Local pain at bite site [80%]
Local swelling [68%]
Pain in regional lymph nodes [55%]
Tender, enlarged lymph nodes [54%]
Spontaneous systemic bleeding [46%]
Hypotension [35%]
Bleeding at bite site [31%]
Vomiting [26%]
Bleeding from distant sites [24%]
Conjunctival oedema [24%]
Bleeding from gums [20%]
Drowsiness [14%]
Haematemesis [11%]

Epigastric pain [8%]
Lower back pain [7%]
Melaena [7%]
Bleeding from incisions [6%]
Subconjunctival hemorrhage [6%]
Epistaxis [2%]
Dizziness/impaired consciousness [2%]

Pain and local bleeding [if present] usually begins within the first few minutes after the bite. Pain may persist for 2 weeks or longer. Swelling is usually greatest 1–4 days after the bite. Unlike the rattlesnakes and other New World pit vipers, tissue necrosis and local blister formation is rarely seen.

*Neurological signs* generally occur during the first 24–48 hours. Neurological manifestations gradually improve and disappear by 5–7 days. Myalgias disappear usually within a few days. Signs include:

Bilateral ptosis and Generalised muscle pain and tenderness [up to 86%]
External ophthalmoplegia [up to 77%]
Dysphagia
Dysarthria

*Haematology*: Generally D. russelii venom shows both pro-coagulant enzyme activity and direct fibrinolytic activity. This presents as a DIC-type coagulopathy, and results in non-coagulating blood and haemorrhage. Fibrinogen, platelet counts, and haemoglobin levels are generally decreased. Fibrin micro-thrombi to renal glomeruli is seen, along with a greater than 50% occurrence of leukocytosis with 70–90% PMNs. A fall in albumin may also be expected secondary to a generalised increase in capillary permeability.

*Urinary Symptoms & Renal Failure*:
Haematuria [72%].
BUN range [14–68%].
Proteinuria [55%].
Oliguria [44%].
Renal-angle tenderness [39%].

Oliguria develops rapidly; usually after 1–3 days in systemic envenomations. Renal-angle tenderness precedes the onset of oliguria in greater than 85% of the patients and can be used as a valuable clinical sign of impending renal failure. Renal failure is usually secondary to acute tubular necrosis [from fibrin micro-thrombi] and is often the main cause of death in Russell's Viper snake bites in Burma. [Davidson, University of California, Snakebite Protocols]

- Symptoms in MM:
∞ Generals, Pain.
∞ Generals, Swelling, general; puffy, oedematous.
∞ Generals, Weakness.
∞ Generals, Wounds bleeding freely.

# DABOIA SIAMENSIS

- Scientific name: Daboia siamensis [Smith, 1917].
- Synonyms: Vipera russelli siamensis [Smith, 1917]. Daboia russelii siamensis [Welch, 1994].
- Common name: Eastern Russell's viper. Siamese Russell's viper. Chain viper.
- Family: Viperidae, subfamily Viperinae.

## Biological Profile
- Highly venomous, stout, heavy-bodied true viper with large, triangular head and strongly keeled scales. Colouration same as that of D. russelii, except that it is more greyish or olive, with small spots between the large spot rows. Belly suffused with grey posteriorly. Average length 1.6 m.
- Range: Southern China, Myanmar, Indonesia, Thailand, Taiwan, Cambodia.
- Habitat: Secondary growth and shrub jungles, eucalyptus plantations, cultivated fields, bushes near marshy areas, grasslands bordering plantations, sandy grounds and rocky hills.
- Tends to avoid dense forests and humid environments, such as marches and swamps.
- Terrestrial.
- Nocturnal; most active in early evening. Crepuscular during cool days.
- May hide in termite mounds or rodent burrows during the hot season.
- Both juveniles and adults use caudal luring.
- Preys on rodents, lizards, birds and frogs.
- When cornered, assumes a defensive posture by swelling its body and hissing forcefully, a 'hiss once heard that is not easily forgotten,' herpetologist Frank Wall once noted. Others have compared the hiss to the sound of air released from a punctured tire. The hiss produced has a mean amplitude of over 82 dB, well above the intensity of most other snake sounds.

## MATERIA MEDICA DABOIA SIAMENSIS

### Sources
1 Effects of bite; endocrine insufficiency.

### Endocrine Insufficiency
Daboia siamensis envenoming is free of neurotoxic manifestations, but there are many reports of pituitary insufficiency following its bites.

Jamie James [2008] has some intriguing things to say about this viper. 'The venom of Vipera russelii is more toxic than that of the cobra [yet less toxic than that of the many-banded krait]; very few victims survive the snake's bite. It's a horribly painful death, typically resulting in massive bleeding from the anus and in the brain, and renal failure. Those who do survive are wrecks: The venom plays havoc with the pituitary gland and reverses adolescence, turning the victim back into a physical 8-year-old. Secondary sexual characteristics recede, leaving the sufferer smooth of body hair, impotent, and sterile.'

Endocrine insufficiency [adrenal and/or anterior pituitary] is part of the chronic phase occurring months to years after the bite, including weakness, loss of secondary sexual hair, amenorrhoea, testicular atrophy, hypothyroidism etc. The syndrome has been particularly observed with envenomation by the eastern subspecies, D. r. siamensis. Results from 5 autopsies showed that the lesion was haemorrhagic anterior pituitary necrosis. An additional mechanism may be direct action of the venom upon the function of anterior pituitary cells.

'Pituitary function was investigated in 9 patients in shock after Russell's viper bites and in 24 individuals who had been severely envenomed 2 weeks to 24 years previously. Three out of 9 patients had hypoglycaemia and inappropriately low serum cortisol, plasma growth hormone, and plasma prolactin concentrations. Four who died had pituitary haemorrhage and 1 had adrenal haemorrhage as well. Of the 24 who had apparently recovered from bites, 7 had clinical features of hypopituitarism and no response in plasma growth hormone or prolactin concentrations to symptom-producing insulin-induced hypoglycaemia.

'Four of these 7 had a sluggish serum cortisol response to 'Synacthen Depot' [synthetic peptide exhibiting the full corticosteroidogenic activity of natural ACTH] and 5 had an abnormal cortisol response to hypoglycaemia. Four men with symptoms who were tested had low serum testosterone concentrations; serum thyroxine was also low in these men but not in 2 women with menstrual disturbances and impaired insulin responses. Of the 17 individuals without clinical evidence of endocrine disease, 4 had pituitary hormonal abnormalities. Russell's viper envenoming may thus produce a disorder resembling Sheehan's syndrome.' [Warrell, 1987]

# ECHIS CARINATUS

## Systematics
- Scientific name: Echis carinatus [Schneider, 1801].
- Synonyms: Pseudoboa carinata [Schneider, 1801]. Echis multisquamatus [Cherlin, 1981].
- Common names: Saw-scaled viper. Little Indian viper.
- Family: Viperidae, subfamily Viperinae.

## Biological Profile
- Stocky venomous true viper with short head, distinctly wider from neck, , and very short tail, abruptly tapering from belly. Snout very short and rounded. Average length 40–60 cm; maximum 80 cm.
- Grey or brownish in colour, patterned with brownish blotches, a wavy white stripe, and a distinctive dark cross or arrow-shaped mark on top of head. Belly whitish to pinkish, uniform in colour or with brown dots that are either faint or distinct.

- Range: Widely distributed from northern Africa, through Middle East, southern former Russia, descending to Iran, Afghanistan, most of Pakistan, India, and Sri Lanka.
- Primarily nocturnal in hot weather; may be active at dusk; sometimes diurnal in cool weather.
- Most active after rains or on humid nights.
- Can bury itself in sand with only the head exposed, or may be found basking during early morning in bushes and shrubs, sometimes as much as 2 m above the ground. When it rains, up to 80% of the adult population will climb into bushes and trees.
- Preys on rodents, lizards, frogs, and a variety of arthropods, such as scorpions, centipedes and large insects.
- Ovoviviparous; 3–15 live young per brood.
- Two recognized subspecies [carinatus and sochureki].

## Behaviour & Temperament
Small but extremely irritable species of snake found close to human habitation. Quick-tempered, nasty disposition, never hesitates to strike when provoked, will attack any intruder. Strikes quickly and repeatedly with considerable reach for a small snake. Coils and twists when threatened, rubbing its serrated scales against each other in a continuous, undulating motion. The result is a chilling rasping noise that sounds like the wind blowing. According to others, the rasping resembles that of a saw cutting wood.

The rasping sound serves a warning prior to fast leaping strikes. It is capable of delivering a lightning fast strike and regaining its position of defiance leaving its challenger perplexed. Its inconspicuous nature, the speed of its strike and its *readiness to bite at the smallest provocation* make it an extremely dangerous snake. Its characteristic pose, a double coil with a figure of 8, with the head poised in the centre, permits it to lash out like a released spring. It has been reported to chase victims aggressively and is said to follow pedestrians for considerable distances. Moves mainly by sidewinding, alarmingly quick.

It can take a jump of 1–2 feet high and can climb into branches of low bushes to avoid heat at the ground, and to feed on nestlings of desert birds. Never likes to be handled but once in captivity may go and coil up in a corner and remain oblivious to external stimuli but almost always turns vicious when attempted to handle.

## Drugs from Venom
'The venom from this species is used in the manufacture of several drugs. One is called echistatin, which is an anticoagulant. Even though many other snake venoms contain similar toxins, echistatin is not only especially potent, but also simplistic in structure, which makes it easier to replicate. Indeed, it is obtained not only through the purification of whole venom, but also as a product of chemical synthesis. Another drug made from E. carinatus venom is called ecarin and is the primary reagent in the ecarin clotting time [ECT] test, which is used

to monitor anticoagulation during treatment with hirudin. Yet another drug produced from E. carinatus venom is Aggrastat [Tirofiban].' [Wikipedia]

Ecarin is moreover an excellent hospital laboratory tool in the analysis of blood from patients with liver diseases or being treated with anticoagulants such as vitamin K antagonists.


## MATERIA MEDICA ECHIS CARINATUS

### Sources
1 Proving Farokh Master [India], 8 provers [6 females, 2 males], 30c; 2004.
2 Effects of bite; clinical manifestations.
3 Effects of bite; acute renal failure.

### Mind
∞ Intense fear of some incurable disease.
∞ Anxiety about health, < at night.
∞ Irritability and anger at trifles.
∞ Impulse to throw things around.
∞ Impulse to do risky things.
∞ Aggressive from contradiction.
∞ Angry outbursts followed by quick repentance.
∞ Dullness; no interest in any activity. Aversion to talking.
∞ Indecisiveness and confusion.

### Generals
∞ Sleeplessness due to anxiety.
∞ Waking up from sleep and sleeplessness from itching in groins.
∞ Fever with intolerance of covering. Forehead, chest and abdomen hot; hands cold.
∞ Thirst for small quantities at long intervals during heat.
∞ No desire to eat or drink.
∞ Wants frequently to have something to eat.
∞ Extreme hunger but cannot eat much at a time.
∞ Desire for ice-cold water and/or frozen food.
∞ Left side more affected.

### Sensations
∞ Dizziness with whirling sensation from right to left.
∞ Heaviness in head < lying on left side; < bending head to left side.
∞ Heaviness of head, esp. at occiput. Heaviness extending to forehead.
∞ Heaviness head & pain at nape of neck.
∞ Heaviness head > pressure on temples.
∞ Something moving in left temple.
∞ Right eye as if pushed into socket, morning on waking.
∞ Heaviness in left ear.

∞ Left ear as if stopped; opening on swallowing.
∞ Reverberating of voices in left ear while talking.
∞ Heat in throat on waking in morning.
∞ Lump in throat.
∞ Tightness and pulling sensation left side cervical region.

## Locals
∞ Dizziness < turning from left to right in bed.
∞ Dizziness < standing, lying on back, lying on right side, closing eyes; > lying on left side with forehead boring into pillow.
∞ Dizziness from sudden movements of head.
∞ Dizziness < movement, esp. of head; > lying down, closing eyes.
∞ Dizziness when getting up from laying down or sitting [postural or orthostatic hypotension].
∞ Dizziness & nausea.
∞ Dizziness with tendency to fall backward.
∞ Burning, pressing pain in right eye, > cold water application.
∞ Blurred vision due to streak in front of right eye.
∞ Hardness of hearing, left ear.
∞ Tinnitus left ear – ringing and sensation of bursting bubbles.
∞ Extreme pulsating pain in left ear in night < lying on affected side, > warmth.
∞ Pulsations in left ear < walking.
∞ Obstruction nose > moist heat.
∞ Burning/dryness in nasopharynx and throat < talking.
∞ Constant urge to clear the throat.
∞ Must first swallow before being able to speak, to prevent voice from getting hoarse.
∞ Pain in enlarged left cervical lymph node < opening mouth.
∞ Eructations < during painless, profuse, gushing diarrhoea.
∞ Offensive, loud, noisy flatulence.
∞ Urging for stool disturbing sleep.
∞ Drawing pain at nape of neck, occiput.
∞ Painful stiffness in left cervical region in morning on waking.
∞ Shooting pain in left gluteal region extending down leg.
∞ Shooting pain at back of left knee joint while walking.
∞ Pain in Achilles tendons while walking.

## Clinical Manifestations
• Smallest of the Big 4 dangerous snakes of India, which are: Indian cobra, Common krait, Russell's viper, Saw-scaled viper. Considered one of the world's most dangerous and deadliest snakes that may cause its victims to bleed "uncontrollably to their death."

'Local symptoms include swelling and pain, which appear within minutes of a bite. In very bad cases the swelling may extend up the entire affected limb within 12–24 hours and blisters form on the skin. The venom yield from individual specimens varies considerably, as does the quantity injected per bite.

About 20% of all bites are fatal. Of the more dangerous systemic symptoms, haemorrhage and coagulation defects are the most striking. Haematemesis, melaena, haemoptysis, haematuria and epistaxis also occur and may lead to hypovolemic shock. Almost all patients develop oliguria or anuria within a few hours to as late as 6 days post bite. In some cases, kidney dialysis is necessary due to acute renal failure, but this is not often caused by hypotension. It is more often the result of intravascular haemolysis, which occurs in about half of all cases. In other cases, acute renal failure is often caused by disseminated intravascular coagulation. In any case, antivenin therapy and intravenous hydration within hours of the bite are vital for survival.' [Wikipedia]

- 115 patients with poisoning caused by its bite were studied in the savanna region of Nigeria, where victims of this snake may occupy 10%b of hospital beds. All patients had local swelling at the site of the bite. Other features included local blistering [13%], local necrosis [11%], incoagulable blood [93%], and spontaneous systemic bleeding [57%]. There was evidence of disseminated intravascular coagulation in all cases; fibrinogen was severely depleted, fibrin degradation products were increased, but significant thrombocytopenia was seen in only 10 severe cases. Clotting factors V, VIII, II and XIII were depleted, while X and VII were usually normal. [Warrell, 1977]

### Acute Renal Failure

Of the 360 cases of E. carinatus envenomation, 62 patients developed acute renal failure. Oliguria occurred in 39 patients [62%], anuria in 21 [34%], and hypotension in 5 [8%]. Intravascular haemolysis present in 49% of cases with acute renal failure was evident from the presence of anaemia, jaundice, reticulocytosis and haemoglobinuria. Thirty-four percent showed evidence of acute disseminated intravascular coagulation [DIC], 47% had compensated DIC and 19% isolated thrombocytopenia.

Most of the patients [90%] developed symptoms and signs of acute renal failure within 48 to 72 hours post bite while 10% of patients developed acute renal failure from 5 to 10 days after the snake bite. Clinically 15 patients had suspicion of acute cortical necrosis. Of the 62 patients with acute renal failure, 44 patients [71%] were dialyzed. 16 patients [25%] died, the remaining 28 patients [45%] on dialysis recovered their renal functions completely and no patient remained dialysis dependent. 46 patients of acute renal failure who survived, recovered their renal functions completely. The duration of recovery ranged from 2 to 6 weeks. All the patients who had acute DIC [21 patients] had evidence of severe renal failure also and this group of patients had maximum mortality; i.e. out of 21 patients 16 patients [76%] died. The leading cause of mortality in these patients was multiorgan failure as evidenced by clotting abnormalities, hepatic dysfunction and acute renal failure. Poor prognostic markers for snakebite-induced acute renal failure are those patients who require dialysis, while as patients who do not require dialysis have better prognosis. [Ali, 2004]

# PROATHERIS SUPERCILIARIS

## Systematics
- Scientific name: Proatheris superciliaris [Peters, 1855].
- Synonyms: Vipera superciliaris [Peters, 1855]. Bitis superciliaris [Kramer, 1961]. Atheris superciliaris [Marx & Rabb, 1965].
- Common names: Swamp viper. Eyebrow viper. Lowland swamp viper.
- Family: Viperidae, subfamily Viperinae.

## Biological Profile
- Heavy-bodied true viper with a greyish-brown dorsum with 3 rows of dark spots separated by yellowish bars that form a broken lateral line on either side of the body. The elongated head has 3 blackish chevrons. Belly whitish with dark blotches, underside of tail orange or yellow. Average length 40–60 cm. Females significantly larger than males.
- Range: Central East Africa – Tanzania, Malawi, Mozambique.
- Habitat: Grasslands near swamps and floodplains.
- Preys on reed frogs and other small amphibians; occasionally takes small rodents.
- Name derives from L. *super*, above, and *cilium*, eyelid, alluding to the snake's large supraocular shields.


## MATERIA MEDICA PROATHERIS SUPERCILIARIS

### Sources
1 Effects of bites; clinical manifestations.

### Clinical Manifestations
- 'On 24 August 1996, during a routine cage maintenance procedure, a keeper was bitten on the left forefinger by a specimen of Proatheris superciliaris approximately 48 cm [19 inch] in length. He managed to return the snake to its container despite it "striking insanely and undulating during the whole process." He immediately experienced severe pain in his hand, which he likened to being splashed by boiling bacon grease. During the next 2 hours the hand experienced necrosis and ecchymosis [purple discolouration] and became covered with blebs. By then he was hospitalised and morphine had been administered for the pain without success. Over the course of the next 2 days he went into massive haemolysis [dissolution or destruction of red blood cells with subsequent release of haemoglobin], experienced complete platelet destruction, and his liver and kidneys began to fail due to the overwhelming amount of protein fragments resulting from the destruction of erythrocytes and platelets. His body turned yellow as a result of the jaundice. A group of leading experts were consulted and there was a belief that he may die due to Haemolytic Uraemic Syndrome. They decided he should undergo plasmapheresis, a process

in which plasma is removed from blood and the remaining components, mostly red blood cells, are returned to the bloodstream.

Fortunately, this individual survived to describe this incident, but not without suffering extreme pain and undergoing extensive and horrible treatment. His recovery from this envenomation took over 6 months. He required 2 surgeries to repair his hand including a cross-flap skin graft. There is some permanent disfigurement to his left forefinger and some reduced mobility. In his words, "I owe those men [the doctors and consultants] my life, my wife was in shreds . . . a very terrible ordeal for a 'supposedly mildly venomous viper'." [Jacobi]

- 'Snake bites caused by viperid snakes of Atheris genus are extremely rare, envenoming of a bite of related viper Proatheris superciliaris was described only once in the literature. The present case study depicts the envenoming of a 57-year-old Czech man, a private herpetologist, who was bitten on his finger. He developed painful local reaction, nausea, haematuria, hypertension, chest and lumbar pain. Coagulopathy and thrombocytopenia subsequently developed as well as acute renal failure, hepatic and lung lesion. Intensive care therapy was purely symptomatic and supportive as no antisera exists. Treatment included haemodialysis, substitution of fresh frozen plasma and platelets. Patient completely recovered in 1 month.' [Valenta, 2008]

### Renal Cortical Necrosis

'Acute bilateral renal cortical necrosis [BRCN] has been reported following envenoming by exotic venomous snakes. Proatheris superciliaris is a rare viper with restricted distribution in East Africa. Very little information is available on envenoming by this species. We herein describe the case of a 60-year-old professional wildlife photographer who was bitten on his thumb while photographing an adult specimen of P. superciliaris that he held at home in France. On admission, physical examination revealed *severe hypertension* and bruising with oedema at the bite site. Within the following 24 h, he developed vomiting, diarrhoea, acute lumbar pain and anuria. Laboratory tests showed acute kidney injury [serum creatinine 4.6 mg/dL], with thrombocytopenia, anaemia and severe coagulopathy. Contrast-enhanced computed tomography scan revealed hypodense areas in the cortex of both kidneys consistent with diffuse BRCN. As no appropriate antivenom existed, only symptomatic care was given to the patient. Coagulation tests returned to normal within 48 h. The patient was placed on chronic haemodialysis, until he underwent successful kidney transplantation 18 months later. . . . Acute kidney injury, including BRCN, is a *classic complication of viper bites*. The present case of end-stage renal failure related to diffuse BRCN illustrates the potentially devastating effects of envenoming by P. superciliaris.' [Pourreau, 2014]

# VIPERA AMMODYTES MERIDIONALIS

## Systematics
- Scientific name: Vipera ammodytes [L., 1758].
- Subspecies: V. a. meridionalis [Boulenger, 1903].
- Synonym: Pelias meridionalis [Reuss, 1930].
- Common name: Eastern nose-horned viper.
- Family: Viperidae, subfamily Viperinae.

## Biological Profile
- Strong, heavy-bodied true viper with triangular head on slim neck. Males commonly less than 85 cm, maximum 95 cm; females smaller.
- Dorsal ground colour dark grey, sometimes silver grey or yellowish grey; with thick dark grey or black zigzag dorsal stripe and longitudinal row of indistinct dark spots along each side. Top of head with irregular dark brown, dark grey, or black markings, with characteristic dark blotch or V marking at back of head often contiguous with dorsal zigzag. Nasal horn vertically erect [obliquely forward in other subspecies]. Underside of tail yellowish-green [red or yellow in other subspecies].
- Range: SE Europe, from Albania to Greece, Corfu [and other islands], and western European Turkey.
- Habitat: Warm, dry areas – relatively barren rocky slopes, forest edges, glades.
- Commonly found abroad both at night and by day, becoming nocturnal in summer or when daytime temperatures become too high. May be active only during warm sunny periods at higher altitudes.
- 'Loafing' behaviour is common during hot weather, with individuals climbing into low branches, remaining motionless for long periods of time.
- Preys on small mammals and adult and nestling birds; juveniles prefer lizards. Large prey is struck, released, tracked and swallowed.
- Death from gluttony has been reported.
- Males engage in combat bouts.
- Ovoviviparous; 4–8 live young per brood.
- Sluggish and lethargic disposition, tending to remain *motionless* while hissing loudly if perturbed. More likely to flee than to bite, unless provoked considerably.
- Three recognized subspecies [ammodytes, meridionalis, montandoni].

## MATERIA MEDICA VIPERA AMMODYTES

### Sources
1 Effects of bite; clinical manifestations.

## Clinical Manifestations

Vipera ammodytes is reputedly the most dangerous of European vipers due to both large size and high venom toxicity. Its bite is potentially more dangerous than any other European viper.

The venom has an exceedingly rapid and devastating effect on mammal prey, which succumb within seconds [small birds] to a couple of minutes [mice and larger birds]. Amphibians, however, may survive a bite. Humans respond rapidly to *V. ammodytes* venom, which is predominantly haemotoxic and proteolytic and causes a dramatic fall in blood pressure. Symptoms generally are immediate; pain is instantaneous and throbbing. The potent blood coagulant properties are similar to and equally powerful as those of pit vipers.

In 147 victims of V. ammodytes admitted to hospital from 1988 to 2003 in Patras, Greece, the most common symptoms and signs included pain [100%], swelling [98.64%], ecchymosis [60.54%], tachycardia [32.65%], fainting or dizziness [29.93%], fever [23.13%], enlargement of regional lymph nodes [17.69%], nausea [16.33%], hypotension [13.61%], and vomiting [12.93%]. The main complications were reduced range of motion, thrombophlebitis, local haemorrhagic blister formation, skin bleeding, rhabdomyolysis, reduced sensation, acute renal failure, necrosis with tissue loss, carpal tunnel syndrome, *compartment syndrome*, Kounis syndrome [concurrence of acute coronary events with allergic or hypersensitivity reactions], and digit amputation. [Frangides, 2006]

- Clinical signs and symptoms of *compartment syndrome* include:
  1 Pain out of proportion to the apparent injury.
  2 Hypoaesthesia in the distribution of nerves passing through the compartment in question.
  3 Pain on passive stretch of the muscles within the compartment.
  4 Tenseness of the compartment on palpation.
  5 Weakness of the involved muscles.
- 'A 60-year-old male was bitten by a venomous snake [Vipera ammodytes] and gradually developed signs of an allergic reaction including generalised itching, generalized rash, and chest discomfort. This was followed by severe retrosternal pain with electrocardiographic evidence of an inferior myocardial ischemia progressing to acute myocardial infarction. Cardiac enzymes and troponin, serum tryptase, and histamine were elevated. Coronary arteriography showed normal coronary arteries. This is a characteristic type I variant of Kounis syndrome, which is the concurrence of acute coronary syndromes with conditions associated with mast cell activation including allergic or hypersensitivity reactions as well as anaphylactic or anaphylactoid reactions. This is the first report to show that viper bites can induce allergic angina and/or allergic myocardial infarction.' [Frangides, 2006]

# VIPERA ASPIS

## Systematics
- Scientific name: Vipera aspis [L., 1758].
- Synonyms: Coluber aspis [L., 1758]. Vipera francisci redi [Laurenti, 1768]. Aspis ocellate [Fitzinger, 1826]. Berus vulgaris [Gray, 1831].
- Common names: Asp viper. European asp. Jura viper.
- Family: Viperidae, subfamily Viperinae.

## Biological Profile
- Small true viper. Body mostly grey, yellowish, light brown, or reddish-brown [Alpine specimens may be black]. Belly may be light grey, yellowish, or dark-grey with lighter flecks. Series of elongated rectangular dark blotches along back from neck to tail, slightly upturned snout, often with dark 'V' or 'X' atop back of head. Tail tip often yellow or orange below. Dorsal scales strongly keeled. Adults usually 50–65 cm long, maximum 75 cm.
- Range: Central and southern Europe.
- Habitat: Most often found in fairly warm dry, hilly areas at lower elevations, on open rocky hillsides exposed to the sun, and which have structured vegetation. Can also tolerate high, wet mountainous regions; found up to 3,000 m elevation.
- Diurnal in cooler months, nocturnal in hot summer months.
- Tolerates very cold weather; observed to move about in temperatures as low as 5°C [41°F].
- Preys on lizards, small mammals, and birds.
- Ovoviviparous; 2–9 live young per brood.
- Usually sluggish and not aggressive. When approached, generally will stop and freeze. Will bite if threatened.
- Five recognized subspecies [aspis, atra, francisciredi, hugyi, zinnikeri].


## MATERIA MEDICA VIPERA ASPIS

### Sources
1 Proving Marie-Claire Boffa and P. Dupin [France], 14 provers, 5c, 9c, 15c; 1970.
2 Degroote, Dream Repertory.
3 Synthesis Repertory Treasure Edition 2009.
4 Effects of bite; clinical manifestations.
5 Effects of bite; periodicity & sequelae.

### Mind
∞ Pessimism. Nervousness. Anxiety.[1]
∞ Irritability. Disposition to contradict. Impatience.[1]
∞ Sadness before menses.[1]

## Dreams
- ∞ Bitten, being, at heel.[2]
- ∞ Blinded by the sun.[2]
- ∞ Child, being a child again.[2]
- ∞ Climbing into a tree.[2]
- ∞ Competition.[2]
- ∞ Criticized, being.[2]
- ∞ Death; dead people.[1]
- ∞ Descending steep stairs.[2]
- ∞ Events, agreeable, long past.[2]
- ∞ Followed by a big black cat.[2]
- ∞ Hide, desire to.[2]
- ∞ House with only one room.[2]
- ∞ Missing the bus.[2]
- ∞ Overpowering and tying down attacker.[2]
- ∞ Snakes, tiny.[2]

## Generals
- ∞ Sleepiness during daytime.[1]
- ∞ Sleepiness during headache.[3]
- ∞ Comatose sleep during convulsions.[3]
- ∞ Comatose sleep with vomiting.[3]
- ∞ Sleeplessness from pain.[3]
- ∞ Left side more affected.[1]
- ∞ Pains throbbing.[1]
- ∞ Intense thirst for cold drinks.[1]
- ∞ During menses >.[1]
- ∞ Gentle motion >.[1]
- ∞ Warm, damp weather <.[1]
- ∞ Warm room <.[1]
- ∞ Heat <.[1]
- ∞ Pressure <.[1]
- ∞ Evening <.[1]
- ∞ Before menses <.[1]
- ∞ Abscesses with foetid pus.[3]
- ∞ Blackness of external parts.[3]
- ∞ Letting limbs hang down <.[3]

## Sensations
- ∞ Worm under skin of forehead.[2]
- ∞ Eyes as if heavy.[1]

## Locals
- ∞ Dazzling when raising eyes.[1]
- ∞ Redness eyes from drinking beer.[2]
- ∞ Dryness of mouth, with pasty tongue, on waking in morning.[1]

∞ Dry mouth before menses.[1]

∞ Pain abdomen > lying on back; < walking.[2]

∞ Menses with small, very dark clots or with big red clots. Menses too short.[1]

∞ Palpitations at night, < lying on left side.[1]

∞ Spontaneous ecchymoses on arms.[1]

∞ Paralysis lower limbs.[3]

∞ Painful heaviness in legs, < walking, > raising legs.[1]

∞ Veins of thighs distended. Marbled, mottled appearance of thighs.[1]

∞ Coldness feet after quarreling/vexation.[2]

## Clinical Manifestations

Venom is mainly haemotoxic, with neurotoxic factors. Symptoms may include pain, swelling and discolouration, necrosis, vomiting, weakened pulse, subnormal body temperatures. Later symptoms may include jaundice, renal impairment, and liver damage. Numerous bites and envenomations of humans by this species and a few [about 4% untreated] subsequent fatalities reported.

Since 1992, cases of neurological envenomation by Vipera aspis snakes have regularly been reported in the southeast of France. All cases involved ptosis, which appears as a characteristic sign of neurotoxic Vipera aspis envenomations. Ophtalmoplegia, diplopia, dysphagia, paraesthesias and drowsiness have also been reported, although less commonly than ptosis. [de Haro, 2002]

## Periodicity & Sequelae

∞ Every year subsequent to the bite, at the first hot weather, he was seized with a painful oedema of the limb, colic and efforts to vomit; digestion became disturbed; he was tormented with somnolence, the gums became fungoid, and his skin had an icteric tint; he was chilly, with great physical and intellectual weariness.

∞ The symptoms subsequent to bite have a periodic character, with tendency of the cachectic symptoms to return. In a large number of cases there is for many years a return of the troubles on a certain day every year, the swelling, pain in the bitten limb, prostration, loss of appetite, nausea, and jaundiced hue of the skin. One girl in Nantes had for years at the period of the bite an eruption of livid spots on the bitten limb. A Young man had for years, at the anniversary of the bite, general malaise, swelling of the limb, and development of spots.

∞ In many cases, after about 18 months to 2 years, there is a marked tendency to apoplexy; the death is due to cerebral congestion or haemorrhage. [Dr. A. Viaud-Grand-Marais, Effects of bites; 1868–69]

# VIPERA BERUS

## Systematics

• Scientific name: Vipera berus [L., 1758].

• Synonyms: Coluber berus [L., 1758]. Coluber prester [L., 1761]. Berus vulgaris [Swainson, 1839]. Pelias berus [Günther, 1859]. Vipera torva [Lenz, 1832].

- Common names: Common European viper. Common adder. Cross adder.
- Family: Viperidae, subfamily Viperinae.

## Biological Profile

- Short but fairly stout-bodied true viper. Body yellow to greyish-green; distinct zigzag dark pattern on back and sides. Can be completely black. Dorsal scales strongly keeled. Average length 55 cm, maximum 90 cm. Females rusty-reddish colour and larger than males.
- Range: Found in suitable habitats throughout most of Europe. Most widespread species of viper in the world.
- Habitat: Found in diverse habitats, like rocky or bushy hillsides, open fields, woods, shady areas, moors, swamps, marshes, and bogs. In northern parts of range, found mainly near sea level; to nearly 3,000 m elevation in southern parts of range.
- Predominantly diurnal in cold months; nocturnal in warm months.
- Cold-adapted in northern range, may crawl over melting snow in spring.
- Preys mainly of small mammals, such as mice, voles, and shrews, as well as lizards, frogs, newts, and salamanders.
- Birds are also reported to be on the menu, esp. nestlings and even eggs, for which they will climb into shrubbery and bushes.
- Males engage in ritual combat during mating season.
- Ovoviviparous; 3–18 live young per brood.
- Four recognized subspecies [berus, bosniensis, nikolskii, sachalinensis].

## Behaviour & Temperament

Basking behaviour is complex. Mainly terrestrial, but climbs low bushes. Generally timid; not aggressive. Tends to freeze when danger presents; but easily alarmed and bites if threatened or stepped on. Usually congregates into groups ['colonies'] during annual hibernation [in rocky dens] during cold months.

## Reproduction & Dancing

'The adder emerges from hibernation in March, with males emerging before females. For the first few weeks after emergence, this species remains fairly inactive and spends much of its time basking. After the male has shed its skin in April it becomes more active and will begin to search for potential mates by following scent trails. The female sheds its skin a month later than the male, and both sexes shed again later on in summer. The adder does not feed until after it has mated, and so during the time before mating, both the male and female adder live off fat reserves that are built up during the previous year.

'Upon discovering a receptive female, the male begins a courtship display in which the tongue is flicked over the female's body. The male and female may vibrate their tails briefly and bouts of body quivering may ensue. If the courtship is a success, copulation takes place, after which the pair may remain together for 2 hours or so. If another male approaches the pair at any point, the first male will defend the female aggressively and a fight may result. These fights are known as 'the dance of the adders' as the males partly raise their bodies off the ground and may become entwined, often repeatedly falling to the ground and rising up again. More than 2 males may be involved in such a contest.

'The female adder usually reproduces once every 2 years, returning to the site of hibernation towards the end of August or early September to give birth. The adder is ovoviviparous, giving birth to between 3 and 18 live young that are initially encased in a membrane. After giving birth the female must feed intensively in order to build up sufficient reserves for hibernation. The young adders do not feed until the following year, but live off the yolk sac and fat reserves that they are born with. The adder reaches sexual maturity at 3 to 4 years of age.' [www.arkive.org]


## MATERIA MEDICA VIPERA BERUS

### Sources
1 Effects of bites collated by Hering as Vipera torva in *Wirkungen des Schlangengiftes* [Effects of snake venoms], 1837.
2 Symptoms, effects of bites, listed in Kent's Repertory.
3 Clinical observations Mangialavori [Italy].
4 Proving Reinhard Flick & Claudia Klun [Austria], 14 provers [11 females, 3 males], 30c; 1998.
5 Degroote, Dream Repertory.
6 Synthesis Repertory Treasure Edition 2009.
7 Effects of bite; clinical manifestations.
8 Effects of bite; clinical features of adder bite.
9 Effects of bite; overview.
10 Effects of bite; specific symptoms of envenomation.
11 Effects of bite; heart block.

### Mind
∞ Restlessness, with headache. Anguish, with vomiting.[1]
∞ Eyes look as if he were raving mad, & staggering and stumbling forward.[1]
∞ Delusion, thinks he is away from home. Desire to go home.[2]
∞ Delusion being pursued.[3]
∞ Suspicious, mistrustful towards doctor.[3]
∞ Forsaken feeling.[3,4]
∞ Increased ambition, competitive.[3]
∞ Ailments from mortification.[4]
∞ Anger at trifles. Hatred and revenge.[4]
∞ Delusion being disrespected, disdained, too little acknowledged as lone fighter, and used by colleagues and husband.[4]
∞ Benevolence.[5]
∞ Clings to mother out of fear.[5]
∞ Desire for the colour red.[5]
∞ Hobby: jigsaw puzzles.[5]
∞ Jealousy.[5]

∞ Aversion to jesting.[5]
∞ Materialistic selfishness.[5]
∞ Likes to talk in verses and use proverbs.[5]
∞ Adulterous.[6]
∞ Ailments from sexual excitement or sexual excesses.[6]
∞ Aversion to change, in children.[6]
∞ Delusion being pursued by the devil.[6]
∞ Discouraged from pain.[6]
∞ Speech hesitating, inarticulate, incoherent, as if intoxicated.[6]
∞ Speech difficult, stammering, thick, wanting.[6]

## Dreams
∞ Accused, falsely, defends himself.[5]
∞ Agility, great.[5]
∞ Amputation of leg.[5]
∞ Attacked and bitten by cats.[5]
∞ Beaten, slap in face.[5]
∞ Bitten, being, by dog; by snake.[5]
∞ Blood, standing up to knees in blood.[5]
∞ Coffins.[4,5]
∞ Danger of falling, with fear.[5]
∞ Death of relatives; own children; mother.[4]
∞ Devils.[5]
∞ Driving a car without brakes.[5]
∞ Escaping from danger by giant jump.[5]
∞ Faithlessness.[5]
∞ Forsaken, being.[4]
∞ Funeral, own.[5]
∞ Hide, desire to, from danger of being attacked.[5]
∞ Hide, desire to, while being pursued.[5]
∞ House, empty, uninhabited.[5]
∞ Ignored, being, by husband.[5]
∞ Incest.[5]
∞ Losing one's way.[5]
∞ Mountains.[5]
∞ Move, cannot, frozen with fear.[5]
∞ Murder, killing, brutal.[4]
∞ Paralyzed arm; legs.[5]
∞ Pursued, being.[5]
∞ Running, being pursued.[5]
∞ Teeth, crumbling into pieces; falling out.[5]
∞ Urination, copious, doesn't stop.[5]

## Generals
∞ Excessive weakness.[1]
∞ Weakness < warm weather.[6]

∞ Fainting fits, & discharge of saliva, or preceded by violent pains, or & violent congestion to heart.[1]
∞ Frequent fainting fits, at night, alternating with vomiting and diarrhoea.[1]
∞ Faintness from pain; < sitting up in bed; > cold water.[6]
∞ Icy-coldness of body.[1]
∞ Cold shivering, & nausea, vomiting, and great thirst.[1]
∞ Chilliness, & paleness of face and thirst.[1]
∞ Unquenchable thirst.[1,4]
∞ Sleep disturbed by nausea, pain, perspiration, vomiting.[6]
∞ Sleepiness during headache.[6]
∞ Sleepiness at first hot weather.[6]
∞ Sleeplessness from anxiety or fear.[6]
∞ Clothing too tight, > loosening it.[3]
∞ Before menses <.[3]
∞ Sexual desire increased during menses.[4]
∞ Desire for alcohol; apples; cheese; coffee; fat and rich food [butter, fat meat]; meat; sweets; tea.[4]
∞ Desire for apples; bananas; broccoli; chicken skin; goat cheese; sweets, during dinner; walnuts.[5]
∞ Aversion to tobacco; smell of coffee; apples.[4]
∞ Aversion to fried food; nuts; water.[5]
∞ Pains burning.[4]
∞ Letting limbs hang down < or >.[6]
∞ Carbuncles with bursting pain.[6]
∞ Paralysis after apoplexy.[6]
∞ Wounds bleeding freely.[6]

## Sensations
∞ Feeling of fullness internally.[6]
∞ Head as if heavy on holding head up.[5]
∞ Objects seem distant during fever.[5]
∞ Objects seem to move to and fro.[5]
∞ Tip of tongue as if burned.[2]
∞ Tip of tongue as if numb.[5]
∞ Band of dryness across tongue, no thirst.[4]
∞ Tongue as if filling whole mouth.[6]
∞ Teeth as if elongated.[2]
∞ Teeth as if large and swollen.[2]
∞ Stone in stomach.[4]
∞ Legs as if bursting.[6]
∞ Legs as if paralyzed.[6]
∞ Varicose veins as if bursting.[6]
∞ Pain in bones as if broken.[6]

## Locals
∞ Dizziness & epistaxis.[6]

- ∞ Dizziness & vomiting.[6]
- ∞ Heaviness of head, & reeling and red face.[1]
- ∞ Headache, stitching pain, on change of weather.[2]
- ∞ Redness of eyes & profuse lachrymation.[1]
- ∞ Protruding eyes & swelling of face.[1]
- ∞ Frequent loss of sight.[1]
- ∞ Chronic deafness.[1]
- ∞ Itching in ears, with sore throat.[5]
- ∞ Perspiration face after wine; when eating; morning on waking.[4]
- ∞ Protruded and pale swollen tongue.[1]
- ∞ Burning pain in tongue or tip of tongue.[4]
- ∞ Dryness of mouth at night, & thirstlessness.[4]
- ∞ Throatache, sore or burning like fire, < swallowing, evening, warm drinks, > eating, cold drinks.[4]
- ∞ External throat < clothing.[5]
- ∞ Swelling of thyroid gland.[6]
- ∞ Burning pain in stomach at night.[4]
- ∞ Stomach pain > sitting erect.[5]
- ∞ Nausea before menses.[4]
- ∞ Nausea on brushing teeth.[5]
- ∞ Vomiting, & stupefaction, or convulsions, or diarrhoea.[1]
- ∞ Vomiting, & headache, or & shuddering and violent thirst.[1]
- ∞ Vomiting after milk.[6]
- ∞ Alternate pains in abdomen and limbs.[1]
- ∞ Asparagus smell to urine.[4]
- ∞ Menses scanty and short, or menses copious at night or beginning at night.[4]
- ∞ Menses when nursing child.[6]
- ∞ Breast milk in women unrelated to pregnancy.[4]
- ∞ Pain nape of neck/cervical region on bending head backward or forward.[5]
- ∞ Pain dorsal region between scapulae > sitting erect.[5]
- ∞ Pain lumbar region extending to feet on sneezing.[5]
- ∞ Pain lumbar region > walking.[5]
- ∞ Excessive swelling of hand and arm, painful when touched.[1]
- ∞ Moving fingers difficult.[6]
- ∞ Pain lower limbs [knees and feet] on change of weather.[2]
- ∞ Large ulcers on tibia, penetrating to the bone, and leaving considerable cicatrices.[1]
- ∞ Deeply-penetrating suppuration after shining swelling, with blue blisters.[1]
- ∞ Heat of soles of feet, uncovers them.[3]

## Constitutional Aspects

'We have had about 10 constitutional cases of Vipera berus, with as main themes and symptoms:

- ∞ Wild sexual excitement.
- ∞ The temptation of adultery.

∞ Everything that is prohibited in this way becomes a temptation.
∞ Simulating death [like the viper in winter].
∞ Coldness [differentiation to other snakes].
∞ Hatred and revenge, rage and fury, jealousy.
∞ Drug addiction especially by injections.
∞ That Satan would be after you.

It seems as if Vipera would be the specifically European and Christian way of "beating dead" the sexual instincts as well as the chaotic female power, which is threatening our cultural order.' [Jürgen Becker]

## Clinical Manifestations
Venom is mainly haemotoxic, with neurotoxic and cytotoxic factors. Envenomation usually causes sharp pain or severe burning at bite site, followed by swelling and inflammation of lymph system. Victim usually develops nausea, headaches, vomiting, chest pains and laboured breathing.

'During 1995 a total of 231 patients were treated for a bite by Vipera berus in Swedish hospitals. The maximum severity of envenomation was as follows: none, 11%; minor, 47%; moderate, 29%; and severe, 13%. Among patients developing severe symptoms, 13 [42%] were less than 10 years old and 10 [32%] were more than 60 years old. In 25 patients the bite did not result in any envenomation. Those with no local swelling and no signs of systemic toxicity within the first 2 hours stayed asymptomatic. Vomiting, abdominal pain, and diarrhoea were the most common systemic symptoms.

'Hypotension and shock as well as CNS depression were frequently observed in severe envenomation. Seven patients were unconscious on admission, and seizures of short duration occurred in 1 case. Angio-oedema developed occasionally. In 1 patient pronounced swelling of lips and tongue partially obstructed the upper airways. Signs of generalised plasma leakage with significant haemorrhagic swelling of the face developed in a 5-year-old boy, bitten in the foot.

'Leukocytosis was a common finding during the first few hours after the bite, particularly in patients initially or subsequently classified as severe. Thrombocytopenia was relatively common in severe poisoning. With a delayed onset, 11 patients developed anaemia.

'A pulmonary oedema supervened on the 5th day in a 4-year-old girl. She had been bitten in the foot and the swelling had progressed to involve the whole extremity and parts of the trunk. Myocardial infarction, presumably related to anaemia, occurred 8 days after the bite in an elderly woman. She died 3 weeks later because of cardiac failure. Autopsy revealed extensive arteriosclerosis.

'Compartment syndrome, requiring surgery, developed in 1 patient. One month later the bitten thumb was still numb and weak. In another patient, persisting loss of tissue was observed after blistering and necrosis in a fingertip. Oedema, worsening after physical exercise, and paraesthesia in the bitten limb persisted 3 years after the bite in an adolescent.' [Karlson-Stiber, 2006]

## Clinical Features of Adder Bite

1 Local [95%]: oedema and haemorrhage spreading over 2–3 days, swelling persistent over 2–3 weeks. Regional lymphadenopathy.
2 Gastrointestinal [24%]: vomiting, abdominal colic, diarrhoea.
3 Cardiovascular: hypotension [20%], sweating, ECG changes [T-wave flattening, arrhythmias 3%].
4 Laboratory: leucocytosis [30%], raised CPK, thrombocytopenia [3%].
5 Fever [5%].
6 Depressed level of consciousness [5%].
7 Pulmonary [3%] bronchospasm, pulmonary oedema, pulmonary haemorrhage. [Harborne, 1993]

• When venom is injected there is usually immediate pain; local swelling starts within minutes. But sometimes local swelling may not appear until at least an hour after the bite, and pain may be minimal or absent despite severe general poisoning. Enlargement and tenderness of regional lymph nodes are often associated with these local effects.

*Vomiting* may start within 5 minutes of the bite and may continue frequently for the next 48 hours. In other cases vomiting does not start until 5 hours after the bite. *Excessive sweating, abdominal colic, and diarrhoea, sometimes with incontinence, often accompany or follow the vomiting. Vomiting, usually with diarrhoea,* occurred in almost all 41 patients with moderate or severe poisoning.

*Shock* – as reflected by weakness, sweating, thirst, collapse, confusion, semi-consciousness, loss of consciousness, coldness, cyanosis, absent pulse, and low or unrecordable blood pressure – may start within 10 minutes of the bite or not until 16 hours after the bite. In at least 12 cases this shock was relatively transient, resolving spontaneously within 2 hours.

*Bleeding* – Generalised bleeding is common in systemic poisoning by many types of viper bite. In adder bites the local oedema is haemorrhagic, as shown by subsequent discolouration, but generalised bleeding is exceptional even in severe adder bite poisoning. Alimentary bleeding has been recorded in an adult victim, in 1 fatal case and in a 14-year-old patient receiving heparin during the first 24 hours after the bite [bleeding promptly ceased when heparin was stopped].

*Swelling* – In 12 of the 29 cases of severe poisoning, swelling of the face and lips or tongue, or both, developed, sometimes immediately after the bite and lasted for up to 2 days. This feature is also common after bites by *Vipera xanthina palaestinae*; it seems to respond well to antihistamines. Oedema of the bitten limb may increase both in amount and extent to reach a maximum 48–72 hours after the bite. The whole limb may be swollen within 5 hours of the bite. In severe poisoning oedema extended to the trunk in two-thirds of cases and affected the whole limb in the remaining third. Initially, the oedema is tense, shiny and non-pitting, and it may be massive. Pain and tenderness in the swollen limb are variable. Sometimes there is remarkably little pain. The oedema starts to resolve 3 to 4 days after the bite and then becomes pitting. Initialy dusky or mottled in appearance, the discolouration of the swelling subsequently changes, as in a bruise.

Apart from the depression of consciousness and dilated pupils associated with shock no abnormal neurological signs were recorded.

Complete recovery in young victims aged 14 years or under was rapid, taking under a week in about a quarter of cases and 1 to 3 weeks in the remainder. Adults took significantly longer to recover, two-thirds taking 3 or more weeks and a quarter taking 1 to 9 months. During these months patients often found *aching pain and intermittent swelling of the bitten limb disabling.*

Non-specific changes in the electrocardiogram [ECG] [mainly T-wave inversions] were recorded in both severe and mild poisoning.

Haemoglobin levels may fall slightly during the first 3 to 4 days. Potassium levels were slightly raised. Electrolytes were otherwise normal. [Reid, 1976]

## Overview of Effects

A review of published reports on the incidence, pathology, and treatment of adder [Vipera berus] bites in man in the United Kingdom and northern Europe produced numerous case studies.

'The main conclusions that can be drawn are: [1] approximately 70% of reported adder bites result in either no or very mild effects; [2] deaths are rare. The principal local effect of adder venom is oedema [sometimes massive], which may be delayed or occur within minutes but which is almost always present within 2 hours. Bruising also occurs and is usually most pronounced in the regions of the main lymphatic trunks and regional lymph nodes. Although the site of the bite is usually painful, pain may be minimal or absent. During the first one to 3 days bruising and tenderness of the tissues increases in extent before slowly subsiding.

'Hypotension is the most important sign of systemic envenoming, usually developing within 2 hours, and may be transient [resolving spontaneously within 2 hours], persistent, recurrent, or progressive and fatal.

'General effects of envenoming may start to appear within the first 10–20 minutes after being bitten. Victims may feel faint, and children in particular may become drowsy or semi-conscious. Nausea is usual and vomiting is a common and prominent feature, which may last for several days. Diarrhoea may also occur.

'Other systemic effects, which may appear within 5 minutes or be delayed for many hours, and which may persist for up to 48 hours, include abdominal colic, incontinence of urine and faeces, sweating, vasoconstriction, tachycardia, and angio-oedema of the face, lips, gums, tongue, throat, and epiglottis, urticaria and bronchospasm.

'Additional features of envenoming include electrocardiographic T-wave inversion or flattening, ST-elevation, second degree heart block and cardiac brady/tachyarrhythmias, atrial fibrillation, and myocardial infarction.

'Uncommon effects of envenoming include defibrinogenation or milder degrees of coagulopathy and spontaneous bleeding into the gastrointestinal tract, lungs, or urinary tract, coma and seizures secondary to hypotension or cerebral oedema, respiratory distress, pulmonary oedema, cerebral oedema, acute renal failure, cardiac arrest, intrauterine death, acute gastric dilatation, and paralytic ileus.

'Laboratory test results include neutrophil leucocytosis, thrombocytopenia, initial haemoconcentration and later anaemia resulting from extravasation into the bitten limb, and rarely haemolysis, elevation of serum creatine phospho-kinase, and metabolic acidosis.' [Reading, 1996]

- The adder [Vipera verus] is the only naturally occurring poisonous snake in Sweden. During one year, 136 patients were hospitalized due to adder bites. Minor local symptoms occurred in 27% of the patients, whereas 46% suffered mild, 15% moderate and 12% severe poisonings. The average duration of hospitalization was 1.6, 3.8, 5.5 and 7.6 days, respectively, for these 4 groups. Shock, CNS disturbances, anaphylactic reactions, extensive oedemas, renal dysfunction and severe anaemia were typical findings in the group with severe reactions. {Persson, 1981]

### Specific Symptoms of Envenomation
Based on authentic cases of Vipera berus envenomation the following symptoms can be regarded as the core of the Vipera berus symptom picture:

1. Overpowering, overwhelming debility to the extent of complete collapse. Loss of muscular power.
2. Extensive swelling.
3. Ecchymoses. Bruising.
4. Vomiting of bile and mucous matter.
5. Epigastric/abdominal pain < pressure.
6. Diarrhoea, which > general symptoms.
7. Coldness; lack of vital heat.
8. Great thirst.

*Swelling Nearly Double Natural Size*
- On the 17th May, 1826, a gardener was bit by a viper, which had been offered to him for sale. This was at 5:30 in the morning. At 7, the part was swollen, with pain tingling in the hand, and sense of coolness, which were followed by vomiting of his ingesta. In a short time afterwards, the swelling increased enor-mously. It seemed to be of the nature of oedema, and its appearance, indicated that gangrene would speedily supervene. The temperature of the part was *lower* than it usually is all over the arm, up to the axilla, to which part, in fact, the swelling had extended. Vomiting of mucous and bilious matter continued now and then; the tongue was natural; the stools were very foetid. Pulsation of the heart feeble; no pulsation was felt in the radial or carotid arteries, whilst that in the crural was very strong. Head and upper extremities were ice cold, the lower members were warm, but not near their natural state. The face was swollen and nearly double its usual size. The neck also participated in the swelling, but there were no spasms. As the patient had 2 wounds on his hand [one of which was not considered by him to be the bite of the animal], it was

thought proper to apply two cupping-glasses, having previously made an incision of 3 lines immediately over the wounds, a quantity of serous fluid, which resembled that in dropsical people, was evacuated. [Revue Médicale, 1826]

*Body Very Cold & Loss of Muscular Power*
- I was called about noon, 17th of April, to Frederick Mann [18 years of age] who in the act of catching an adder was bitten on the middle finger of the left hand and arrived within an hour from the time of the accident. The *whole body was very cold*, with trembling, and much swelling about the face, neck, eyelids, and tongue; the left hand and arm were also much swelled, but without pain. Pulse scarcely perceptible and the heart's action very slow, not exceeding 36 beats in the minute. Vision indistinct and the muscular power of the lower extremities much diminished. On various parts of the body, particularly about the neck, were broad livid patches, resembling *extravasated* blood into the cellular membrane from *bruises*. Now and then slight vomiting. These symptoms began to appear about 10 minutes after the bite was inflicted and continued to increase to the above state in which I found him; and so sudden was the *depression of muscular power that he had to be carried home* from the field where the accident occurred.

  . . . On the 20th he was walking about and doing so well that I did not see him till the evening of the 22d, when I was again sent for. The pulse 96, full and hard, skin hot; great restlessness; breathing oppressed, but no pain. He complained of a sense of constriction, upon swallowing, referable to the upper part of the larynx, but showed no aversion to swallow anything given to him. Tongue brown and furred, considerably swelled, and on each side of the frenum were dispersed a number of pellucid vesicles, the size of large pin heads. On the left side, where the swelling appeared greater, was a large vesicle extending along the under edge of the tongue. These, excepting the large one, were round, and unyielding to pressure. The left submaxillary gland was also very much swelled. The bowels not very free; urine of a dark colour and depositing a rosy mucus. [Cocks, 1827]

*Extreme Lassitude, Hardly Able to Walk*
- A young, robust man was in the summer of 1827 bitten by a viper. . . . He suddenly felt a bite in the index of the right hand. He immediately returned home, but had hardly gone a hundred paces when he felt a violent pain in the throat, giddiness, and *extreme lassitude, so that he could hardly walk*; fortunately there was a house at about a 100 paces from the spot where he had been bitten and *after extreme efforts* succeeded in reaching it; on his arrival he felt so faint that he was obliged to lie down; he felt sick; had a slight fit of syncope, and vomited a large quantity of bile; at the same time his tongue began to swell, so that he could not articulate. About an hour after the accident a silk thread had been placed around the finger, but was afterwards taken off by a surgeon, who cauterised the wound; the hand, arm, and even the whole of the right side of the trunk, began to swell under violent pain, so that the

patient repeatedly fainted away. The application of a hundred leeches to the hand and arm, as well as the use of embrocations and poultices, were without any effect, and the pain and swelling still continued, and increased to such an alarming extent that a physician, who meanwhile had been sent for, advised the sulphate of quinine in large doses, which having been administered, the patient felt immediately relieved, and under the continued use of quinine perfectly recovered on the 8th day, with the exception of stiffness in the arm, which, however, also gradually subsided. [Beaumont, 1830]

*Burning Pain & Abdominal Tenderness*
- About 5:15 p.m. on August 7, 1839, a private in the 2nd Battalion East Yorkshire Regiment was placing an adder, which he had just found in the grass on Strensall Common, into his pocket when he was bitten on the tip of the index finger of the right hand. . . . He then became faint, fell down, and soon began to froth at the mouth. He walked to the hospital with the assistance of 2 men. When brought to the hospital he was only partially sensible, with pallid face and bloodless lips, and very convulsed.

   He was seen by me in about 15 minutes after being bitten; he was then in bed on his back with the knees drawn up and groaning with pain, which he referred to his belly. The face was lived and features swollen, with profuse perspiration running off forehead. The lips were now swollen and bright red in colour, with saliva frothing out of the mouth. Eyes open, pupils widely dilated. Sensible, and complaining of *much pain in pit of stomach*, and of great dryness of throat and month. On examining the mouth the tongue was found to be greatly swollen in front and of bright scarlet colour, and the whole mouth in much the same condition.

   The skin cyanosed, cold to the hand, and bathed in a profuse clammy perspiration. Also lessening of the sensibility of the skin. Absolutely pulseless at the wrist, not even the slightest fluttering could be made out. Breathing was regular, but light. Temperature less than 96.8°F [36°C]. Inclined to vomit, retching frequently, flatulent.

   On admission to the Station Hospital, York, he was still prostrate and *unable to walk without assistance*. He complained of a *burning pain* referred to the back of the sternum, and general abdominal tenderness. The pain, he said, was unlike colic or soreness produced by vomiting. Its severity was such that he begged to be afforded some relief. . . . The right upper limb from the shoulder to the hand was much increased in size, hard, brawny, and discoloured. The axillary glands were enlarged and tender on pressure. . . . The only subjective symptoms connected with the arm were feelings of weakness and stiffness. [Cree, 1888]

*Extreme Pain at Epigastrium from Least Pressure*
- John Burr, aet. 20, of moderate muscular make, when first seen was suffering from a state of collapse and gave the following history of himself. On endeavouring to catch a viper, it became enraged and flew at his hand. He immediately felt a prick, as of a needle. . . . This feeling of a prick was immediately

followed by intense pain in the wounded part, in a short time extending along the forearm to the middle of elbow, and thence to axilla. He describes this pain as being of a *burning* character, and almost directly followed by great swelling of the hand and wrist. Simultaneously with its reaching axilla, a pain or *feeling of constriction was experienced about the head, throat, and right side of tongue*, accompanied also with a sense of heat about these parts. He also complained of having had great difficulty in attempting deglutition. To these symptoms were added nausea [no actual vomiting], dyspnoea, faintness, and a sudden attack of severe pain at scrobiculus cordis [*epigastrium*], with considerable thirst.

Countenance pallid, extremely anxious, and covered with drops of perspiration; hands, feet, as well as body, pretty natural as to temperature; pulse small, nearly 100, no irregularity. . . . Great swelling and tension of the part, having an oedematous appearance, which extends to a considerable distance beyond wrist: great pain, although less severe than at first, extends from the punctures along the anterior part of forearm to axilla. But very moderate pressure can be borne along this track; pressure over the 4 or 5 ribs of the right side also causes pain; an *extreme degree of pain at epigastrium, the least pressure there causing him great suffering;* no swelling of the right side of face; the tongue, however, has a swollen appearance; it can be protruded but slowly and in a small degree, and is evidently directed to the side affected. The voice hesitating and thick, and somewhat resembling that of a man suffering from slight intoxication, but, otherwise, he is certainly quite collected and rational; there is also a *troublesome thirst and craving for cold drinks*, nausea, and slight attempts at vomiting, which appear to aggravate the suffering. [Owen, 1840]

*Unable to Move a Limb, Lacking Strength to Speak*
- A man, aged 26, of short stature, and weakly constitution, was bit by a viper on the inner ankle. Immediately he felt as if something moved upwards along his thigh; he became *heavy and drowsy and was scarcely able to make the 10 paces necessary* to carry him out of the wood into a field. His *strength then entirely failed him*; he was sick, and vomited, first alimentary matter, then *bile*, the last repeatedly; violent pain in the belly, with bilious purging, followed; in this state he lay 3 hours. In another hour he was seen by M. Gaspard, who found him in a state of extreme weakness, *unable to move a limb*, having barely strength to speak; his pulse a thread scarcely perceptible, with great thirst, and *extreme soreness of the hypochondria*. The bitten part was not swelled and presented only 2 slight ecchymoses. The patient swallowed some ammonia in water, and brandy and water, and gradually rallied. The next day he was almost well, having nearly regained his strength; there was trifling swelling of the ankle, which soon disappeared. [Mayo, 1841]

*Sore All Over, Black & Blue*
- Paul D., aged 51, was bitten on the right thumb by an adder. . . . The part looks sloughy and inflamed and swelling extends from this point throughout the entire limb, terminating at the shoulder. Lividity commences on the posterior aspect of the thumb, prevails upon the inner side of the dorsum of the hand,

where it becomes of a bluish tint, and gradually assumes the appearance of ecchymosis as it approaches the forearm. Here, and upon the upper arm, the ecchymosis is general, of a bright red colour in places, in others blue and black, and everywhere tinctured with livid spots. . . . The discolouration and tumefaction terminate at the axilla. He complains of pain on pressing the thumb. He states that a *general feeling of soreness* extends over the extremity, not aggravated, however, by pressure. . . . The tongue is generally white, slightly tremulous; pulse 96, soft; the bowels have acted 5 times since last night. Respiration is natural; the heart's impulse remarkably feeble. He at times experiences a *sensation of uneasiness about the epigastrium.*

He experienced, instantly, a sensation of *burning* and smarting, and, squeezing the part, he washed the blood off upon the grass. . . . He now experienced sensations of great depression; his surface became cold; he had nausea, and faintness and diarrhoea prevailed for nearly an hour. . . . During the evening, stiffness, which had been present slightly, began to increase; the arm became swollen, and lividity became permanent. These conditions becoming aggravated during the night, in the morning, on examining his arm, the ecchymoses were apparent, as described above. [Pemberton, 1849]

### Feeling Cold & Sick

- George R., aged 23, weaver, was admitted into the London Hospital, May 18, 1851, under the care of Mr. Adams. On attempting to catch a viper he was bitten on the ring finger of the ring hand. He was much alarmed at the time and about 20 minutes afterwards vomited a large quantity of bitter yellow fluid; was much purged; had desire to micturate, but could not; felt very faint and sleepy, and seemed as though he were deprived of sight. . . . Appearance when admitted. The patient *feels cold and sick*; great anxiety expressed in the countenance and the pulse small. The finger was white, but little swollen; the back of the hand very much swollen; red lines reaching to the elbow; forearm not much swollen or discoloured, but rather tender.

  Next day. Has not slept; suffers no pain; pulse improved; arm much swollen and ecchymosed, the discolouration extending to the axilla; the glands in that region also much swollen and inflamed. Nine days later: The forearm and elbow feel very hard, and the patient complains of pain and stiffness on attempting to bend the elbow. The discolouration and stiffness gradually disappeared and the patient was discharged cured, June 3.

  The circumstances that are the most worthy of remark in this case are the *extreme prostration of strength* and the extensive ecchymosis, which exceeded in intensity of colour and extent anything I have ever seen. [Lambert, 1851]

### Constant Vomiting of Bilious Matter

- Samuel S., aged 31, a vermin hunter, was brought to the General Hospital, Birmingham, on Sunday, June 16th, 1850, at 12 noon, having been bitten on the cheek by an adder. . . . He described the bite as being instantly followed by acute pain and by a *burning* sensation of heat and tumefaction. He experienced also nausea and faintness in his walk to the hospital. Upon his admission the entire face presented a swollen appearance and the part immediately adjacent to the bite were discoloured, of a livid hue. The pulse was imperceptible, the respiration difficult, the surface cold and clammy.

He complained of *intense pain about the umbilicus, greatly augmented on pressure*, and there was constant vomiting of bilious matter; he *appeared wandering as if drunk and answered questions in a mumbling incoherent manner*. The bowels acted frequently and involuntarily, and both blood and mucus were mingled with the motions. He also complained of pain in the throat, and there was some difficulty in deglutition. On examination, a copious secretion of viscid mucus was seen to be adherent to the pharynx.

. . . The pulse is still imperceptible, and the pain unrelieved. He appears to be sinking, and sickness and diarrhoea continue, together with great thirst. . . . Copious, dark, and watery motions have taken place; the pulse is 104, full, and incompressible. . . . The parts adjacent to the bite are assuming the departing and varying hues of an ecchymosis. . . . Complains of pain and soreness in the chest. [Pemberton, 1851]

*Feeling as if Dying*
- On August 19th, 1858, about midday, I came upon a large, nearly black snake, which, from its size and colour, I took to be one of the common harmless species. I seized it by the tail, held it up to show my companions and was instantly bitten in the last joint of the forefinger of the right hand. . . . Very little blood flowed, but the pain was acute. . . . In about 10 to 15 minutes after the bite, the finger became swollen and painful; a sense of numbness and rigidity gradually extended up the hand and arm, succeeded by *giddiness and confusion in the head*, with an acrid, *burning* sensation in the lips, mouth, and throat. I told my wife I wished to get home as quickly as possible; but before we had accomplished half the distance [about half a mile] the *power of locomotion began to fail me*, my speech became thick and inarticulate, the giddiness increased to loss of vision, violent retching came on, and I was led, or rather dragged, *like a drunken man staggering home*.

  By the time we had reached our destination, all the previous symptoms were greatly increased in intensity; the lips and tongue were livid, swollen, and protruding; the mouth and throat so parched and swollen that to swallow any liquid was impossible. . . . The pain at the pit of the stomach and in the bowels was excruciating and was accompanied with severe cramps in the lower extremities, profuse cold clammy perspirations, faintness, and extreme prostration. *I felt as if I were dying* and was quite unable to direct those around me what to do until the arrival of the nearest medical man. . . . Incessant vomiting continued, of a viscid greenish fluid, in colour and taste like *inspissated bile*, followed by a severe attack of bilious diarrhoea, about 2 hours after the bite, which greatly relieved my sufferings, and I was then able to take repeated draughts of sal volatile in soda water.

  Towards evening the hand and arm became painfully inflamed and swollen to 3 or 4 times their natural size. Spots of *purpura haemorrhagica* appeared the next day in various parts of the body and limbs. The inflammation, which was of an erysipelatous character, gradually spread from the arm to the shoulder, integuments of the neck, chest, abdomen, and back, on the right side, as low down as the hip. For 3 or 4 nights I suffered much from sleeplessness, thirst, and exhaustion, requiring the frequent administration of wine with soda water, and strong beef-tea. The bright-red hue of the skin began to fade after the fourth day, leaving it of a mottled livid colour, with patches of ecchymosis. The oedema of the limb, which was very considerable, was much relieved by finely puncturing with a lancet. At the end of a week I was able to leave my bed, but the hand and arm were quite useless and did not recover their former powers until 6 or 8 weeks after the accident; the right leg also remained weak for some time, *causing me to drag it in walking*. [Weston, 1859]

## Heart Block

- A 69-year-old man, with a history of myocardial infarction 10 years previously, attended the Accident and Emergency Department of Morriston Hospital, Swansea, Wales, 30 min. after being bitten on the right thumb by a common adder [V. berus]. He immediately felt unwell and, on arrival at hospital, he was complaining of abdominal pain and vomiting. Diarrhoea developed within minutes of arrival. On examination, he was in shock [pulse 60/min with decelerations, blood pressure 80/50 mmHg] and there was some discolouration of the tip of the right thumb at the site of the bite. There was epigastic tenderness and guarding but no other evidence of peritonism. The electrocardiogram showed intermittent 2: 1 second degree heart block [Mobitz type 2].

  Early features of Vipera berus envenomation include abdominal pain, vomiting, diarrhoea, shock and swelling of the bitten part. Non-specific ECG changes, such as T-wave inversion, have been reported in al degrees of envenomation by Vipera berus, but this appears to be the first report of heart block associated with adder bite. . . . The patient had a confirmed history of ischaemic heart disease but had been asymptomatic for the preceding 10 years. Moreover, there was no evidence of myocardial damage on this admission. [Moore, 1988]

- T-wave inversion on electrocardiogram [ECG] is often associated with myocardial ischemia or ventricular strain. In people with heart block, also called AV [atrioventricular] block, the electrical signal that controls the heartbeat is partially or completely blocked from reaching the ventricles. In second degree heart block [Mobitz type I] the electrical impulses are delayed further and further with each subsequent heartbeat until the heart actually skips a beat. This type of block most often is physiological and is seen in a highly relaxed state and during sleep. It rarely causes symptoms. It sometimes causes dizziness and/or other symptoms.

  In second degree heart block [Mobitz type II] some of the electrical impulses are unable to reach the ventricles. The pattern is irregular. Individuals with this type of heart block may have a heartbeat that is slower than normal. This condition is less common than type I and is more serious. Second degree Mobitz type II heart block is likely to induce symptoms such as light-headedness, fainting, chest pain [worse during physical activity], shortness of breath, tiring easily when undertaking physical activity, and sudden dizziness when standing up from a lying or sitting position. Mobitz type II heart block is more common in people with certain heart conditions. Examples of heart disease that can lead to heart block include heart failure, coronary heart disease, and cardiomyopathy [heart muscle diseases]. An estimated 1 in 30 people with heart disease will develop Mobitz type II heart block.

# CASE

'This is an interesting case, because I think, it is impossible to be solved by repertorising: a lady of 30 years of age, married, 1 daughter, came with dysplasia of cervix, Pap IV. The main problem in her life was, that when she was 12, she found out that her father, a well-known gynaecologist, had been giving sleeping pills to her mother and secretly going off to another woman at night.

'The patient must have had a special sense for this and found out about it. So she was sneaking after him, setting traps for him. For example she put things in front of the basement door to make a big noise when he would open it at night so that her mother would find out about it. She became a real threat to the double life of her father. He started to hate her for it and forbid her to open her mouth at home unless she would be asked. 'This was the main story of her life. She did shocking things at school in order to do something against his good and clean reputation. She took drugs, dropped out of school, left home very early and had a wild life. She did not see her father for many years. Later on she had a relationship of the same kind: her boyfriend was going off with other women at night, when she was exhausted from so much work, earning money for the 2 of them, bringing up his daughter and doing the household. He came back early in the morning, when she was still sleeping, just like her father.

'So far I understood this story as I understand the life of a snake: the sneaking, the setting traps, the sleeping pills, the secret sexual thing, the double morality. But it was not Lachesis, because she was not loquacious at all. Instead she was talking in a peculiar way: little short sentence, long pause, staring in the air. So what other snake could it be?

'Now it just so happens that a few years ago we were proving Vipera berus, the German viper. The patient and I talked about this snake and about her life. After 2 hours we ended up with the theme of the modern gynaecological clinic with controlled birth, where all the power is taken away from women and midwives by male doctors. Everything is controlled by injections and infusions. The natural process of birth is in the hands of men, they take over.

'When I asked her if she had anything to do with this, she was very astonished: both her father and her brother are strong followers of this kind of gynaecology. Both of them had been studying in the same hospital with the same professor who is the biggest interventionist in all of Germany. She herself has been born in this way, but due to some problem her mother had to be anaesthetised and she was borne blue. Her father nearly fainted.

'So I had only these symptoms, the snake things in her and her parents life, the birth incident and her father practicing exactly the same kind of birth method we were talking about when proving Vipera.

'In this proving we understood Vipera as the force which is subconsciously threatening our world. So much so that if we see a snake we immediately beat it to death. Her story bore some similarities; she became the threatening force for her father so he prevented her from talking anymore. There is the same deadly hostility between our culture and the snake as between her father and her.

'So I gave her Vipera berus C 200. She said, it was the strongest drug she ever took. She went through her entire life again. She even had a dramatic dream of her birth, where some horrible device overwhelmed her. All the memories of her youth with her father came up again. She only wanted to be alone in her bed, far away from any people, just like the viper lives far away from any people. She had an immense hatred for her father. When she met her former boyfriend again she could see everything very clearly and could tell him. Nothing could be denied. The feelings about an abortion she had had came up again. Her migraines returned, which reminded her of her birth. She treated her daughter as badly as her father had treated her. She fell into a staring rigidity for weeks, scolding at everybody who came near, just like a viper. After many months of this psychological process she came back to social life again with a much better relationship to her father.'
[Jürgen Becker, Vipera; HL 1991]

# VIPERA LEBETINA

## Systematics

- Scientific name: Macrovipera lebetina [L., 1758].
- Synonyms: Coluber lebetinus [L., 1758]. Vipera lebetina [Wall, 1908].
- Common names: Blunt-nosed viper. Levant viper. Kufi viper.
- Family: Viperidae, subfamily Viperinae.

## Biological Profile

- Medium to large, very robust true viper with broad, triangular head distinct from neck and blunt, rounded snout. Average length 1.2 m, maximum 2.2 m. Females and males of similar size.
- Body usually light grey, khaki or buff to reddish-brown, with double row of opposing or alternating dorsal spots from head to tail. Dark lines usually form a V-mark, pointing forward, on top of head. Females usually darker, background

colour brownish; males usually lighter, background colour greyish. Belly light grey to yellow, with small dark brown spots. Tail short, tapers abruptly, underside of tip yellow.
- Range: Southern Europe, northern Africa, Middle East, Asia to Iran and northern parts of India.
- Habitat: Brushy, overgrown, rocky hillsides, ravines, and valleys.
- Frequently found associated with human activity, such as in and around agricultural fields, farmyards, gardens, and villages.
- Oviparous; up to 22 eggs per clutch.
- Active in evening and night during the warm season.
- Preys on birds and small mammals. Favours birds [adults, chicks, eggs]; will climb trees and shrubs to forage. May be found in association with dense populations of partridges and quail and will raid henhouses for chicks and eggs.
- Tendency to overfeed in captivity, often becoming 'unhealthily obese'.
- Five recognized subspecies [lebetina, cernovi, obtusa, transmediterranea, turanica].

## Behaviour & Temperament
Most active and alert at night, usually very slow-moving and almost oblivious to stimuli during day, but temperament unpredictable and may suddenly strike quickly and savagely, accompanied by loud hissing. One author observed that it usually bites only after sunset.

Its ability to survive, indeed to prosper, around human habitations may affect human activity to the extent that people often time their activities to take advantage of the snake's quiescent periods.

The subspecies Macrovipera lebetina lebetina [available from homeopathic pharmacies under the name Vipera lebetina lebetina] is the only venomous snake on the island of Cyprus and found almost everywhere. Well camouflaged and often waiting near small water pits for birds to approach, the Cyprus blunt-nosed viper usually doesn't move, not even when passed close by, which makes it easily overseen by hikers.


## MATERIA MEDICA VIPERA LEBETINA

### Sources
1 Effects of bite; clinical manifestations.

### Clinical Manifestations
Venom haemotoxic – haemorrhagic, necrotic and proteolytic. Proteolytic activity is high, approaching the level of pit vipers, which have the most active protease systems known.

Envenomation causes sharp pain at site of bite, followed by local swelling, red spots on the skin, reduced blood-clotting capability and necrosis. Breathing quickly becomes rapid, pulse rate increases, and there is extreme thirst. Additional early systemic symptoms also include weakness, faintness, sweating, nausea, vomiting, and frequently diarrhoea. Numerous serious envenomations and deaths of humans reported each year over much of its range.

# VIPERA PALAESTINAE

## Systematics
- Scientific name: Daboia palaestinae [Werner, 1938].
- Synonyms: Vipera palaestinae [Werner, 1938]. Vipera xanthina palaestinae [Mertens, 1952].
- Common name: Palestine viper.
- Family: Viperidae, subfamily Viperinae.

## Biological Profile
- True viper with elongate, triangular head distinct from neck and many small keeled scales dorsally. Average length 70–90 cm, maximum 130 cm.
- Body grey, reddish-brown, beige, olive, or yellowish, usually with a wide central zigzag band of dark grey, blackish, brown, or reddish.
- Range: Israel, Syria, Jordan, Lebanon. Mediterranean coastal plains to inland hills of Lebanon and Israel, and adjoining regions of Syria and Jordan.
- Habitat: Rocky slopes, pastures, fallow and planted fields, wetlands; agricultural settlements – barns, stables, animal pens, along canals and irrigation ditches.
- Favoured habitats are associated with humans and water.
- Generally nocturnal, due largely to extremely high daytime temperatures; may be found during daylight hours basking in morning in early spring. Basking often occurs in branches of shrubs or trees.
- Oviparous; 7–22 eggs per clutch.
- Prefers warm-blooded prey, esp. birds and small mammals. Mammals are struck, released, then followed via the scent trail for consumption. Birds are held until venom takes effect.

## Behaviour & Temperament
'Daboia palaestinae is not usually aggressive, preferring to flee even when provoked. It exhibits a characteristic coiling and hissing threat display, ceasing to hiss when uncoiling to escape. If disturbance continues, the display increases until the forward part of the body is held off the ground in the pre-strike coil and flattened by rib spreading. The animal may continue elevating and hissing when retreating from this posture. There are reports of aggressive individuals pursuing people who disturbed them during the mating season.' [Mallow, 2003]

## MATERIA MEDICA VIPERA PALAESTINAE

## Sources
1 Effects of bite; clinical manifestations.

## Clinical Manifestations

Over a 7-year period in Israel [1969–1975], 92% of snakebites where the offending animal was identified were *V. palaestinae*. Men were found to be at greater risk than women. The extremely toxic venom has anti-coagulant, pro-coagulant, protease, lecithinase, and L-amino acid oxidase fractions in addition to major neurotoxic and haemotoxic components. Zinc and copper contents are very high, although it is not fully understood what role these trace metals play in envenomation.

*Hypotension* is a characteristic symptom. It is induced primarily by neurotoxic effects on vasoregulatory centres in the brain. Neurotoxic fractions in the venom reduce blood pressure by reducing control centre function in the medulla oblongata. Hypotension occurs secondarily as a result of extravasation due to vessel wall disruption.

'Immediately after the bite, which in the majority of cases on the hands or feet, a local tender swelling appears, which spreads proximally during the first few hours. The swelling may extend further over the homo-lateral half of the body within a period of hours to a few days and in severe cases it may extend even to the opposite side of the body. The swelling is accompanied by the appearance of haemorrhagic or serous blisters at the site of the bite, while subcutaneous haemorrhages may occur with the oedema; large ecchymoses and haematomata may be seen. Lymphangitis and regional lymphadenitis are frequently observed.

'In more severe cases an almost immediate generalised reaction consisting of nausea, vomiting, abdominal pain, diarrhoea, and signs of peripheral shock may occur within the first hour. Gastrointestinal disturbances may persist for many hours and cause severe dehydration. In not a few cases, urticaria and Quincke's oedema [angioedema], swelling of lips and face, and fever will appear. The patient often becomes severely anaemic after extensive haemorrhages in the internal organs and sometimes after melaena, haematemesis, and epistaxis. Slight jaundice may appear. Haematuria occurs rather infrequently.

'The swelling may recede and the haemorrhages may be absorbed and the patient may recover in a few days. In severe cases the patient may die in shock during the first 24–48 hours, or he may recover gradually. In some of these patients delayed shock may suddenly develop after a week of subjective and objective improvement. The patient becomes restless and sweats profusely; the respiration is rapid and the temperature rises. Very soon tachycardia develops and the blood pressure falls to shock levels. Renewed oedema spreads centripetally from the site of the bite and new subcutaneous haemorrhages appear, while in some cases dark red urine and sanguinolent diarrhoeas are seen. The patient may recover after a relatively long interval, but some die in a few hours to 2 days of the onset of delayed shock.

'Pathological findings . . . include internal haemorrhages, especially subendocardial, myocardial, pericardial, pleural, and intestinal bleeding, as well as bleeding in the brain and the adrenals. . . . Late sequelae of *V. palaestinae* bite have been described, such as lymphoedema of the bitten extremity, Dupuytren's peripheral neuritis [sic], an osteolysis.' [Bücherl & Buckley, Vol. I, 1968]

# VIPERA REDI

## Systematics
- Scientific name: Vipera aspis francisciredi [Laurenti, 1768].
- Synonyms: Vipera redi [Sonnini & Latreille, 1801]. Vipera aspis var. redi [Calabresi, 1924].
- Common name: Central Italian asp viper.
- Family: Viperidae, subfamily Viperinae.

## Biological Profile
- Subspecies of V. aspis endemic to Italy, differing from V. aspis in having much more apparent white or cream coloured spots near outer edge of ventral scales. Background colour can range from dull grey to maroon to dark brown with darker blotches. Average length 60 cm; maximum 80 cm.
- Head distinctly swollen behind eyes and upper lips
- Range: South Switzerland, north-central Italy, Austria, Slovenia, NW Croatia.
- Habitat: Woodlands of average humidity and mountainous areas at elevations of 1200–1900 m.
- Forms small groups in winter and spring. Tends to stay in one area in spring but disperses towards new localities in summer.
- Displays rather reduced activities in March and the first third of April, coiling up in sunny spots with dry grass and leaves. Inactively halts in shade of bushes at temperatures of 30°C or above. Females may climb up bushes as high as 30–70 cm above ground level, coiling up in suitable sunny spots.
- Ovoviviparous; 4–12 live young per brood.
- Preys on small mammals and, rarely, lizards.
- Named for the Italian empiricist Francesco Redi [1626–1697], who was the first to bring scientific method to bear on venomous snakebite.
- Venom mixed haemotoxic and neurotoxic.

## MATERIA MEDICA VIPERA REDI

### Sources
1 Effects of bites collated by Hering in *Wirkungen des Schlangengiftes* [Effects of snake venoms], 1837.
2 Effects of bite; sleeping into aggravation.

### Mind
∞ Restlessness increasing to despair, & disposition to sleep, violent headache, glistening eyes, yellow complexion with red cheeks.

### Generals
∞ Paralysis of single limbs, or of one-half of body.
∞ Fainting, & vertigo, nausea, and stinging pain about heart.
∞ Stiffness and coldness of body, & clammy sweat.

∞ Profuse perspiration.

∞ Great drowsiness, & languor, loss of sight, difficult breathing, retching, vomiting, spasms, violent pain in umbilical region, tension of abdomen, and small frequent pulse.

∞ Violent thirst.

## Locals

∞ Frequent vertigo, to fainting, particularly during the nausea and vomiting.

∞ Heat in eyes and profuse lachrymation.

∞ Protruded eyes.

∞ Dark-yellow eyes.

∞ Weakness of one eye.

∞ Obscuration of sight.

∞ Swelling of face, or particularly of lips and eyelids.

∞ Tongue swollen, protruding, turning blackish-brown.

∞ Difficulty of speech, & swelling of tongue, or lockjaw.

∞ Diarrhoea and vomiting, with profuse emission of urine.

∞ Difficulty of breathing, & cold sweat.

∞ Oppression of chest, & anguish, or & chills and vertigo.

∞ Reddish-black, lentil-sized spots all over, even in face.

### Sleeping Into Aggravation

Josephina Poggi, 20 years old, of a strong constitution, in the spring of last year, was bitten by a viper, at the external ankle of the right foot. The wound having been immediately cleaned with saliva, by which the small quantity of blood covering it was wiped off, she began to walk towards her village, when she was *suddenly seized with a sensation of extreme debility*, violent pain in the epigastrium, and vomiting, and the tongue began to swell in an extraordinary manner. Dr. Marianini, who saw the patient 1½ hour after the accident, found her in the following state: The features were considerably altered; the cheeks puffed; the lips and tongue enormously swelled, but not painful, covered with saliva, and very pale. The swelling of the tongue rapidly increased, so that it at last *almost filled the cavity of the mouth*, and caused great difficulty of breathing; the voice was inaudible, but the patient expressed, by signs, that she suffered much from *pain in the epigastrium and stomach*; she had frequent attacks of syncope; the pulse was intermittent, and very weak; the limbs were in a state of relaxation; the whole body was very pale, and from time to time agitated by *fits of shivering*.

The wounded part was neither swelled nor tender on pressure. M. Marianini endeavoured to administer a dose of liquor ammonia in peppermint water, but the swelling of the tongue, and the continual flow of saliva, prevented him from attaining his object and he was at last forced to inject it through the nose. After an hour, the swelling of the tongue and face having a little subsided, the vital powers being somewhat restored, and the pulse having acquired more force, and in the same proportion the wound having begun to swell and become painful, M. Marianini applied a cupping-glass to the wound, and, after having taken about 2 ounces of blood, covered it with the empl. opii.

The internal use of the ammonia, with the addition of some opium, having been continued for about 6 hours, the face and tongue regained their natural size and appearance, and the patient felt an excessive inclination to sleep; *she had not, however, slept more than an hour when the swelling of the tongue and the general symptoms of debility returned with such violence as to place her life again in danger*; it was therefore necessary to rouse her from her sleep and to keep her awake; the above medicine being at the same time administered in full dose. The swelling of the tongue, as well as the general symptoms, then gradually disappeared, and, after perseverance in the use of the ammonia for about 24 hours, did not return again.

The swelling of the wounded foot, from this time, increased to such a degree, that very active antiphlogistic means were resorted to and after some weeks the patient was perfectly cured. [Marianini, 1829]

# VIPERA XANTHINA

## Systematics
- Scientific name: Montivipera xanthina [Gray, 1849].
- Synonyms: Daboia xanthina [Gray, 1849]. Vipera xanthina [Strauch, 1868].
- Common names: Ottoman viper. Rock viper. Near East viper. Turkish viper.
- Family: Viperidae, subfamily Viperinae.

## Biological Profile
- Large, stout-bodied true viper. Average length 70–90 cm; maximum 1.3 m.
- Body often grey, but can be yellow, olive, reddish-brown or dark grey. Dark brown or blackish wavy dorsal stripe along midline from back of head to tail. Series of dark circular or rectangular spots along each flank. Pattern more vivid in males than females. Belly grey to yellowish, often with black or dark greyish mottling. Snout rounded and blunt, covered with small keeled scales. Tail slender, short, underside of tip may be yellow.
- Range: Northeastern Greece and Turkey, incl. Greek and Turkish Aegean islands.
- Habitat: Swamps, rocky hillsides and open grassy areas with few bushes or trees. Most often found in areas with ample water, moisture and vegetation. Found from near sea level to 2,500 m elevation.
- Often found in populated areas in yards, fields, irrigation ditches, and gardens.
- Mainly nocturnal, but active at daytime during cooler months. Mainly terrestrial but can climb into small trees and bushes.
- Preys on small mammals, birds, and possibly lizards. Seeks out and robs nests of birds and small mammals in late spring and early summer.
- Ovoviviparous; 2–15 live young per brood.
- Four recognized subspecies [xanthina, nilsoni, dianae, occidentalis].

## Behaviour & Temperament

Lethargic and slow-moving but can move rapidly and strike quickly. Not aggressive and shy; avoids human confrontation, but easily agitated, and will defend itself if molested.

## MATERIA MEDICA VIPERA XANTHINA

### Sources

1 Effects of bite; clinical manifestations.

### Clinical Manifestations

Moderately potent haemotoxin and some neurotoxic factor[s]. Envenomation causes sharp pain and local swelling, which may spread. Discolouration, blisters, and pus-filled or fluid-filled vesicles may appear within hours. Other symptoms may include dizziness, weakness, vomiting, and cold sweats.

# TURTLES AND TORTOISES

## Once a Turtle, Always a Turtle

'There are snakes that look like lizards, lizards that look like snakes, lizards that look like crocodiles, and the tuatara, which is always taken for a lizard. In contrast to all this confusion, the turtles stand alone among reptiles by always looking like turtles. . . .' [Pope, 1971]

## BIOLOGICAL PROFILE

### Names

British English normally describes testudines as turtles if they live in the sea; terrapins if they live in fresh or brackish water; or tortoises if they live on land. American English tends to use the word turtle for all freshwater species, as well as for certain land-dwelling species [e.g. box turtles]. Oceanic species are usually referred to as sea turtles and tortoise is restricted to members of the true tortoise family, Testudinidae.

The name terrapin is typically reserved only for the brackish water diamond-back terrapin. The word 'terrapin' is also often taken to mean edible turtle. But to the Algonquin Indians, from whom the word originated, a terrapin was any kind of turtle.

Australian English uses turtle for both the marine and freshwater species but tortoise for the terrestrial species. Veterinarians, scientists, and conservationists prefer the name *chelonians*.

Turtle in Dutch is 'schildpad' and in German 'Schildkröte'. Both mean, literally, 'shielded toad'.

## Shell

Testudines are characterised by a special bony or cartilaginous shell developed from their ribs that acts as a shield. The upper portion of the shell is called the *carapace* and covers the back and sides; the lower portion of the shell is called the *plastron* and covers the belly. Carapace and plastron are joined on each side by a bony bridge. Both the carapace and the plastron are fusions of bones; the carapace of about 50 bones – the ribs and vertebrae; the plastron of the clavicles, bones between the clavicles, and portions of the ribs. The shell is covered in horny scales [called scutes] consisting of keratin, with the exception of the leatherback sea turtle and soft-shelled turtles, in which the shell is covered with leathery skin.

The shell shapes of turtles differ with each species and are often related to habitat. Most aquatic turtles are generally flatter, allowing them to move faster through the water. Terrestrial species, on the other hand, have carapaces that are dome-shaped.

In strong contrast to snakes and lizards, among which we find many bluffers, turtles have *little bluffing ability* and equally little necessity to bluff since their shell provides them ample protection. Numerous turtles can *close up so completely* that the thinnest blade of a knife cannot be forced into any of the cracks between the carapace and plastron.

The shell greatly enhances the turtle's chances of survival. Apart from protection against predators, turtles have been found to survive wildfires, presumably by withdrawing tightly within their shell and pushing as deeply into the ground as possible.

## Feet

Turtles appear inept, ungainly, awkward, and sluggish due to their *'caged' construction*, their shell being an extended ribcage holding all internal organs as well as bony structures normally placed outside the ribcage such as clavicles, shoulder blades and pelvis. Turtle feet make up for this confinement. Highly significant to turtle anatomy, their feet provide insight into the ecological niche occupied by any given species.

Some of the many necessary functions performed by the turtle's feet include climbing, swimming, walking amid rocky cliffs, providing propulsion while swimming, digging tunnels, burrows and nests, securing a grip onto the female's shell while mating, stroking the female's face, covering the own face, and maintaining traction in slippery mud.

## Respiration

'The rigid shell means that turtles can't breathe as other reptiles do, by changing the volume of their chest cavity via expansion and contraction of the ribs.

Instead, turtles breathe in 2 ways. First, they employ buccal pumping, pulling air into their mouth then pushing it into the lungs via oscillations of the floor of the throat. Secondly, by contracting the abdominal muscles that cover the posterior opening of the shell, the internal volume of the shell increases, drawing air into the lungs, allowing these muscles to function in much the same way as the mammalian diaphragm.' [Wikipedia]

'Breathing in a turtle is far from the simple and regular taking in and forcing out of air as in man. There are cycles of partial and complete expirations, and periods of pause during which the lungs are only partly filled. These pauses may last from a minute or less to several hours. This ability to "hold the breath" is due to 3 factors: very thorough ventilation of the lungs, low consumption of oxygen and a *low unloading tension for haemoglobin*, the part of the red blood cells that carries oxygen. The holding of the breath referred to here occurs in land turtles that have no chance to supplement their oxygen supply by getting any from water.' [Pope, 1971]

## Eating & Fasting
Turtles use their jaws to cut and chew food. They have no teeth, but instead horny ridges on the upper and lower jaws. In carnivorous turtles these ridges are sharp as knives and slice through their prey. Herbivorous turtles have serrated-edged ridges that help them cut through tough plants. Turtles use their tongues to swallow food, but they cannot, unlike most reptiles, stick out their tongues to catch food.

The turtle's method of getting and swallowing food is extremely simple and shows none of the complexities found among snakes. Lizards and crocodilians hold an intermediate position in this respect. To put it briefly, turtles *chop down their food*, in combination with front legs for tearing off mouthfuls and a strong tongue for working it into the throat.

'Although, like other reptiles, turtles can comfortably fast for months on end, they will feed almost as often as mammals, and grow very obese. Digestion is slow and its rate varies with the body temperature, which is always about the same as that of the surroundings. . . .

'Specialisation in choice of food is rare among turtles. Many kinds eat both plant and animal matter; not a few devour carrion. Succulent leaves and stems and delicate blossoms are always chosen. Even certain species that have powerful jaws with greatly expanded surfaces for crushing hard-shelled animals do not confine themselves to such, but eat soft-bodied animals as well. . . . In short, a turtle will probably consume any animal that it can readily capture.' [Pope, 1971]

## Sexual Selection
Sexual selection can result in intra-sexual competition for mates, usually in the form of male-male combat, or inter-sexual choice, usually in the form of female choice of a mate. Abundant evidence is available to suggest the existence of both forms of sexual selection in turtles.

1 In most terrestrial species, males engage in combat with each other. Males typically grow larger than females. Copulation is often a *brutal* affair.
2 In semi-aquatic and bottom-walking aquatic species, male combat is less common, but males often *forcibly* inseminate females. As in terrestrial species, males are usually larger than females.
3 In strictly aquatic species, male combat and forcible insemination are rare. Instead, males utilise elaborate pre-coital displays, and *female choice is highly important*. Males are usually smaller than females.

Female green sea turtles [Chelonia mydas] have been shown being capable of avoiding copulation with a variety of behavioural patterns incl. biting, avoidance, and refusal. Females are *completely in control* whether mating occurs or not.

Female slider turtles [Trachemys scripta scripta] assume an active role in courtship including the use of proceptive behaviours that actively solicit male attention and may communicate receptivity.

## Courting & Caring

In some species, temperature determines whether an egg develops into a male or a female: higher temperature produces females, lower temperature causes males.

Large numbers of eggs are deposited in holes dug into mud or sand. They are then covered and left to incubate by themselves. When the turtles hatch, they squirm their way to the surface and head toward the water. There are no known species in which the mother cares for the young.

'In strong contrast to meticulous nest construction is the female's blissful unconcern with what may be taking place while she is nesting; once the mechanism has been released, a person may sit behind and put the eggs in a bucket as they appear; later she will turn and cover up the empty nest just as thoroughly as if it were full of eggs. . . . Courtship in turtles may be little more than pursuit of the female or it may take the form of harmless biting and pushing of her as well. Some of the giant tortoises violently pound their mates, using the body like battering rams, uttering resounding roars all the while. . . . Differences in colour are rare. By far the most constant mark of the male is the longer tail.' [Pope, 1971]

'The excitation of the males during their attempts to copulate can, at least in captivity, lead to their completely ignoring the species of the other turtle. Thus there are often "mismatches" between members of quite different species. Testudinids even court shoes and other objects having roughly the shape of a turtle shell. Because they are constantly ready to mate, sometimes copulating even in the autumn, and are so vigorous in their courtship, turtles are actually considered in eastern Asia to be a symbol of *sexual prowess and the intensified enjoyment of life*.' [Grzimek]

Mark Twain [1909] held a completely opposite opinion regarding the turtle's lust and sex life: '. . . the tortoise, that cold calm puritan, that takes a treat only once in 2 years and then goes to sleep in the midst of it and doesn't wake up for 60 days . . . neither the gentleman tortoise nor the lady tortoise is ever hungry enough for solemn joys of fornication to be willing to break the Sabbath to get them.'

## Senses

For the most part, turtles are *visually oriented* animals that rely heavily on their eyesight to identify con-specifics, food, and potential danger. They are thought to have exceptional night vision due to the unusually large number of rod cells in their retinas. They have colour vision with a wealth of cone subtypes with sensitivities ranging from the near ultraviolet [UVA] to red. Their range of colour perception approximates that of humans, but certain colours seem to be more interesting to them than others. Normally, *the colours red, orange, and yellow elicit investigative responses* from turtles that are looking for a meal.

Although turtles lack an ear opening, a fleshy membrane called the tympanum covers their eras. Within the middle ear, the columnella bone translates airborne vibrations into sound. Turtles also lack vocal chords, yet many of them are capable of produce sounds, most often by forcing air from the lungs.

The sense of smell is good at close range, given the fact that pet turtles, for example, often appear to smell objects before eating or rejecting them.

The skin and shell of turtles are surprisingly sensitive. Hulking horny-skinned testudines reportedly can feel the tip of straw dragged along their skin. Their well-developed sense of touch allows turtles to thermoregulate, select ideal refuge sites, detect climatic changes, locate prey, and detect vibrations transmitted across the ground by approaching organisms.

## Solitary

Turtles are essentially *solitary* animals. There is not much family life per se among turtles, and *not much territorial or dominance behaviour*, in contrast to lizards and crocodilians. Land turtles may have home ranges. Home ranges of box turtles frequently overlap, sharing common space, regardless of age and sex. Range- or burrow-sharing turtles show no antagonism towards each other. Certain aquatic turtles may live in small, stable groups. Some sea turtles, particularly Lepidochelys olivacea [Olive Ridley turtle], will form immense assemblages, or *arribadas*, as a manifestation of group nesting.

## Temperature

Like other reptiles, turtles are ectotherms – varying their internal temperature according to the ambient environment, commonly called cold-blooded.

Most species live in or around water; the largest turtles are strictly aquatic [their immense weight is much less cumbersome in water].

## Distinct Sense of Time

'Since turtles have a definite sense of time, their daily schedule is fairly well regulated. Most land turtles are most active in the late morning, after they have thoroughly sunned themselves to bring their bodies to an adequate "opening temperature." Then they run about, looking for food or mating, until the sun is at its maximum elevation at noon. In order not to become overheated, the animals seek out shady places, creeping into shrubbery or other protected spots, for there is an upper limit to the desirable body temperature.

'If one keeps such a turtle in the open and offers it no shade, it runs a serious risk of succumbing to heatstroke. In the early afternoon the turtles resume their activity and wander about, though not quite as briskly as in the morning. Toward evening, when the sun noticeably loses strength, they turn to their resting places, often selecting particular spots to which they return every evening. . . .

'The daily rhythm of the aquatic turtles is not so pronounced, for such large temperature fluctuations do not occur in their habitat. Whereas most aquatic turtles are active by day and spend much time sunning themselves on the shore or on tree trunks in the water, certain species such as the Argentinean snake-necked turtles and the matamata, are active at night or at least during the hours of twilight. The marine turtles, on the other hand, are definitely diurnal [daytime] animals; at night they drift about, asleep, on the surface of the water.' [Grzimek]

### Turtles with Tumours

Sea turtle fibropapillomatosis [FP] was first discovered in 1938 in a green turtle from Florida. Reports of the disease were relatively rare until after 1980; now FP occurs around the globe, causing an epidemic amongst sea turtles. The condition has the highest incidence in green turtles and occurs to a much lesser degree in loggerhead and olive ridley turtles, and incidentally in the remaining 4 species of sea turtles.

FP is a disease marked by proliferation of benign but debilitating cutaneous fibropapillomas and occasional visceral fibromas. What distinguishes FP from other forms of neoplasm is the proliferation of both the epidermal and dermal skin layers. The most visible manifestation of FP is the presence of large tumours on the skin, eyes, and corners of the mouth. The appearance varies from smooth to cauliflower-like with small spiky projections. The colour of tumours can be white, pink, red, grey, purple or black. The number of tumours per turtle can be as many as 70. In some instances, the tumours can become very large and occlude vision. Growths of fibropapillomas can also adversely affect locomotion, swallowing, and breathing. Blood analyses have indicated that turtles with many tumours are typically anaemic.

About 25% of turtles with FP also have internal tumours, most commonly in the lungs, heart, and kidney. On histology, these tumours are universally composed of a connective tissue matrix and fibroblasts. In the case of skin tumours, these have been characterised as fibropapillomas, while tumours in internal organs have been classed as fibromas, myxofibromas, or fibrosarcomas of low-grade malignancy.

Hawaiian green turtles also have tumours in the glottis, and as expected, such animals are prone to getting pneumonia and other respiratory inflammatory problems. Green turtles with FP from Florida, strangely enough, do not get tumours in the glottis.

Fibropapillomatosis is caused by a herpes-type virus. In one recent sample from the Hawaiian Islands more than 90% of green turtles showed symptoms of the illness. In the 1990s, it was thought that this was a deadly condition for sea turtles and would quickly lead to the extinction of all sea turtles. New research shows that larger species can and will recover from the disease.

Interestingly, long-term studies have shown that pelagic [living in open oceanic waters] turtles recruiting to near shore environments appear to be free of the disease.

## POWER TO THE SHELL

### Venerable Upholder of the World

'Though a creature to laugh over when we see it creeping stealthily about on tip-toe, as if it were abroad for the purpose of picking pockets, it has a very notable place in myth, and was almost universally reverenced. The East believes that the world rests upon a tortoise, which rests upon nothing – and what a grand old testacean it is, this Vedic turtle, standing simply on its own dignity, and yet upholding upon its Atlantean carapace all the burdens of the round world and of them that dwell therein! Here is a subject for Walt Whitman himself, the self-sufficient, democratic, thewy-and-sinewy, double-sexed, bully-for-you, old tortoise. More power to your shell, sir! We creeping things take off our hats to you, testudinous ancient. And how splendidly the deliberate thing looms out of Hindu myth as the hereditary foe of the mystical elephant, the Darkness.

'The Red Indian to this day says that in the beginning of things there was nothing but a tortoise. It brooded upon space: covered Chaos as with a lid. But after a while it woke up: its solitary existence was irksome to it, and it sank splendidly into the abysmal depths; and lo! when it re-emerged, there was the terrestrial globe upon its back! For something to do, it had fished up our earth from the depths in the protoplasmic fluids, and, rather than be idle, it still keeps on holding it up. But some day it will sink again, and then will come the End – with Ragnarok and Armageddon.

'In Greek and Roman fancies, the tortoise hardly fares so well. It is the form to which a bright nymph, who had jested at the nuptials of Zeus and Hera, was turned into by Mercury; and ridicule falls upon the greatest of the Greeks when a tortoise falls upon his head. Yet they, too, knew of the tradition of the world-supporting thing and did reverence to it. And so from East to West, from antiquity to today, the creature, vast, ponderous, inert, has commanded and commands the homage of men.' [Robinson, 1893]

### Turtle Symbolism & Associations

- Key words: Strength; patience; endurance; stability; slowness; longevity; fecundity; wisdom under duress.
- Caspari [2003] sums up the key features of turtles/tortoises thus: 'Wondrously self-contained, ponderously slow and proverbially steady.'
- In the Far East, the carapace symbolised the vaulted Heaven and the plastron stood for the Earth. The turtle was an animal whose magic united Heaven and Earth.

- In ancient China the turtle was associated with the north, water, and winter. It appeared also on imperial banners as the Black Warrior, which protected against fire as well as in war.
- Associated by Native American with female strength and fertility.
- Represent steadfastness and longevity, the ability to withstand whatever misfortunes life may bring.
- A creature that lives in a box of its own making.
- Tortoises have been described as Tanks with Attitude.
- The turtle withdrawing into its shell is a sign of cowardice in some Far East cultures, a refusal to confront a situation head-on; whereas to Hindus it indicates turning away from the world and into oneself, a spiritual concentration, a return to the primal state.
- For the Aztecs, the turtle represented cowardice and boastfulness – hard on the outside, soft on the inside.
- 'The turtle in general is a dull, heavy, stupid animal, its brain being no bigger than a small bean, though the head is very large.' [Richard Brookes, 1790]
- In Christian symbolism the turtle represents modesty in marriage and morality; women living in the seclusion of the home as the turtle in its shell.
- In most cultures the turtle is a symbol of material existence and not of any aspect of transcendence since both its square and round forms allude to the forms of the manifest world and not to the creative forces. In view of its slowness, it might be said to embody natural evolution as opposed to spiritual evolution, which is rapid or discontinuous to a degree. In alchemy, the turtle symbolises matter at the beginning of the evolutionary process.
    Chinese alchemists likewise regarded the tortoise as the starting point of development.
- 'The contrast between worldly materialism and domestic bliss was particularly brought out in the Netherlands in the 17th century. In *Van de Uutnementheyt des Vrouwelicken Geslachts* [On the Excellence of the Female Sex], Johan van Beverwijck depicted the ideal wife not as a figure standing on top of the world but on a tortoise. Still bearing a torch in her left hand, she has resolved the conflict between the attractions of the wider world and the call to homely duties by the compromise of a mobile home. Behind her Adam delves in the garden while Eve spins within the cottage. The tortoise was adopted as an emblem of morality. If a wife had to leave home then she should conduct herself as though she had never left it.' [Young 2004]
- 'A large, heavy-bodied, slow-minded and slow-moving middle-aged woman, without a gleam of intelligence or sympathy in her big expressionless face, a sort of rough-hewn pre-Adamite lump of humanity, or gigantic land-tortoise in petticoats.' [William Henry Hudson, 1906]

## Turtle Sayings & Proverbs
- Contempt penetrates even the shell of the tortoise. [Iran]
- A turtle travels only when it sticks its neck out. [Korea]

- A turtle can't walk if doesn't push his head out of his shell. In life, you cannot make any kind of progress if you do not take risks. Also, the first steps must be made. [Guyana]
- The turtle lays thousands of eggs without anyone knowing, but when the hen lays an egg, the whole country is informed. [Malaysia]
- It is not only the hare, the tortoise arrives also at the destination. [Nigeria]
- It is the fear of what tomorrow may bring that makes the tortoise carry his house along with him wherever he goes. [Nigeria]
- The biting fly gets nothing by alighting on the back of the tortoise. [Ashanti, Ghana]
- The child who breaks a snail's shell cannot brake a tortoise's shell. There are certain things any human being can do and others he cannot because his powers are limited, therefore one must know the limit of one's abilities.
- The tortoise is said always to travel with its musical instrument in case it meets other musicians. Maintaining a state of preparedness. [Nigeria]
- A snake that bites a tortoise, bites only a shell. [Nigeria]

[Summarised from Health Sciences Libraries, Turtle Derby, University of Minnesota]

### The Wisest of All

Very old spurred tortoise males have the fifth vertebral scute almost vertical, giving them the appearance of a chair or seat, on which ancient Dogon sages may sit to pass out decrees and sentences. This link of the tortoise with wisdom in the Republic of Mali is common to various other traditions in western Africa, in particular Senegal and Nigeria. There the tortoise features in such legends as the following:

The tortoise was known to be the wisest of animals. He had many visitors who sought his wisdom, and they gave him many gifts. The tortoise was wise enough to want to become wiser. Then he decided to collect all the wisdom in the world, keep it for himself in a hollow gourd, or calabash, and to hang the calabash on a tree for safekeeping. For a long time the tortoise went about in the world, collecting all the wisdom that could be found and stuffing it into his calabash. When he could find no more, he tied the calabash around his neck and found a tree that he thought he could climb. Every time the tortoise started up the tree, the calabash got caught between him and the tree trunk and he fell down.

This happened many times. A man came by and watched the tortoise. Then the man suggested, "Why don't you hang the calabash on your back, so that it will not be in the way?" The tortoise did so and then it was able to climb the tree. Before hanging the calabash on a branch, he thought about how foolish he had been, even though he had so much wisdom in his calabash. Then he realised that the man could not have shown any wisdom unless the tortoise had missed some in his travels. With no hope of getting all the wisdom there was to be had, the humbled tortoise broke his calabash and let all the wisdom go back into the world again.

There are various slightly different endings to this tale. In one the tortoise in his unwise attempts to climb the tree becomes the laughing stock to some children witnessing the scene and commenting on its lack of common sense. Feeling angry for being rectified by little kids the tortoise breaks his calabash in pieces, revealing the moral of the story as that one is never too old to learn.

In another version, the tortoise's cunning deceit defeats itself. Here the tortoise steals from the gods a calabash containing all the wisdom in the world. Then, when failing to scale an obstacle on the road due to the calabash getting in his way, he smashes the calabash in a fit of irritation, and so, ever since that day, wisdom has been scattered all over the world in tiny pieces.

Somewhat different also is the version in which the tortoise is intent on keeping all gathered wisdom to himself. He is looking for a tree to hang the calabash where it would not be easily accessible to anyone else, so that he would remain the best and the only custodian of wisdom in the whole wide world. When it takes the advice of a little boy to move the calabash to his back in order to climb the tree, it dawns on the tortoise that the plan to keep all the world's wisdom to himself was a mission impossible and the height of foolishness.

In Nigeria also a version is told where the tortoise sets about in trying to monopolise the world's wisdom, in order to make everyone dependent upon him. Like in the other tales, this tortoise also tries hanging the wisdom-filled calabash high up in a tree to no avail. But this time it is a snail snickering at him, suggesting the only sensible solution we now know so well. Bottom-line: anyone, large or small, smart or dull, slow or quick, may possess a share of the world's wisdom.

## Festina Lente – Make Haste Slowly

The Roman emperors Augustus and Constantine had 'festina lente' as their motto. The Italian merchant prince and the founder of the Medici political dynasty, Cosimo de' Medici [1389–1464] adopted the adage and prided himself on his ability to 'hurry slowly', by which he meant to think deeply and decide quickly. It became the motto of the Medicis. The double tomb for Giovanni and Piero de' Medici, Cosimo's sons who died in 1463 and 1469, respectively, was rested on the backs of tortoises as a visual form of the Medici maxim.

Much favoured during the Renaissance, the motto was often accompanied by various depictions or emblems, the best known of which are a tortoise with a hosted sail attached to its back, and an anchor entwined by a dolphin. Giorgio Vasari and Doceno's fresco of 1555, *The Fruits of the Earth Offered to Saturn* shows on the right side Fortuna rising from the sea and offering the tortoise with sail to Saturn. The implication is that careful and determined application will achieve better results than rushing at the same problem unprepared.

The Dutch Renaissance humanist Desiderius Erasmus [c. 1466–1536] made 'festina lente' the subject of his scholarly commentaries in *Adagia*, his compilation of classical proverbs and commonplaces. Erasmus dubs it the 'royal proverb' and remarks that it advocates 'a *wise promptness together with moderation*, tempered with both vigilance and gentleness, so that nothing is done rashly and then regretted, and nothing useful to the common weal omitted out of carelessness.' It represents, in short, the *reining of passion by reason*.

Although Erasmus alludes to the dolphin curled around the anchor, it historically fits the turtle/tortoise equally well. Dutch humanist and physician Hadrianus Junius [1511–1575], born Adriaen de Jonghe, added several dozens of adages not yet found in Erasmus. Number 32 portrays a half-naked woman sitting on a stool with one foot firmly on the ground and the other foot somewhat raised. In her right hand is a pair of wings, in her left a tortoise. The woodcut illustration is accompanied by a Latin motto and epigram, meaning 'Less haste, more speed. Delay your speed and this will keep the delay under control in turn.'

## From Slowness to Stagnation

'Hasten slowly. It is one of those 2-faced maxims that have a great deal to answer for. . . . When I was a boy I suffered many things at the hands of a fable entitled, "The Hare and the Tortoise," which still dwells, though perhaps a little imperfectly, in my recollection. As a check upon the rapidity of my movements, I was recommended to get it by heart, and I did so. . . . But [the fable] does not prove that "slow and steady" is better than "swift and steady." All this I used to represent when I was a youngster, but I was only assured in return that when I was older I should be wiser. . . .

'If we only succeed in impressing mankind with the notion that they are moving too fast, they will go from slowness to slowness till at last they stand clean stock-still. This might be agreeable to certain evil-disposed persons, but it would never do for those who believe in progress and love it. If we have a goal to reach, the quicker we go the sooner we shall get there. All we need take care of is that we move in the right direction. . . .

'I maintain that the natural tendency of the general run of mankind to be slow is so serious a matter that any man who furnishes them with epigrammatic excuses for going slower still is a common enemy. Much more, if he tells them that they will have heart-disease, or go mad, if they live so fast. True, there is in this matter the same sort of unequal distribution that there is in others. That is, if some poor devils appear too quick, it is because all the rapid work is devolved upon their shoulders. . . .

'The poet Longfellow has lamented that at the end of every day there is something left undone. That is because the slow people will not co-operate with the swift. Otherwise we might all go to bed tomorrow night like Christians and get up next morning with nothing else to do for the rest of our lives. The Hare might lie down with the Tortoise and the Idle Apprentice eat air with the Industrious. *Hoc age* [Do This] would be an idle legend and a deserving universe would have its holiday. At all events, I shall do my share, and be as quick as ever I can.' [Browne, 1871]

## Unmasked Affection for Rugged Sturdiness

Wondering why almost everyone likes turtles and why so many people have such a warm fascination for them, Whit Gibbons [1983] knows beyond doubt 'that turtles are nowhere near "all bad" and scientists like myself are not the only ones who have an unmasked affection for these senior citizens of the reptile world. . . . Turtles are like pet rocks that move. . . . Turtles are the only reptiles that automobile drivers will not try to hit. . . . I think it is because turtles possess traits we admire in ourselves and others – *patience, perseverance, and the quality of being assertive without being too aggressive*. Turtles are really tough, too. Many seem to be more resistant to various environmental abuses than are other vertebrates, having the ability to live in the chemically charged effluents from paper mills, coal-fired power plants, or other industries. Such environmental conditions may be completely inhospitable to fish and waterfowl. Turtles even have been found to be some of the most resistant animals in the world to radiation exposure. Turtles are also surprisingly rugged when it comes to accepting physical punishment such as from automobile and tractor tires, forest fires, and the assaults of predators like alligators, raccoons, and dogs. Although some do not make it, the tales of the scars and scrapes on the shells of the survivors would make true adventure stories.'

## Toughing It Out

'Turtles are built for hard times. Through famine, flood, heat wave, ice age, a predator's inspections, a paramour's rejections, turtles *take adversity in stride*, usually by striding as little as possible. "The tale of the tortoise and the hare is the turtle's life story," said Mr. Cover, who calls himself a card-carrying member of the "turtle nerds" club. "Slow and steady wins the race."

'With its miserly metabolism and tranquil temperament, its capacity to forgo food and drink for months at a time, its redwood burl of a body shield, so well-engineered it can withstand the impact of a stampeding wildebeest, the turtle is one of the longest-lived creatures Earth has known. Individual turtles can survive for centuries, bearing silent witness to epic swaths of human swagger. Last March, a giant tortoise named Adwaita said to be as old as 250 years died in a Calcutta zoo, having been taken to India by British sailors, records suggest, during the reign of King George II. In June, newspapers around the world noted the passing of Harriet, a Galapagos tortoise that died in the Australia Zoo at age 176 – 171 years after Charles Darwin is said, perhaps apocryphally, to have plucked her from her equatorial home.

'Behind such biblical longevity is the turtle's stubborn refusal to senesce – to grow old. Don't be fooled by the wrinkles, the halting gait and the rheumy gaze. Researchers lately have been astonished to discover that in contrast to nearly every other animal studied, a turtle's organs do not gradually break down or become less efficient over time.

'Dr. Christopher J. Raxworthy, the associate curator of herpetology at the American Museum of Natural History, says the liver, lungs and kidneys of a centenarian turtle are virtually indistinguishable from those of its teenage counterpart, a Ponce de Leonic quality that has inspired investigators to begin examining the turtle genome for novel longevity genes.

"Turtles don't really die of old age," Dr. Raxworthy said. In fact, if turtles didn't get eaten, crushed by an automobile or fall prey to a disease, he said, they might just live indefinitely. *Turtles resist growing old and they resist growing up.*' [Angier, 2006]

## Two Sides to a Turtle

American author Herman Melville [1819–1891], best known for his novel *Moby Dick* [1851], gave a masterly portrayal of testudines in *The Encantadas*, a series of sketches about the Galapagos, or 'Enchanted' Islands.

'Everyone knows that tortoises as well as turtles are of such a make that if you but put them on their backs you thereby expose their bright sides without the possibility of their recovering themselves and turning into view the other. But after you have done this and because you have done this, you should not swear that the tortoise has no dark side. . . . The tortoise is both black and bright.

'. . . three huge antediluvian-looking tortoises, after much straining, were landed on deck. . . . behold these really wondrous tortoises – none of your schoolboy mud turtles, but black as widower's weeds, heavy as chests of plate, with vast shells medallioned and orbed like shields, and dented and blistered like shields that have breasted a battle, shaggy, too, here and there, with dark green moss, and slimy with the spray of the sea. These mystic creatures, suddenly translated by night from unutterable solitudes to our peopled deck, affected me in a manner not easy to unfold. They seemed newly crawled forth from beneath the foundations of the world. Yea, they seemed the identical tortoises whereon the Hindu plants this total sphere. . . . I no more saw 3 tortoises. They expanded – became transfigured. I seemed to see 3 Roman Coliseums in magnificent decay. . . .

'The great feeling inspired by these creatures was that of age: dateless, indefinite endurance. What other bodily being *possesses such a citadel wherein to resist the assaults of Time?* . . .

'As I lay in my hammock that night, overhead I heard the slow weary draggings of the 3 ponderous strangers along the encumbered deck. Their stupidity or their resolution was so great that they never went aside for any impediment. One ceased his movements altogether just before the mid-watch. At sunrise I found him butted like a battering ram against the immovable foot of the foremast, and still striving, tooth and nail, to *force the impossible* passage. That these tortoises are the victims of a penal, or malignant, or perhaps a downright diabolical enchanter, seems in nothing more likely than in that strange *infatuation of hopeless toil* which so often possesses them. I have known them in their journeyings ram themselves heroically against rocks, and long abide there, nudging, wriggling, wedging, in order to displace them, and so *hold on their inflexible path.* Their crowning curse is their *drudging impulse to straightforwardness in a belittered world.* . . .

'I then pictured these 3 straightforward monsters, century after century, writhing through the shades, grim as blacksmiths; crawling so slowly and ponderously that not only did toadstools and all fungus things grow beneath their feet, but a sooty moss sprouted upon their backs.'

## Turtles, says Melville

- Resist the assaults of Time.
- Perpetually strive to force the impossible passage.
- Are possessed by that strange infatuation of hopeless toil.
- Heroically attempt to displace rocks.
- Hold on to their inflexible path.
- Are bedeviled by a drudging impulse to straightforwardness in a belittered world.

## No Place Like Home

'Concerning the tortoises found here, most mariners have long cherished a superstition, not more frightful than grotesque,' Herman Melville wrote after visiting the Galapagos Islands on a whaler boat. 'They earnestly believe that all wicked sea-officers, more especially commodores and captains, are at death [and, in some cases, before death] transformed into tortoises; thenceforth dwelling upon these hot aridities, sole solitary lords of Asphaltum.'

Melville most likely knew that ancient mythmakers had pictured the creation of the turtle as retaliation for the water nymph Chelone's rejection to attend the wedding of Zeus and Hera.

The Roman grammarian Maurus Servius Honoratus presented the Roman version of Chelone's transgression: 'For his wedding with Juno [Hera], Jupiter [Zeus] ordered Mercurius [Hermes] to invite all the gods, the men and the animals to the wedding. Everyone invited by Mercurius [Hermes] came, except for Chelone who did not deign to be there, mocking the wedding. When Mercurius noticed her absence, he went back down to the earth, threw in the river the house of Chelone that was standing over the river and changed Chelone in an animal that would bear her name. "Chelone" is said "testudo" [tortoise] in Latin.'

In Aesop's Fable the tortoise is a home-loving tortoise instead of a haughty nymph: 'Zeus invited all the animals to his wedding. The tortoise alone was absent and Zeus did not know why, so he asked the tortoise [khelone] her reason for not having come to the feast. The tortoise said, "Be it ever so humble, there is no place like home." Zeus got angry at the tortoise and ordered her to carry her house with her wherever she went.'

## Calling the Turtle

To the people of Nacamaki Village in Koro Island, the sixth largest island of Fiji, turtles are their sacred ancestral god. There is one group of family descendants that perform a special ritual to summon the turtles to the surface. Australian writer, anthropologist and biologist Elliot Lovegood Grant Watson [1885–1970] once witnessed the ritual [emphasis added]:

'About 30 of the local tribesmen were already awaiting me when I had climbed along the cliff path. After a ceremonial drinking of *yangona* [kava kava, Piper methysticum] they led me to a yet higher cliff-top, and there after a good deal of conversation, which I could not understand, began to sing in their resonant voices, bidding the turtles come up, and show themselves.

TURTLES AND TORTOISES

'Turtles are usually solitary reptiles that do not move in social groups, but, lo and behold! after a few minutes, before the hymn was by any means finished, 8 turtles appeared far below. They stayed on the surface in close assembly through-out the remainder of the chanting. Interested though incredulous, and a little excited, I raised an arm to point. Immediately one of the Fijians seized it and pushed it down explaining that it was unlucky to point, but that I might nod with my head, thus showing a right respect.

'No question of any utilitarian purpose in the ritual! The turtles were a long way off and no attempt to hunt them was possible. They answered to the psychic call. The turtle-element in man called to the turtles, and they responded. A relationship had been established, and what Dr Martin Buber would call a *Thou* relation formed a link between man and reptile. How far back in time such bond has been established the contemporary Fijians had no conception. No problem presented itself. They drank the ceremonial *yangona*, sang the traditional hymns, and the turtles, whether they heard or not, answered. *Like is only understood by like.* Thus it is that myths are made, and verities of the soul revealed.' [Grant Watson, 1966]

## May My Life Be Like A Tortoise

'As I walk through life, may my steps be like those of a tortoise, sure and steady.

'No matter what obstacle is placed in his path, he will eventually find a way round, over or under it.

'And if any unthinking person should pick him up and put him down again facing the opposite way, he will always turn round, find his original path and head for his ultimate goal.

'May I be covered like the tortoise with a hard, round waterproof shell, to protect me from the knocks and bruises of life and give me shelter from the storms, and should I ever fall flat on my back, may a friend always be there to turn me gently on my feet again.

'May my skin be like that of a tortoise, thick and leathery, so that harsh words spoken in anger will not pierce my heart.

'May my heart be like the legs and claws of a tortoise, sturdy and strong, and no matter how hard, dry or stony the ground may be, I shall always be able to dig in it and plant the seeds of happiness, peace and contentment, and may all the seeds that I plant in my life grow and flower and bear wondrous fruits.

'And lastly, may my eyes be like those of the tortoise, shiny and bright, never looking back at the storm clouds gathered behind, but always looking ahead to a bright and shiny future.' [British Chelonia Group Newsletter, cited in Young 2003]

| Homeopathic name | Common name | Abbreviation | Symptoms |
|---|---|---|---|
| Chelonia mydas | Green turtle | Chelon-my. | + |
| Chelydra serpentina | Snapping turtle | Chelyd-se. | ++ |
| Cholos terrapini[1] | bile of freshwater turtles | Cho. | + |
| Eretmochelys imbricata | Hawksbill turtle | Eret-im. | + |
| Geochelone sulcata | African spurred tortoise | Geoch-sc. | ++ |
| Lepidochelys olivacea | Olive Ridley turtle | Lepi-ol. | – |
| Terrapene carolina | Eastern box turtle | Terr-ca. | – |
| Testudo hermanni[2] | Hermann's tortoise | Test-h. | – |
| Trachemys scripta elegans | Red-eared slider | Trach-se. | + |

1 = Misspelled in Boericke and repertories as Cholas terrapina. 2 = Remedy name: Tortoise shell.

# CHELONIA MYDAS

## Systematics
- Scientific name: Chelonia mydas [L., 1758].
- Synonyms: Testudo mydas [L., 1758]. Testudo marina vulgaris [Lacépède, 1788]. Chelonia midas [Link, 1807]. Euchelus macropus [Girard, 1858]. Mydas viridis [Gray, 1870].
- Common names: Green turtle. Soup turtle.
- Family: Cheloniidae.

## Biological Profile
- Large sea turtle with a carapace length of 96 to 116 cm. Average weight 130–180 kg. Males larger than females.
- Largest green turtle ever found was 152 cm in length and 395 kg.
- 'By all odds the most valuable of reptiles,' according to Pope [1971], the world-famous soup turtle is also called green turtle because its sub-dermal fat is greenish [due to its diet of sea-grasses and algae].
- Head small and blunt with serrated jaw. Can't pull head inside shell. Carapace bony without ridges and with large, non-overlapping scutes; only 4 lateral scutes. Carapace colour varies from pale to very dark green and plain to very brilliant yellow, brown and green tones with radiating stripes. Plastron colour varies from white, dirty white or yellowish in the Atlantic populations to dark grey-bluish-green in the Pacific populations. Flippers have one visible claw.
- Easily distinguished from other sea turtles by a single pair of prefrontal scales [scales in front of its eyes], rather than 2 pairs as found on other sea turtles.
- Range: Subtropical and tropical waters of Atlantic, Indian and Pacific oceans where water temperature does not fall below 20°C [68°F].
- Habitat: Fairly shallow waters [except when migrating] inside reefs, bays, and inlets. Prefers lagoons and shoals with an abundance of marine grass and algae.

- Oviparous; 75–200 eggs per clutch. May lay as a many as 9 clutches within a nesting season [overall average is about 3.3 nests per season] at about 13-day intervals. Nesting occurs nocturnally at 2, 3, or 4-year intervals.
- Only sea turtle that is strictly herbivorous; adults feed chiefly on marine grasses and algae. Juveniles feed on jellyfish, mollusks, crustaceans, sponges and worms.
- Males almost never leave the water; females swim to the shore to lay their eggs.
- Can rest or sleep underwater for several hours at a time but submergence time is much shorter while diving for food or to escape predators.
- Breath-holding ability is affected by activity and stress, which is why turtles drown in shrimp trawls and other fishing gear within a relatively short time.
- Three recognized subspecies [mydas, agassizi, japonica].

## Migration – Finding your Wave

When it is time to mate green turtles migrate from several hundred to over a thousand miles across the ocean to their place of birth. Female green turtles use the same beaches to nest as their mothers and grandmothers. They exhibit an extraordinary capacity for memory and migration, unerringly navigating a thousand miles or so to particular nesting sites. Not only do they appear on the same beach, they often emerge within a few hundred yards of where they last nested. Along with other species of sea turtles, green turtles are believed to retain their bearings primarily by 'reading' wave motion.

'Sea turtles are among the most impressive navigators in the animal kingdom. As hatchlings, turtles that have never before been in the ocean are able to establish unerring courses towards the open sea and then maintain their headings after swimming beyond sight of land. Young turtles follow complex migratory pathways that often lead across enormous expanses of seemingly featureless ocean. After completing their years in the open sea, juvenile turtles take up residence in coastal feeding grounds and show *great fidelity to their feeding sites, homing back* to specific locations after long migrations and experimental displacements. Similar navigational abilities exist in adult turtles, which migrate considerable distances between specific feeding areas and nesting beaches.

'Hatchlings embark on an impressive transoceanic migration, but they do not navigate to targets more specific than broad oceanic regions. In contrast, older turtles acquire an ability to pinpoint specific geographic locations such as feeding areas and nesting beaches. Recent experiments have demonstrated that sea turtles possess a remarkable ability to exploit positional information in the Earth's magnetic field as a kind of navigational map that can be used to guide movements toward specific goals.' [Lohmann Lab, University of North Carolina]

Hatchlings do not rely on magnetic cues during the initial phase of the offshore migration. Instead, they use waves as an orientation cue, consistently swimming directly *into* approaching waves. Because waves and swells reliably move towards shore in shallow coastal areas, swimming into waves usually results in movement towards the open sea. Since hatchlings enter the sea at night, they swim under water in darkness. Experiments by K.J. Lohmann &

C.M.F. Lohmann of the University of North Carolina indicate that young turtles detect wave direction by monitoring the circular movements that occur as waves pass above.

Intriguingly in accord with the navigation skills of turtles was a belief among Japanese fishermen working in Hawaii at the end of the 19th century. They scratched Japanese characters into turtles' carapaces, then set the turtles free in the belief that turtles so treated would guide them back to land should they be lost at sea.

## Exploration – Finding your Way

The green turtle was an important factor in the colonisation of the Americas. The British Navy counted on the green turtle to extend its cruising in the New World. The Spanish fleets took on turtles for the voyage back home to Cadiz. A green turtle fed a host of people and to some of them it became a dish of almost ceremonial stature.

'The Tortugas [Turtle Island] of Columbus became the *Caymanes* – the Cayman Islands – and for 300 years the vast "flotas" there – the fleets of breeding green turtles – were a prime factor in the growth of the Caribbean. As the settlements grew and got hungry, ships of half a dozen flags converged on the untended islands in June. They took away as many as their holds and decks would carry. The turtle flotas were as infinite as the herring schools. Or so it seemed.

'The vitamin hunger of sailors, which came from nowhere and made men's gums grow over their teeth, and could send a corpse a day sliding over the rail, practically disappeared in the Caribbean after the discovery of *Chelonia*, the green turtle. No other edible creature could be carried away and kept so long alive. Only the turtle could take the place of spoiled kegs of beef and send a ship on for a second year of wandering or marauding. All early activity in the new world tropics – exploration, colonisation, buccaneering and the maneuverings of naval squadrons – was in some way dependent on the turtle. Salted or dried it everywhere fed the seaboard poor. It was at once a staple and a luxury – a slave ration, and in soup and curries the pride of the menus of the big plantation houses. More than any other dietary factor the green turtle supported the opening up of the Caribbean.

'*Chelonia* had all the qualities needed for a role in history. It was big, abundant, available, savory and remarkably tenacious of life. . . . They grew fat and numerous and succulent, and in every way a blessing.' [Carr, 1954]

## Whatever Her Own Fate Might Be

'The one flaw in the green turtle resource was that the females came ashore to lay their eggs. At breeding time, when survival is in most delicate balance, all sea turtles leave the familiar safety of the sea, where they have grown to a size that makes them almost immune to predation, and lumber ashore and expose themselves and their offspring to the hazards of the land.

'A green turtle on shore is almost defenceless. She weighs on the average nearly 300 pounds but seems almost wholly unable to use her bulk and strength in active self-defense. She is awkward of gait, myopic of vision, and *single-track of mind*. Once the nesting has started, she will go on doggedly through the hour-long ceremony with a pack of dogs digging out her nest beneath her, or with drunken Indians drumming on her back. It is as if she were sure that this last legacy to her race must be left, whatever her own fate might be.' [Carr, 1954]

### Green Turtle Tumours
Of all 7 species of sea turtles, green turtles appear to be most susceptible to fibropapillomatosis [FP], a benign to moderately malignant neoplastic disease. In Hawaii, FP is the most significant cause of stranding morbidity [resulting from exhaustion and starvation] and mortality in green turtles. The prevalence of disease in juvenile turtles far exceeds that found in adults and given that juveniles are an important life stage for long-lived species like sea turtles, the disease may have demographic effects in the longer term.

Green turtles with moderate to severe FP are over-represented on strandings and are less likely to be recaptured. Green turtles with moderate to severe FP are also lymphopenic [abnormal low blood level of lymphocytes], suffer from chronic inflammation, are immuno-suppressed, and are prone to systemic bacterial infections. All this indicates that FP is more than a mere cosmetic disease and has detrimental impacts on the survival of affected animals. To top it all off, 100% of turtles that strand with FP have concomitant infections with blood flukes that resemble the human disease Schistosomiasis.

Many causes for FP have been proposed including pollutants, blood flukes, marine toxins, ultraviolet light, and viruses. Recent evidence from Hawaii and Florida implicates an alpha herpes virus as closely associated with FP. Whether this herpes virus is the cause of FP or just happens to be found associated with tumoured tissue remains unknown. Attempts to culture the virus in the laboratory have been unsuccessful as yet. [Work, 2005]

*See* also above, Turtles with Tumours.


## MATERIA MEDICA CHELONIA MYDAS

### Sources
1 Clinical observations Karl-Josef Müller [Germany], in Wissmut Materia Medica Müller 2.0, 2009.
2 Poisoning symptoms.

### Symptoms
∞ In great need of safety and security, lives in restraint.
∞ Aversion to change. Wants things to remain the same.
∞ Unconditional acceptance of own limitations; ruled by common sense.
∞ Fixated on parents' planning of life and schooling. Wants to remain in parental home.
∞ Home-bound, rarely goes out. Only dares looking further than own nose in safe world of books.
∞ Likes tight clothing [cf. *Trillium pendulum*].

∞ Sea sickness.

∞ Chilly. Prone to cold, sweaty hands and feet.

∞ Chilliness and tendency to fixation and conservation give rise to Silicea as a first differential diagnosis; also *Kali carbonicum* and *Calcium carbonicum*. The dreams of floating in air and the sympathy for turtles, however, tip the scales in favour of Chelonia.

### Green Turtle Poisoning

'Symptoms commence a few hours to several days after ingestion of the turtle; they include anorexia, nausea, vomiting, abdominal pain and diarrhoea in many cases; abnormal sensation around the lips, mouth, tongue, throat, etc., may extend to include dryness or increased salivation and difficulty in swallowing, mouth ulcers and inflammation may supervene and become extensive – lasting for weeks or months before healing is completed.

'Other symptoms include weakness, sweating, pallor, vertigo, headache; a generalised red itchy rash may later peel; difficulty in breathing or tightness in the chest, may extend to severe respiratory distress, central cyanosis [bluish tinge to lips] and death.

'Liver damage may result in jaundice, liver enlargement and tenderness, coma and death. Other manifestations may mimic ciguatera [fish] poisoning. Renal failure may result in a decreased urinary output and then the development of uraemia over the next few days.' [Edmonds, 1995]

*See* also Eretmochelys imbricata, Hawksbill Poisoning.

# CHELYDRA SERPENTINA

### Systematics

- Scientific name: Chelydra serpentina [L., 1758].
- Synonyms: Testudo serpentina [L., 1758]. Chelonura serpentina [Say, 1824]. Macroclemys lacertina [Rhoads, 1895]. Devisia mythodes [Ogilby, 1905].
- Common names: Snapping turtle. Snapper. Mossback. Mud turtle.
- Family: Chelydridae.

### Biological Profile

- Freshwater turtle with a total length, head and tail outstretched, of 71 cm. Average weight 19.5 kg; gigantic individuals weighing up to 30 kg have been reported.
- Head rough, covered with soft skin. Snout short, pointed. Eyes superior. Carapace chestnut brown to black; rough, with 3 tubercular keels, becoming gradually smoother with age. Plastron whitish or yellowish; small, leaving the limbs exposed and providing *'greater flexibility for aggression'*. Bridge very narrow. Feet broad and webbed. Toes 5, all with nails except outer one. Fingers 5, all with nails. Tail long and pointed, three-fourths the length of the carapace in adults. Skin of neck, lower jaw, limbs and tail rough and wrinkled, covered with large and small warts.

TURTLES AND TORTOISES

- Range: From Canada in North America to Ecuador in South America.
- Habitat: Slow-running, muddy rivers and streams, ponds and marshes. Prefers muddy water.
- Oviparous; 20–30 eggs per clutch.
- Omnivorous; feeds on both plant and animal matter, the latter consisting of fish, crayfish, frogs, small rodents, small and young waterfowl, as well as carrion.
- Becomes obese rapidly.
- Solitary in summer, but collecting in considerable numbers in autumn and early winter in order to hibernate.
- Males engage in battle, biting and butting at each other like rams, backing a short distance to give greater force to the blows.

### Snake-like Snapping & Striking

'Sinister in appearance and equally vicious as its looks imply, the Snapping Turtle is one of the most familiar of the North American reptiles. . . . Very old specimens are sometimes so bloated and overburdened with fat that the fleshy parts protrude beyond the margin of the shell and so hinder the progress of the limbs that the reptile is almost helpless when removed from the water. Specimens in this condition are said to be excellent as food.

'With the exception of the soft-shelled turtles [genus *Amyda*], the snapping turtles are rather unique among chelonians, in defending themselves in a like fashion to snakes: namely by "striking" at the object of anger. The rapidity with which the head is lurched forward rivals the dexterity of the rattlesnake. So *quick is the movement that the eye is barely able to follow it*. Backed up by a pair of keen-edged, cutting mandibles and jaw muscles of tremendous power, the stroke of these dangerous brutes may be followed by anything but superficial injury.

'The amputation of a finger by a medium-sized specimen, or a hand by a very large individual would be an accomplishment of no difficulty to the reptile. As in their native state these turtles lie partially embedded in the mud of the river-bottom, the rapid movements of the head and neck are important in the capture of fish which form the larger portion of the food.

'But the snapping turtle is an *exceedingly voracious brute* and is not particular as to its fare. Young water fowl are stalked from beneath the surface, seized by a dart of the jaws and pulled below to drown and be quickly torn to pieces by the keen mandibles assisted by the front limbs. The turtle is entirely carnivorous. It never feeds unless under water, but it will sometimes seize its prey on the bank of a stream, then retreat into the necessary element. To keep one of these reptiles in water so shallow that it is unable to entirely immerse its head and supply it regularly with the most tempting food would ultimately result in its starvation. It appears that the reptile is unable to swallow unless the head is under water.

'As a captive the snapping turtle feeds readily and lives for many years. It will take food from the hand that feeds it, but most specimens *resent undue familiarity and snap viciously when handled*. The safest way to handle a large specimen is to pick it up by the tail and hold it well off from one's body. As the animal is able to throw the head well back over the shell and to strike a considerable distance sideways, it is altogether dangerous to hold a large specimen by the shell.

'In the early summer, the female leaves the pond or stream so persistently haunted at all other times and prowls about for a place to deposit her eggs. She often wanders many feet from the water and, selecting a damp spot, scoops away the earth to form a hollow into which she crawls and moves about until the loose soil falls back over her. Thus she is hidden until the eggs are deposited and to the number of about 2 dozen. As she crawls forth the shell is reared to a sharp degree and the earth that has fallen upon it is left covering the eggs.

'As the snapping turtle is persistently aquatic the shells of many specimens become coated with moss. As they lie partially buried in the mud, in shallow water, they look much like flat stones. In such places they remain for hours, poking the extreme tip of the snout from the water to breathe. They are able to remain for long periods entirely submerged and will dive to the deepest portions of rivers where they prowl along the bottom in search of food.' [Ditmars, 1907]

## Dual Personality

Perhaps the most cosmopolitan of the *true grouches* of the reptile world, snapping turtles are frequently encountered on land, a place where they feel insecure and act in a very *hostile* manner to intruders.

'The ferocity of the snapper is proverbial. Hatchlings not yet free of their shells will bite, and an aroused adult, the *very picture of impotent rage*, will even advance to the attack. The forward thrusts of the head may be violent enough to lift the turtle from the ground if the target is missed. Once the jaws close on a victim, they retain their grip until the thunder rolls or the sun sets; at least that is the folk belief, which of course must be taken with a grain of salt.

'If anyone wants to witness a remarkable phenomenon of turtle behaviour, let him pick up by the tail an enraged snapper and hold it in water. The minute it becomes submerged, all the ferocity will vanish and it will think only of escaping. Here is evidence that a snapper has a dual personality, one for the land, the other for the water.' [Pope, 1971]

The use of the term 'dual personality' is worthy of note in light of endearing red-eared turtle youngsters turning into adult pond terrorists encountered in the section on Trachemys scripta elegans; *see*.

## MATERIA MEDICA CHELYDRA SERPENTINA

### Sources

1 Proving by Eric Sommermann and Teresa Stewart, Northwestern Academy of Homeopathy [Minnesota, USA], 12 provers, 6c, 12c, 30c, 2004.

### Mind

∞ Determined and motivated; feeling very upbeat, positive and hopeful; as if surrounded by great possibilities and potential for success. Task oriented and industrious.

- ∞ Curious and detail oriented; craning one's neck in order to see better.
- ∞ Irritability with children, co-workers, family members, pets.
- ∞ Extreme irritability and annoyed with everything.
- ∞ Irritability when coerced; when expectations not met; when not appreciated.
- ∞ Anger, fury, rampage, rage, extremely ill-tempered and irritable, with unfiltered aggression.
- ∞ Dictatorial. Impatient. Overreacting.
- ∞ Desire to hide and rest; wanting to stay home and inside the house.
- ∞ Sensation that time is running out. Hurried.
- ∞ Feeling light-hearted and happy. Almost a little euphoria. Wants to sing all day. "Feel my heart is open and want to express love to everyone."
- ∞ Easily angered, < noise.
- ∞ Anxiety about not enough food.
- ∞ Blunt and direct, speaks his mind.
- ∞ Delusions: Being forgotten; ignored; left out; unappreciated; worthless, if not accomplishing.
- ∞ Delusion others move in slow motion.
- ∞ Fears: Being taken advantage of; being trapped.
- ∞ Desires home; desires to stay inside, where it is warm and safe.
- ∞ Deceit, lying, stealing, taking advantage of another, and treachery.
- ∞ Long held guilt and shame.
- ∞ Possessiveness.

**Dreams**
- ∞ Abandoned child.
- ∞ Bloody.
- ∞ Cave.
- ∞ Cold, being.
- ∞ Dismemberment of body.
- ∞ Deceit.
- ∞ Dismissed.
- ∞ Disoriented.
- ∞ Dwarves.
- ∞ Examinations, failure.
- ∞ Excluded.
- ∞ Giants.
- ∞ Hopelessness.
- ∞ Lost and on the wrong track.
- ∞ Pool of water.
- ∞ Ridiculed.
- ∞ Scorned.
- ∞ Shunned, being.
- ∞ Trapped.

## Generals
∞ Pain sharp – sharp pain ear; pain eye as from a nail; sticking pain bridge of nose; stitching pain bladder; shooting pain lower back.
∞ Thirst upon awakening, water does not >.
∞ Cold <.
∞ Wet, damp weather <.
∞ Cold to the bone.
∞ Sleep impossible on right side due to too loud heartbeat; feels forceful. Better from sleep left side.
∞ Symptoms come on quickly, intense, and leave quickly.
∞ Appetite absent during day, increased at night.
∞ Cravings for anything and everything and nothing satisfies. Go from one food to the other. Worse late at night. Feeling of wanting to keep sinking teeth into something.
∞ Craving for raw meat.
∞ Catnaps between 1–6 p.m.

## Sensations
∞ Strange sensation when driving through a tunnel at night, when illuminated. Felt like I was a cell or something very small passing through a blood vessel.
∞ Head as if squeezed during vertigo.
∞ Head as if having ice pressed in on it; skin as if paper-thin.
∞ Back of head as if pulled down, from tightening of neck muscles.
∞ Nail in eye.
∞ Inner ear as if being pushed out, & whale-like underwater sounds in ears.
∞ Upper lip as if swollen.
∞ Lips as if swelling.
∞ Sensation of a hair on cheek.
∞ Twitching face.
∞ Teeth as if hollow.
∞ Fullness stomach after eating ever so little.
∞ Stomach as if knotted.
∞ Pylorus as if squeezed.
∞ Something alive moving in abdomen, sometimes regular like a heartbeat, sometimes irregular.
∞ Menstrual pain, as if something turning or tumbling in uterus. Better from placing a round hard object against uterus, like a fist.
∞ Heart feels tight and full.
∞ Heart pounding, feels full and anxious.
∞ Heaviness and gradual tightening of muscles between shoulder blades.
∞ Cold, wet feeling on left shin.
∞ Limbs as if trembling internally.

## Locals
∞ Head hot when angry.
∞ Heat rushes upward to head in waves.

∞ Toothache < honey, sweets.

∞ Dry patches of acne around lips.

∞ Trouble sleeping due to abdominal pain and flatulence. "Waking up every half hour, tossing from side to side, belching and farting all night, tired by morning."

∞ Loose stool during menses.

∞ Speech thick, slurred.

∞ Desire to stretch neck.

∞ Waking in early morning with violent itching between shoulder blades.

∞ Cramping pain in nates at night.

∞ Restless movement of legs and feet, while practicing music.

∞ Patches of desquamating acne.

• This individual's reactions are often out-of-proportion for the situation. The patient appears slow, dazed and confused. The person needing this remedy is almost always defensive. They will experience tightness throughout their bodies, esp. tightness of their jaws, grinding of their teeth, and have a great sensitivity on their necks. From clinical experience it has been observed that there is a long history of abuse, deceit, and treachery, as one patient reported, "no one has your back, so you've got to hunker down and protect yourself." Finally, these patients will report, "I practically raised myself . . ." as their parents seemingly abandon them to work, or use drugs, or are off partying. [Jason-Aeric Huenecke]

# ERETMOCHELYS IMBRICATA

## Systematics

• Scientific name: Eretmochelys imbricata [L., 1766].

• Synonyms: Testudo imbricata [L., 1766]. Chelonia imbricata [Schweigger, 1812].

• Common names: Hawksbill turtle. Shell turtle. Comb turtle. Spectacled turtle.

• Family: Cheloniidae.

## Biological Profile

• Small sea turtle, up to 76–91 cm in carapace length, and weighing between 40 and 60 kg.

• Distinguished from other sea turtles by loosely overlapping [*imbricate*] scutes of carapace. Carapace dark brown or black, richly marbled with yellow. Plastron yellow. Structure of plastron is like that of the green turtle. Head, limbs, and flippers covered with scutes. Scutes of head and limbs dark brown or black, margined with yellow. Head elongated; upper mandible terminating in a pronounced hook or beak [hence *hawksbill*]. Two claws on each front flipper.

• Range: Pantropical

- Habitat: Coastal reefs, bays, estuaries and lagoons in tropical and subtropical Atlantic, Pacific and Indian Oceans. Deemed the most tropical of all sea turtles.
- Omnivorous; feeds on plants and preys on fish, crustaceans, sponges and mollusks.
- Oviparous; lays eggs on isolated sandy beaches, above the tide line. Solitary nester.
- Females disturbed by light and moving shadows [persons, animals, trees] in early stages of nesting; disturbed females rapidly return to the sea.
- May be fairly sedentary, remaining in the proximity of nesting areas year-round, or may migrate considerable distances.

## Making for the Open Ocean

A baby sea turtle successfully hatching from its egg must survive several years in the ocean before reaching maturity. No one knows exactly where baby sea turtles spend their time between leaving the laying beach and turning up once again as young turtles. What is known is that they must face numerous hardships and dangers in this so-called 'lost year'.

Scientific studies show that just 0.02 to 0.2% of every 10,000 turtle offspring survive to adulthood and breeding age. Being small, defenceless, and too slow-moving to evade predators, young turtles rely on orientation mechanisms that guide them quickly and reliably to the relative safety of the open ocean along paths that approximate straight lines. Experiments indicate that young turtles use specific cues to find the sea, such as the light reflected from large water bodies, downward motion on sloping beach, and possibly the sound [vibration?] of waves breaking on the shore.

'Upon emergence, hatchlings orient phototropically, which is presumed to be an innate behaviour to guide them to the sea. Mrosovsky found this orientation is an uncomplicated type of tropic reaction, and Philibosian observed that hatchlings can become disoriented by artificial light sources, which result in mortality from automobiles.

'The hatchlings undergo a frenzy of activity lasting several hours after emergence, occasionally all stopping simultaneously to rest for several seconds. This frenzy is presumably a survival mechanism whereby newly emerged hatchlings can rapidly escape the violent, predator-infested shoreline environment to the relative safety of the open ocean. The hatchlings initially swim by simultaneous strokes of the fore flippers and diving is reportedly difficult due to the presence of buoyant egg yolk material.

'Hawksbill hatchling mortality is high, resulting from physical hardships and predation. Hatchlings were unable to dig their way out of the nest through heavy soil or root masses, and emergences above ground during the day may lead to immediate immobilisation, rapidly followed by death by desiccation.' [Witzell, 1983]

## Truculent Turtle

'The hawksbill turtle has been called an *aggressive and pugnacious* species, an unfair accusation considering that this behaviour apparently refers to individuals that were just harpooned, netted, or otherwise molested in their natural environment. True [1893] reported that United States fishermen had to be careful because capture hawksbills bit severely, inflicting painful wound. Deraniyagala found that hawksbills defended themselves by biting with vigorous snaps in Sri Lanka. Caribbean turtles also snap and bite furiously when captured and must be subdued with clubs before being boated. In Malagasy, Loveridge and Williams [1957] found that fishermen protect their fragile craft from considerable damage by holding out a piece of wood for harpooned hawksbills to fasten their jaws into. Female hawksbills, on the other hand, are docile when laying eggs.

'Captive West African specimens of unknown size were said to be touchy, irascible and viciously attacked and bit all other animals, even their own species. Juveniles kept in Sarawak were reported to quarrel over food but were otherwise amiable. They were reported to be cannibalistic in Indonesian culture ponds. Several authors found that young hawksbills could be raised in captivity, but must be of similar size and not be overcrowded to mitigate injuries due to their aggressiveness.' [Witzell, 1983]

## MATERIA MEDICA ERETMOCHELYS IMBRICATA

### Sources
1 Poisoning symptoms; chelonitoxism.

### Hawksbill Poisoning
Biotoxins that accumulate in the flesh of sea turtles may cause chelonitoxism, a type of food poisoning with a high mortality rate in humans. The exact nature of the toxins has not been established as yet, although the general consensus leans toward the opinion that the toxins are derived from poisonous marine algae eaten by turtles. Recent study of trace element accumulation in hawksbill turtles from Yaeyama Islands, Japan, on the other hand, indicates a possible link with the extreme high concentrations of copper in the liver and cadmium in the kidneys of hawksbills, whereas the levels of mercury in liver were low in comparison with those of other marine animals. Similar results were found for the green turtle, Chelonia mydas.

Halstead [1970] reviewed the cases of sea turtle poisoning, summarising all pertinent information on species reported as poisonous to eat. Most poisoning cases are associated with ingestion of hawksbill or, less frequently, green turtles [Chelonia mydas], leatherbacks [Dermochelys coriacea], loggerheads [Caretta caretta], and Asian giant softshell turtle [Pelochelys bibroni]. Halstead notes that the hawksbill turtle in the Caribbean was reputed to have 'a special purgative quality'.

'Symptoms generally develop within a few hours to several days after eating the turtle. In one large outbreak involving 100 persons, most of the victims developed symptoms about 12 hours after eating the turtle. The initial signs and symptoms usually consist of nausea, vomiting, diarrhoea, facial tachycardia, pallor, severe epigastric pain, sweating, coldness of the extremities, and vertigo.

There is frequently reported an acute stomatitis consisting of a dry, burning sensation of the lips, lining of the mouth, tongue, and throat. Some victims complained of a sensation of tightness of the chest. The victim frequently becomes *lethargic* and unresponsive. Swallowing becomes very difficult and hyper-salivation is pronounced.

'The oral symptoms may be slow to develop but become increasingly severe after several days. The tongue develops a white coating, the breath becomes foul and later the tongue may become covered with multiple, pinhead-size, reddened pustular papules. The pustules may persist for several months, whereas in some instances they break down into ulcers. *Desquamation of the skin* over most of the body has been reported. Some victims develop a severe hepatomegaly with right upper quadrant tenderness. The conjunctivae become icteric. Headaches and a feeling of "heaviness of the head" are frequently reported. Deep reflexes may be diminished. *Somnolence* is one of the more pronounced symptoms present in severe intoxications and is usually indicative of an unfavourable prognosis. At first the victim is difficult to awaken and then gradually becomes comatose, which is followed rapidly by death. The symptoms presented are typical of a hepato-renal death. The overall case fatality rate on reported outbreaks is about 28 percent.'

Deraniyagala, who has written a monograph on the tetrapod reptiles of Ceylon, offered the opinion that if a poisonous hawksbill should be eaten, the resulting sickness could be cured by dosing the patient with soup made from the carapace and plastron of the green turtle, Chelonia mydas!

*See* also Chelonia mydas, Green Turtle Poisoning.

# GEOCHELONE SULCATA

## Systematics
- Scientific name: Centrochelys sulcata [Miller, 1779].
- Synonym: Testudo sulcata [Miller, 1779]. Testudo calcarata [Schneider, 1784]. Geochelone sulcata [Pritchard, 1967].
- Common names: African spurred tortoise. Grooved tortoise. Sulcata. Sahel tortoise.
- Family: Testudinidae.

## Biological Profile
- Large land tortoise, the world's largest mainland species, with recorded carapace lengths to 83 cm and exceptionally large individuals weighing up to 100 kg.
- Distinct features include sandy-ivory or golden yellow-brown and very thick skin, and 2 or more very large and prominent tubercles [or spurs] on the rear legs. Carapace broad, oval, flattened, yellow to brown in colour. Plastron light tan to ivory coloured without markings. Scutes outlined by brown growth rings. Head moderate in size, with a slightly hooked upper jaw and non-protruding snout.

- Range: Sub-Sahara, from Senegal in the west across to Ethiopia and Eritrea in the east of Africa.
- Habitat: Hot, arid environments ranging from desert fringes to dry savannahs.
- Oviparous; 15–30 eggs per clutch.
- Largely herbivorous, but also eats dead animals and detritus.
- Voracious eater, growing very fast and heavy.
- Goes underground in periods of intolerable heat and drought. Burrows are cooler and supply enough humidity to prevent it from dehydrating. Will flip mud on its back if mud is available. Salivates when temperatures reach more than 40°C [104°F] and smears the saliva on its forelimbs to help with cooling.
- Does not tolerate damp or cold.

### Behaviour

'Able to run and burrow quite well. Get excited just before it rains, running around. Become *inactive when very hot or very cold*. Can survive extended drought periods in self-dug burrows or "pallets." Digs permanent sleeping burrows, which may be shared by 2 or more tortoises. Sides slant steeply down at 45-degree angles. Adult males hiss when approached too closely and retreat into their shell or burrow, where they wedge themselves in. Females do the same, make croaking noises and throw the rear part of their shell violently about. Females may raise their shell up off the ground and drop it with a thud. Have been instances where adults "conversed" with each other through a series of croaks, grunts and whistles. This may have been challenge or threat behaviour. Males are frequently *aggressive, ramming and biting each other*.' [website Honolulu Zoo]

### Burrowing

'The rest of the animal is totally dedicated to the burrowing role: powerful scaly plaques on the forelimbs, deep grooves on each scute, multiple long spurs on the thighs, head wide and covered with heavy scales, and enormous muscular strength. . . . In order to protect itself from the heat and aridity, this tortoise digs very long burrows, where it spends the hot hours of the day and also the entire dry season. These galleries have a cross section identical to that of the tortoise itself, with various wide chambers for resting and turning around, where it finds a little humidity during the dry season and perhaps even some dead animals upon which it might feed. 'Tortoises have even been seen to push clumps of grass into their chambers, using the forked gulars as a bulldozer, to provide for the long months when no fresh food is available. . . . The juveniles share the burrows of the adults during the early years, or they retreat to natural cavities in the sand. They do not start to dig a personal burrow until they have reached an age of 5 to 6 years. Each tortoise digs one or several burrows each year, according to the size of its home range. Some burrows become flooded during the rainy season, and others may collapse. But a tortoise is able to excavate several metres of burrow in a single day, in a substrate of compact sand and often under trees and bushes that keep the soil coherent and well drained.' [Bonin, 2006]

## Nesting

'Sulcatas exhibit a degree of nest protection. The behaviour isn't as intense as what is seen with Manouria emys, but it is more than what is observed in other tortoises. I have seen a female continue to work soil over her nest up to 3 days after nesting. Many females in my collection become aggressive, to varying degrees, if they find you or another tortoise around their nests the first few days. When digging up nests, I have had females come speeding [for a tortoise] 30 to 40 yards across a pen to confront me, and they returned numerous times after being relocated. Some have attempted biting, but most just pull their head into their shell and begin ramming whatever is closest. A 60- to 100-pound tortoise attempting to push the front edge of its shell into your body is definitely an attention getter. Once I withdraw, they immediately recover their nests, even if they are empty. Each female is different, and some skip the aggression and just begin methodically closing the nest as you attempt to dig it up.' [www.Reptile Channel.com]

## Battering, Ramming & Bulldozing

Sulcatas are very aggressive toward each other, esp. during breeding time, although aggression starts from the day they hatch. Males ram each other repeatedly, trying to flip the opponent over, and sometimes end up with bloody limbs and heads. There is a projection on the plastron that makes an effective battering ram during territorial scuffles. A male sulcata with the apt name Bulldozer in Seneca Park Zoo in Rochester, New York, 'rams any new object in the exhibit, including the keepers.' Its muscular strength is so enormous and its violence so brutal that it can hit a person with the front of its carapace and break his leg.

Sulcatas are active and like to burrow, climb and roam about, often in search of food. They are extremely strong animals and have been known to break down fences and even walls. Highly inquisitive, they are very attracted to items with bright colours and will *attempt to move through anything* between the attraction and themselves.

## MATERIA MEDICA GEOCHELONE SULCATA

### Sources

1 Proving Todd Rowe [USA], 13 female and 3 male provers, 30c; 2006.

### Mind

∞ Emotions felt in stomach, particularly empty or hollow sensation that must be filled, & feelings of loneliness and anxiety.
∞ Sentimental. Lovesick. Makes verses; listens to love songs. Teenager feeling.
∞ Sensitive to sensory impressions – smells; light; noise [of someone eating].
∞ Sensitive to heights; can't get close to the edge; looking down is difficult.
∞ Sudden shifts between being energetic and inability to move. "I move in spurts, like a burst of energy, need to move and go forward. When I stop, I cannot move. Sudden shifts."

∞ Confrontational; very blunt with everything. "Saying all I want to say without feeling bad about hurting someone's feelings."
∞ Irritability about not moving fast enough; needing to get to the point; don't want to take a long time; hurry up and get it done.
∞ Snappy irritability.
∞ Suicidal or desiring death, from pains [head; throat; face; teeth]; & feeling weak, helpless, depressed; feeling of giving up; world as if falling apart or as if flipped upside down.
∞ Anxiety > eating.
∞ Co-dependency.
∞ Contemptuous of self.
∞ Desire for darkness.
∞ Delusion being able to go out of body and walk around, looking down upon.
∞ Delusion head separated from body.
∞ Delusion being confined and restricted.
∞ Feeling of helplessness.

## Dreams
∞ Biting.
∞ Bitten by animals.
∞ Circle.
∞ Fights.
∞ Food.
∞ Kill, desire to.
∞ Killing.
∞ Large, growing.
∞ Protecting babies and others.
∞ Shots.
∞ Stool.

## Generals
∞ Night <.
∞ Warm, hot flushes.
∞ Tendency towards injuries, weight gain, swelling, and lassitude.
∞ Insatiable appetite.
∞ Appetite, increased at night; ravenous in evening.
∞ Great thirst, unquenchable, for cold drinks.
∞ Extreme thirst; very dehydrated; cannot get enough water; lips chapped, hands dry.
∞ Right side more affected.
∞ Pains pressing.
∞ Pains burning – eyes; ears; nose; face; lips; tongue; teeth; throat; abdomen; rectum; feet.
∞ Wandering burning sensations.
∞ Excessive energy; must do something; aggressive when exercising; pushing oneself.

∞ Motion sickness; in car when driving; in airplane during descent.

∞ Lactose intolerance.

∞ Direct sunlight <; needs to be in the shade.

∞ Downward motion <.

## Sensations

∞ Empty feeling mentally, like someone passed away.

∞ As if contained in a shell.

∞ Headache on top of head and forehead; like a steel cap or helmet; tight and compressed.

∞ Head as if full of swishing water.

∞ Head as if compressed, jammed, squeezed.

∞ Oesophagus as if constricted when eating.

∞ Bloated stomach; stomach feels too big and in the way.

∞ Stomach fat as if going to burst; liver hurts; < lying on back.

∞ Stomach as if empty.

∞ Bubbles in stomach.

∞ Puffy, full-chested, outward pressure at sternum at xyphoid process.

∞ Sensation of being an upside down turtle; as if on back and unable to turn over.

∞ Anxiety in shoulders, as from a heavy weight in shoulders.

∞ Aching in arms as if being grasped very hard.

∞ Hands as if enlarged.

∞ Foot as if broken.

## Locals

∞ Heaviness head, desire to lean on or against something.

∞ Headache < light, > pressure; pain extending to face and/or chest.

∞ Lachrymation and burning pains. Eyes heavy and discoloured red; profound photophobia and pressing pains, & foreign body sensation. Rubbing eyes often.

∞ Extreme photophobia; eyes hurt with the light; headache from the light. "I could go in a cave for a while; I like it dark; or a hole; where it is dark and cool."

∞ Pain in eyes < closing eyes; < change of weather.

∞ Pressing pain in inner canthi at night.

∞ Earache extending to jaw.

∞ Itching tip of nose.

∞ Clenching of teeth.

∞ Throat pain extending to chest.

∞ Nausea < brushing teeth, eating, turning head quickly.

∞ Cough < cold drinks.

∞ Crushing pressure in right breast radiating to sternum and down arm to wrist.

∞ Intense pain in tailbone, < lying, at night, > standing.

∞ Stiffness & swollen sensation, right wrist, right knee, right ankle, < morning, > limbering up.

## Summary of Proving

*Sensations.* The core sensation for this proving was related to the sensation of tingling/prickling/burning as if something was coming alive. This was experienced in the head, chest, stomach and upper extremities.

Most strongly expressed in the stomach area, many provers described a numbness or emptiness in this area, which was followed by a tingling prickling excitement. When this sensation was most strong it was accompanied by a feeling of anxiety and agitation.

The opposite of this sensation was that of numbness, which was experienced by several provers, worse at night. This was primarily located in the extremities.

Other sensations noted during the proving included, fullness, heaviness, burning pains, stitching pain, pressing pains and biting sensations.

*Lovesick.* Several provers experienced lovesickness during the proving. The feeling was one of romantic excitement. The feelings were intense. One prover described it as originating from the stomach and associated with numbness and tingling in that region.

*Compression.* Another prominent sensation during the proving was that of compression by a circular band. This was accompanied by a hand gesture of circular tightening. Many of the provers described pressing pains in the head as if someone was pressing their finger or a band tightly on them. The compression tended to be circular. One prover described it as compression of the head like an iron helmet. Band like constrictions around the abdomen and feet were also noted. One prover could not tolerate shoes around the feet because of the compression. There was also an emotional component to the compression-a feeling of emotional restriction and an accompanying intolerance to this.

*Reptile themes.* Reptile themes present in this remedy include constriction and compression, attack and defense, violence, conspiracy, suspicious, antagonism with himself, sexuality, loquacity, sudden unpredictable attack, fear of death, desire to kill and lethal. There was a strong theme of killing, particularly around cutting off the head. Turtles are particularly vulnerable in the head area.

*Desert themes.* Many desert themes were seen throughout the proving. These included water themes, distension and contraction, violence, attack and defense, photophobia, large and small, wandering, restlessness, isolation, death and dying, and excitement and hurry following a prolonged period of torpor. The presence of a strong thirst, without a desire to drink is characteristic of desert remedies. Formication is also typical of desert remedies. [Todd Rowe, American Medical College of Homeopathy]

# LEPIDOCHELYS OLIVACEA

## Systematics
- Scientific name: Lepidochelys olivacea [Eschscholtz, 1829].
- Synonyms: Chelonia olivacea [Eschscholtz, 1829]. Caretta olivacea [Rüppell, 1835]. Thalssochelys olivacea [Strauch, 1862].
- Common names: Olive Ridley turtle. Pacific Ridley turtle.
- Family: Cheloniidae.

## Biological Profile
- Smallest and most numerous sea turtle, between 50 and 70 cm in carapace length, and weighing up to 45 kg.
- Carapace round, smooth, olive to greyish-green. Carapace distinctive in having a variable and often uneven number of lateral scutes, between 6 and 10 pairs. Plastron light greenish-yellow or whitish. Head large and triangular. Skin grey. Males have longer thicker tails than females and well-developed curved claws on the forelimbs.
- Range: Tropical waters of the Pacific and Indian Oceans.
- Habitat: Found well out to sea and in protected, relatively shallow bays and lagoons and the shallow water between reefs and the shore.
- Oviparous; 50–200 eggs per clutch.
- Nests both individually and in large nesting aggregations.
- Mostly carnivorous; eats mollusks, crustaceans, jellyfish, sea urchins, crab, fish, sea urchins, snails, jellyfish, and occasional plant material – algae, seagrass, and seaweed.
- Strong diver, known to dive up to 150 m in search of crabs, sea urchins and other bottom-dwelling creatures. Also roams widely in the open ocean in search of jellyfish.
- Little is known about Olive Ridley behaviour other than nesting behaviour. Unlike most sea turtles that migrate among their breeding ground and foraging areas, Olive Ridleys resemble *nomadic migrants* that swim hundreds of thousands of kilometers over vast oceanic stretches.
- Name from Gr. *lepido*, scaled, and *chelys*, turtle.

## Nesting & Crying
Olive Ridleys nest together in synchronised mass nesting called "arribadas", which may consist of thousands of females nesting at the same time. From 20,000 to 200,000 females may visit a nesting beach in one season. Tropical beaches and barrier islands, often near river mouths, are preferred. Many females reproduce every year, but some nest every 2–3 years, usually from 1–2 times per season, every 14–30 days.

Nesting occurs mostly at night, but diurnal nesting also occurs. A female crawls onto the nesting beach, scoops a body pit, then digs a nest and lays a clutch of 30–170 eggs, which she covers with sand before crawling back into the ocean. The whole procedure takes less than an hour. Nests are robbed by a variety of predators incl. humans, pigs, opossums, raccoons, coyotes, caimans, and snakes. The eggs hatch in 45–70 days depending on the weather and temperature. Hatchlings emerge and begin a frantic race to the sea, chased by predators such as crabs, vultures, and seabirds. Once they reach the water they are still in danger from predators such as sharks, fish and crocodiles. [www.californiaherps.com]

Carr observed in 1947 what he called 'crying' in nesting females on the Pacific coast of Honduras. 'The curious "crying" by nesting females, apparently a device to keep the eyes free of sand, has been noted in other species. The present turtle began secreting copious tears shortly after she left the water, and these continued to flow as the nest was dug. By the time she had begun to lay, her eyes were closed and plastered over with tear-soaked sand and the effect was doleful in the extreme. Her behaviour as the eggs were deposited heightened the melancholic atmosphere. Each time, just before eggs were laid, her head was elevated at an unnatural angle and her mouth was slightly opened, frequently allowing a loud gasp or sigh to escape. With the contraction which pushed out the eggs came a rapid lowering of her head until her chin pressed into the sand, after which she lay for a while heaving slightly. It was difficult to believe that she was not suffering acutely, but impossible to explain why.' [cited in Pope, 1971]


## MATERIA MEDICA

• No symptoms.


# TERRAPENE CAROLINA

### Systematics
• Scientific name: Terrapene carolina [L., 1758].
• Synonyms: Testudo carolina [L. 1758]. Cistudo carolina [Duméril & Bibron, 1835].
• Common names: Box turtle. Closed turtle. Locked turtle.
• Family: Emydidae.

### Biological Profile
• Small land turtle up to 15 cm in carapace length. Carapace high-domed; pattern extremely variable, but generally consisting of short yellow bands arranged in irregular groups in each shield, or of bands that run together on the sides to form broad E-like markings. Front and rear margins of upper shell of males flare outward or sometimes curl upward; less so in females. Plastron dark brown, black, or blotched with yellow. Plastron tightly closing shell, no bridge. Four claws on each slightly webbed hind foot. Head brightly blotched or speckled with yellow. Upper jaw hooked. Lower jaw turned upward at tip. Limbs and feet scaly. Short tail.
• Range: Eastern USA; New England States south to the Gulf, westward to Mississippi River.

- Habitat: Thin woodland, brushy areas, pastures, marshy meadows; often near streams and ponds.
- Oviparous; 3–8 eggs per clutch. Most nests are started at twilight and finished during the night. Nests are usually dug in sandy or loamy soil, using the hind legs. Sex determination is temperature dependent – nests between 22–27°C [71.6–80.6°F] tend to be males, nests above 28°C [82.4°F] tend to be females.
- Diurnal, active during all daylight hours in spring and fall, but largely restricts its activity to mornings and after rain in heat of summer.
- Omnivorous; eats snails, insects, berries, fungi, slugs, worms, roots, flowers, fish, frogs, salamanders, snakes, birds, and eggs indiscriminately. Has been observed eating carrion, feeding on dead ducks, amphibians, assorted small mammals, and even a dead cow.
- Juveniles primarily carnivorous while growing during first 5–6 years. Adults tend to be mostly herbivorous, but they eat no green leaves.
- When resting, partially imbeds itself by successively shoveling with anterior limbs and hind feet, followed by twisting and forcing its shell into the loosened soil, covering its marginal area.
- Hibernates; burrows as much as 50–60 cm deep into loose earth, mud, stream bottoms, old stump holes, or mammal burrows.
- Males have characteristic bright, red eyes. Based upon observations on captive box turtles, the brilliance fades from the male's eyes immediately after mating, suggesting that this colour trait has a hormonal basis and provides a visual signal to females that the male is ready to mate.
- Shy and timid, the box turtle, when harassed, will promptly withdraw its head, legs and tail within its shell, closing it tightly with hinges at the front and rear of its plastron.
- Four recognized subspecies [bauri, carolina, major, trionguis].

### Courtship & Going Belly Up

'Based on 72 observations of mating, Evans suggested that the behaviour could be divided into 3 phases but that there was considerable variation among the phases in the courtship sequence. The entire process may last 6 hours. In phase 1, the male moves toward the female but stops about 10 cm away from her. He keeps his legs straightened and his head held high, although one leg may be raised above the ground. The female watches the male and may retract her head, legs, and tail into her shell. The male then approaches the female, circles her, and at the same time bites at her shell. He may push her shell as he bites at it, a movement that can be repeated many times, or he may bite her shell, seize it, and drag her toward him as he moves backward. He may or may not lunge at her shell. If he does, he retracts his head before he hits her and pokes it out after *ramming* her. He then may repeat the charge. The female seems to hunker down to await the next charge or attempts to walk away, usually without success. Ernst reported that the male "smells' his perspective mate, especially in the inguinal region, around the tail, and at the head. This part of phase 1 can last from several minutes to an hour.

'During the second part of phase 1, the male mounts the female. The posterior part of her plastron may or may not be open during initial mounting. If it is not, he attempts to induce her to open it, sometimes after considerable *pushing and shoving*. As the male mounts the female, he tries to hook his rear claws into the inner surface of her plastron. Initially, he might be too high on her carapace, which causes his claws to scrape against the posterior portion of her shell. This causes a scratching vibration, which may help to stimulate her and make her receptive to his intentions. Eventually he finds the right height, where he again uses his claws, this time to scratch the plastron as he gropes for a foothold. . . .

'In phase 3, the male abandons his biting and grasping and leans back, thus resting on his rear ankles and carapace. His imprisoned rear claws hold him firmly to the female. At this point he is almost vertical in relation to the ground. Meanwhile the female rocks back on her ankles, bringing their tails into parallel position and their cloacae into apposition. . . .

'Copulation ends as the female relaxes her plastron, thus causing the male's rear claws to break free of their hold. He slides off her carapace onto the ground. Cloacal apposition is thus broken, and copulation ceases. At this time the male may tumble onto his back and must right himself. Because of his intense exertions, fatigue may cause him to be unable to turn over easily. Cahn and Conder [1932] and Evans [1953] noted that rear leg strength in males seems to decrease substantially after copulation because of their inability to right themselves if they land in soft leafy debris.' [Dodd, 2002]

## Dog Appeal

'Box turtles hold a strange fascination for dogs, esp. hunting dogs. An otherwise flawless pointer – rabbit-proof and staunch as a rock – will often freeze in a rigid point at the near scent of a *Terrapene* and then droop in bewildered humiliation when his error is shown to him. The only other creature I have seen deceive a bird dog so utterly is a little ground-dwelling bird [presumably a sparrow, though I never have had a good look at one] that is so often mistaken for quail that it is known throughout the southern states as stink-bird.

'Hounds, too, are demoralised by box turtles, but in a different way. Whether because of the scent or the challenge of the unassailable shell, hounds often drop whatever business is at hand to attend to a box turtle. One dog may stop and lie quietly, muzzle between paws, to regard a disinterested tortoise with un-accountable emotion, or even raise his head from time to time to voice his feeling in the low, soft, eerie moan of a bereaved oboe. Another may bury the turtle at once, and another simply [may] carry it about for the rest of the day.

'I have several times known the depths of frustration when on a deer hunt a star hound left the drive to trot brightly up and show me a box turtle he had found, confident of applause and pained when it failed. Occasionally a dog tries his hand at gnawing into the shell, but I have no recollection of seeing a success-ful assault of this kind unless the unfortunate turtle had been cracked on the highway to begin with.' [Carr, 1996]

## Homeward Bound

During the summer and fall of 1956, Edwin Gould conducted experiments with over 100 box turtles to test the hypothesis that box turtles employ a means of orientation on the sun similar to that found in birds in finding their way home. The results demonstrated that most turtles start to walk in the homeward direction within a few minutes after being released in unfamiliar territory. The sun proved to be one of the cues on which orientation was based.

Homing ability of the box turtle had been reported earlier by Breder [1927] and by Nichols [1939], who recorded several returns to the home territory after transportation to distances as great as 1,3 km. Stickel [1950] estimated the average diameter of the range of this species to be about 350 feet, basing his estimate on 440 recoveries of 55 turtles. Home ranges of individual turtles overlap, and longer journeys may be made to lay eggs or for other reasons. Some turtles have 2 home ranges.

Alternating sunny- and cloudy-weather releases at irregular intervals resulted in *correct orientations in sunny weather and in poor orientations in cloudy weather*. Turtles released in cloudy weather headed in the direction opposite from home more frequently than would be expected by chance. Others had a strong tendency to go in the direction they were faced when first released and in most cases this was opposite to the homeward direction. Facing the turtle in different directions in sunny weather had no effect, although very active turtles moving off immediately upon being released will often start in the direction faced and then veer off to the homeward direction after a short distance.

While the turtle is moving on its course the head is held high and is directed forward so that if it is walking in a direction opposite to the sun's position it is necessary for the turtle to turn its head in order to see the sun directly. This was frequently observed. The turtles would stop, look about them for 30 seconds to a minute or more and then continue on their way. These stops were often made every 2 to 4 minutes, varying considerably with the individual turtle. Many turtles showed ability to maintain a straight course. Seven turtles released before sunrise moved but little until the sun was visible. Turtles released just before sunset either stopped after the sun had set or changed to a wrong direction after having followed the correct course while the sun was visible. [Gould, 1957]


## MATERIA MEDICA

- No symptoms.


# TESTUDO HERMANNI

## Systematics
- Scientific name: Testudo hermanni [Gmelin, 1789].
- Synonyms: Testudo graeca bettai [Lataste, 1881]. Testudo graeca [Boulenger, 1889].

- Common name: Hermann's tortoise.
- Family: Testudinidae.

## Biological Profile
- Small to medium-sized land tortoise; 18–26 cm in carapace length and 3–4 kg in weight. Carapace black and yellow patterned in juveniles and some adults, fading to a less distinct grey, yellow or straw colouration with age. Plastron yellow with 2 dark longitudinal bands. Limbs scaly, greyish to brown, with some yellow markings. Tail of males long, thick and tipped with a large horny scale. Females larger than males.
- Range: SE Europe.
- Habitat: Densely wooded hillsides and coarsely vegetated gentle slopes at elevations between 500 and 700 m.
- Oviparous. Preferred nesting sites include sunny slopes, deserted terraced olive groves or woodland openings.
- Females can store sperm for as long as 3–4 years.
- Males are notoriously indiscriminate breeders, trying to copulate with any tortoise-like object.
- Largely vegetarian; feed on leguminous plants [beans, clovers, and wild lupines], fruits and flowers, as well as snails, slugs, carrion, and even animal faeces.
- Two recognized subspecies [hermanni, boettgeri].

## Behaviour
'Southern California, with its mild Mediterranean climate, offers ideal conditions for keeping and breeding Testudo hermanni. . . . In my experience, Hermanns are among the bright stars as far as turtle intelligence is concerned. Captives quickly become very tame and often show distinct individual characteristics and behaviour patterns. My adults, some of which are free to wander about my backyard, often follow me when I am out gardening or doing yard work, just in case I should happen to have a treat for them or should happen to uncover a tasty slug or snail. During the summer "barbecue" months the Hermanns may hang around the patio, patiently waiting for food to appear. They have learned that if nothing falls to the ground within a reasonable span of time, a quick nip of someone's toes will often produce results.

'Hermanns are very active tortoises. In mornings and late afternoons throughout the spring, summer and fall my males are out patrolling the yard *looking for a fight or a chance to court a female*. Here in southern California they may remain active even during the winter months, occasionally digging themselves into loose soil or the piles of straw or leaves provided in their "house" during cold spells.

'The males frequently interact with each other and often engage in combat among themselves or with other animals they come across. This male-male interaction may be important in conditioning the males for breeding. During courtship and breeding the males may become even more aggressive than usual, and more than once have inflicted nasty bites on the flanks of the females. Because of this aggressive tendency, Hermanns should be examined regularly so that any wounds are dealt with promptly, particularly during the breeding season.

'Because Hermann's tortoises lead very active life styles for chelonians they should be given as large and as varied an area as possible. They should be able to run, forage, hunt, dig, climb, sun bathe, hide and have access to drinking water within their enclosure.' [Connor, 1993]

### Display Behaviour & Clamorous Copulation

'When compared to lizards or snakes, signals related to warning and threat are not very important in land tortoises. Within social and sexual contexts, tactile and chemical signals seem more important than visual, and certainly than auditory ones. Colour patterns are rarely, if ever, sexually discriminatory. Seasonal colour differences are rare. In general, positional signals are rather limited, chiefly because of the shell. However, shell positional changes are an important part of the visual and tactile signal repertory of all land tortoises. Head movements are also important in several groups. Audible signals are poorly developed. They are largely concerned with courtship and their role is not understood. Chemical signals are pronounced, esp. in displays related to sex identification, largely based on scents associated with the cloaca. Tactile displays are important particularly during courtship. They include biting and esp. shell ramming by the male. The tail is used as a tactile organ during courtship of some species.' [Auffenberg, 1997]

Courtship of Hermann's tortoise males consists of elaborate chasing, ramming and biting behaviours, which can be both incessantly persistent and aggressive to the point of injuring the females. This courtship behaviour is energetically costly and may represent a cue females use to assess partner endurance, based on the presumption that female mate-choice relies on signals that reliably indicate male quality to sire fit offspring. As soon as the male mounts the female he becomes very vocal, emitting regular series of peeping, which sound like whimpers or wailings and are highly stereotyped within an individual. Males vocalise chiefly at the time of copulation.

### MATERIA MEDICA

- No symptoms.

# TRACHEMYS SCRIPTA ELEGANS

### Systematics
- Scientific name: Trachemys scripta [Thunberg in Schoepff, 1792].
- Subspecies: T. s. elegans [Wied, 1838].
- Synonyms: Emys elegans [Wied, 1839]. Trachemys lineata [Gray, 1873]. Chrysemys scripta var. elegans [Boulenger, 1889]. Pseudemys elegans [Force, 1928].

- Common name: Red-eared slider..
- Family: Emydidae.

## Biological Profile

- Semi-aquatic turtle with conspicuous reddish-orange to red stripe on each side of head behind the eye. Carapace up to 28 cm long in females, and 20 cm in males. Carapace domed in females, relatively flat in males. Males have a longer tail and long curved claws on front legs [which are used in mating rituals]. Carapace green with black and cream stripes; plastron cream with black markings.
- Range: Eastern USA, west to Texas, and adjacent areas of NE Mexico. Has established feral populations worldwide due to release of pet turtles in the wild, and consequently has been banned from import in many countries.
- Habitat: Both fresh and brackish waters, incl. lakes, water courses, wetlands and coastal marsh ponds. Prefers larger bodies of quiet water with soft bottoms, an abundance of aquatic plants and suitable basking sites.
- T. s. scripta can tolerate a period of progressive pollution, under which circumstances the population increases.
- After complex courtship behaviour in the water, involving e.g. titillation by the male's elongated foreclaws, the male mounts the female as he grasps her carapace with the claws. Copulation may last up to 15 minutes.
- Oviparous; 2–23 eggs per clutch.
- Omnivorous; feeds on insects, crayfish, shrimp, worms, snails, amphibians, tadpoles, small fish, as well as aquatic plants. Juveniles more carnivorous, adults more herbivorous.
- Seems to target invertebrates such as dragonflies and their larvae, as well as nesting birds and their young. Sits and basks on bird nests and presses nest into the water, thereby killing any eggs. Also preys on young birds by pulling them under water and drowning them [in crocodilian fashion].
- Often carrier of Salmonella spp.
- Three recognized subspecies [elegans, scripta, troostii].

## Pet Trade & Turtle Farms

The majority of turtle species can become quite aggressive and quickly outgrow most aquariums or outlast the owner's commitment to care for them. As a result, some pet owners are unwilling to care for their turtles and release them into nearby bodies of water. This scenario is particularly likely for *Trachemys scripta*, which is the most common turtle in the pet trade.

'By the end of the Second World War the demand for pet turtles increased dramatically, which resulted in a high pressure on the natural populations due to collection in the wild. For that reason several turtle farms were established in southern USA in the late 1950s and during the 1960s. Commercial farming began around 1957 and by 1960 more than 150 farms were in operation. However, in 1975 the U.S. Food and Drug Administration banned the sale of turtles under 4 inches [10 cm] carapace length in the United States and Canada because they transmitted salmonellosis by bacteria of genera Salmonella and Arizona. In spite of major exports to Old World countries, an annual market of some 10 million individuals was lost and as a result only about 50 farms were left in business. The vast majority was formed by the subspecies Trachemys scripta elegans.

'Through the 1980s the annual exports of T. s. elegans from USA amounted to roughly 1–2 million, and during the first half of the 1990s approx. 3–4 million per year. In 1996 the total exports of T. s. elegans from USA were 7,884,634 individuals, of which 2,240,172 individuals [28%] were imported by Europe. . . .

'Trachemys scripta is introduced to European nature because pet turtles are released by their owners. The vast majority of turtles are imported individuals, bred in farms in USA. Previously T. s. elegans was imported in huge quantities, but after the EU ban of that particular subspecies in December 1997, other North American freshwater turtles have partly replaced it in the pet market. T. s. scripta is one of the replacement species.' [Bringsøe, 2006]

### Dumped Heroes & Pond Terrorists

Red-eared sliders dumped in London ponds and waterways have been terrorising ducklings. Adult reptiles were seen emerging from the ponds to drag young birds beneath the water. Children are warned not to dip their fingers in the ponds as the terrapins have a strong bite capable of severing a finger, and could also be carrying diseases such as salmonella.

'They're *aggressive*, impart a painful nip, and chomp their way through other pondlife. Hundreds of dumped terrapins are terrorising Hampstead Heath's pools – and now rangers are racing against time to round them up. . . . "It's the Steve McQueen of terrapins," sighs Rob Renwick, one of the heath's conservation team leaders. Hampstead has a problem. These American reptiles began life as cute little critters when they were kept as pets during the first Teenage Mutant Ninja Turtle-inspired craze of the early 90s. But when they outgrew their owners, scores were dumped into Hampstead's waters. Life in the heath's lush ponds agreed with them and they grew some more. Now up to 150 cruise up and down almost all the 25 main ponds on the 792-acre heath, incl. the men's and women's bathing pools.

'Many have swelled to the size of dinner plates, chomping their way through our native species: fish, newts, toads, frogspawn, dragonfly larvae and, possibly, the occasional great crested grebe, coot, moorhen or mallard. There are a growing number of tales of aggressive, illegally released terrapins – "terrorpins" as the tabloids call them – bringing death and destruction to ponds and waterways across the country. . . .

'Two years ago, schoolchildren were reduced to tears at a pond in Mill Hill, London, when they apparently saw ducklings being consumed by a group of ravenous terrapins. A mallard was later found with its legs bitten off. . . .

"Dear little things about the size of a 50p piece grow to be as big as the bottom of a bucket," says Don Freeman, chairman of the British Chelonia Group. "When they are that size they are a bit of a problem unless you are a devotee – they make a terrible smell, they bite, and they are not terribly friendly animals. If they are put into a small environment like a village pond they will soon decimate all the wildlife in it."' [Barkham, 2007]

## Not Letting Go
In his book *Their Blood Runs Cold*, American herpetologist Whit Gibbons recounts with zest and wit a number of his adventures with reptiles and amphibians. In *Once Upon A Bushmaster* he stumbles upon a large Lachesis species in the Costa Rican jungle, whilst in *How to Catch an Alligator in One Uneasy Lesson* he finds out that big alligators are remarkably fast runners on land, to be outrun solely by technicians, graduate students, and research ecologists faced with speedy reptiles. In Chapter 3, Gibbons goes on a nocturnal river turtle hunt, along with 2 co-workers. This time a 'lesson of another danger was brought home to all river workers in the most dramatic way by Bob Webb.' . . .

'Webb's hand motions gave evidence of turtles. The boat roared forward and Webb scrambled. He flipped a small ringed sawback turtle back into the middle of the boat and went after something else. Legs kicking to keep himself in the boat, he grappled over the front end with something in the water. Then came the scream. Even the big bobcat that had been on the high bank half a mile downstream probably stopped dead still when he heard Bob Webb scream. Rather than fall back in the boat immediately, Webb continued to hang over the bow. Finally he rolled back onto the floor of the boat, and the problem was obvious. Attached to his Adam's apple was a large female slider turtle.

'Bob had grabbed the big turtle in the brush pile, pulled her in toward the boat and then got her too close to his neck. The turtle's grip was a solid one, deep into the flesh of his neck. And true to reputation, she was not letting go. In fact, 10 minutes passed before Bob was free. A surgical operation at night on the Pearl River with only a greasy pair of pliers and a screwdriver takes time. Webb still has a scar on his neck, the turtle is permanently catalogued in the Tulane Museum Collection, and all of us now know to be extra careful when we lean over the front of a boat while catching turtles at night.' [Gibbons, 1983]

## Cholos terrapini – Turtle Bile
Dr. Jacob Jeanes [1800–1877], an associate of Hering in Philadelphia, introduced a number of remedies into the homeopathic materia medica. Only a few of these became well established and frequently used remedies, such as Benzoicum acidum, Pix liquida and Juglans cinerea. Most others never caught on, among them some eccentric ones like Cholos terrapini, the potentised bile of freshwater turtles.

Since North America has about 50 native species of turtles, there is no telling of which species the bile was obtained and used. There is also very little to find about Jeanes' turtle bile in the homeopathic literature. Misspelling it as Cholas terrapina, Boericke lists it under the Relationship of Cuprum metallicum as good for 'cramps in calves and feet; rheumatism, with cramp-like pains.'

E.A. Farrington gave it some more text in his *Lesser Writings with Therapeutic Hints*, 1880: 'Whatever may be said against the class of remedies, or remedies of which this is a sample, I, for the one, will ever feel grateful towards Dr. Jeanes for introducing this bile of the Terrapin, *Cholos Terrapin*. He recommends it for "cramps in the calves," a symptom it has often removed. Quite recently I gave it in a case of secondary syphilis with these cramps as a prominent symptom. In

3 weeks the sore throat, pains in bones and cramps disappeared, and 4 or 5 vesicles formed at the site of the old chancre. These have disappeared, leaving the patient apparently well. In olden times, *Terrapin* was used in venereal diseases.'

## MATERIA MEDICA TRACHEMYS SCRIPTA ELEGANS

### Sources
1 Clinical observations Uta Santos [Austria], Homeopathic Links 3/07.

# CASE

### Symptoms – Case summary
8-year-old girl with severe headaches, intense shyness, slowness, and difficulties falling asleep at night. Never sweats, however hot she may feel. Dreamy and slow, needs tranquility lest she gets headache and bellyache. Never gets things done in time. Refuses to talk on the telephone, covering her ears whenever it rings and saying that voices sound different on the telephone. Fear of ghosts and darkness. Very social. Deliberate, wants to say things correctly or else won't talk. Favourite fairytale is Little Red Riding Hood. Sensitive to odours; smells all food before eating; likes lemons, peppermint, and salads; dislikes fish and milk. Water is her element; loves the sea and jumps into the water even if it is ice cold.

Prescription *Astacus fluviatilis* 30c, after which the headaches are reduced to once a week.

Returns 16 months later; retake of case. Headaches worse again, but not as strong as before Astacus. A peculiar new symptom is her face suddenly turning white, which is accompanied by apparent exhaustion and a cold sensation in the neck.

Criticised at school for not participating actively enough. Homework takes ages. Likes to learn about animals; turtles are her favourites.

'I ask her to tell me about turtles and her whole physiognomy changes as she describes them in a very tender and sympathetic way. What she especially loves is that they can pull in their heads and are therefore better protected.'

Prescription *Chrysemys* [Trachemys] *scripta elegans*. Prescription based on signatures. In addition, both the mother and Dr. Santos had the distinct impression that the girl in describing turtles 'was clearly talking about something very similar to herself, something she could identify with very well.'

*Follow-ups:*

'Some weeks later I got a phone call from the mother who said the headaches had slowly become better. . . . Another telephone call [about 1 year later] revealed that Mary had only needed the remedy 3 times during the last year. She has changed school and was now really blossoming. In February 2007 Mary had a very high fever that persisted even after taking anti-pyretics. Then her mother remembered to give the remedy and within half an hour the fever came down to normal. Mary fell asleep and woke up in good health. At school Mary feels well, even if she doesn't participate very actively. She only answers when asked. She loves geography and mathematics. There is still a fear of robbers. The only physical complaint is a dry skin.' [Santos, 2007]

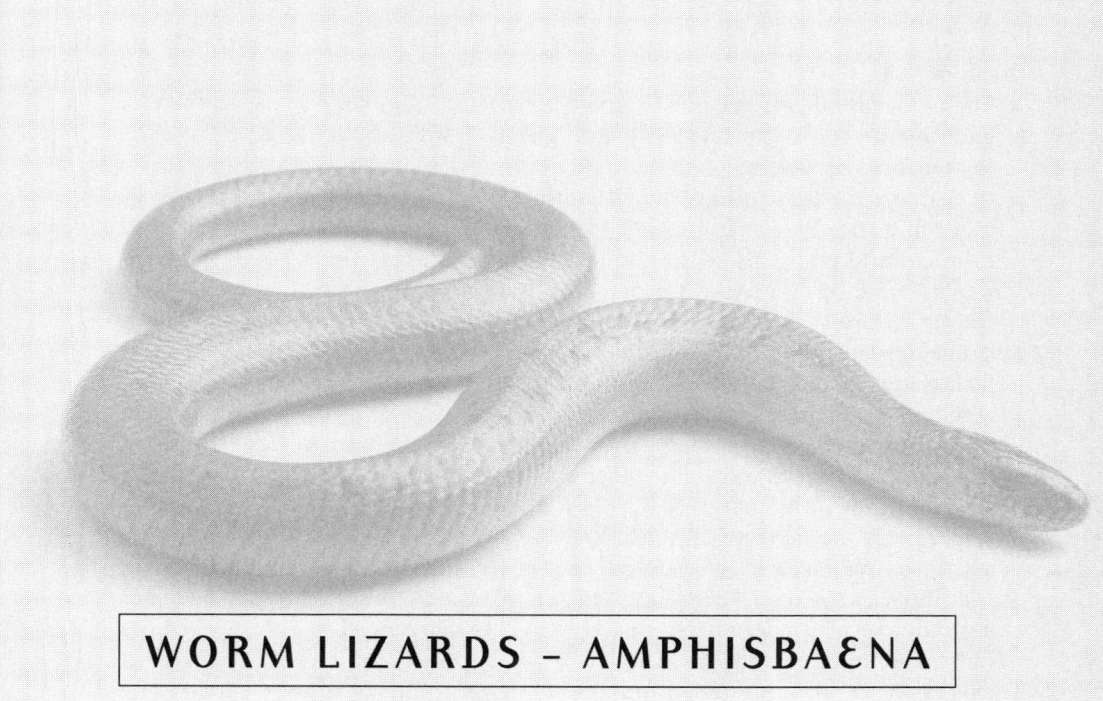

# WORM LIZARDS – AMPHISBAENA

## Biological Profile

- Highly specialised, burrowing reptiles that are neither worms nor true lizards but certainly are related to the latter. They have elongated, cylindrical bodies of nearly uniform diameter, and lack any trace of external limbs, except for 3 species in the genus Bipes that have small front legs with toes. With soft skin divided into numerous rings, and eyes and ears hidden under skin, the amphisbaenians superficially resemble earthworms. Most species are less than 15 cm long.
- Four families, 24 genera, and 196 species are recognized within this distinct group of subterranean lizards. Amphisbaenians have an extensive distribution in South America and tropical Africa.
- Due to their secretive habits, spending most of their time under leaf litter or burrowing through the soil, very little is known about the ecology of amphisbaenians. Most species construct burrows as they move, using their heads as a digging tool. Neck and body muscles are well developed to accommodate head-first burrowing, with forward thrust generally resulting from rectilinear locomotion.
- Amphisbaenians eat invertebrates, primarily arthropods, but may also take small vertebrates.

## Head or Tail

- The name 'amphisbaena' means 'to go both ways' from Gr. *amphis*, both ways, and *bainein*, to go, in allusion to the animal's scales allowing them to slide forward and backward.
- 'When threatened, amphisbaenians move their short tails around in a very menacing, headlike manner. If a potential predator is fooled by such head mimicry and grabs the reptile by its tail [tails of many are scarred], its head remains free to bite back. If a predator grabs an amphisbaenian by its head, the lizard presses its blunt tail hard against the attacker, perhaps making it think the tail is the lizard's head and causing the predator to release it, thus facilitating escape. Tails of many amphisbaenians autotomise, but they do not regenerate.' [Pianka, 2006]
- According to Greek mythology, the amphisbaena was spawned from the blood that dripped from the Gorgon Medusa's head as Perseus flew over the Libyan Desert with it in his hand. Cato's army then encountered it along with other serpents on the march. Amphisbaenae fed off of the corpses left behind. The amphisbaena has been referred to by the poets, such as Nicander, John Milton, Alexander Pope, Lord Tennyson, and A.E. Housman, and the amphisbaena as a mythological and legendary creature has been referenced by Lucan, Pliny the Elder, Isidore of Seville, and Thomas Browne, the last of whom debunked its existence. Of this harmless and useful reptile, Pliny seriously wrote: 'The amphisbaena has 2 heads; that is, it has a second one at its tail, as though one mouth were too little for the discharge of all its venom!' Even at the present day this belief in '2 heads' or '2 tails' and 'death at both ends' is not wholly eradicated.

Thus Amphisbaena, I have read,
At either end assails;
None knows which leads or which is led,
For both heads are both tails.
   Alexander Pope

## Differences with other Reptiles

'Despite a superficial resemblance to some primitive snakes, amphisbaenians have many unique features that distinguish them from other reptiles. Internally, their *right* lung is reduced in size to fit their narrow bodies, whereas in [other limbless lizards and] snakes, it is always the left lung. Their skeletal structure and skin are also different from those of other squamates.

'The head is stout, not set off from the neck, and either rounded, sloped, or sloped with a ridge down the middle. Most of the skull is solid bone and they have a distinctive single median tooth in the upper jaw. They have no outer ears, and the eyes are deeply recessed and covered with skin and scales. The body is elongated, and the tail truncates in a manner that vaguely resembles the head.

'The skin of amphisbaenians is only loosely attached to the body and they move using an accordion-like motion, in which the skin moves and the body seemingly just drags along behind it. Uniquely, they are also able to perform this motion in reverse just as effectively.

'Amphisbaenians are carnivorous, able to tear chunks out of larger prey with their powerful, interlocking, teeth. Like lizards, some species are able to shed their tail [autotomy]. Most species lay eggs, although at least some are known to be viviparous.' [Wikipedia]

## WORM LIZARDS IN HOMEOPATHY

| Homeopathic name | Common name | Abbreviation | Symptoms |
|---|---|---|---|
| Amphisbaena alba | White worm lizard | Amph-a. | – |
| Amphisbaena vermicularis | Wagler's worm lizard | Amph. | ++ |

# AMPHISBAENA ALBA

### Systematics
- Scientific name: Amphisbaena alba [L., 1758].
- Synonyms: Amphisbaena rosea [Shaw & Nodder, 1791]. A. flavescens [Wied, 1825].
- Common names: White worm lizard. White-bellied worm lizard.
- Family: Amphisbaenidae.

### Biological Profile
- Burrowing ringworm-like amphisbaenian, 45–85 cm long, with ringed scales around body, small and square dorsal scales, and a rounded head with 1 large tooth and 6 smaller ones in front of upper jaw.
- Range: Central America, Caribbean, South America.
- Habitat: Almost always stays in its underground tunnels, buried under dead leaves, or inside the nests of leaf-cutter ants. It is thought to forage in the ants' deep galleries where the insects deposit their waste.
- Secretive.
- Solitary.
- Skull and jaw bones heavy and fused together for strength, allowing for a powerful bite to effectively crush prey
- Preys on spiders, beetle larvae, ants, termites, crickets, and other insects and invertebrates.
- Oviparous; 8–16 eggs per clutch, probably once a year during the dry season.
- It is believed that as it moves inside tunnels, the secretion plugs from glands in the femoral or cloacal region are abraded against the substrate, releasing a secretion trail. Many authors assume that these glands are mainly associated with reproduction and demarcation of territory, constituting an efficient means of intraspecific communication inside the tunnels.

- Cannot drop its tail, unlike many other amphisbaenians; instead curls up its body so the head and tail are next to one another and then raises its head and opens wide its mouth while lifting up and swaying its tail, producing the impression of having 2 heads. Effectiveness of tail display may have offset the advantages of tail loss in this species.

## MATERIA MEDICA

- No symptoms.

# AMPHISBAENA VERMICULARIS

### Systematics
- Scientific name: Amphisbaena vermicularis [Wagler, 1824].
- Synonym: Amphisbaena spixi [Schmidt, 1936].
- Common name: Wagler's worm lizard.
- Family: Amphisbaenidae.

### Biological Profile
- 'This species moves either backwards or forwards, as occasion may require, and is quite frequent in the woods of Brazil. Its body is cylindrical, from 2 feet to 2½ long, terminated by a very obtuse tail. It has no scales properly speaking, but its skin is divided into quadrilateral compartments disposed in rings round the body; 228 on the trunk and 26 on the tail. The lower lip is divided into 6 long and narrow plates; the head is small, rather sharp, protected by scales, and not distinguished from the neck. It has small eyes; the jaw is not dilatable, the teeth are conical, bent, unequal and distinct from each other; the nostrils are on the sides, and pierced in a single naso-rostral plate. The amphisbaena is of a brownish colour above, and a pinkish-white under the belly. The poison was taken from the living animal by cutting off part of its jaw, which was triturated immediately.' [Mure]
- Range: Brazil, Bolivia.
- Oviparous.

## MATERIA MEDICA AMPHISBAENA VERMICULARIS

### Sources
1 Proving Mure [France-Brazil], 1847; no further details.

### Mind
∞ Sadness and lassitude in morning, > while walking.
∞ Tender sadness disposing one to be gentle and meek.
∞ Depression. Ennui. Impatience.

## Generals
∞ Wakes at midnight, for 10 consecutive nights. Disturbed sleep.

## Sensations
∞ Vertigo as if one would fall towards one side and is then impelled towards opposite side by a contrary oscillation.
∞ Weight in forehead and parietal regions.
∞ Repeated beating at right side of forehead as if hail-stones fell upon it.
∞ Horrible headache, with sensation as if feet were in brain.
∞ Pain at inner canthus of right eye as if a stye would form.
∞ Constriction of right eye as if strung together with a cord.
∞ Air as if rushing into ear.
∞ Teeth as if elongated and set on edge, esp. right lower molars.

## Locals
∞ Constant twitching at upper eyelids, especially left.
∞ Weariness of eyes, in evening, & pain and pricking when looking at light.
∞ Painful and large pimple on the side of upper lip, suppurating.
∞ Pains in right lower jaw, and considerable swelling < open air and dampness.
∞ Swelling of tonsils; swallowing difficult, unable to swallow saliva.
∞ Red miliary eruption extending over chest, elbows, and back, & itching < morning and > evening.
∞ Violent pain in whole spinal column, < walking, moving arms or stooping.
∞ Swelling of arm with great pain.
∞ Cramp in left leg; it remains behind in walking as if paralysed.
∞ Cramps in left leg accompanied by insensibility of same.

## Forward or Backward
What is particular for Amphisbaena are the sensations of always feeling dizzy and unstable. He doesn't know whether he is going forward or backwards. This characteristic sensation for Amphisbaena is noted in the following rubric: Mind; delusions: body parts, feet are in brain, with headache. Which end is his head and which is his feet? Among all the other typical Lizard themes, Amphisbaena, will be dizzy, not knowing which end is up, esp. when having to make decisions.

# REFERENCES

- Agarwal R. et al. 2006. *Is the patient brain-dead?* Emergency Medicine Journal 2006 Jan; 23(1): e5.
- Alberts A. 1993. *Lizard Tough Guys.* The Vivarium, Sept./Oct. 1993; www.anapsid.org.
- Alexander G.J. & Marshall C.L. 1998. *Diel activity patterns in a captive colony of rinkhals, Hemachatus haemachatus.* African Journal of Herpetology 47(1):29–32, January 1998.
- Ali G. et al. 2004. *Acute renal failure following Echis carinatus (saw-scaled viper) envenomation.* Indian Journal of Nephrology, 2004; 14: 177–181.
- Allen B. 1987. *Into the Crocodile Nest: A Journey Inside New Guinea.* London: Faber and Faber.
- Allen G.E. 2012. *Clinical Effects and Antivenom Dosing in Brown Snake (Pseudonaja spp.) Envenoming – Australian Snakebite Project (ASP-14).* PLoS One, Vol. 7, No. 12, 2012.
- Al-Sadawi M. et al. 2019. *Cerebrovascular Accident and Snake Envenomation: A Scoping Study.* International Journal of Clinical Research & Trials 2019, 4: 133.
- Anadure R.K. et al. 2018. *Two Cases of Early Morning Neuroparalytic Syndrome (EMNS) in the Tropics – Masquerading as Brain Death.* Journal of the Association of Physicians of India, Vol. 66, Jan. 2018.
- Andrews T. 1993. *Animal-Speak: The Spiritual & Magical Powers of Creatures Great & Small.* St. Paul: Llewellyn Publications.
- Angier N. 1995. *The Beauty of the Beastly.* Boston: Peter Davidson.
- Angier N. 2006. *All but Ageless, Turtles Face Their Biggest Threat: Humans.* New York Times, December 12, 2006.
- Anitha M.S. 2017. *A prospective study regarding cardiovascular manifestations following snake bite.* International Journal of Advances in Medicine, 2017 Feb.; 4(1):152–155.
- Anthony L. 2008. *Snakebit: Confessions of a Herpetologist.* Vancouver: Greystone Books.
- Ariaratnam C.A. et al. 2008. *Distinctive Epidemiologic and Clinical Features of Common Krait (Bungarus caeruleus) Bites in Sri Lanka.* Am. J. Trop. Med. Hyg. 79(3), 2008.
- Armstrong B.L. & Murphy J.B. 1979. *The Natural History of Mexican Rattlesnakes.* Lawrence: University of Kansas.
- Aronson V. & Szejko A. 2010. *Iguana Invasion! Exotic Pets Gone Wild in Florida.* Sarasota: Pineapple Press.
- Attenborough D. 1981. *Life On Earth: A Natural History.* Glasgow: Fontana/ Collins.
- Attenborough D. 2005. *Life in the Undergrowth.* Princeton: Princeton University Press.
- Auffenberg W. 1997. *Display Behavior in Tortoises.* Integrative and Comparative Biology, Vol. 17, No. 1, February 1977.
- Avins M. 2002. *Prelude to a Hiss in the L.A. Foothills.* L.A. Times, April 26, 2002.
- Azad C. et al. 2013. *Locked-in Syndrome as a Presentation of Snakebite.* Indian Pediatrics 2013; 50: 695–696.
- Backshall S. 2007. *Venom: Poisonous Animals in the Natural World.* London: New Holland Publishers.
- Badger D. 2002. *Lizards.* Osceola: Voyageur Press.
- Baeckens S. et al. 2016. *Chemical communication in the lacertid lizard Podarcis muralis: the functional significance of testosterone.* Acta Zoologica, 17 December 2016.

- Bailey J.D. 2001. *The Biogeography of Sceloporus occidentalis.* San Francisco State University: Department of Geography.
- Barkham P. 2007. *Horror in a half-shell: Terror of the Terrapins.* blog Beasts of London, 13 May, 2007.
- Barringer P.B. 1892. *The Venomous Reptiles of the United States, with the Treatment of Wounds Inflicted by them.* Gaillard's Medical Journal, Vol. 55.
- Bauchot R. [ed.]. 2006. *Snakes: A Natural History.* New York: Sterling Publ.
- Bear J.B. 2008. *Accounts of My Two Venomous Snake Bites.* Southwestern Center for Herpetological Research.
- Beaumont. 1830. *Effects of the Bite of a Viper.* The Lancet, December 11, 1830.
- Beck D.D. 2004. *Venomous lizards of the desert.* Natural History, July-August, 2004
- Beck D.D. 2005. *Biology of Gila Monsters and Beaded Lizards.* Berkeley: University of California Press.
- Beddard F.E. 1905. *Natural History in Zoological Gardens.* London: Archibald Constable & Co.
- Benn K.M. 1951. *A Further Case of Snake-bite by a Taipan Ending Fatally.* The Medical Journal of Australia, Vol. 1.
- Bennett D. 1995. *Little Book of Monitor Lizards: A Guide to the Monitor Lizards of the World and Their Care in Captivity.* Aberdeen: Viper Press.
- Benyus J.M. 1997. *Biomimicry: Innovation Inspired by Nature.* New York: William Morrow.
- Bernheim et al. 2001. *Three cases of severe neurotoxicity after cobra bite [Naja kaouthia].* www.world-snake.ch.
- Blanchard F.N. 1921. *A revision of the King Snakes: Genus Lampropeltis.* Bulletin 114, U.S. National Museum.
- Blaylock R.S. et al. *Clinical manifestations of Cape cobra [Naja nivea] bites.* South African Medical Journal, Vol. 68, 31 August 1985.
- Bonin F., Devaux B. & Dupré A. 2006. *Turtles of the World.* Baltimore: Johns Hopkins University Press.
- Bosak A.R. et al. 2014. A *Case of Neurotoxicity Following Envenomation by the Sidewinder Rattlesnake, Crotalus cerastes.* Journal of Medical Toxicology, 2014 June; 10(2): 229–231.
- Brandt A. 1956. *Treasury of Snake Lore.* New York: Greenberg.
- Bringsøe H. 2006. *Trachemys scripta.* Nobanis Invasive Alien Species Fact Sheet; 2006.
- Brown D.E. & Carmony N.B. 1999. *Gila Monster: Facts and Folklore of America's Aztec Lizard.* Salt Lake City: University of Utah Press.
- Browne M. 1871. *Festina Lente.* Saint Pauls Magazine, Vol. 8, 1871.
- Bryson P.D. 1997. *Comprehensive Review in Toxicology for Emergency Clinicians [3rd ed.].* Washington, DC: Taylor & Francis.
- Bucaretchi F. et al. 2002. *Snakebites by Crotalus durissus ssp. in Children in Campinas, São Paulo, Brazil.* Revista do Instituto de Medicina Tropical de São Paulo, Vol. 44, No. 3, 2002.
- Bucaretchi F. et al. 2016. *Coral snake bites (Micrurus spp.) in Brazil: a review of literature reports.* Clinical Toxicology, Vol. 54, No. 3, 2016.
- Bücherl W. & Buckley E.E. [eds.]. 1968. *Venomous Animals and Their Venoms,* Vol. 1 and II, Venomous Vertebrates; Vol. III, Venomous Invertebrates . New York: Academic Press.
- Buckland F.T. 1858. *Curiosities of Natural History.* London: R. Bentley.
- Cadbury D. 2001. *Terrible Lizard: The First Dinosaur Hunters and the Birth of a New Science.* New York: Henry Holt and Company.
- Cairo da Silva N. 1910. *Lachesis lanceolatus (Bothrops lanceolatus, Fer de Lance, Jararaca).* The Hahnemannian Monthly, Vol. 45, April 1910.
- Calmette A. 1908. *Venoms; Venomous Animals and Antivenomous Serum-Therapeutics.* New York: William Wood & Co.

- Cann J. 2001. *Snakes Alive!* Seymour Lansing: ECO.
- Cantrell F.L. 2003. *Envenomation by the Mexican Beaded Lizard: A Case Report.* Clinical Toxicology, Vol. 41, No. 3, 2003.
- Caras R. 1974. *Venomous Animals of the World.* Englewood Cliffs: Pentrice-Hall.
- Caras R. 1977. *Dangerous to Man.* South Hackensack: Stoeger Publishing Company.
- Carr A.F. Jr. 1954. *The Passing of the Fleet.* American Institute of Biological Sciences, 1954.
- Caspari E. & Robbins K. 2003. *Animal Life in Nature, Myth, and Dreams.* Wilmette: Chiron Publications.
- Charbonneau-Lassay L. 1991 [orig. 1940]. *The Bestiary of Christ.* New York: Parabola Books.
- Chermel R. 2018. *Basilisk Lizard Information and Care.* www.reptilesmagazine.com.
- Chevalier J. & Gheerbrant A. 1994. *The Penguin Dictionary of Symbols.* London: Penguin.
- Chevers N. 1856. *A Manual of Medical Jurisprudence for Bengal.* Calcutta: F. Carbery, Bengal Military Orphan Press.
- Ciolek J. et al. 2016. *Green Mamba peptide targets type-2 vasopressin receptor against polycystic kidney disease.* Proceedings of the National Academy of Sciences of the United States of America.
- Cirlot J.E. 1995. *A Dictionary of Symbols.* New York: Philosophical Library.
- Clark R.W. 2005. *Social Lives of Rattlesnakes.* Natural History, Vol. 114, No. 2.
- Clarke R.W. 1838. *Dreadful Effort to Cure Elephantiasis and Leprosy by Receiving the Bite of a Rattlesnake.* The Lancet, Vol. I, December 15, 1838.
- Cocks T. 1827. *Case of Viper Bite.* The Lancet, May 16, 1827.
- Cogger H.G. & Zweifel R.G. [eds.]. 2003. *Encyclopedia of Reptiles & Amphibians.* San Francisco: Fog City Press.
- Colagrande J. 2000. *In the Presence of Dinosaurs.* Time Life.
- Cole M. 1996. *Cerebral Infarct After Rattlesnake Bite.* Archives of Neurology, Vol. 53 No. 10, Oct. 1996.
- Connor M.J. 1993. *Hermann's Tortoise, Testudo hermanni.* Tortuga Gazette 29(8):1–3, August 1993.
- Cree H.E. 1888. *Case of Snake Bite.* Report of the Army Medical Department, Great Britain, Vol. 30.
- Danforth L.L. 1881. *Naja tripudians.* American Homeopath, Vol. VII, No. 8, August 1881.
- Das M. 2011. *Hemidactylus flaviviridis Rüppell,* 1835 (Sauria: Gekkonidae) an invasive gecko in Assam. North-Western Journal of Zoology, Vol. 7, No. 1, pp. 98–104.
- Dickens C. [ed.] 1882. *The influence of music on the lower animals.* All the Year Round, Dec. 30, 1882.
- Ditmars R.L. 1907. *The Reptile Book.* New York: Doubleday, Page & Company.
- Ditmars R.L. 1910. *Reptiles of the World.* New York: Sturgis & Walton Co.
- Ditmars R.L. 1934 (reprint 1970). *Confessions of a Scientist.* Freeport: Books for Libraries Press.
- Ditmars R.L. 1937a [orig. 1907]. *The Reptiles of North America.* New York: Doubleday & Co.
- Ditmars R.L. 1937b. *Snakes of the World.* New York: Macmillan.
- Dodd K.C. 2002. *North American Box Turtles: A Natural History.* University of Oklahoma Press.
- Donovan P. 2019. *The Boomslang Snake of Africa.* Reptiles Magazine, March 2019.
- Edmonds C. 1995. *Dangerous Marine Creatures.* Flagstaff: Best Publishing Company.
- Ernst C.H. 1999. *Venomous Reptiles of North America.* Washington, D.C.: Smithsonian Institution Press.

- Erulu V.E. et al. 2018. *Revered but Poorly Understood: A Case Report of Dendroaspis polylepis (Black Mamba) Envenomation in Watamu, Malindi Kenya, and a Review of the Literature.* Tropical Medicine and Infectious Diseases, 2018, 3, 104.
- Evans L. 2002. *Poisonous Geckos: The Validity of an Ancient Egyptian Belief.* Bulletin of the Australian Centre for Egyptology, (2002), p.47–55.
- Faiz M.A. 2017. *Bites by the Monocled Cobra, Naja kaouthia, in Chittagong Division, Bangladesh: Epidemiology, Clinical Features of Envenoming and Management of 70 Identified Cases.* American Journal of Tropical Medicine and Hygiene, Vol. 96, No. 4, April 2017.
- Finn F. 1905. *Putting on Frills: The Extraordinary Effects of Animal Emotions.* The Country-Side: A Wildlife Magazine, Vol. 1, May 20, 1905.
- Fitch G. 1916. *Vest Pocket Essays.* New York: Barse & Hopkins.
- Fitch H.S. 1960. *Autecology of the Copperhead.* Lawrence: University of Kansas.
- Fitzsimons F.W. 1912. *The Snakes of South Africa: Their Venom and the Treatment of Snake Bite.* Cape Town: T. Maskew Miller.
- Font E. 2012. *Social behavior, chemical communication, and adult neurogenesis: Studies of scent mark function in Podarcis wall lizards.* General and Comparative Endocrinology 177 (2012) 9–17.
- Fowler M.E. & Cubas Z.S. 2001. *Biology, Medicine and Surgery of South American Wild Animals.* Ames: Iowa State University Press.
- Frangides C.Y. et al. 2006. *Snake venom poisoning in Greece. Experiences with 147 cases.* European Journal of Internal Medicine, Vol. 17, No. 1, 2006.
- Frangides C.Y. et al. 2006. *Hypersersensitivity and Kounis syndrome due to a viper bite.* European Journal of Internal Medicine, Vol. 17, No. 3, 2006.
- Franklin C.J. 2007. *Turtles: An Extraordinary Natural History 245 Million Years in the Making.* St. Paul: Voyageur Press.
- Frazer, J.G. 1966. *The Golden Bough: A Study in Magic and Religion.* New York: St. Martin's.
- Freiberg M. 1984. *The World of Venomous Animals.* Neptune City: TFH Publications.
- Freitas A.C.N. & de Lima M.E. 2017. *Animal Venom Components: New Approaches for Pain Treatment.* Approaches in Poultry, Dairy & Veterinary Sciences.
- Frembgen J. 1996. *The Folklore of Geckos: Ethnographic Data from South and West Asia.* Asian Folklore Studies, Vol. 55, No. 1 (1996), pp. 135–143.
- Fry B.G. et al. 2009. *A central role for venom in predation by Varanus komodoensis (Komodo Dragon) and the extinct giant Varanus (Megalania) priscus.* PNAS June 2, 2009, vol. 106 no. 22.
- Fry B.G. 2015. *Venom Doc.* Sydney: Hachette Australia.
- Garnett S. & Ross C.A. 1989. *Crocodiles and Alligators.* New York: Facts on File.
- Gibbons W. 1983. *Their Blood Runs Cold: Adventures with Reptiles and Amphibians.* Tuscaloosa: University of Alabama Press.
- Gibbons W. & Gibbons A.R. 1998. *Ecoviews: Snakes, Snails, and Environmental Tales.* Tuscaloosa: University of Alabama Press.
- Giuliani C. & Peri A. 2014. *Effects of Hyponatremia on the Brain*; Journal of Clinical Medicine, Dec. 2014.
- Goleman D. 1985. *'Social Chameleon' May Pay Emotional Price.* New York Times, March 12, 1985.
- Gopalakrishnakone P. [ed.] 1994. *Sea Snake Toxinology.* Singapore: Singapore University Press.
- Gorzula S. & Oduro W. 1997. *Survey of the status and management of the Royal python (Python regius) in Ghana.* Genève : Secrétariat CITES.
- Gould E. 1957. *Orientation in Box Turtles, Terrapene c. carolina (Linnaeus).* Biological Bulletin 112(3), June 1957.

- Gourlay W. 1811. *Observations on the Natural History, Climate, and Diseases of Madeira: During A Period Of Eighteen Years.* London: J. Callow.
- Graham A.D. & Beard P.H. 1973. *Eyelids of Morning: The Mingled Destinies of Crocodiles and Men.* New York: A & W Visual Library.
- Graham J.B. et al. 1971. *Temperature physiology of the sea snake Pelamis platurus: An index of its colonization potential in the Atlantic Ocean.* Proceedings of the National Academy of Sciences of the United States of America, Vol. 68, No. 6, June 1, 1971.
- Grant M.L. & Henderson L.J. 1957. *A Case of Gila Monster Poisoning with a Summary of Some Previous Accounts.* Proceedings of the Iowa Academy of Science, Vol. 64, Article 91.
- Grant Watson E.L. 1966. *Animals in Splendour and Decline.* British Homeopathic Journal, Vol. 55, No. 1, January 1966.
- Greene H.W. 1997. *Snakes: The Evolution of Mystery in Nature.* Berkeley: University of California Press.
- Greene H.W. 2006. *Parental Behavior in Anguid Lizards.* South American Journal of Herpetology, Vol. I, No. 1, 2006, 9–19.
- *Grzimek's Animal Life Encyclopedia,* Vols. 1–13. 1984. New York: Van Nostrand Reinhold Co.
- Gubernatis A. de. 1978 (orig. 1872). *Zoological Mythology.* New York: Macmillan.
- Hannay J.B. 1922. *Sex Symbolism in Religion.* London: The Religious Evolution Research Society.
- Harborne D.J. 1993. *Emergency treatment of adder bites: case reports and literature review.* Archives of Emergency Medicine, 1993, 10, 239–243.
- Hardy J. 2000. *Two Cases of Cenchris contortrix, the Copperhead Snake.* Homeopathic Links 1/2000.
- Haro L. de. 2002. *Unusual neurotoxic envenomations by Vipera aspis aspis snakes in France.* Human & Experimental Toxicology (2002) 21, 137–145.
- Hartwig G. 1877. *The Polar and Tropical Worlds: A Description of Man and Nature in the Polar and Equatorial Regions of the World.* Springfield: C.A. Nichols.
- Hay O.P. 1892. *The Batrachians and Reptiles of the State of Indiana.* Indianapolis: Wm. B. Burford.
- Hayes A.W. [ed.] 2007. *Principles and Methods of Toxicology.* Boca Raton: CRC Press.
- Hermon Slade Foundation. *Conservation ecology of a nationally threatened reptile, the Green Python, Morelia viridis.*
- Higgins S.B. 1873. *Ophidians.* New York: Boericke & Tafel.
- Hill R. & Mackessy S.P. 2000. *Characterization of venom (Duvernoy's secretion) from twelve species of colubrid snakes and partial sequence of four venom proteins.* Toxicon, Vol. 38, December 2000.
- Hilligan R. 1987. *Black mamba bites: A Report of 2 Cases.* South African Medical Journal, Vol. 72, Aug. 1987.
- Hilton Jr. B. 2002. *This Week at Hilton Pond.* Hilton Pond Center for Piedmont Natural History, 8–14 May 2002.
- Hodgson P.S. & Davidson T.M. 1996. *Biology and treatment of the mamba snakebite.* Wilderness and Environmental Medicine, 2, 133–145 (1996).
- Hopley C.C. 1882. *Snakes: Curiosities and Wonders of Serpent Life.* London: Griffith & Farran.
- Hopley C.C. 1888. *British Reptiles and Batrachians.* London: Swan Sonnenschein, Lowrey, & Co.
- Hornaday W.T. 1904. *The American Natural History; a Foundation of Useful Knowledge of the Higher Animals of North America.* New York: C. Scribner's Sons.
- Houston E.J. 1907. *The Wonder Book of the Atmosphere.* New York: Frederick A. Stokes Co.

- Hudson W.H. 1919. *The Book of a Naturalist*. New York: George H. Doran Co.
- Hung H.T. et al. 2009. *Clinical Features of 60 Consecutive ICU-Treated Patients Envenomed by Bungarus multicinctus*. Southeast Asian Journal for Tropical Medical Public Health, May 2009.
- Ionides C.J.P. 1969. *Mambas and Man-Eaters: A Hunter's Story*. London: Mayflower.
- Ireland J.P. *The Eclectic Repertory and Analytical review*, Vol. III, No. III, April 1813.
- Isbister G.K. et al. 2012. *Tiger snake (Notechis spp) envenoming: Australian Snakebite Project (ASP-13)*. Medical Journal of Australia, 2012; 197 (3): 173–177.
- Jackson K. 2008. *Mean and Lowly Things: Snakes, Science, and Survival in the Congo*. Cambridge: Harvard University Press.
- Jacobi M.A. *Notes on a serious envenomation by Proatheris superciliaris*. www.kingsnake.com.
- James J. 2008. *The Snake Charmer: A Life and Death in Pursuit of Knowledge*. New York: Hyperion.
- Jeyarajah R. 1984. *Russell's Viper Bite in Sri Lanka*. American Journal of Tropical Medicine and Hygiene, Vol. 33, No. 3, May 1984.
- John J. 2008. *Snakebite mimicking brain death*. Cases Journal 2008, June 12;1(1):16.
- Johnson J. & Johnson H.J. 1834. *The Medico-chirurgical review and Journal of Practical Medicine*; Oct. 1834, p. 522–523.
- Karlson-Stiber C. et al. 2006. *A Nationwide Study of Vipera Berus Bites During One Year – Epidemiology and Morbidity of 231 Cases*. Clinical Toxicology, Vol. 44, No. 1, 25–30, 2006.
- Keatley H.W. 1914. *Epilepsy and Its Treatment: Illustrating the Use of Snake Venom*. American Journal of Clinical Medicine, June 1914.
- Kelly L. 2006. *Crocodile: Evolution's Greatest Survivor*. Crows Nest: Allen & Unwin.
- Kervran L. 1998. *Biological Transmutations*. Magalia: Happiness Press.
- Keyler D.E. et al. 2016. *Local envenomation from the bite of a juvenile false water cobra*. Toxicon, Vol. 111, March 1, 2016.
- Khaldun A. et al. 2017. *Locked-in Sundrome Following a King Cobra (Ophophagus hannah) Envenomation*. Medicine & Health, Dec. 2017; 12(2):357–362.
- Kiem Xuan Trinh et al. 2010. *Hyponatraemia, rhabdomyolysis, alterations in blood pressure and persistent mydriasis in patients envenomed by Malayan kraits (Bungarus candidus) in southern Viet Nam*. Toxicon, Nov. 2010.
- Kitajima T. 1908. *On 'Habu' Venom and its Serum Therapy*. The Philippine Journal of Science, Vol. 3, 1908.
- Kitto J. 1841. *Palestine: The Physical Geography and Natural History of the Holy Land*. London: Charles Knight & Co.
- Klauber L.M. 1982. *Rattlesnakes: Their Habits, Life Histories & Influence on Mankind*. Berkeley: University of California Press.
- Klotzsch B. 2001. *The Mystery and Power of Python Regia: A Proving*. Bergisch Gladbach.
- Kularatne S.A.M. 2002. *Common krait (Bungarus caeruleus) bite in Anuradhapura, Sri Lanka: a prospective clinical study, 1996–98*. Postgraduate Med. Journal 2002;78:276–280.
- Kularatne S.A.M. 2003. *Epidemiology and Clinical Picture of the Russell's Viper (Daboia Russelii Russelii) Bite in Anuradhapura, Sri Lanka: A Prospective Study of 336 Patients*. Southeast Asian Journal for Tropical Medical Public Health, Vol 34, No. 4, December 2003.
- Kularatne S.A.M. et al. 2011. *Revisiting saw-scaled viper (Echis carinatus) bites in the Jaffna Peninsula of Sri Lanka: Distribution, epidemiology and clinical manifestations*. Transactions of The Royal Society of Tropical Medicine and Hygiene, Vol. 105, No. 10, October 2011.
- Kularatne S.A.M. et al. 2014. *Revisiting Russell's Viper (Daboia russelii) Bite in Sri Lanka: Is Abdominal Pain an Early Feature of Systemic Envenoming?* PLoS One, February 26, 2014.
- Lacina S. 2000. *Natural History of the Wagler's Viper*. www.kingsnake.com.

- Lalloo D.G. 1997. *Electrocardiographic abnormalities in patients bitten by taipans (Oxyuranus scutellatus canni) and other elapid snakes in Papua New Guinea.* Transactions of The Royal Society of Tropical Medicine and Hygiene, Vol. 91, No. 1, Jan.–Feb. 1997.
- Lambert G. 1851. *Poisoning by the Bite of an Adder.* The London Lancet, Vol. 2, No. 6, Dec. 1851.
- Lane M. 1963. *The Snake Man.* London: Hamish Hamilton.
- Lapidus R. 2006. *Snake Hunting on the Devil's Highway.* Indianapolis: Dog Ear Publishing.
- Lappin A.K. 2006. *Showing Off Your Weapons In The Animal Kingdom: Threat Displays May Prevent Serious Physical Harm.* ScienceDaily, 21 June 2006.
- Lauridsen L.P. 2016. *Toxicovenomics and antivenom profiling of the Eastern green mamba snake (Dendroaspis angusticeps).* Journal of Proteomics, 136, 248–261.
- Lee D. 1996. *Black Mamba!* International Wildlife, 1996.
- Leighton G.R. 1903. *The Life History of British Lizards.* London: Wm. Blackwood & Sons.
- Leite dos Santos G.G. 2012. *Antinociceptive properties of Micrurus lemniscatus venom.* Toxicon. 2012 Nov; 60(6):1005–12.
- Linville S.E. 2004. *History Films, Women, and Freud's Uncanny.* Austin: University of Texas Press.
- Lizardlover H. 1993. *Iguana Owner's Manual.* Los Angeles: Prymal Pig Publishing.
- Lloyd C.N.V. 1974. *Some Observations on Egg-Laying Behaviour in the Green Mamba, Dendroaspis angusticeps.* Journal of the Herpetological Association of Africa, Vol. 12, No. 1, 1974.
- Lockley M. 2009. *Tracking Dinosaurs: A New Look at an Ancient World.* Cambridge University Press.
- Louw J.X. 1967. *Specific Mamba antivenom – Report of survival of 2 patients with black mamba bites treated with this serum.* South African Medical Journal, 2 Dec. 1967.
- Lovic V. 2017. *Venomous Snakebites and Near Misses; SE Asia Edition.* ThailandSnakes.com.
- MacLean P.D. 1985. *Brain Evolution Relating to Family, Play, and the Separation Call.* Archives of General Psychiatry, Vol. 42, April 1985.
- MacLean P.D. 1990. *The Triune Brain in Evolution: Role in Paleocerebral Functions.* New York: Springer.
- Madden R.R. 1829. *Travels in Turkey, Egypt, Nubia and Palestine in 1824, 1825, 1826 & 1827.* London: Henry Colburn.
- Mahendra B.C. 1936. *Contributions to the Bionomics, Anatomy, Reproduction and Development of the Indian House-Gecko, Hemidactylus flaviviridis Rüppel. Part I.* Proceedings of the Indian Academy of Sciences – Section B, September 1936, Vol. 4, No. 3, pp 250–281.
- Mallow D. et al. 2003. *True Vipers: Natural History and Toxinology of Old World Vipers.* Malabar: Krieger.
- Mao Y-C. et al. 2017. *Bungarus multicinctus multicinctus Snakebite in Taiwan.* American Journal of Tropical Medicine and Hygiene, Vol. 96, No. 6, June 2017.
- Marais J. 2004. *A complete guide to the snakes of southern Africa.* Cape Town: Struik Publishers.
- Marianini P. 1829. *Singular Effect of the Bite of a Viper.* The Lancet, February 7, 1829.
- Marques O.A.V. 1996. *Reproduction, seasonal activity and growth of the coral snake, Micrurus corallinus (Elapidae), in the southeastern Atlantic forest in Brazil.* Amphibia-Reptilia 17(3):277–285; January 1996.
- Marques O.A.V. et al. 2006. *Activity Patterns in Coral Snakes, Genus Micrurus (Elapidae) in South and Southeastern Brazil.* South American Journal of Herpetology, 1(2), 2006, 99–105.
- Mascarenhas N. 2009. *The revenge of the cobra.* www.saligaoserenade.com.
- Master F. 2008. *Snakes to Simillimum.* Assesse: B. Jain Archibel.

- Mattingly J. & Bosse G. *Snake Bite in the State of Kentucky; Crotalid Envenomation.* Website Kentucky Regional Poison Center
- Mattison C. 2002. *The Encyclopaedia of Snakes.* London: Cassell.
- Mattison C. 2004. *Lizards of the World.* New York: Facts on File.
- Maughan R.C.F. 1914. *Wild Game in Zambezia.* New York: Charles Scribner's Sons.
- Mayo H. 1841. *Of the Bites of Venomous Serpents.* London Medical Gazette, Vol. 29, Dec. 24, 1841.
- McCarthy K.M. 1998. *Alligator Tales.* Sarasota: Pineapple Press.
- McElroy E.J. 2008. *Functional Morphology of Lizard Locomotion.* Dissertation presented to the faculty of the College of Arts and Sciences of Ohio University; 2008.
- McIlhenny E.A. 1987 [orig. 1935]. *The Alligator's Life History.* Berkeley: Ten Speed Press.
- McNair Wright J. 1895. *Sea-side and Way-side.* Boston: D.C. Heath.
- Means D.B. 2008. *Stalking the Plumed Serpent.* Sarasota: Pineapple Press.
- Mebs D. et al. 1998. *Severe coagulopathy after a bite of a green bush viper (Atheris squamiger): case report and biochemical analysis of the venom.* Toxicon, Vol. 36, No. 10, Oct. 1998.
- Meenakshisundaram R. et al. 2013. *Severe hypertension in elapid envenomation.* Journal of Cardiovascular Disease Research, 2013 Mar; 4(1): 65–67.
- Meier J. & White J. 1995. *Handbook of Clinical Toxicology of Animal Venoms and Poisons.* Boca Raton: CRC Press.
- Merchant M.E. et al. 2003. *Antibacterial properties of serum from the American alligator.* Comparative Biochemistry and Physiology – Part B: Biochemistry & Molecular Biology, 2003 Nov.; 136(3):505–13.
- Milani Jr. R. 1997. *Snake bites by the jararacucu (Bothrops jararacussu): clinicopathological studies of 29 proven cases in Sao Paulo State, Brazil.* QJM 1997 May; 90(5):323–34.
- Minton S.A. 2001. *Life, Love, and Reptiles: An Autobiography of Sherman A. Minton.* Malabar: Krieger.
- Mirtschin P. & Davis R. 1995. *Dangerous Snakes of Australia.* Sydney: Landsdowne Publ.
- Mitchell A. 1873. *Bite of the Diamond Rattlesnake (Crotalus adamanteus).* Boston Medical and Surgical Journal, October 2, 1873.
- Mocino-Deloya E. et al. 2009. *Cannibalism of nonviable offspring by postparturient Mexican lance-headed rattlesnakes, Crotalus polystictus.* Animal Behaviour, Vol. 77, No. 1, Jan. 2009.
- Monckton C.A.W. 1921. *Taming New Guinea: Some Experiences of a New Guinea Resident Magistrate.* New York: John Lane Company.
- Monteiro H.S.A. et al. 2001. *Actions of Crotalus durissus terrificus venom and crotoxin on the isolated rat kidney.* Brazilian Journal of Medical and Biological Research, Oct. 2001, Volume 34(10) 1347–1352.
- Moore G.M. [ed.]. 1962. *Poisonous Snakes of the World.* Washington, D.C.: Department of the Navy, Bureau of Medicine and Surgery 1962.
- Moore R.S. 1988. *Second-degree heart block associated with envenomation by Vipera berus.* Archives of Emergency Medicine, 1988, 5, 116–118.
- Moquin-Tandon A. & Hulme R.T. 1861. *Elements of Medical Zoology.* London: H. Baillière.
- Morgan D. 2009. *Exploring Self Immunization With A Bush Viper Venom.* www.normal-benoit.com.
- Morris D. & R. 1968. *Men and Snakes.* London: Sphere Books.
- Müller G.J. et al. 2012. *Snake bite in southern Africa: diagnosis and management.* Continuing Medical Education, Vol 30, No 10 [2012].
- Murphy J.B. 1998. *A Glimpse in the Life of a Zoo Herpetologist.* Herpetological Review 29(2), 1998.
- Murphy M.J. 1996. *A Field Guide to Common Animal Poisons.* Ames: Iowa State University Press.

- Myers P.Z. 2005. *Hot-blooded crocodiles?* Pharyngula Science, 19 April 2005.
- Nagami P. 2004. *Bitten: True Medical Stories of Bites and Stings.* New York: St. Martin's Griffin.
- Nayak K.C. et al. 1990. *Profile of cardiac complications in snake bite.* Indian Heart Journal, 1990 May-June; 42(3):185–8.
- Neill W.T. 1971. *The Last of the Ruling Reptiles.* New York: Columbia University Press.
- Nichol J. 1989. *Bites and Stings: The World of Venomous Animals.* New York: Facts on File.
- Nisbet W. 1795. *An Inquiry into the History, Nature, Causes, and Different Modes of Treatment hitherto Pursued in the Cure of Scrophula and Cancer.* Edinburgh: Thomas Kay.
- Numeric P. et al. 2002. *Multiple Cerebral Infarctions Following a Snakebite by Bothrops caribbaeus.* American Journal of Tropical Medicine and Hygiene, 67(3), 2002, pp. 287–288]
- Owen H.K. 1840. *Bite of a Viper.* London Medical Gazette, Vol. 26, May 22, 1840.
- Pandya S.S. 2004. *The First International Leprosy Conference, Berlin, 1897: the Politics of Segregation.* Indian Journal of Leprosy, Jan-March, 76(1):51–70, 2004.
- Papanagnou D. 2008. *Sea Snake Envenomation.* emedicine.medscape.com.
- Parves N. & Alam S.M.I. 2015. *Hemidactylus flaviviridis (Reptilia: Gekkonidae): Predation on Congeneric Hemidactylus frenatus in Dhaka, Bangladesh.* The Herpetological Bulletin 132, 2015: 28–29.
- Pe T. et al. 1997. *Envenoming by Chinese krait (Bungarus multicinctus) and banded krait (B. fasciatus) in Myanmar.* Transactions of the Royal Society of Tropical Medicine and Hygiene (1997) 91, 686–688.
- Pemberton O. 1849. *Bite of the Thumb by the Common Adder, Followed by Prostration of the Vital Powers, Swelling and Extensive Ecchymosis of the Right Upper Extremity.* The London Lancet, Vol. 1, No. 3, March 1850.
- Pemberton O. 1851. *Bite of the Face by the Common Adder, Followed by Vomiting, Diarrhoea, and Extreme General Prostration.* The Lancet, August 16, 1851.
- Persson H. & Irestedt B. 1981. *A study of 136 cases of adder bite treated in Swedish hospitals during one year.* Acta Medica Scandinavica, 1981; 210:433–439.
- Phelps T. 2007. *Observations of the Cape cobra, Naja nivea in the DeHoop Nature Reserve.* Herpetological Bulletin, Number 99, 2007.
- Pianka E.R. 1994. *The Lizard Man Speaks.* Austin: University of Texas Press.
- Pianka E.R. & Vitt L.J. 2006. *Lizards: Windows to the Evolution of Diversity.* Berkeley: University of California Press.
- Plumwood V. 2000. *Being Prey.* In: The Ultimate Journey: Inspiring Stories of Living and Dying. San Francisco: Travelers' Tales.
- Pochanugool C. et al. 1997. *Spontaneous recovery from severe neurotoxic envenoming by a Malayan krait Bungarus candidus (L.) in Thailand.* Wilderness and Environmental Medicine, 8, 223–225.
- Pope C.H. 1958. *Fatal Bite of Captive African Rear-Fanged Snake [Dispholidus].* Copeia, Vol. 1958, No. 4, Dec. 22, 1958.
- Pope C.H. 1971. *The Reptile World: A Natural History of the Snakes, Lizards, Turtles, and Crocodilians.* New York: Alfred A Knopf.
- Poppelbaum H. 1961. *A New Zoology.* Dornach: Philosophic-Anthroposophic Press.
- Pourreau F. 2014. *Bilateral renal cortical necrosis with end-stage renal failure following envenoming by Proatheris superciliaris: a case report.* Toxicon, 2014 June; 84:36–40.
- Quammen D. 1998. *The Flight of the Iguana: A Sidelong View of Science and Nature.* New York: Scribner.
- Quammen D. 2003. *Monster of God: The Man-Eating Predator in the Jungles of History and the Mind.* New York: W.W. Norton & Company.
- Quarch V. et al. 2017. *An Unexpected Case of Black Mamba (Dendroaspis polylepis) Bite in Switzerland.* Case Reports in Critical Care, Vol. 2017.

REFERENCES

- Rand A.S. 1967. *Running Speed of the Lizard Basiliscus basiliscus on Water.* Copeia, Vol. 1967, No. 1. [Mar. 20, 1967], pp. 230–233.
- Raskova H. 1971. *Pharmacology and Toxicology of Naturally Occurring Toxins.* Oxford: Pergamon Press.
- Rasmussen A.R. & Elmberg J. 2009. *Venomous Sea Snakes Play Heads Or Tails With Their Predators.* ScienceDaily, August 6, 2009.
- Reading C.J. 1996. *Incidence, pathology, and treatment of adder (Vipera berus L.) bites in man.* Journal of Accident & Emergency Medicine, Vol. 13, No. 5, Sept. 1996.
- Redfield J.W. 1854. *The Bite of a Copperhead Snake.* American Journal of Homeopathy, Vol. 9, No. 2, June 1854.
- Rehabi H. 2014. *Severe Envenomation by Cerastes cerastes Viper: An Unusual Mechanism of Acute Ischemic Stroke.* Journal of Stroke & Cerebrovascular Diseases, Vol. 23, No. 1, January 2014.
- Reid H.A. 1976. *Adder bites in Britain.* British Medical Journal, 1976, 2, 153–156.
- Reid P.F. 2007. *Alpha-cobratoxin as a possible therapy for multiple sclerosis: a review of the literature leading to its development for this application.* Critical Reviews in Immunology, Vol. 27, Issue 4, 291–302.
- Revue Médicale. 1826. *Case of the Bite of a Viper Treated Successfully by the Application of the Cupping Glass.* The Lancet, Vol. 11, 1826]
- Ripa D. 2001. *Bushmasters and the Heat Strike.* VenomousReptiles.org.
- Ripa D. 2002. *The Bushmasters (Genus Lachesis Daudin, 1803): Morphology in Evolution and Behavior.* Wilmington: Cape Fear Serpentarium.
- Ripa D. 2004. *Resurrecting Garcia's Botrops (Lachesis) acrochordus.* Bulletin of the Chicago Herpetological Society, 39(7):122–134, 2004.
- Ripa D. 2015. *The Bushmaster: Silent Fate of the American Tropics.* Cape Fear Serpentarium.
- Rittenberg M. 1913. *Swirling Waters.* New York: G.W. Dillingham Company.
- Rivas J.A. & Burghardt G.M. 2005. *Snake Mating Systems, Behaviour, and Evolution.* Journal of Comparative Psychology, Vol. 119, No. 4, 2005.
- Robinson P. 1893. *The Poets and Nature: Reptiles, Fishes, and Insects.* London: Chatto & Windus.
- Rosen B.C. 2001. *Masks and Mirrors: Generation X and the Chameleon Personality.* Westport: Praeger Publishers.
- Rubio M. 1998. *Rattlesnake: Portrait of a Predator.* Washington, D.C.: Smithsonian Institution Press.
- Russell F.E. 1980. *Snake Venom Poisoning.* Philadelphia: Lippincott.
- Sano-Martins I.S. et al. 2001. *Coagulopathy following lethal and non-lethal envenoming of humans by the South American rattlesnake [Crotalus durissus] in Brazil.* QJM. 2001 Oct. 94(10):551–9.
- Santos-König U. 2007. *They Can Pull In Their Head: A Case of Chrysemys Scripta Elegans.* Homeopathic Links 3/07.
- Scalise K. 1998. *Lizards slay Lyme disease spirochetes.* California Agriculture 52(2): 4–4, March–April 1998.
- Schneemann M. et al. 2004. *Life-threatening envenoming by the Saharan horned viper [Cerastes cerastes] causing micro-angiopathic haemolysis, coagulopathy and acute renal failure: clinical cases and review.* QJM Vol. 97, No. 11, 2004.
- Scop J. et al. 2009. *Sixteen years of severe Tiger snake (Notechis) envenoming in Perth, Western Australia.* Anaesthesia and Intensive Care, Vol. 37, No. 4, July 2009.
- Seal J. 2001. *The Snakebite Survivors' Club: Travels Among Serpents.* San Diego: Harvest, Harcourt.

- Selous P.S. 1900. *Notes and observations regarding the habits and characteristics of the Massasauga, Sistrurus catenatus, during captivity.* Michigan Academy of Science.
- Shine R. 1994. *Sexual Dimorphism in Snakes.* Copeia, May 16, 1994
- Shukla C. 1999. *A Gigantic Black Skeleton: A Case of Crotalus cascavella.* Homeopathic Links 2/99.
- Silva A. et al. 2016. *Neuromuscular Effects of Common Krait (Bungarus caeruleus) Envenoming in Sri Lanka.*
- Silva-de-França F. et al. 2019. *Naja annulifera Snake: New insights into the venom components and pathogenesis of envenomation.* PLOS, Neglected Tropical Diseases, January 18, 2019.
- Singh L.A.K. et al. 1984. *Observations on the Reproductive Biology of the Indian Chameleon, Chamaeleo zeylanicus (Laurenti).* Journal of the Bombay Natural History Society, Vol. 81.
- Singh S. et al. 2019. *Study of electrocardiographic changes pattern in cases of snake bites in a tertiary care hospital of Mahakaushal area of central India.* International Journal of Research in Medical Sciences, 2019 May; 7(5):1450–1454.
- Souza de R.C.G. et al. 2007. *The Enigma of the North Margin of the Amazon River: Proven Lachesis Bites in Brazil, Report of Two Cases.* Bulletin of the Chicago Herpetological Society, 42[7]:105–115.
- Sprackland R.G. 1992. *Giant Lizards.* Neptune City: TFH Publications.
- Stackhouse J. 1972. *Australia's Venomous Wildlife.* Sydney: Paul Hamlyn.
- Stahnke H.L. 1966. *The Treatment of Venomous Bites and Stings.* Tempe: Arizona State University.
- Stephenson J. 1832. *Medical Zoology and Mineralogy.* London: John Churchill.
- Stewart J.P. & Strathern A. 2005. *Expressive Genres and Historical Change: Indonesia, Papua New Guinea and Taiwan.* Farnham: Ashgate Publishing.
- Strover H.M. 1967. *Report on a Death from Black Mamba bite.* Central African Journal of Medicine, Vol. 13, No. 8, August 1967.
- Stutesman D. 2005. *Snake.* London: Reaktion Books.
- Sutherland S.K. 1983. *Australian Animal Toxins.* Melbourne: Oxford University Press.
- Switalski J. & Smit M. 2007. *The Black Mamba: Some insight into Africa's most notorious serpent.* www.venomousreptiles.org/articles/336.
- Tien-Yow Chuang et al. 1996. *Guillain-Barré Syndrome: An Unusual Complication After Snake Bite.* Archives of Physical Medicine and Rehabilitation. July 1996.
- Tilbury C.R. 1982. *Observations on the bite of the Mozambique spitting cobra (Naja mossambica mossambica).* South African Medical Journal 1982 Feb 27; 61(9):308–13.
- Tinkham E.R. 1957. *I Was Bitten By A Gila Monster.* Desert Magazine, Sept. 1957.
- Tongpoo A. et al. 2018. *Krait Envenomation in Thailand.* Therapeutics and Clinical Risk Management, Vol. 14, 2018.
- Topsell E. 1608. *The History of Serpents.* London: William Haggard.
- Tosney K.W. 2004. *Caring for an Australian Bearded Dragon.* http://www.bio.miami.edu.
- Toso E. 2007. *Zero at the Bone: Rewriting Life after a Snakebite.* Tucson: University of Arizona Press.
- Tout du D.M. 1980. *Boomslang Bite: Case Report and Review of Diagnosis and Management.* South African Medical Journal; 29 March 1980.
- Tresidder J. 1998. *Dictionary of Symbols.* San Francisco: Chronicle Books.
- Twain M. 1909. *Letters from the Earth.*
- UC Davis. 2007. *Lizards 'Shout' Against A Noisy Background.* ScienceDaily, February 27, 2007.
- U.S. Department of the Navy. 1991. *Poisonous Snakes of the World.* New York: Dover Publications.

- Valenta J. 2008. *Envenoming by the viperid snake Proatheris superciliaris: A case report.* Toxicon, Vol. 52, No. 2, 1 August 2008.
- Vincent M.R. 1887. *Word Studies in the New Testament.* New York: Charles Scriber's Sons.
- Vinod K.V. & Dutta T.K. 2013. *Snakebite, dysautonomia and central nervous system signs.* QJM: An International Journal of Medicine, Vol. 106, No. 9, Sept. 2013, pp. 865–866.
- Vinton K.W. 1956. *The Jungle Whispers.* New York: Pageant Press.
- Virmani S.K. 2002. *Cardiac Involvement in Snake Bite.* Medical Journal Armed Forces India. 2002 April; 58(2): 156–157.
- Wagner R. & Wagner M. 2006. *Tread Lightly: Venomous and Poisonous Animals of the Southwest.* Tucson: Rio Nuevo Publishers.
- Wake C.S. 1888. *Serpent Worship and Other Essays.* London: G. Redway.
- Wall A.J. 1873. *Report on the Physiological Effects of the Poisons of the Naja Tripudians and the Daboia Russellii.*
- Walt v.d A.J. & Müller G.J. 2019. *Berg adder (Bitis atropos) envenoming: an analysis of 14 cases.* Clinical Toxicology, Vol. 57, No. 2, Febr. 2019.
- Warrell D.A. et al. 1975. *Bites by puff-adder (Bitis arietans) in Nigeria, and value of antivenom.* British Medical Journal, 1975, 4, 6, 97–700.
- Warrell D.A. et al. 1977. *Poisoning by bites of the saw-scaled or carpet viper (Echis carinatus) in Nigeria.* Quarterly Journal of Medicine, 1977 Jan.; 46 (181):3 3–62.
- Warrell D.A. et al. 1983. *Severe neurotoxic envenoming by the Malayan krait, Bungarus candidus*; British Medical Journal vol. 286, 26 Feb. 1983.
- Warrell D.A. et al. 1987. *Acute and chronic pituitary failure resembling Sheehan's syndrome following bites by Russell's viper in Burma.* The Lancet, October 3, 1987.
- Werler J.E. & Dixon J.R. 2000. *Texas Snakes: Identification, Distribution, and Natural History.* Austin: University of Texas Press.
- Weston P. 1859. *On the Poison of the Common Adder.* The Lancet, May 21, 1859.
- Wium C.A. et al. 2017. *Berg adder (Bitis atropos): An unusual case of acute poisoning.* South African Medical Journal, Vol. 107, No. 12, Dec. 2017.
- World Health Organization. 2010. *Guidelines for the Prevention and Clinical Management of Snakebite in Africa.*
- Wilson C. 2006. *The Occult.* London: Watkins Publishing.
- Wise A. 2001. *Leaving the Crocodile: The Story of the East Timorese Community in Sydney.* Casula, NSW : The Liverpool Regional Museum, 2001.
- Witzell W.N. 1983. *Synopsis of Biological Data on the Hawksbill Turtle, Eretmochelys imbricata.* FAO, Roma 1983.
- Woolcott I. 2015. *Lizard, Power Animal, Symbol of Dreaming and Conservation.* www.shamanicjourney.com.
- Work T.M. 2005. *Cancer in Sea Turtles.* Hawaii Medical Journal, Vol. 64, January 2005.
- Wüster W. et al. 2002. *Origin and phylogenetic position of the Lesser Antillean species of Bothrops (Serpentes, Viperidae): Biogeographical and medical implications.* Bulletin of the Natural History Museum Zoology, 68(02):101–106, November 2002.
- Wykes A. 1961. *Snake Man: The Story of C.J.P. Ionides.* New York: Simon and Schuster.
- Yang D.C. et al. 2016. *The snake with the scorpion's sting: novel three-finger toxin sodium channel activators from the venom of the long-glanded blue coral snake (Calliophis bivirgatus).* Toxins 2016, 8(10), 303.
- Závada J. et al. 2011. *Black Mamba Dendroaspis Polylepis Bite: A Case Report.* Prague Medical Report / Vol. 112 (2011) No. 4, p. 298–304.

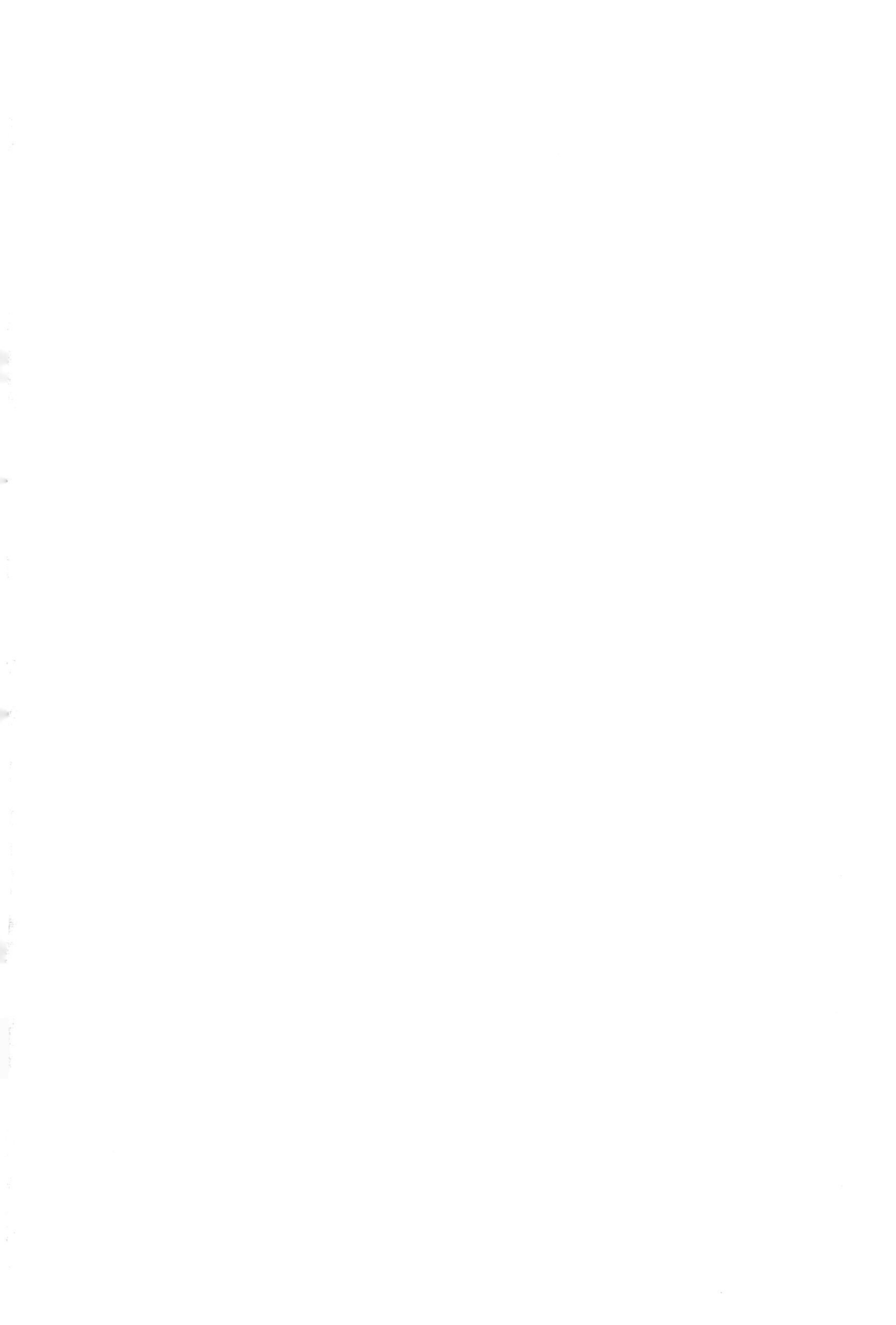